QV 4 MAC   £21.42

ERS

Drugs in
Nursing Practice

For Churchill Livingstone:

Senior Commissioning Editor: Ninette Premdas
Project Development Manager: Katrina Mather
Designer: Judith Wright

Drugs in Nursing Practice

An A–Z Guide

A M MacConnachie BSc(Hons) MSc MRPharm S

*Principal Pharmacist, Tayside Medicines Information Service,
Ninewells Hospital and Medical School, Dundee, UK
Honorary Lecturer, Department of Clinical Pharmacology, University of
Dundee, Dundee, UK
Part-time Lecturer in Nursing Studies, University of Abertay Dundee,
Dundee, UK*

Joan Hay BSc(Hons) MSc MRPharm S

*Senior Pharmacist, Tayside Medicines Information Service,
Ninewells Hospital and Medical School, Dundee, UK*

Jane Harris MSc BNurs RGN RM RHV NDNCert RDNT PWT

*Senior Lecturer in Nursing, School of Nursing and Midwifery,
University of Dundee, Dundee, UK*

Sheila Nimmo MEd BSc RGN DN RNT PWT

Lecturer in Nursing, University of Abertay, Dundee, UK

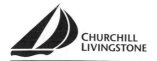

CHURCHILL
LIVINGSTONE

EDINBURGH LONDON NEW YORK PHILADELPHIA ST LOUIS SYDNEY TORONTO 2002

CHURCHILL LIVINGSTONE
An imprint of Harcourt Publishers Limited

© Longman Group Limited 1995
© Harcourt Publishers Limited 1999
© Harcourt Publishers Limited 2002

 is a registered trademark of Harcourt Publishers Limited

First edition 1982
Second edition 1986
Third edition 1989
Fourth edition 1993
Fifth edition 1995
Sixth edition 2002

ISBN 0 443 05946 2

British Library Cataloguing in Publication Data
A catalogue record for this book is available from the British Library

Library of Congress Cataloging in Publication Data
A catalog record for this book is available from the Library of Congress

Note
Medical knowledge is constantly changing. As new information becomes
available, changes in treatment, procedures, equipment and the use of drugs
become necessary. The authors and the publishers have, as far as it is
possible, taken care to ensure that the information given in this text is
accurate and up to date. However, readers are strongly advised to confirm
that the information, especially with regard to drug usage, complies with the
latest legislation and standards of practice.

The
publisher's
policy is to use
**paper manufactured
from sustainable forests**

Printed in China by RDC Group Limited

Contents

About this book and how to use it

The sections of this book include the following.

Drug notes listing over **600** drugs in common use arranged alphabetically.
Appendix 1 Nurse Prescribers' Formulary
Appendix 2 Drugs in pregnancy and lactation
Appendix 3 Analgesic and related drug therapy
Appendix 4 Metric weights and other measures
Index of drugs by proprietary (trade) name

DRUG NOTES

This is the main part of the text consisting of a description of drugs in common use listed in alphabetical order by approved name or, where appropriate, arranged under a group name (e.g. ACE Inhibitors). Once the individual drug has been located the relevant information is set out under a series of headings as follows:

a. Presentation This describes the various formulations and strengths which are available for each drug e.g. tablets, capsules, injections, ointments, creams, suppositories, etc.

b. Actions and uses This section is aimed at providing the nurse with a brief therapeutic background to the drug which explains its indication(s) in practice. It is hoped that an appreciation of how drugs act may enable more effective monitoring of the patient's response and help to inform decisions about its relative effectiveness.

c. Dosage The doses provided in the text are those commonly prescribed for the different dosage forms and listed indications. It should be appreciated that, for various reasons, there may be a need to treat patients outwith the stated dosage range. For example, the elderly and the very young are often particularly sensitive to medicines which requires that they be administered in modified dosage; in fact not all medicines are licensed for use in children but nevertheless their use may be warranted on clinical grounds. There may also be a lack of information on suitable dosages for patients who are unable to inactivate or excrete drugs normally either because they have impaired liver or kidney function or both. Also, the results of new research may dictate that a medicine be used for a new indication in practice before a change in the licensed dosage can follow. In any event, advice on dosages prescribed outwith that stated can be obtained by referring any questions to the hospital or community pharmacist.

d. Nursing implications This section highlights the important contribution that nurses can, and increasingly do, make in achieving the most effective and safe use of medicines in their patients. It deals for example with the possible unwanted side effects of drugs and may be consulted to ascertain the signs and symptoms of adverse drug reactions, the detection of the most severe of which may require prompt intervention and even discontinuation of treatment. On the other hand nurses may be prompted to alert doctors to lack of effect as well as possible adverse effects so that drug dosage can be modified or alternative therapy commenced. This section also highlights those patients for whom individual drugs are contraindicated or should not be used and cases in which extra precautions e.g. closer than normal patient monitoring, should follow.

e. Storage This section advises on the appropriate storage conditions for individual drug formulations and provides extra advice on stability when necessary.

APPENDICES

Appendix 1 *Nurse Prescribers' Formulary.* This consists of a series of monographs providing information on products listed in the Nurse Prescribers' Formulary section of the 41st edition of the British National Formulary. The information is set out as for that in Drug Notes (above) in order to provide consistency in accessing and using the text. Although it is anticipated that there will be a substantial increase in the range of pharmacy-only and prescription-only medicines which nurses will eventually be able to prescribe, it is hoped that those currently qualified to prescribe medicines from the existing list will benefit from publication of this information.

Appendix 2 *Drugs in pregnancy and lactation.* Nurses are often put on the spot, perhaps more than any other healthcare professionals, by concerned pregnant women who are prescribed medicines or else discover that they are pregnant whilst already taking medication. Likewise, lactating mothers often request advice on the safety of their medication in relation to breast feeding. This Appendix aims to put the risks of drugs in pregnancy and lactation in perspective and in addition give advice on specific drugs in a series of Tables. Whilst ultimately it is not possible to give absolute assurances on the safety of medicines in these situations, it may be possible to reassure patients or highlight potential concerns within the clinical team.

Appendix 3 *Analgesic and related drug therapy.* The management of chronic pain and related symptoms presents a major challenge and is at the heart of palliative care. All too often this area of therapy is poorly managed, often because the effect of uncontrolled pain and other symptoms on day to day quality of life is not appreciated by clinicians who only see patients from time to time throughout their illness. This being the case, nurses have a vital role to play in the delivery of palliative care simply because they are best placed to monitor patient need and the effect of treatment on an ongoing basis. This is the reason for including this Appendix which is intended as a ready reference to analgesia and co-analgesia, or adjuvant therapy. The reader is provided with the principles on which pain is assessed and managed and offered a range of choice of drugs for use in practice. Information is also provided on the preparation and administration of parenteral medicines by continuous subcutaneous infusion.

The authors gratefully acknowledge the important contribution by Dr Barbara Dymock at Roxburghe House in Dundee in the preparation of this Appendix. The text has been reproduced by kind permission of the Scottish Partnership Agency for Palliative and Cancer Care.

Appendix 4 *Metric weights and other measures.* This section is included to allow nurses to refer to units of weight and other measures which they meet in everyday practice and to enable them to make relevant calculations when preparing drug dosages. A nomogram for calculation of body surface area, on which basis some drug dosages are calculated, is also included.

Index of drugs by proprietary (trade) name The proprietary name of a drug denotes a trade name by which a given manufacturer's product can be identified e.g. Zantac® brand of ranitidine manufactured by GlaxoSKB. Not surprisingly, it is this name that often appears in large or bold print on the manufacturer's pack and in promotional material so that many doctors are influenced to prescribe using such names. If a drug does not appear in the text setting out drugs by approved name in alphabetical order then it is possible that the trade name has been used in which case this index should be consulted. Finally, it should be noted that numerous combinations of two or more drugs in a single tablet, capsule, etc., may exist under one proprietary name. It is not possible to cover all such combinations here and the reader must first determine what approved name drugs are included in such combinations then refer to each one separately in the text.

Preface

The aim of *Drugs in Nursing Practice*, since its first edition, has been to provide preregistration nursing students and postregistration nurses with a compact though comprehensive guide to aspects of modern drug therapy relevant to their practice. This, the 6th, edition also includes the Nurse Prescribers' Formulary, which we hope will not only be useful for nurse prescribers but will also serve to inform all nurses of this important development in the delivery of nursing care.

Those readers familiar with previous editions will recognize the easy-to-use A–Z format of the 6th edition, which comprises the largest section of the book. An updated selection of drugs, which reflects the authors' experience as being those most important to nurses, is included. Some of these have been included in previous editions, some are new therapies, whilst others have become more closely aligned with modern nursing practice and responsibility. A feature of this section continues to be the emphasis on the implications of drug therapy from the nurse's perspective. Each monograph clearly identifies the possible effect of therapy on patients and the nurse's subsequent responsibilities surrounding safety, concordance, efficacy, and patient education. Additional information to support the drug notes is provided in the appendices and finally drugs are indexed by proprietary name.

New for the 6th edition is the Nurse Prescribers' Formulary (NPF). Since the previous edition of *Drugs in Nursing Practice*, published in 1994, nurse prescribing has become established practice for a specific group of community-based nurses, namely district nurses, health visitors and some practice nurses. We therefore regard the inclusion of the NPF an essential addition and a key feature of the book particularly for the nurse prescriber. However, government plans to extend the formulary considerably are likely to be implemented within the next 12 months and it is beyond the scope of this edition to predict accurately the contents of this new formulary. The NPF is presented in A–Z format, providing the framework for a detailed monograph of all items included in the formulary. Each monograph again highlights the implications of therapy for patients and the responsibilities of nurses, particularly in a prescribing role. We have also described in this edition important aspects of the background of nurse prescribing which set this development within its past, present and future contexts.

Nursing practice is constantly developing to meet the challenges posed by changing health care needs, the structure of health care delivery and advances in technology and treatment, to name a few. Many roles which were new to nurses in the 1990s, and included as specific sections in the previous edition of the book, are now part of everyday practice. This is not to say that they are no longer important but that the emphasis has changed. Where specific sections were given to issues such as intravenous and parenteral feeding and the nurse's role in the management of AIDS, HIV and infectious diseases in the previous edition, these are now included within the drug notes section in relation to individual drugs.

Drugs in Nursing Practice has been designed to be both portable and practical and a ready reference to drugs in common use. We hope that the 6th edition will continue to provide a useful pocket guide to those aspects of modern drug therapy which are important to pre- and postregistration nurses, including nurse prescribers.

Dundee 2002

A.M. MacConnachie
Joan Hay
Jane Harris
Sheila Nimmo

Nurse prescribing

Nurse prescribing became a reality in the UK in England in 1994, when it was piloted by a small group of community nurses in eight sites around the country. Despite the apparent success of this scheme, it was not until 1998 that a national UK roll-out got under way, with a target to give all eligible nurses prescribing authority by the end of 2001. Nurse prescribing was introduced to enable nurses to prescribe a limited range of items which were viewed as integral to routine nursing care rather than part of the medical management of the patient's condition. However, recent government proposals which have been accepted by the nursing, medical and pharmaceutical professions are set to change this original position.

The legislation enabling nurses to prescribe from a limited formulary, passed in 1992, restricts prescribers to qualified and practising district nurses and health visitors or practice nurses holding either qualification who have successfully completed a course of preparation for prescribing approved by one of the four national nursing boards. Other conditions include the nurse's attachment to a general practice and employment by the local NHS trust. Since 1999, initial programmes of preparation for district nurses and health visitors/public health nurses have included nurse prescribing so that these newly qualified practitioners also have prescribing authority once the above conditions are met.

The current Nurse Prescribers' Formulary (NPF) is listed as an appendix in the British National Formulary (BNF), which is revised and updated twice a year. Nurse prescribers are issued with the NPF, which presents the formulary in itemized format followed by the complete BNF to enable cross-referencing. However, the current NPF has remained largely the same since it was issued in 1994 and reflects the practice of the community nurses eligible to prescribe. The majority of the items included in the NPF are General Sales Listed (GSL) and therefore readily available for purchase over the counter. However, many judge the success of nurse prescribing to date in terms of its convenience for nurses and patients and the prompt commencement of treatment rather than the scope of the formulary.

Government and professional bodies in all UK countries are currently devising the mechanisms which will take nurse prescribing forward. Prescribing authority will be extended to include a wider range of nurses. The NPF will be revised to include all GSL and pharmacy items and more prescription-only items. There are also plans to differentiate nurse prescriber status. This will result in some nurses having independent prescribing status and others supplementary prescribing status (i.e. relying on another practitioner for the initial diagnosis). This heralds a new era in nurse prescribing, with nurses prescribing independently for minor injuries, minor ailments, health promotion and palliative care. There are implications for education and continuing professional development, monitoring, and role development. Over the next few years, these will clearly impact on nurses in many settings other than those currently working in the community.

This edition of *Drugs in Nursing Practice* includes the most up-to-date version of the NPF (at time of going to press). As with any other formulary, items will be added and omitted in response to new information. Nurse prescribers therefore have a professional responsibility to keep updated and access relevant sources of information, including the BNF and the Medicines Control Agency.

We therefore stress that nurse prescribers use this book to supplement other sources of information and do not use it as their only prescribing guide.

Acknowledgements

The authors gratefully acknowledge the contributions of Dr Barbara Dymock and the Scottish Partnership Agency, which were invaluable in the preparation of the text relating to chronic pain and symptom control.

DRUG NOTES
(arranged alphabetically by approved name)

A

ABCIXIMAB (Reopro)

Presentation
Injection – 10 mg in 5 ml

Actions and uses
This drug is a monoclonal antibody which binds to specific sites on the surface of the platelet, so preventing platelet aggregation and the subsequent binding of fibrinogen leading to thrombus formation. It has a specialist use in conjunction with heparin and aspirin for patients undergoing percutaneous transluminal coronary angioplasty (PTCA) in which there is a high risk of platelet clotting and thrombus formation. It is included here in recognition of the extent of coronary heart disease in society and the frequency of PTCA as a result.

Dosage
A loading dose 0.25 mg/kg is administered by bolus IV injection 10 minutes before the procedure and immediately followed by maintenance IV infusion 10 microgram/minute for the following 12 hours.

Nursing implications
- Abciximab is intended for single use only.
- Intravenous infusions are prepared in glucose 5% or sodium chloride 0.9% injection and administered via an infusion pump. Transfer of solution and ultimate injection is via a sterilizing, non-adherent filter. Seek advice from pharmacy.
- Abciximab use is associated with a significant risk of bleeding and should be restricted to those at high risk of coronary thrombosis.
- Facilities for dealing with anaphylactic reactions should be available.

Storage
Abciximab is stored in a refrigerator between 2 and 8°C.

ACARBOSE (Glucobay)

Presentation
Tablets – 50 mg, 100 mg

Actions and uses
This drug is an inhibitor of an intestinal enzyme (alpha-glucosidase) responsible for the 'digestion' of complex carbohydrates to monosaccharides (sugars) which are then absorbed across the gut wall. Since the diet is normally a rich source of carbohydrates, acarbose inhibits their utilization to the extent that it induces a 'low' carbohydrate diet. This makes it potentially useful as an adjunct to dietary therapy in type II (non-insulin dependent) diabetes mellitus.

Dosage
In adults: initially 50 mg three times a day, either chewed with the first mouthful of food or swallowed whole directly before a meal. If there is an inadequate response after 1–2 months the dose may be doubled or re-doubled.

Nursing implications
- Acarbose should be avoided in patients with inflammatory bowel disease, intestinal obstruction or chronic digestive or absorptive disorders.

A

- Acarbose is potentially hepatotoxic so liver function should be monitored, especially in patients receiving full doses.
- As carbohydrate is retained in the gut patients should be advised of the possibility of flatulence, a feeling of fullness, abdominal discomfort and diarrhoea.
- As acarbose reduces carbohydrate absorption it may be abused by patients as an aid to dieting to achieve cosmetic weight loss.

Storage

Acarbose tablets are stored at room temperature.

ACE INHIBITORS (ACEIs)

Presentation

See individual drugs.

Actions and uses

ACE stands for angiotensin-converting enzyme, a substance present in the circulation which is responsible for the formation of angiotensin. Under normal circumstances angiotensin is formed in response to falling blood pressure and when there is excessive sodium loss. This it counteracts by causing direct generalized vasoconstriction and promoting the retention of sodium by the kidney (through stimulation of aldosterone release). The net result is to provide circulatory support. As the name suggests, the ACE inhibitors are a group of drugs which block the actions of ACE in situations where the enzyme is inappropriately overactive. These drugs have two main uses.

- Hypertension which is often associated with vasoconstriction and sodium retention. ACE inhibitors result in normalization of the blood pressure and are especially suitable for patients with diabetes and others who are unable to tolerate the metabolic and related side effects of other first-line antihypertensives.

- Heart failure in which the peripheral arterial dilatation which they produce is associated with a significant reduction in the work which the heart is required to do in order to expel blood into the circulation during systole. This effect is often referred to as an 'unloading' of the heart or 'afterload' reduction. Further, since patients with heart failure are prone to sodium retention, the loss of sodium which the ACE inhibitors induce is also beneficial. ACE inhibitors have had a major impact on quality of life and survival in heart failure and are now considered first-line drugs together with the diuretics in such patients.

Other, more recent uses, include:

- myocardial infarction in which the prognosis is improved by ACE inhibitors in patients with obvious or asymptomatic left ventricular impairment
- diabetic nephropathy in which preservation of renal function has been noted.

Although the mechanism is not yet clear, many diabetologists believe that the ACE inhibitors have a protective action on the kidney and use them as first-choice antihypertensives in this group.

Dosage

See individual drugs.

Nursing implications
- Within a few hours of the administration of an ACE inhibitor there may be a sudden and precipitous fall in blood pressure, especially when patients have previously been treated with diuretics or are otherwise salt depleted. Patients should therefore be commenced on the lowest possible dose and carefully monitored during the first 24 hours of treatment.
- The concentration of potassium in the blood may rise in patients receiving ACE inhibitors, particularly if already taking potassium supplements or

potassium-sparing diuretics. A high blood potassium (hyperkalaemia) may result in serious cardiac arrhythmias and should be avoided.

- All drugs of this type can produce a persistent dry cough (especially in women) which may be quite disabling for some patients. The reason appears to be that the enzyme (ACE), which is also present in lung tissue, is blocked, leading to the accumulation of irritant substances called kinins (ACE is also responsible for inactivation of tissue kinins). It may be possible to control cough using an antiinflammatory drug including oral ibuprofen or inhalation of sodium cromoglycate.
- The use of an ACE inhibitor is associated with a reduction in filtration pressure in the kidney. Normally this has few consequences but in patients with renal impairment, particularly those with renal artery stenosis, renal failure may result. The monitoring of serum creatinine is essential so that early renal failure can be detected. Elderly patients, in particular, may already have a degree of renal impairment and are especially sensitive to this side effect.
- Some ACEIs are excreted largely by the kidney and need to be given in reduced dosage if kidney function is impaired. Others are to a greater extent excreted by the liver and may be preferred in such cases.
- The use of ACEIs should be avoided in patients who are likely to become pregnant and is contraindicated in pregnancy.

Storage
See individual drugs.

ACEBUTOLOL (Sectral)

Presentation
Capsules – 100 mg, 200 mg
Tablets – 400 mg

Actions and uses
Acebutolol is a cardioselective beta-adrenoreceptor blocking drug and the section on beta-blockers (p. 51) should be consulted for a full account of its actions.

It is converted in the body to a metabolite which is, in fact, non-cardioselective and this explains why some patients develop side effects consistent with beta-2 receptor blockade.

In practice, acebutolol is used in the treatment of:

- angina pectoris
- cardiac arrhythmias
- hypertension.

Dosage
Adult dose range:

- angina pectoris: 200–600 mg twice daily
- cardiac arrhythmias: 200–600 mg twice daily or 200–400 mg three times daily
- hypertension: 200–400 mg twice daily.

Nursing implications
The section on Beta-blockers (p. 51) should be consulted for a full account of the nursing implications which apply to this drug.

Storage
Acebutolol capsules and tablets are stored at room temperature.

ACECLOFENAC (Preservex)

Presentation
Tablets – 100 mg

Actions and uses
Aceclofenac is a non-steroidal anti-inflammatory drug and the section on NSAIDs (p. 250) should be consulted for a full account of its actions.

In practice aceclofenac is licensed for use in the treatment of:

- ankylosing spondylitis
- osteoarthritis
- rheumatoid arthritis.

Dosage
Adult dose (all indications): 100 mg twice daily.

> **Nursing implications**
> The section on NSAIDs should be consulted for a full account of the nursing implications which apply to this drug.

Storage
Aceclofenac tablets are stored at room temperature.

ACEMETACIN (Emflex)

Presentation
Capsules – 60 mg

Actions and uses
Acemetacin is a non-steroidal anti-inflammatory drug and the section on NSAIDs (p. 250) should be consulted for a full account of its actions.

In practice acemetacin is used in the treatment of:

- low back pain
- osteoarthritis
- postoperative inflammatory pain
- rheumatoid arthritis.

Dosage
Adult dose (all indications): 60 mg two or three times daily, as required.

> **Nursing implications**
> - The section on NSAIDs should be consulted for a full account of the nursing implications which apply to this drug.
> - Side effects may include tinnitus and dizziness which may affect performance of skilled tasks such as operating machinery and driving.

Storage
Acemetacin capsules are stored at room temperature.

ACETAZOLAMIDE (Diamox)

Presentation
Tablets – 250 mg

Capsules – 250 mg sustained release

Injection – 500 mg vials

Actions and uses
Acetazolamide inhibits the action of an enzyme called carbonic anhydrase which acts as a catalyst for the reaction which leads to hydration of carbon dioxide in the cells of the body through carbonic acid and ultimately to bicarbonate and hydrogen ion. Chemically the reaction is as follows:

$$CO_2 + H_2O = H_2CO_3 = HCO_3^- + H^+$$

This is, amongst other things, an important chemical reaction whereby the body regulates acid/base balance. Acetazolamide has one major use.

- Glaucoma in which oral administration is associated with a decrease in the flow of aqueous humour within the chamber of the eye, thus reducing intraocular pressure. Formation of bicarbonate, and water secreted along with it, is an important step in determining the volume of aqueous humour produced. Acetazolamide is also administered by injection in the preoperative preparation of patients with closed-angle glaucoma.

Other rare uses for acetazolamide include:

- as a weak diuretic in mild oedematous states, though its action is self-limiting and much less pronounced than that of the thiazide or loop diuretics. This action comes about as a result of impaired bicarbonate formation and hence renal tubular reabsorption
- as a second- or even third-line anticonvulsant in atypical absence, tonic or clonic seizures, usually in childhood and often associated with cerebral damage or mental retardation. The mechanism is unclear but probably related to metabolic change within the central nervous system.

Dosage
Treatment of glaucoma in adults.

- Oral: using standard tablets the dose varies from 125 mg twice daily up to 250 mg four times a day. It is often more convenient to take a

single daily dose in the form of slow-release capsules.
- Parenteral: 500 mg, preferably by IV injection (but IM route if necessary) reconstituted with 5 ml of water for injection immediately before use.

As a diuretic in adults: a single morning dose (or alternate morning dose) of 250–375 mg by the oral, IV or IM route.
As an anticonvulsant.

- Adult dose is in the range 125–500 mg twice daily.
- Children's dose is 4–15 mg/kg twice daily to a maximum of 750 mg per day.

Nursing implications
- Side effects, which occur most often in the initial stages of treatment, include flushing, thirst, headache, drowsiness, dizziness, fatigue, paraesthesia, ataxia, hyperventilation and gastrointestinal upset (anorexia, nausea and vomiting). Elderly patients are more sensitive to the side effects of this drug.
- Much more rarely, hypersensitivity reactions occur leading to skin, kidney and bone marrow damage. Acetazolamide is, in fact, a sulphonamide derivative and, as such, can affect the skin, kidney and bone marrow in much the same way.
- Prolonged use may lead to stone formation in the kidneys with resultant ureteric colic.
- Acetazolamide may produce an abnormality in blood biochemistry known as acidosis which is potentially serious. Symptoms include altered consciousness with, initially, drowsiness and later coma and deep irregular respiration.

Storage
Acetazolamide tablets, capsules and injection vials are stored at room temperature. Solution for injection should be prepared immediately before use and any unwanted residue discarded.

ACETYLCYSTEINE (Ilube, Parvolex)

Presentation
Eye drops – 5% with hypromellose 0.35%
Injection – 2 g in 10 ml

Actions and uses
Acetylcysteine has three main uses.

- It is a specific antidote in paracetamol poisoning, a major cause of acute (and often fatal) self-poisoning worldwide. It acts by blocking the binding of the toxic paracetamol metabolite to liver cells, thus preventing the hepatotoxicity which otherwise results.
- It has a viscous (slimy) consistency in solution and therefore it is used with hypromellose (a thickening agent) in eye drops. Drops are reserved for treatment of excessively dry eyes associated with overproduction of mucus and unresponsive to treatment with hypromellose solutions alone.
- Concentrated solutions of acetylcysteine are also administered orally to chemically break down and mobilize the thick mucous secretions (meconium ileus) which build up and block intestinal transit of foodstuffs (nutrients) in patients with cystic fibrosis and which, in doing so, contribute to malnutrition in this group.

Dosage
- Paracetamol overdosage, when indicated (i.e. by suspected amount of paracetamol ingested, time in relation to overdose, elevation of serum transaminases, etc.): 150 mg/kg body weight by IV infusion over 15 minutes (in 200 ml glucose 5% injection) followed by an infusion of 50 mg/kg (in 500 ml glucose 5%) over 4 hours. Thereafter a dose of 100 mg/kg is administered (in 1 litre glucose 5%) over the next 16 hours. This provides a total dose of 300 mg/kg in 20 hours.
- Dry eye associated with mucus excess: one or two drops instilled in the eye three or four times daily, as required.

A

- Cystic fibrosis: for oral use, special solutions are available from the pharmacy. Seek advice on preparation and dosage.

Nursing implications
- When administered orally, side effects, though uncommon, include nausea, vomiting, heartburn, tinnitus, headache and skin rashes (urticaria).
- Acetylcysteine, by injection, is an effective antidote to paracetamol if administered up to 8–10 hours after poisoning. Its effectiveness rapidly diminishes thereafter. It is therefore important, if possible, to determine the time of poisoning in relation to hospital admission.
- Note that the drug is incompatible with rubber and metals and for this reason plastic cannulae are used when doses are administered.
- The drug is generally well tolerated but a few patients develop hypersensitivity manifest as skin rashes. Rarely, acute anaphylaxis has occurred.

Storage
- Acetylcysteine preparations are stored at room temperature.
- Solutions for injection should be used immediately.
- Eye drops should be used within 4 weeks of opening or within · 1 week if used in hospital.

ACICLOVIR (Zovirax)

Presentation
Tablets – 200 mg, 400 mg, 800 mg
Suspension – 200 mg in 5 ml, 400 mg in 5 ml
Injection – 250 mg, 500 mg vials
Eye ointment – 3%
Cream – 5%

Actions and uses
Aciclovir is an antiviral agent which acts by blocking the synthesis of viral DNA. It is itself inactive but becomes activated (phosphorylated) by a viral enzyme called thymidine kinase to form aciclovir phosphate. Aciclovir is therefore only active within host cells which have become virally infected. Aciclovir has potent activity against herpes simplex virus (HSV) and is, to a lesser extent, active against herpes zoster virus (varicella). In clinical practice it is used for the following.

- Treatment of varicella (chickenpox) and herpes zoster (shingles) infections. Acute pain of shingles is alleviated and possibly also the pain associated with postherpetic neuralgia.
- Treatment and long-term suppression of HSV infections of the skin and mucous membranes.
- Prevention of recurrent HSV infections in susceptible (immunocompromised) patients.
- Treatment and long-term suppression of genital herpes and prophylaxis of genital herpes in the immunocompromised.
- As topical cream, for the treatment of HSV infections of the skin, including genital herpes.
- As ophthalmic ointment applied in the treatment of herpes simplex keratitis.

Dosage
Treatment of HSV infection (oral route).

- Adults and children >2 years: 200 mg (400 mg if immuno-compromised) five times a day, usually for a period of 5 days.
- Child <2 years: 100 mg (200 mg if immunocompromised) five times a day, as above.

Treatment of HSV and recurrent varicella zoster infection (IV route).

- Adults: 5 mg/kg (or 10 mg/kg if primary and recurrent varicella zoster infection in the immunocompromised and in herpes simplex encephalitis) administered every 8 hours and continued for at least 10 days.
- Child <3 months: 10 mg/kg administered every 8 hours.
- Child >3 months: 250 mg/m^2 body surface area administered every 8 hours.

NB: Children's doses (above) are doubled in the immunocompromised and in herpes simplex encephalitis and continued for at least 10 days.

Prevention of recurrence of HSV infection (oral route).

- Adults and children >2 years: 200 mg four times a day or 400 mg twice daily.
- Children <2 years: half the above dose.

Prophylaxis of HSV infection in the immunocompromised (oral route).

- Adults and children >2 years: 200–400 mg four times a day, preferably at strict 6-hourly intervals.
- Children <2 years: half the above dose.

Treatment of varicella and herpes zoster infection (oral route).

- Adults: 800 mg five times a day for 1 week.
- Chickenpox in children based on 20 mg/kg four times a day, preferably at strict 6-hourly intervals. Treat for 5 days. This approximates to:
  - children >5 years: 800 mg four times a day, as above
  - children 2–5 years: 400 mg four times daily, as above
  - children <2 years: 200 mg four times a day, as above.

Topical treatment in herpes virus infection of the eye, skin and genitalia.

- Apply cream or eye ointment five times a day (approximately 4-hourly). Treat skin lesions for 5 days and continue for a further 5 days if not completely healed. Continue application of eye ointment for at least 3 days after healing has taken place.

Nursing implications

- Note that the spelling has changed from *acyclovir* in recent years. This may cause unnecessary confusion but only serves to bring the official name, aciclovir, in line with European and US standards.
- The importance of compliance with the oral dosage regimen must be stressed in view of the relative frequency of dosing and need for prolonged therapy, even after initial healing is apparent. Note that early commencement of treatment is vital to ensure efficacy.
- A reversible increase in blood urea and serum creatinine may occur after intravenous infusion. This effect is less marked if patients are well hydrated before treatment is administered. Hydration can be assessed by noting the blood urea level in the normal range.
- Patients with severe renal impairment (creatinine >200 micromol/litre) should receive a reduced dosage and advice regarding dosage should be sought from pharmacy.
- Aciclovir for infusion is irritant and inflammation and ulceration may arise at injection sites, if extravasation occurs. Bolus injection or rapid infusions should therefore be avoided.
- Topical application may be associated with skin irritancy which is usually described as a burning sensation. Creams should not be used on mucous membranes.
- The irritant nature of aciclovir is also reflected in the occurrence of gastrointestinal upsets in some patients.
- Dizziness, fatigue and headache are potentially signs of neurotoxicity due to aciclovir.
- The drug is only contraindicated in patients who have displayed previous hypersensitivity, usually manifest as a generalized skin rash.
- Aciclovir for IV infusion is initially reconstituted by addition of water for injections or sodium chloride 0.9% to the vial to yield a solution containing 25 mg/ml. This can be administered over 1 hour via an infusion pump. Usually, the solution is further diluted to a final concentration 5 mg/ml

A

(minimum volume 50 ml) in sodium chloride 0.9%, glucose 5% or glucose/saline injection and administered over 1 hour. NB: Aciclovir which has been prepared for IV use should not be administered orally.

Storage
- Preparations containing aciclovir are stored at room temperature.
- Solution for IV infusion should be used immediately.
- Eye ointment should be discarded 1 month after first opening.

ACIPIMOX (Olbetam)

Presentation
Capsules – 250 mg

Actions and uses
Acipimox is chemically related to nicotinic acid (a member of the vitamin B group). Nicotinic acid itself lowers both cholesterol and triglyceride levels but, at the doses required, is limited by the pronounced side effects (particularly flushing and gastrointestinal upsets) which it produces. Derivatives such as acipimox have been developed in an attempt to improve tolerability but, while successful up to a point, they are used much less often than more modern lipid-lowering drugs.

Acipimox reduces cholesterol and triglyceride synthesis by a direct action on the liver and is occasionally used in the treatment of hypercholesterolaemia and mixed hyperlipidaemias as an alternative to first-line drugs.

Dosage
The usual adult dose is 500–750 mg daily taken in two or three divided doses with meals, up to a maximum of 1200 mg per day.

Nursing implications
- Nicotinic acid produces severe gastrointestinal upset including heartburn, epigastric pain, nausea and diarrhoea, and although derivatives such as

acipimox are designed to reduce this risk, such an effect cannot be ruled out. It is therefore important to monitor patients for signs of gastrointestinal disturbances, especially in those with a history of peptic ulcer disease.
- Other side effects common to nicotinic acid derivatives include flushing, nausea and diarrhoea.

Storage
Acipimox capsules are stored at room temperature.

ACITRETIN (Neotigason)

Presentation
Capsules – 10 mg, 25 mg

Actions and uses
Acitretin is a chemical derivative of vitamin A. It therefore belongs to the family known as the retinoids. It is used in the treatment of severe psoriasis which is unresponsive to other first-line drugs. Other uses include congenital ichthyosis (a skin condition characterized by hyperkeratinization) and Darièr's disease. The mechanism of action of acitretin (and related vitamin A compounds) is their antikeratitic (antimitotic) activity which results in inhibition of the abnormally rapid turnover of cells in the skin's thick outer keratin layer which underlies the conditions for which they are used.

Dosage
Adults only: an initial dose of 25–30 mg is taken once daily for up to 4 weeks, then gradually adjusted according to the response. Up to 75 mg daily may be given but the lowest possible maintenance dose should be used.

Nursing implications
- Treatment with acitretin is suppressive rather than curative and the patient should

understand that long-term therapy is required.

- Vitamin A derivatives are strongly teratogenic and fetal malformations are likely in the event of pregnancy. Pregnancy must therefore be excluded in women of child-bearing age at the outset and patients must be actively counselled thereafter to ensure that adequate contraceptive measures are always taken. Therapeutic abortion is generally offered in the event of pregnancy. Furthermore, pregnancy must be avoided for at least 2 years after treatment is discontinued since acitretin metabolites are stored for prolonged periods in the body's fat tissues.
- It is important to note that treatment with acitretin must be arranged through a specialist clinic and supplies of the drug are therefore restricted to hospitals only.
- Vitamin A compounds are poorly tolerated by some patients, hence the need for careful dosage adjustment. Dryness of the skin, erythema, pruritus and alopecia are common and erosion of mucous surfaces is possible. Other side effects include headaches, nausea, drowsiness, joint pain and myalgia.
- Hepatotoxicity may occur and liver function tests should be carried out regularly to detect early liver damage. Concurrent use of hepatotoxic drugs and alcohol should be discouraged and treatment avoided in the event of existing liver impairment.
- A further metabolic effect results in an unfavourable shift in the blood lipid profile with possible hyperlipidaemia. This can have important consequences for patients who have a history of angina, myocardial infarction and other risk factors for coronary heart disease.

- Caution is also required in patients with diabetes in whom glucose tolerance may be altered.
- Abnormal bone formation and calcification of non-osseous tissues may occur during long-term use and should be monitored by occasional X-rays.
- Acitretin should be avoided in patients with significant renal impairment.

Storage

Acitretin capsules are stored at room temperature and protected from light.

ACRIVASTINE (Semprex)

Presentation

Capsules – 8 mg

Actions and uses

This drug is an antihistaminic (histamine H1 receptor antagonist) which is less likely than older antihistamines to produce significant sedation and drowsiness. It is licensed for use in the treatment of allergic rhinitis and urticaria.

Dosage

Adults: 8 mg three times daily.

Nursing implications

- The section on antihistamines (p. 33) should be consulted for a full account of the nursing implications which apply to this drug.

Storage

Acrivastine capsules are stored at room temperature and protected from light.

ACROSOXACIN (Eradacin)

Presentation

Capsules – 150 mg

Actions and uses

Acrosoxacin is a member of the quinolone group of antibiotics (i.e. it chemically resembles ciprofloxacin, the first drug in this series). However, unlike ciprofloxacin, the use of this

A

drug is restricted to the treatment of acute gonorrhoeal infection in both men and women. As a result of its long action, single-dose therapy is all that is required.

Dosage

Adults only: 300 mg is administered, under supervision, as a single dose.

Nursing implications

- Compliance with drug treatment is a major problem in patients attending the genitourinary clinic. For this reason, drugs which only require to be taken in one, two or otherwise few doses are favoured **but** supervision is recommended and dosing is preferably carried out before the patient leaves the clinic.
- Since it is given as a single dose, acrosoxacin is unlikely to cause persistent side effects. However, gastrointestinal upsets, headache, dizziness and drowsiness, albeit short-lived, may be experienced.
- As acrosoxacin may cause drowsiness, the performance of skilled tasks such as driving may be impaired.
- Patients with liver and/or kidney impairment are more likely to report prolonged side effects.

Storage

Acrosoxacin capsules are stored at room temperature and protected from light.

ACTINOMYCIN D (Cosmegen, Lyovac)

Presentation

Injection – 500 microgram (0.5 mg) vial

Actions and uses

Actinomycin D is one of a group of antibiotics subsequently shown to have cytotoxic activity. A simplified version of its action is as follows. All mammalian cells have a nucleus composed of two strands made up of proteins known as DNA which contain all the (genetic) information necessary for the cell to divide (replicate) and subsequently mature. Actinomycin D combines with DNA to effectively block this process and cell death inevitably ensues. It is used mainly in the treatment of cancers affecting children including:

- Wilms' tumour of the kidney
- choriocarcinoma
- testicular teratomas.

There is evidence to suggest that the drug is more effective if patients receive concurrent radiotherapy.

Dosage

Actinomycin D is administered by the intravenous route. The dose of cytotoxic drugs used in chemotherapy regimen is regularly changing as experience dictates the optimum use of these drugs. For up-to-date information and advice, current dosage schedules should be consulted.

Nursing implications

- Note that this drug is often referred to as dactinomycin.
- It is **VERY** important that current dosage schedules for a given cytotoxic drug be **DOUBLE CHECKED** before chemotherapy proceeds. The consequences of dosage error are potentially very severe and may even be life threatening.
- Actinomycin D is highly irritant to surrounding tissues if allowed to escape from the vein (extravasation). Good injection technique is therefore essential.
- During treatment course abdominal pain, anorexia, nausea and vomiting may occur.
- Side effects, which may be delayed for days or even weeks after finishing a course, include bone marrow depression with anaemia, leucopenia and thrombocytopenia and resultant increased risk of severe infection and haemorrhage. Ulcerative stomatitis and dysphagia, alopecia, erythema, fever, hypocalcaemia, myalgia, malaise and gastrointestinal symptoms can also occur.

- Skin reactions may occur with this drug, more often at sites where simultaneous or prior radiotherapy has been given.
- Actinomycin D should never be given to patients with chickenpox as a severe or fatal generalized reaction may result.
- It should also be avoided during pregnancy.
- Adverse effects are particularly severe when given to children under the age of 1 year.
- Nurses should be aware of the risks posed by cytotoxic drugs. Some are irritant to the skin and mucous surfaces and care must be exercised when handling them. In particular, spillage or contamination of personnel or the environment must be avoided. If cytotoxic drugs are handled regularly, it is theoretically possible that repeated skin contact or inhalation may produce systemic toxic effects in nurses who have developed hypersensitivity to them. Most hospitals now operate a centralized (pharmacy-organized) additive service. While this reduces the risk of exposure to cytotoxic drugs, it is essential that nurses recognize and understand the local policy on their safe handling and disposal. The Health and Safety Executive has decreed that such a policy should be in place wherever cytotoxic drugs are administered. These should be adapted, wherever possible, to care of patients in the community.

Storage
- Vials containing sterile actinomycin D powder for injection are stored at room temperature under dry conditions.
- Solutions for IV injection or infusion are prepared by adding 1.1 ml water for injection to each vial to give a final solution containing 0.5 mg in 1 ml. This may be injected directly or via the drip tube of a 5% dextrose or 0.9% sodium chloride

infusion. Any unused solution must be discarded immediately.

ADENOSINE (Adenocor)

Presentation
Injection – 6 mg in 2 ml

Actions and uses
Adenosine is an antiarrhythmic agent. When administered by rapid intravenous injection, it slows conduction via the atrioventricular (AV) node, so interrupting reentry circuits involving this pathway (including those associated with Wolff–Parkinson–White syndrome) and restoring sinus rhythm in patients with paroxysmal supraventricular tachycardia. A further use is in assisting interpretation of atrial activity in the ECG by transiently slowing the rate of cardiac conduction.

Dosage
Adults: 3 mg administered by rapid intravenous injection, i.e. over 2 seconds followed by further doses of 6 mg and 12 mg if arrhythmias are not abolished within 1–2 minutes. Children: doses of between 0.0375 and 0.25 mg (37.5 and 250 microgram)/kg body weight have been used as above.

Nursing implications
- Facial flushing, chest tightness or dyspnoea, nausea and lightheadedness are common side effects. Others include sweating, palpitations, hyperventilation, headache, anxiety, burning sensation, bradycardia, chest pain, dizziness, arm/back/neck pain and metallic taste.
- Severe bradycardia has been reported. It is not reversed by atropine administration but some patients may require pacing.
- Adenosine should be avoided in patients with second- or third-degree heart block and sick sinus syndrome (unless a functioning pacemaker is in situ).
- Note that dipyridamole inhibits the inactivation of adenosine,

A

so potentiating its action. On the other hand, its activity is inhibited by theophylline and caffeine.

Storage

Adenosine injection is for immediate use, undiluted. Do not retain any residual solution.

ADRENALINE (Eppy, Simplene)

Note that the above-named products are only two of the many forms in which this drug is administered. It is most often recognized by its approved name of adrenaline.

Presentation

Injection – 1 in 1000 = 0.1% solution or 1 mg (1000 microgram) in 1 ml
– 1 in 10 000 = 0.01% solution or 0.1 mg (100 microgram) in 1 ml (10 ml ampoule)
Eye drops – 0.5% and 1%

Actions and uses

Adrenaline is the hormone secreted by the adrenal medulla in order to 'boost' the sympathetic nervous system in times of stress. Once in the circulation, its effects are widespread and complex.

It increases cardiac output by stimulating the rate and force of contraction of the heart and produces generalized vasoconstriction by its action on vascular smooth muscle. This is the basis for its use in cardiology and in acute anaphylaxis when circulatory support must be maintained. In the eye, adrenaline is only a weak mydriatic but it also reduces aqueous humour production and increases its outflow. Since it causes marked local vasoconstriction in the microcirculation, topical adrenaline solutions and ointments have been used to arrest bleeding.

In clinical practice adrenaline is used in:

- asystolic cardiac arrest in combination with calcium chloride to provoke ventricular fibrillation
- anaphylactic shock or other manifestations of severe allergy (e.g. angiooedema)

- open angle (chronic simple) glaucoma.

Dosage

Acute coronary care: 10 ml of a 1 in 10 000 solution by IV injection. Anaphylaxis and other allergic emergencies in adults: 0.5–1 ml of a 1 in 1000 solution by IM injection should be administered and repeated every 10 minutes until there is an improvement in blood pressure and pulse. Some use the subcutaneous route but absorption from this site in shock is less predictable.
Anaphylaxis and other allergic emergencies in children: <1 year: 0.05 ml; 1–2 years: 0.1 ml; 2–3 years: 0.2 ml; 3–5 years: 0.3 ml; 5–6 years: 0.4 ml; 6–12 years: 0.5 ml.
Glaucoma: one drop is instilled in the eye once or twice daily.

Nursing implications

- Adrenaline is not used in heart failure or cardiogenic shock since it possesses both alpha and beta actions. The former carries a risk of precipitating cardiac arrhythmias. This is accepted in asystole, however, since it is intended that ventricular fibrillation (subsequently responsive to cardioversion) be produced.
- Adrenaline injection may cause tachycardia, anxiety, tremors, dry mouth and a feeling of intense cold affecting the extremities (particularly the digits). It also raises blood pressure and inadvertent intravenous administration (particularly if combined with a local anaesthetic) has resulted in a precipitous rise in blood pressure and resulting haemorrhage.
- Adrenaline should be used with caution in situations where its stimulant action on the cardiovascular system and endocrine function may pose problems, e.g. ischaemic heart disease, hyperthyroidism, diabetes mellitus and hypertension.

- Adrenaline solutions may produce slight irritation when applied to the eye.

Storage
- Adrenaline eye drops may be stored at room temperature (or refrigerated when not in use) but must be protected from light. Any darkening in colour indicates a light-accelerated degradation of the solution which should be discarded.
- Eye drops, once open, can be used for 1 month in the community or 1 week in hospital wards.
- Adrenaline injection solutions are stored at room temperature but they too should be protected from light. Degradation may be detected as a slight pink discolouration of the solution.

ALCLOMETASONE (Modrasone)

Presentation
Cream – 0.05%
Ointment – 0.05%

Actions and uses
Alclometasone is a corticosteroid for topical use. The section on Corticosteroids, Topical (p. 107), should be consulted for a full account of its actions.

Alclometasone is a moderately potent steroid for use in the treatment of the dermatoses.

Dosage
Cream and ointment should be applied to affected areas 2–3 times daily.

Nurse monitoring
See the section on Corticosteroids.

Storage
Tubes of alclometasone cream and ointment are stored at room temperature. Dilution with other creams and ointments is not recommended.

ALENDRONATE (Fosamax)

Presentation
Tablets – 10 mg

Actions and uses
Alendronate is classed as a bisphosphonate or diphosphonate, a group of drugs which alter the metabolic activity of bone. Bone is metabolically very active, being constantly destroyed and rebuilt in a process known as remodelling which maintains fresh bone throughout life. In some circumstances, however, the breakdown of bone (which is influenced by the activity of cells called osteoclasts) is relatively greater than new bone synthesis (which is influenced by cells called osteoblasts). Alendronate inhibits osteoclast activity and so redresses this balance.

Alendronate by its action inhibits the release of calcium from bone and is used therefore when this occurs excessively, such as after the menopause when oestrogen (which is an important stimulant of osteoblast activity) is in rapid decline. Thus the current indication for alendronate is in the treatment of established osteoporosis in postmenopausal women in whom it reduces the risk of fracture at all skeletal sites.

Dosage
A single daily dose 10 mg is usually taken in the morning, swallowed whole with a generous amount of water.

Nursing implications
- It is essential to stress the need to swallow tablets intact and with a generous portion (whole glass) of water. This advice has been issued as a result of several cases of serious oesophageal irritation and ulceration due to the irritant nature of alendronate. Patients should avoid lying down immediately after taking alendronate to enhance the passage of tablets through the oesophagus.
- The above advice is especially important since the majority of patients will be relatively elderly and therefore have poor oesophageal motility. Alendronate is, in fact,

A

contraindicated in those with established oesophageal stricture or swallowing difficulty.
- Tablets must never be crushed or chewed before swallowing.
- Patients should avoid all food for at least 30 minutes before and after treatment. This particularly applies to calcium-containing foods and drinks such as milk and mineral water.
- Abdominal pain and discomfort may occur. Patients must be advised to report any swallowing difficulty or sensation of heartburn.
- It remains to be seen whether or not drugs of this group can effectively prevent (as well as treat) osteoporosis. They may nonetheless be tried in younger patients for whom hormone replacement therapy (the recognized preventive therapy) is poorly tolerated or otherwise contraindicated.

Storage
Alendronate tablets are stored at room temperature.

ALFACALCIDOL (Alfa D, One-Alpha)

This drug is also known as 1-alpha hydroxycholecalciferol.

Presentation
Capsules – 0.25 microgram and 1 microgram
Oral solution – 0.20 microgram in 1 ml
Injection – 1 microgram in 0.5 ml
— 2 microgram in 1 ml

Actions and uses
Naturally occurring vitamin D is a mixture of ergocalciferol and chole-calciferol (vitamins D2 and D3 respect-ively). These are, in fact, prohormones which require further conversion by the kidney and liver to produce the active compounds, one of which is alfa-calcidol. Most patients can adequately utilize natural vitamin D but in some it is necessary to administer the active compounds directly. Alfacalcidol is used in the treatment of the following.

- Renal osteodystrophy, a bone-wasting condition in patients with severe renal impairment and vitamin D deficiency. In such cases, conversion of natural vitamin D by the kidney is impaired.
- Severe vitamin D deficiency such as that which occurs in nutritional malabsorption and resistant vitamin D rickets and osteomalacia.
- Hypoparathyroidism (associated with reduced plasma calcium) and hyperparathyroidism in patients with bone disease.
- Neonatal hypocalcaemia.

Dosage
All indications.

- Adults and children >20 kg: initially 1 microgram (0.5 microgram in the elderly) with subsequent adjust-ments to avoid hypercalcaemia.
- Children < 20 kg: initially 0.05 microgram/kg per day initially with subsequent adjustments as above.
- Premature infants: initially 0.05–0.1 microgram/kg per day initially with subsequent adjustments as above.

Nursing implications
- The above doses are administered once daily by oral or IV route over 30 seconds.
- It is important to note that alfacalcidol is a very active form of vitamin D. Serum calcium must be regularly checked to ensure that hypercalcaemia does not result.
- Note that the risk of hypercalcaemia is increased when thiazide diuretics (e.g. bendrofluazide), which them-selves reduce calcium excretion, are given concurrently.
- Note that the following symptoms are evident in cases of overdose: anorexia, nausea and vomiting, weakness, weight loss, polyuria, sweating, headache, thirst and raised concentrations of calcium and phosphate in plasma and urine.

Storage

- Alfacalcidol capsules, oral solution and injection should be stored preferably in a refrigerator.
- Protect from light.

ALFENTANIL (Rapifen)

Presentation

Injection – 1 mg in 2 ml
 – 5 mg in 1 ml
 – 5 mg in 10 ml

Actions and uses

Alfentanil is a narcotic (morphine-like) analgesic which has a characteristically brief action (i.e. approximately 30–45 minutes duration). It is widely used as an analgesic for short operative procedures, e.g. in an outpatient setting when pain control can be readily adjusted by altering the rate of administration. Alfentanil is also used to enhance anaesthesia and reduce respiratory drive in ICU patients receiving assisted ventilation.

Dosage

Administered by intravenous bolus injection with spontaneous respiration.

- Adults: 50–200 microgram with further doses of 50 microgram as required.
- Children: 3–5 microgram/kg with additional doses of 1 microgram/kg as required.

Administered with assisted ventilation.

- Adults: 300–3500 microgram followed by 100–200 microgram as required.
- Children: 15 microgram/kg with additional doses of 1–3 microgram/kg as required.

Nursing implications

- It is important to note that alfentanil is a potent respiratory depressant and patients not receiving assisted ventilation must be closely monitored.
- It should be used with caution in situations where the occurrence of respiratory depression may pose a particular risk,

e.g. in myasthenia gravis, the elderly and debilitated, chronic respiratory disease, hypothyroidism, chronic liver disease and obstetrics.
- Other common side effects include transient hypotension, bradycardia, nausea and vomiting.
- Skilled tasks such as driving should be avoided as drowsiness may be experienced.
- Alcohol should be avoided.

Storage

Alfentanil is a Controlled Drug and as such it must be stored in a locked cupboard, ordered by special requisition and its use recorded dose by dose, in line with current legislation.

ALGINIC ACID (Gastrocote, Gaviscon)

Presentation

Combined with various antacids in tablet, liquid and granular (sachet) form.

Actions and uses

Alginic acid forms a protective coating on the surface of gastric juice and therefore prevents reflux of gastric acid and bile into the oesophagus, so reducing associated symptoms of oesophagitis. It is used for the treatment of heartburn and dyspeptic pain when these are caused by hiatus hernia and reflux oesophagitis.

Dosage

Adults: 1–3 tablets or 10–20 ml (Gaviscon) after meals and at bedtime.
Children: one tablet or 5–10 ml liquid after meals and at bedtime.
Infants: a special formulation of infant Gaviscon is available for the very young. The dose is $\frac{1}{2}$–1 sachet mixed with water or with made-up feeds.

Nursing implications

- Tablets and granules should be thoroughly chewed before swallowing. The liquid may be

A

diluted with up to an equal amount of water for ease of administration.

- This drug is not normally associated with troublesome side effects though it may be unpalatable for some. Hence the value of different available preparations and dosage forms.
- It does, however, contain sugar which therefore, if given to diabetics, should be taken into account when formulating low sugar diets.

Storage

Tablets, granules and liquid preparations containing alginic acid are stored at room temperature.

ALLOPURINOL (Zyloric)

Presentation

Tablets – 100 mg, 300 mg

Actions and uses

If uric acid accumulates in excess in the blood, gout may be produced with subsequent arthritis, skin lesions and impairment of renal function. Increased blood urate occurs most commonly in patients suffering from classic gout and in patients with malignant disease who are treated with cytotoxic drugs or radiotherapy. In the latter case the increased urate is due to an increased destruction and turnover of cells. A less common cause of raised blood uric acid is diuretic therapy which can, in fact, precipitate gout in susceptible individuals.

Allopurinol is used to prevent raised blood uric acid (hyperuricaemia) and in the prophylaxis of gout and associated complications. It acts by inhibiting an enzyme (xanthine oxidase) which takes part in the production of uric acid from its chemical precursors (collectively termed xanthines), thereby reducing the total amount of uric acid produced.

Dosage

Prophylaxis of gout (adults): initially 100 mg once daily increasing to a maintenance dose of 300 mg (occasionally higher doses) per day. Usually administered once (or perhaps twice) daily.

Treatment of hyperuricaemia in adult leukaemic patients: 200 mg three times a day for 3 days prior to treatment, then adjusted as required to a maintenance dose of 300 mg per day. Treatment of hyperuricaemia in childhood leukaemia: maintenance 20 mg/kg per day.

Nursing implications

- When allopurinol treatment is commenced, the blood urate is likely to fall. It has been found that any change in blood urate may lead to an acute attack of gout. Therefore, an antiinflammatory analgesic drug (NSAID) or colchicine is often given concurrently for up to 1 month to counter such an effect.
- Poor compliance with allopurinol treatment may give rise to acute attacks of gout. Patient education regarding regular dosing is therefore an important part of the nurse's role. However, in practice the pain of gout is so severe that patients are usually amenable to advice.
- Side effects which occasionally occur with this drug are nausea, vomiting and skin rashes.
- Rarely severe skin reactions, fever, joint pain and eosinophilia may occur as a general hypersensitivity to allopurinol. Treatment must be discontinued in such cases and alternative therapy substituted.
- Side effects are more common in patients with kidney or liver disease and the dose should be reduced by an appropriate amount in patients with renal failure.
- Allopurinol inhibits the liver metabolism of cytotoxic drugs such as mercaptopurine and azathioprine. The dosage of these drugs must therefore be reduced substantially in order to avoid serious toxicity.

- Allopurinol also inhibits the metabolism of aminophylline and theophylline and severe theophylline toxicity may result. Anticoagulant control should similarly be closely monitored in patients receiving warfarin.

Storage
Allopurinol tablets are stored at room temperature.

ALPROSTADIL (Caverject, Prostin VR)

Presentation
Injection (intracavernosal) – 10 microgram and 20 microgram + diluent/syringe
Injection (intravenous in neonates) – 500 microgram in 1 ml

Actions and uses
Alprostadil is prostaglandin E1. It has two main uses.

- It increases blood flow in the corpus cavernosum (the spongy tissue of the shaft) of the penis and is used to induce erection in men with erectile impotence associated with vascular impairment.
- It prevents closure of the ductus arteriosus in neonates with congenital heart defects (e.g. atrioventricular septum deformity) and is used therefore to maintain patency prior to corrective surgery.

Dosage
Impotence in males: a single dose of 2.5 microgram is injected directly into the corpus cavernosum. If a partial response only is achieved, a second dose of 5 microgram is then injected or, if no response to the initial dose, this is increased to 7.5 microgram. Further dosage increments of 5 microgram may be required but no more than 60 microgram in total in any one day should be used.
Congenital heart defects in neonates: by intravenous infusion, 0.05–0.1 microgram/kg/min reduced thereafter to lowest possible maintenance dose.

Nursing implications
- The nature of use in erectile impotence is such that careful patient education and instruction are essential to the appropriate use and safety of alprostadil.
- Intracavernosal injection may be associated with painful and prolonged erection. If erection is sustained beyond 1 hour and up to 4 hours or if priapism occurs, then aspiration or intervention with vasoconstrictor drugs may be necessary in which case medical help must be sought immediately.
- It is possible that some patients can be taught to self-inject the antidote (adrenaline, phenylephrine, etc.) but only if unlikely to be compromised by the increase in blood pressure which might result.
- A number of side effects are associated with the use of alprostadil in the treatment of erectile dysfunction; these may include penile pain, oedema, rash and irritation. Systemic effects include testicular pain and swelling, changes in micturition and localized pain (head, buttocks, pelvis, back).
- The vascular effects of alprostadil may manifest as flushing, bradycardia, hypotension (even tachycardia) and arrhythmias in neonates.

Storage
- Alprostadil (Prostin VR) injection is stored in a refrigerator.
- Solutions for infusion prepared in glucose 5% or sodium chloride 0.9% should be used within 24 hours.
- Do not allow concentrated injection solution to remain in contact with plastics. Discard such solutions if they turn hazy.
- Alprostadil intercavernosal injection (Caverject) is refrigerated during prolonged storage. Once dispensed, it can be kept at room temperature for up to 3 months.

A

A

- Once reconstituted, solution should be used immediately.

Patients weighing <65 kg should receive a reduced dosage.

ALTEPLASE (Actilyse)

Presentation
Injection – 20 mg and 50 mg dry powder vials

Actions and uses
Alteplase is a genetically engineered form of human tissue type plasminogen activator (tPA), a protease enzyme which, as the name suggests, activates plasminogen. Plasminogen is a natural antifibrinolytic substance found in body tissues which converts fibrin (deposited in thrombi) into a soluble form. As a result, preformed blood clots are dissolved and the blockage which they create is removed. Thrombolytics are often described as 'clot busters' as a result. They are used in the following.

- Treatment of acute myocardial infarction (coronary thrombosis) in which they produce early reperfusion (recanalization) of the coronary arteries with consequent reduction in infarct size, reduced mortality and improved prognosis.
- Dissolution of intravascular thrombus in pulmonary embolism. They may also be used in extensive deep venous thrombosis, acute or subacute occlusion of peripheral arteries and central retinal venous or arterial thrombosis but such uses are, as yet, unlicensed.

Dosage
Acute myocardial infarction (within 12 hours): initially 15 mg is administered by bolus IV injection. This is followed by IV infusion of 50 mg over 30 minutes, then 35 mg over 1 hour. A total dose of 100 mg alteplase is therefore given. In cases where more than 12 hours have elapsed since myocardial infarction, individual coronary units should be consulted for advice regarding the most beneficial administration. Pulmonary embolism (use as a guide to treatment of other intravascular thrombus formation): initially, 10 mg by bolus IV injection followed by an IV infusion of 90 mg over 2 hours.

Nursing implications
- Experience has shown that the earlier thrombolytic therapy is administered, the better the outcome. Best results are obtained if given within 6 hours of myocardial infarction but later administration is still warranted. An accurate history on admission may therefore be helpful in determining likely prognosis.
- The incidence of hypersensitivity reactions and failure of treatment due to antibody formation (as seen with streptokinase and its derivatives) does not apply in the case of this drug. It is, as a result, generally reserved for patients with a history of intolerance to streptokinase or in whom streptokinase has been administered within the previous 12 months.
- The cost of alteplase, however, dictates that its use is generally limited to reinfarction in the above situations.
- Careful control by pressure of the site where the drug or other intravenous therapy may be administered is essential to control bleeding.
- The nurse may play an important role in identifying contraindications to thrombolytic therapy, as a result of the risk from bleeding. These include:
  - recent (i.e. within 3 months) cerebrovascular accident
  - uncontrolled or uncontrollable hypertension
  - known bleeding diathesis
  - active peptic ulceration
  - aggressive CPR with possible internal bleeding
  - recent (i.e. within 3 months) major surgery or trauma
  - severe liver disease with impaired clotting mechanism.
- Check individual coronary care units for local policy on

contraindications to thrombolytic therapy.
- Vials of alteplase are reconstituted with water for injection to provide a concentration of 1 mg in 1 ml. This may be infused directly or further diluted in sodium chloride 0.9% injection to a final concentration *not less than* 200 microgram (0.2 mg) in 1 ml.
- Do not dilute using glucose injection.

Storage
- Alteplase injection is stored below 25°C but reconstituted solution may be stored for up to 24 hours in a refrigerator (between 2 and 8°C) and up to 8 hours at room temperature.
- Unopened vials should be kept in their original package until preparation.

ALUMINIUM HYDROXIDE (Alu-Cap)

Presentation
Tablets – 500 mg
Suspension/gel – 3.5/4.4% as aluminium oxide
Capsules – 475 mg

Actions and uses
Aluminium hydroxide has two main uses.

- It is a simple antacid used for the relief of mild to moderate indigestion and heartburn as a result of chemical neutralization of gastric acid excess.
- It is used as a phosphate-binding agent in chronic renal failure where there is reduced phosphate excretion by the kidney. Aluminium hydroxide binds to phosphate in the gut, so reducing the amount absorbed and its subsequent accumulation in the circulation (hyperphosphataemia).

Dosage
Indigestion/heartburn in adults: two tablets are chewed or 10 ml suspension taken over a few hours as required.

Prevention of hyperphosphataemia in chronic renal failure: the dosage must be individualized to meet the needs of each patient. However, up to 20 Alu-Cap capsules (taken with meals) may be necessary to achieve adequate control of the serum phosphate level.

Nursing implications
- Constipation may occur. If used in combination with magnesium salts (e.g. magnesium hydroxide, magnesium trisilicate), which tend to cause diarrhoea, this effect may be offset.
- Neurological toxicity (including dementia) may arise in patients who regularly ingest large quantities of aluminium hydroxide and is a particular problem in patients with chronic renal failure. Others should be discouraged from overuse of the drug for prolonged periods. This is often a sign that upper gastrointestinal problems (e.g. oesophagitis, peptic ulceration) exist and require thorough investigation. More suitable (effective) treatments are available in such cases.
- The clinical effectiveness of drugs such as digoxin and some antibiotics (notably the tetracyclines) may be impaired by concurrent administration of aluminium hydroxide. If relevant, at least 1–2 hours should be allowed to elapse before or after dosing with such drugs.
- Tablets should be chewed before swallowing and the suspension/gel thoroughly shaken before each dose is taken. Capsules are swallowed whole.

Storage
Aluminium hydroxide preparations are stored at room temperature.

AMANTADINE (Symmetrel)

Presentation
Capsules – 100 mg
Syrup – 50 mg in 5 ml

A

Actions and uses

Amantadine was developed as an antiviral agent for the prevention and treatment of influenza and is still used, albeit very rarely, to reduce the complications of influenza. It is also used in the treatment of herpes zoster (shingles) infection. An additional benefit, discovered by chance in patients with Parkinson's disease who received the drug, was improvement in symptoms. Although the mechanism of action is not clearly understood, amantadine is still (and generally only) used as part of the treatment of Parkinson's disease.

Dosage

Parkinson's disease: 100 mg once daily for first week then 100 mg twice daily. Treatment of influenza (adults and children >10 years): 100 mg daily for up to 5 days.
Prophylaxis of influenza (adults and children >10 years): 100 mg daily for as long as protection is deemed necessary, usually up to 6 weeks, or for 2–3 weeks after influenza vaccination. Treatment of herpes zoster (shingles) infection (adults only): 100 mg twice daily for up to 1 month.

Nursing implications

- This drug should be used with caution in patients with a history of convulsions, peptic ulceration and in severe renal impairment and is contraindicated in pregnancy and breastfeeding.
- Side effects involving the central nervous system may be severe and include: nervousness, insomnia, dizziness, convulsions, behavioural disturbances and hallucinations.
- It should be noted that the beneficial effects of amantadine in the treatment of Parkinson's disease may be short-lived (limited to a few months only) and this should be taken into account when assessing patient expectation of their treatment.

Storage

Amantadine capsules and syrup are stored at room temperature.

AMIKACIN (Amikin)

Presentation

Injection – 100 mg in 2 ml vial
– 500 mg in 2 ml vial

Actions and uses

Amikacin is a member of the aminoglycoside group of antibiotics. Drugs of this type are notably active against Gram-negative bacilli including the often troublesome pathogen *Pseudomonas aeruginosa*. They are widely used in the treatment of Gram-negative sepsis, which is a particular problem in elderly hospitalized patients and in the immunocompromised. Aminoglycoside antibiotics also have an important role in the management of severe, recurring respiratory infections (often due to Pseudomonas), in cystic fibrosis and in bronchiolitis. They are also used together with broad-spectrum penicillins and cephalosporins in the prevention and treatment of infections in at-risk groups when broad-spectrum cover is required.

The aminoglycosides are specifically bactericidal. They act by inhibiting the synthesis of essential proteins after binding to the bacterial ribosome. Some resistance does occur, either as a result of reduced penetration and transport across the bacterial cell membrane or the production by resistant organisms of enzymes which destroy the drugs by a chemical action. Resistance is, however, relatively uncommon.

Dosage

The dosage for adults and children is calculated on a basis of 15 mg/kg per day in total, usually given in two divided doses by intravenous injection. The maximum daily dose may be as high as 1.5 g.

Nursing implications

- Experience with the aminoglycosides suggests that once-daily (rather than two or three times daily) dosing may be most effective since the bactericidal effect seems to be related to the initial

---

(peak) blood levels which are reached after IV administration.

- Aminoglycoside antibiotic therapy is associated with two major side effects. It is potentially toxic to the tissues of the kidney (nephrotoxicity) and the inner ear (ototoxicity). For this reason it is necessary to monitor blood levels, especially predose (trough levels), in order to limit the possibility of such toxicity. The pharmacy can advise on target blood levels.
- As a result of the above, it is essential that patients who develop hearing loss or difficulty or unexpected loss of balance and coordination be evaluated for possible aminoglycoside toxicity.
- Amikacin injection is administered by direct IV bolus injection or added to 50–100 ml sodium chloride and infused over 30 minutes to 1 hour.
- Penicillin and cephalosporin antibiotics should never be mixed in the same IV infusion system since they are chemically incompatible.

Storage

Amikacin injection is stored at room temperature.

AMILORIDE (Midamor)

Presentation

Tablets – 5 mg
Also combined with other diuretics, e.g. frusemide, bumetanide, hydrochlorothiazide, in combination products.

Actions and uses

Amiloride has a mild diuretic action. Its site of action is the distal tubule where it inhibits active sodium reabsorption at the expense of potassium. Although of little value as a diuretic alone, it may be usefully combined with the thiazide and loop diuretics because of its potassium-conserving action. Amiloride is therefore used to prevent the hypokalaemia which is commonly

encountered in patients treated with thiazide and loop diuretics when otherwise used alone.

Dosage

The usual adult dose is 5–10 mg taken as a single dose in the morning.

Nursing implications

- Hyperkalaemia may occur, particularly in patients with impaired renal function. It is clinically undetectable, and extremely dangerous as it may lead to sudden death due to cardiac arrest. Plasma potassium levels should therefore be checked regularly.
- Possible side effects include anorexia, nausea, vomiting, abdominal pain, constipation (or diarrhoea), dry mouth, thirst, paraesthesia, dizziness, weakness, lethargy and muscle cramps.
- Skin rashes, itching, mental confusion and visual disturbances may occur.
- Some of the above effects are related to overenthusiastic use of diuretic therapy leading to dehydration and loss of electrolytes.

Storage

Amiloride tablets are stored at room temperature.

AMINOPHYLLINE (Phyllocontin)

Presentation

Tablets, slow release – 100 mg, 225 mg, 350 mg
Injection – 250 mg in 10 ml

Actions and uses

Aminophylline is a water-soluble form of theophylline (to which it is converted in the body), hence its availability in injectable form. Its action in the lung is thought to result from direct relaxation of bronchial smooth muscle and indirectly from stabilization of mast cells. By injection, aminophylline has a special role in the

A

management of acute, severe asthma in which it is a third-line treatment for patients uncontrolled by oral/intravenous steroid and nebulized salbutamol/terbutaline. Similarly, it is used in the treatment of respiratory disease associated with right-sided heart failure (chronic hypoxic cor pulmonale) in which it exerts a positive inotropic (cardiac stimulant) action.

Dosage

Adults.

- Oral: slow-release tablets are taken twice daily in a dose of 225–450 mg.
- Intravenous: 250–500 mg administered very slowly (over 10–15 minutes) by bolus injection. Alternatively, an intravenous infusion is given in sodium chloride 0.9% or glucose 5% at a rate of 500 microgram (0.5 mg) to 1 mg per kg per hour.

Children.

- Oral: slow-release tablets for children aged 3–5 years or more, in a dose of 100–200 mg twice daily or as a single dose at bedtime for nocturnal wheeze.
- Intravenous: a loading dose of 5 mg/kg body weight by bolus injection (over 20 minutes) is used. This may be followed if necessary by maintenance infusion at a rate of 1000 microgram (1 mg)/kg per hour (up to 9 years) or 800 microgram per kg per hour in older children. Intravenous infusion has also been administered in the management of apnoea in prematurity.

Nursing implications

- The above doses are for guidance only. In practice, patients should have their blood theophylline (aminophylline is converted to theophylline) levels monitored. The precise dose is that which maintains the blood theophylline level within the therapeutic range of 55–110 mmol/litre. Higher levels are associated with CNS toxicity, including a risk of convulsions.
- It should be noted that certain factors can alter theophylline blood levels and might explain an apparent lack of effect or the sudden development of toxicity. Drugs such as allopurinol, cimetidine, erythromycin, clarithromycin and ciprofloxacin inhibit the liver metabolism of theophylline and their introduction may be associated with a sudden increase in level and the occurrence of associated side effects. Cigarette smoking and the use of barbiturates will reduce blood levels of theophylline.
- It is important to note the risk of severe toxicity after intravenous injection in patients already taking oral aminophylline or theophylline. Intravenous loading doses should be avoided and maintenance infusions given with extreme caution in such cases. It is therefore important to determine in advance any patient's current drug therapy.
- Gastrointestinal irritation is a major problem with oral therapy. Patients who complain of dyspepsia may benefit from a change of theophylline preparation.
- The other major side effect associated with blood levels in excess of the target range is CNS overstimulation. This results in anxiety, confusion and restlessness. Patients may complain of vertigo and show marked hyperventilation.

Storage

Aminophylline tablets and injection are stored at room temperature.

AMIODARONE (Cordarone X)

Presentation

Tablets – 100 mg, 200 mg
Injection – 150 mg in 3 ml

Actions and uses

Amiodarone is used for the treatment of cardiac dysrhythmias including paroxysmal supraventricular, nodal and ventricular tachycardias, atrial flutter and atrial fibrillation. It may also be effective in dysrhythmias resistant to more commonly used drugs. It is thought to be of particular value in the treatment of paroxysmal arrhythmias associated with the Wolff–Parkinson–White syndrome.

Dosage

Adults: the initial loading regime is 200 mg three times a day for 1 week. This may be extended if a response is not achieved. To decide the maintenance dose, the initial regime is gradually reduced until the lowest dose that will maintain control is obtained, usually 200 mg once daily.

Nursing implications

- During prolonged therapy patients have developed microcrystalline deposits of the drug in the cornea, occasionally producing visual impairment. Regular ophthalmic examinations are therefore advised.
- Peripheral neuropathy and tremor have occurred which may be diminished or resolved by a reduction in dosage. If they persist, however, discontinuation of treatment may be necessary.
- Photosensitivity and skin pigmentation are reported. Other common side effects include headaches, dizziness, nausea, vomiting and a metallic taste in the mouth.
- Sleep disturbances (including nightmares) also occur although more often at the outset and tend to diminish as maintenance doses are achieved.
- Amiodarone should be avoided or used with caution in:
  - the presence of sinus bradycardia or AV block
  - cardiac failure uncontrolled by digoxin and diuretic therapy
  - patients currently receiving beta-blockers or verapamil
  - those with a history of thyroid disease (amiodarone is a rich source of iodine)
  - pregnancy and breastfeeding
  - iodine sensitivity.
- It is important to recognize that amiodarone may increase the serum level of digoxin and such patients should be carefully monitored for evidence of digoxin toxicity.

Storage

Amiodarone tablets and injection are stored at room temperature but must be protected from light.

AMITRIPTYLINE (Tryptizol, Lentizol)

Presentation

Tablets – 10 mg, 25 mg, 50 mg
Capsules – 25 mg, 50 mg (both as sustained release)
Syrup – 25 mg in 5 ml, 50 mg in 5 ml
Injection – 100 mg in 10 ml

Actions and uses

For an account of the actions and uses, see Antidepressant Drugs (p. 31). Amitriptyline is one of the tricyclic and related antidepressants.

Dosage

- Orally for the treatment of depression: the usual dose range is 75–150 mg or higher in resistant cases. The drug may be taken in three divided doses or as a single evening dose, especially in slow-release form, on retiring.
- If given by the intramuscular or intravenous routes: 20–30 mg four times daily is the usual required dose.
- Doses in the lower range, as above, are used in the treatment of neurogenic pain.

Nursing implications

See Antidepressant Drugs (p. 31).

A

Storage
- Preparations containing amitriptyline are stored at room temperature.
- The injection solution and oral syrup should be protected from light.
- For ease of administration amitriptyline syrup may be diluted with Syrup BP before use but such dilutions must be used within 14 days.

AMLODIPINE (Istin)

Presentation
Tablets – 5 mg, 10 mg

Actions and uses
Amlodipine is a calcium antagonist and has the actions and uses described for this group on p. 67.

Dosage
All indications (adults): 5 mg once daily which may be doubled depending upon the individual patient's response.

Nursing implications
See Calcium Antagonists (p. 67).

Storage
Amlodipine tablets are stored at room temperature.

AMOXAPINE (Asendis)

Presentation
Tablets – 25 mg, 50 mg, 100 mg

Action and uses
Amoxapine is an antidepressant which is chemically unrelated to the tricyclic antidepressants (e.g. amitriptyline, imipramine, etc.) but nevertheless shares many of their properties. Like other antidepressants (see p. 31), it acts in the brain to boost levels of the neurotransmitter noradrenaline. However, amoxapine also has central actions consistent with those of the neuroleptics or major tranquillizers and may therefore be of particular value in the treatment of psychotic depression which is unresponsive to an antidepressant drug alone.

Dosage
- Adults: initial doses of 100–150 mg daily are used and increased up to 300 mg depending upon clinical response. Amoxapine may be taken in divided doses throughout the day or, if preferred, as a single night-time dose.
- Lower initial doses are recommended for elderly patients, e.g. 25 mg twice daily increased gradually over a period of 1 week to a maximum of 50 mg three times daily.

Nursing implications
- Although not strictly a tricyclic drug, the nursing implications for these drugs (see Antidepressant Drugs, p. 31) apply to amoxapine.
- Early loss of efficacy, e.g. within 3 months of starting therapy, has been reported to occur in some patients treated with amoxapine. Regular supervision is essential in order to detect this, but non-compliance remains the likeliest cause of loss of effect.

Storage
Amoxapine tablets are stored at room temperature.

AMOXYCILLIN (Amoxil)

Presentation
Capsules – 250 mg, 500 mg
Tablets, dispersible – 500 mg
'Fiztab' (buccal dispersible) – 125 mg, 250 mg, 500 mg
Sachets – 750 mg and 3 g
Syrup – 125 mg in 5 ml, 250 mg in 5 ml
Drops – 125 mg in 1.25 ml
Injection – 250 mg, 500 mg vials

Actions and uses
Amoxycillin is a broad-spectrum antibiotic of the penicillin group with activity against common Gram-positive and Gram-negative organisms. It is widely used in the treatment of infections of the upper and lower respiratory tract and urinary tract due to, e.g., *Strep. pneumoniae* (Pneumococcus), *E. coli,*

Haemophilus influenzae, etc. Amoxycillin has actions and uses identical to ampicillin but can be given less frequently since it is much better absorbed by the oral route.

Dosage

Oral.

- Adults and older children: 250–500 mg three times a day.
- Children aged 1–7 years: 125–250 mg three times a day.
- Children less than 1 year: 62.5 mg three times a day.
- Single (high) 3 g oral doses are available and may be repeated once at a 12-hourly interval. (These are used for short-term treatment of respiratory and urinary tract infections.)

Injection.

- The parenteral and oral dosages are the same. May be given by intra-muscular or intravenous injection.

Nursing implications

- Skin rashes associated with amoxycillin are relatively common, especially when used inappropriately to treat a viral respiratory infection. The occurrence of skin rash does not necessarily confirm allergy to drugs of the penicillin group generally.
- Nevertheless, it is important to recognize that cross-allergy does exist between different penicillins. Allergic reactions vary from skin rashes and fever to more serious angiooedema and even anaphylaxis.
- Allergy apart, drugs of the penicillin class are remarkably free from side effects. Broad-spectrum drugs such as amoxycillin may, however, produce diarrhoea as a result of disturbance of the normal bacterial flora of the bowel.

Storage

- Preparations containing amoxycillin are stored in dry powder form at room temperature.

- When reconstituted for injection such solutions should be used immediately and any unused portion discarded.
- Intravenous infusions are given over 15–30 minutes in 100 ml sodium chloride 0.9%, glucose 5% or glucose/saline mixtures.
- Oral mixtures, once prepared, should be used within 7 days or 14 days if kept in a refrigerator.

AMPHOTERICIN B (Abelcet, AmBisome, Amphocil, Fungilin, Fungizone)

Presentation

Oral suspension – 100 mg in 1 ml
Lozenges – 10 mg
Injection – 50 mg, 100 mg vials

Actions and uses

- This drug is an effective antifungal agent useful against a wide variety of yeasts and yeast-like fungi, including Candida albicans. It is important to note that absorption from the gut is negligible, even with very large doses, and that intravenous therapy is necessary if treating systemic fungal infections.
- Intravenous preparations are available which are effective against cryptococcosis (Torulopsis), North American blastomycosis, the disseminated forms of candidosis, coccidiomycosis and histoplasmosis and also aspergillosis and other extremely rare fungal infections.
- Conventional amphotericin injection is limited by dose-related toxicity. As a result, newer preparations which 'encase' amphotericin within a protective colloid or lipid layer have been introduced. These products, called 'liposomal' or 'colloid complex' amphotericin, are much less toxic and can be given in higher dosage. They are unfortunately vastly more expensive than conventional injection.

Dosage

In oral candidiasis (thrush) infection: oral drops are instilled four times daily. The usual dose for babies, children or adults is 100 000 unit (100 mg) but up

A

to 500 000 unit (50 mg) may be required for extensive lesions. Lozenges are sucked four times daily. Parenteral therapy (conventional): for adults and children the total daily dose should be administered by slow intravenous infusion over a period of 6 hours. The dosage is calculated on the basis of initially 0.25 mg/kg body weight, gradually increasing to a level of 1 mg/kg body weight depending on individual response and tolerance. Parenteral therapy (liposomal/colloid complex): the above dosage can be extended up to a maximum of 4 mg/kg. While these newer preparations are undoubtedly safer, there is no evidence that they are more effective than conventional amphotericin injection.

- Reduction in serum potassium (hypokalaemia) and serum magnesium (hypomagnesaemia) is associated with amphotericin and replacement therapy may be warranted.

Storage
- Amphotericin topical liquid and lozenges are stored at room temperature.
- Injection vials are stored in a refrigerator. Reconstituted solutions for injection must be freshly prepared.
- The preparation of individual intravenous forms should be carried out in the pharmacy. Special conditions are required.

Nursing implications
- The main problems are associated with systemic toxicity, especially after intravenous administration of conventional amphotericin. Strict attention to dosage, concentration of the infusion and rate of administration is essential to limit the likelihood of toxicity.
- Systemic therapy is associated with fever, rigor, headache, anorexia, weight loss, nausea, vomiting, malaise, painful muscles and joints, dyspepsia and cramping stomach pains, diarrhoea, anaemia and hypokalaemia.
- Irritation and thrombophlebitis are relatively common injection site reactions. If severe, the infusion may need to be stopped and recommenced using an alternative site. Extravasation must be avoided.
- Intravenous infusion may cause renal failure, disturbance of cardiac rhythm, visual and auditory defects and convulsions.
- Amphotericin should be used with great caution in patients who are known to have kidney disease. Renal function can be checked by monitoring serum creatinine level.

AMPICILLIN (Penbritin)

Presentation
Capsules – 250 mg, 500 mg
Syrup and suspension – 125 mg in 5 ml, 125 mg in 1.25 ml, dropper 250 mg in 5 ml
Injection – vials containing 250 mg and 500 mg

Actions and uses
Ampicillin is a broad-spectrum antibiotic of the penicillin group with activity against common Gram-positive and Gram-negative organisms. It has been widely used in the treatment of infections of the upper and lower respiratory tract and urinary tract due to, e.g., *Strep. pneumoniae* (Pneumococcus), *E. coli* and *Haemophilus influenzae*. However, amoxycillin, which has actions and uses identical to ampicillin, is now generally preferred. It is much better absorbed by the oral route and can be given less frequently as a result.

Dosage
Oral.

- Adults and older children: 250–500 mg four times a day.
- Children aged 1–7 years: 125–250 mg four times a day.
- Children less than 1 year: 62.5 mg four times per day.

Injection.

- The parenteral and oral dosages are the same. May be given by intramuscular or intravenous injection.

Nursing implications
- Skin rashes associated with ampicillin are relatively common, especially when used inappropriately to treat a viral respiratory infection. The occurrence of skin rash does not necessarily confirm allergy to drugs of the penicillin group generally.
- Nevertheless, it is important to recognize that cross-allergy does exist between different penicillins. Allergic reactions vary from skin rashes and fever to more serious angiooedema and even anaphylaxis.
- Allergy apart, drugs of the penicillin class are remarkably free from side effects. Broad-spectrum drugs such as ampicillin may, however, produce diarrhoea as a result of disturbance of the normal bacterial flora of the bowel.

Storage
- Preparations containing ampicillin are stored in dry powder form at room temperature.
- When reconstituted for injection, such solutions should be used immediately and any unused portion discarded.
- Intravenous infusions are given over 15–30 minutes in 100 ml sodium chloride 0.9%, glucose 5% or glucose/saline mixtures.
- Oral mixtures, once prepared, should be used within 7 days or 14 days if kept in a refrigerator.

AMSACRINE (Amsidine, m-AMSA)

Presentation
Injection – 75 mg ampoule

Actions and uses
Amsacrine is a cytotoxic drug which blocks the synthesis of DNA and hence cell proliferation by binding DNA through a mechanism known as intercalation. A toxic effect on the cell membrane is also likely to explain its action. It has been used mainly in the treatment of acute leukaemia in adults, either as remission induction or maintenance therapy.

Dosage
This is largely determined by specific indications and current dosage schedules which may change from time to time. The existing schedule should be consulted for up-to-date details of dosage and route of administration. Courses of 90–120 mg/m^2 daily have been given for induction up to a total dose of 450 mg/m^2 and maintenance doses of about one-third of this used thereafter.

Nursing implications
- Myelosuppression with pancytopenia leading to infection and haemorrhage is the major toxic effect of this drug, which limits the total dose which can be given. This also makes patient education regarding control of infection and enhanced bleeding tendency an important aspect of the nurse's role. Treatment can be monitored by the use of a bone marrow biopsy.
- Frequent side effects include nausea (but not necessarily vomiting) and ulceration of the buccal mucosa and oesophagus. Therefore, nurses should pay particular attention to oral hygiene, fluid and dietary intake.
- CNS toxicity has resulted in generalized seizures requiring treatment with an anticonvulsant drug.
- Amsacrine is also potentially toxic to the liver, kidney and heart and has produced jaundice, acute renal failure and cardiac failure.
- The incidence of alopecia with this drug is relatively high.
- Severe local irritation and phlebitis result from

A

extravasation of amsacrine and care is required when siting the needle. The infusion site should be closely examined during and following intravenous administration. Amsacrine must be diluted before use; see below.

- Nurses should be aware of the risks posed by cytotoxic drugs. Some are irritant to the skin and mucous surfaces and care must be exercised when handling them. In particular, spillage or contamination of personnel or the environment must be avoided. If cytotoxic drugs are handled regularly, it is theoretically possible that repeated skin contact or inhalation may produce systemic toxic effects in nurses who have developed hypersensitivity to them. Most hospitals now operate a centralized (pharmacy-organized) additive service. While this reduces the risk of exposure to cytotoxic drugs, it is essential that nurses recognize and understand the local policy on their safe handling and disposal. The Health and Safety Executive has decreed that such a policy should be in place wherever cytotoxic drugs are administered. These should be adapted, wherever possible, to the care of patients in the community.

Storage
- Amsacrine is stored at room temperature and protected from light.
- Glass syringes only should be used when preparing intravenous infusions. The drug must be diluted in 500 ml glucose 5% and infused over 60–90 minutes. It must not be diluted in sodium chloride solutions.
- Infusions must be used within 8 hours of preparation and be protected from light.

ANASTROZOLE (Arimidex)

Presentation
Tablet – 1 mg

Actions and uses
Anastrozole represents a new treatment for advanced postmenopausal breast cancer. It is an inhibitor of the enzyme aromatase which is responsible for the conversion of androgen to oestrogen at peripheral (non-ovarian) sites, so removing the stimulus for growth of oestrogen-dependent tumours. Unlike earlier aromatase inhibitors, anastrozole is not itself a steroid. Its action is very specific, it does not interfere with adrenocorticosteroid synthesis and it can be administered by the oral route.

Dosage
1 mg single tablet once daily.

Nursing implications
- Side effects are similar to those reported for other antioestrogen therapy (e.g. tamoxifen). They include hot flushes, vaginal dryness, hair thinning, GI upsets, weakness and tiredness. Feelings of weakness and tiredness usually diminish with time. At the commencement of treatment, however, drowsiness may interfere with the ability to drive and perform skilled tasks.
- Anastrozole is not intended for treatment of premenopausal women. If in doubt, menopausal status should be checked before initiating therapy.
- Slight increase in blood cholesterol level may be noted. Occasional checks are therefore warranted.

Storage
Anastrozole tablets are stored at room temperature and protected from light.

ANISTREPLASE (Eminase)

Presentation
Vials containing 30 units

Actions and uses
This drug, previously known as APSAC or anisoylated plasminogen streptokinase activator complex, binds selectively to a preformed blood clot

after which the streptokinase portion of the molecule is released. Streptokinase in turn activates plasminogen, the natural antifibrinolytic substance found in body tissues which converts fibrin (deposited in thrombi) into a soluble form. As a result, preformed blood clots are dissolved and the blockage which they create is removed. Thrombolytics are often therefore described as 'clot busters'.

Anistreplase is used in the treatment of acute myocardial infarction (coronary thrombosis) in which it produces early reperfusion (recanalization) of the coronary arteries with consequent reduction in infarct size, reduced mortality and improved prognosis.

Dosage
- Acute myocardial infarction (within 12 hours): a single IV dose 30 units by slow bolus injection over 4–5 minutes.
- Individual coronary care units should be consulted for optimum administration beyond 12 hours of myocardial infarction.

Nursing implications
- Experience has shown that the earlier thrombolytic therapy is administered, the better the outcome. Best results are obtained if given within 6 hours of myocardial infarction but later administration is still warranted. An accurate history on admisson may therefore be helpful in determining likely prognosis.
- There is a risk of hypersensitivity reactions to streptokinase since most people have been exposed to the substance during earlier streptococcal infections. Early reactions include flushing, bradycardia and transient hypotension. Other, more severe allergic reactions such as bronchoconstriction and anaphylaxis are uncommon in practice and usually reversible.
- Treatment failure may follow early reexposure due to formation of streptokinase-inactivating

antibodies. Treatment of reinfarction within this period should therefore be carried out using alteplase (p. 20) as thrombolytic drug of choice.
- The most common complication associated with thrombolytic therapy is bleeding; this can be controlled by local pressure at the sites of intravenous cannulae.
- The nurse may play an important role in identifying contraindications to thrombolytic therapy, as a result of the risk from bleeding. These include:
  - recent (i.e. within 3 months) cerebrovascular accident
  - uncontrolled or uncontrollable hypertension
  - known bleeding diathesis
  - active peptic ulceration
  - aggressive CPR with possible internal bleeding
  - recent (i.e. within 3 months) major surgery or trauma
  - severe liver disease with impaired clotting mechanism.
- Check individual coronary care units for local policy on contraindications to thrombolytic therapy.

Storage
- Alteplase injection is stored below 25°C but reconstituted solution may be stored for up to 24 hours in a refrigerator (between 2 and 8°C) and up to 8 hours at room temperature.
- Unopened vials should be kept in their original package until preparation.

ANTIDEPRESSANT DRUGS

See also: Tricyclic Antidepressants p. 371.

Presentation
See individual drugs.

Actions and uses
These drugs are used in the treatment of depressive illness. Their pharmacology is complex and poorly understood but for practical purposes they can be subdivided into three main types

A

depending upon their action on neurotransmission within the CNS.

Tricyclic and related drugs (p. 371)

These are the traditional antidepressants which have been in use for almost 50 years. They appear to enhance catecholaminergic neurotransmission by blocking reuptake and hence removal of transmitter substances including noradrenaline, 5-hydroxytryptamine (serotonin) and dopamine, so leading to their accumulation in brain tissues. This action is associated with elevation of mood and neuropsychiatric 'activation'.

Selective reuptake inhibitors

This group includes the modern range of antidepressants, introduced in the last few years, which continue to be developed by the pharmaceutical industry. They have very specific effects on particular neurotransmitters, especially 5-hydroxytryptamine (serotonin). The reuptake and hence inactivation are duly blocked, hence the terms *selective serotonin reuptake inhibitor (SSRI)* and *selective serotonin/noradrenaline reuptake inhibitor (SSNRI)*. The reasons for the apparent popularity of these newer drugs are their (allegedly) improved efficacy and lesser degree of toxicity, especially in overdosage.

Monoamine oxidase inhibitors

Drugs of this type increase the concentration of neurotransmitters (for example, noradrenaline) by blocking their metabolism in brain tissue via the enzyme monoamine oxidase. This action has special importance for their safety, particularly in relation to interactions with other drugs and foodstuffs.

A further use for antidepressants (usually the traditional agents) is in the treatment of neurogenic pain, i.e. shooting or stabbing pain associated with nerve damage or as a result of trauma (e.g. amputation, tumour infiltration, etc.) or infection (e.g. herpes virus/shingles) in which conventional analgesics are of limited use. Antidepressants appear to reduce transmission via pain pathways in the spinal cord, so abolishing the sensation of pain.

Dosage

See individual drugs.

Nursing implications

- It is important that patients realize from the outset that the full benefits of antidepressant therapy may not be apparent for several weeks after treatment is commenced. During this period, the nurse has an important role in supporting and educating patients to ensure good compliance with treatment.
- Note that the main reasons for therapeutic failure are poor patient compliance or underdosage, both of which can arise from fears over toxicity or the occurrence of side effects.
- Many traditional antidepressants and monoamine oxidase inhibitors have anticholinergic and sedative properties. Elderly patients, in particular, should be advised of the likelihood of side effects, including dry mouth, blurred vision, constipation and urinary hesitancy, but may be reassured that such effects become less troublesome as treatment continues.
- Sedation, on the other hand, is potentially useful for those with sleeping difficulty and related anxiety. For this reason the daily dose is often taken on retiring. Note, however, that some newer antidepressants may cause anxiety and sleep disturbances.
- The possibility of severe, acute urinary retention should be considered when older antidepressants are prescribed for men with prostatic hypertrophy.
- Drugs which have anticholinergic activity are contraindicated in patients with glaucoma associated with acute angle closure.
- Older antidepressants are markedly cardiotoxic in overdosage and should be used with caution in coronary heart disease, including within 3–6 months of myocardial infarction.

This arises because of their tendency to produce ectopic ventricular arrhythmias within the ischaemic myocardium.

- Many drugs are also proconvulsant and must be avoided or used with caution in patients with a history of epilepsy, especially if poorly controlled.
- All drugs are potentially hepatotoxic, causing direct injury to the liver cells or cholestatic jaundice. Such an effect is more likely in patients who develop abnormal liver function test results during treatment.
- The occurrence of impotence in some men treated with antidepressants can be anticipated. Though patients are understandably reluctant to volunteer this information, referral to the andrology specialist may be appropriate. Women too may develop sexual dysfunction, often reported as lack of orgasm.
- Weight gain is a frequent side effect noted by women, in particular, who may interrupt treatment as a result. If compliance is in doubt, careful counselling and sensible dietary advice can help. Fluoxetine is the exception. It can actually cause weight loss.

Storage
See individual drugs.

ANTI-D IMMUNOGLOBULIN (Partobulin)

Presentation
Injection – 1250 international units (IU) in 1 ml

Actions and uses
Anti-D immunoglobulin is administered to rhesus-negative women to prevent sensitization and formation of antibodies to fetal rhesus-positive cells which may mix with maternal blood during childbirth or abortion. In this way any subsequent child is protected from the danger of haemolytic disease of the newborn.

Dosage
1250 units is administered by intramuscular injection immediately or within 72 hours of childbirth or abortion. The same dose may be given at weeks 28 and 34 of pregnancy but this does not replace its use following birth.

Nursing implications
- Rubella vaccination can be carried out at the same time that anti-D is administered but different syringes and injection sites should be used and a test for rubella antibodies should follow 2 months or more later.
- MMR vaccine should not be administered within 3 months of a dose of anti-D.

Storage
This product has a shelf life of 3 years when stored in a refrigerator.

ANTIHISTAMINES

This group comprises many different chemicals with a common action.

Presentation
See individual drugs.

Actions and uses
Antihistamines (more precisely, histamine H1 receptor antagonists) block the effect of histamine at specific sites in the body. Histamine is released as part of the allergic/inflammatory response and is therefore partly responsible for the production of inflammation, erythema and pruritus which accompanies such reactions. The antihistamine group of drugs have, in addition, effects on the autonomic nervous system and the central nervous system. In clinical practice they are used for the treatment of the following.

- To suppress generalized minor allergic responses to allergens such as foodstuffs and drugs.
- To suppress local allergic reactions, e.g. inflammatory skin response to insect stings and bites, contact allergens and urticaria.

A

- Orally and in eye drops for allergic occular inflammatory conditions, e.g. due to hay fever and allergic rhinitis.
- As nasal decongestants, e.g. in the treatment of allergic rhinitis and hay fever. They are also added to a few proprietary cough preparations because of their decongestant action.
- In the treatment of nausea and vomiting, particularly motion sickness.
- As an antipruritic agent.
- They are also used for the treatment of vertigo and the symptoms of vertigo and nausea due to Menière's disease.

Dosage
See individual drugs.

Nursing implications
- The older antihistamines have a sedative effect and may cause marked drowsiness, while some newer agents (e.g. astemizole, terfenadine) do not. In some clinical situations sedative antihistamines are actually used for this effect but, more often, drowsiness may prove a troublesome side effect.
- Nurses can contribute to patient management by reemphasizing the dangers of driving or using industrial machinery while receiving sedative drugs.
- Common side effects include headache, blurred vision, tinnitus, sleep disturbance, gastrointestinal upset and, in susceptible patients, urinary retention.
- Topical applications of antihistamines may produce skin sensitization and subsequent eczematous and other eruptions.

Storage
See individual drugs.

ASPARAGINASE

Presentation
Injection – 10 000 units per vial

Actions and uses
Asparaginase is a cytotoxic drug. It is an enzyme obtained from cultures of Erwinia. It interferes with the synthesis of a specific amino acid required for the growth of malignant cells and therefore reduces the capacity of those cells to both grow and multiply. Its major use is in the induction of remission of acute lymphoblastic leukaemia. It has also occasionally been used in the treatment of acute myeloid leukaemia.

Dosage
It is important to note that a proportion of patients display hypersensitivity to the drug. Therefore all patients should receive an initial intradermal test dose of 50 IU and the injection site observed for 3 hours for signs of tissue reaction. If a tissue reaction occurs this is a contraindication to using asparaginase in standard dosage.

The usual initial dose is 200 units/kg body weight daily by slow intravenous injection or infusion over 20–30 minutes. Doses are then increased to a maximum of 1000 IU/kg according to individual response.

It is recommended that the course of treatment should be continuous as interruption and recommencement of treatment increase the risk of sensitivity reactions.

Nursing implications
- As noted above, all patients should receive an intradermal test dose prior to commencing full treatment.
- Gastrointestinal side effects include anorexia, nausea and vomiting.
- Suppression of bone marrow function may result in anaemia and increased risk of infection due to suppression of white cell function.
- In addition, bone marrow suppression may result in thrombocytopenia. If fibrinogen levels and clotting factors are also suppressed, there is a marked risk of haemorrhage during treatment.

- Impaired liver function, pancreatitis and hyperglycaemia have also been observed during treatment with this drug.
- Nurses should be aware of the risks posed by cytotoxic drugs. Some are irritant to the skin and mucous surfaces and care must be exercised when handling them. In particular, spillage or contamination of personnel or the environment must be avoided. If cytotoxic drugs are handled regularly, it is theoretically possible that repeated skin contact or inhalation may produce systemic toxic effects in nurses who have developed hypersensitivity to them. Most hospitals now operate a centralized (pharmacy-organized) additive service. While this reduces the risk of exposure to cytotoxic drugs, it is essential that nurses recognize and understand the local policy on their safe handling and disposal. The Health and Safety Executive has decreed that such a policy should be in place wherever cytotoxic drugs are administered. These should be adapted, wherever possible, to the care of patients in the community.

Storage

- Vials for injection should be stored in a refrigerator.
- The vials are reconstituted using the accompanying 10 ml sodium chloride 0.9% ampoules.
- The prepared solution is administered by slow intravenous injection or as a rapid infusion (20–30 minutes) in 0.9% sodium chloride solution.

ASPIRIN

Presentation

Tablets – 75 mg, 100 mg, 300 mg (including enteric coated)

Actions and uses

- Aspirin relieves pain and reduces inflammation in a variety of conditions affecting the joints, tendons, cartilages and muscles. To produce a significant anti-inflammatory effect, however, it has to be given in high regular dosage. Effective and better tolerated drugs exist for this purpose.
- It is an effective simple analgesic for minor painful disorders such as headache, toothache or muscle strain.
- It may also be used as an antipyretic to lower the temperature of fevered patients.
- The antiplatelet action of aspirin has long been recognized and probably accounts for its major use today. Aspirin irreversibly blocks the synthesis of a prostaglandin, thromboxane A2, by the platelet in response to injury to the vascular epithelium. In the presence of this substance, platelets adhere to form a platelet plug which under normal circumstances reduces bleeding and promotes blood clotting. Aspirin is so potent in this respect that it can inhibit platelet aggregation and prevent clotting at very low concentrations. This has led to the widespread use of aspirin in the following situations:
  - prevention of a first or subsequent stroke in patients with transient ischaemic attacks thought likely to be due to microembolization following platelet aggregation or thrombotic stroke
  - acute myocardial infarction in which aspirin adds considerably to the effectiveness of thrombolytic therapy in increasing survival
  - primary prevention of myocardial infarction in patients with symptoms of coronary heart disease and secondary prevention of reinfarction and sudden death in the period following myocardial infarction
  - to improve prognosis after coronary artery bypass graft surgery and vascular surgery of the lower limbs

– prevention of stroke in patients with non-rheumatic atrial fibrillation who are otherwise considered unsuitable for oral anticoagulant therapy.

Adults only.

- The usual antiinflammatory dose range is 2.4–4.8 g daily taken in divided doses, often with or after meals in an attempt to reduce gastric irritation.
- As a simple analgesic, 600 mg taken 4–6 hourly as required.
- When used as an antithrombotic drug, single daily doses of 75 mg, 150 mg or 300 mg are taken.

Nursing implications

- Aspirin is notably irritant to the gastric mucosa and is poorly tolerated by many patients. Severe gastrointestinal upset and gastric bleeding are not uncommon even with modest antiplatelet doses.
- In patients who do not tolerate even the lowest (single 75 mg tablet) dose, this can be further reduced by halving tablets irrespective of how accurately this can be done. Even 'minute' doses provide effective antiplatelet levels.
- The use of aspirin in children under 12 years of age is no longer recommended. This follows the observation that Reye's syndrome, a potentially fatal condition affecting the central nervous system, occurred in a number of young children with febrile illness who received aspirin. Although a clear association was not shown, safer alternatives exist and should be used.
- The use of aspirin is not recommended in pregnancy and during breast feeding.
- Symptoms of toxicity after overdosage with aspirin are as follows.
  - Mild symptoms of intoxication include dizziness, tinnitus, sweating, nausea, vomiting, mental confusion.
  - More serious signs of toxicity include fever, ketosis, hyperventilation, respiratory alkalosis and metabolic acidosis. This may lead to shock, respiratory failure and coma.
- It must be remembered that the early features of toxicity as described above may not occur in children who may present initially with the more serious effects described.
- Aspirin is readily available in many 'over-the-counter' preparations.
- About 10% of patients with asthma may develop bronchospasm on exposure to aspirin. Caution is therefore warranted in those with obstructive airways disease.

Storage

Aspirin tablets are stored at room temperature. However, if stored in a 'moist' atmosphere (i.e. in the bathroom cabinet), conversion to acetic acid and hence inactivation is likely.

ASTEMIZOLE (Hismanal)

Presentation

Tablets – 10 mg
Oral suspension – 5 mg in 5 ml

Actions and uses

Astemizole is an antihistamine, the actions and uses of which are described under Antihistamines (see p. 33). Note that astemizole is long acting and lacks the marked sedative effect of the majority of drugs of this type. In practice, it is used in the management of hay fever, allergic rhinitis and allergic skin disorders.

Dosage

Adults: 10 mg taken once daily before one of the main meals.
Children (over 5 years): 5 mg once daily as above.

Nursing implications
- See Antihistamines (p. 33).
- During 1992 the Committee on Safety of Medicines drew attention to the possibility that serious cardiac dysrhythmias may arise in patients who receive excessive doses or in whom plasma concentrations are otherwise likely to be raised. The latter may arise if erythromycin and clarithromycin are co-prescribed with astemizole.
- The drug is best avoided in patients with heart disease who may be predisposed to hypokalaemia and/or ventricular rhythm disturbances.

Storage
Astemizole tablets and suspension are stored at room temperature.

ATENOLOL (Tenormin)

Presentation
Tablets – 25 mg, 50 mg, 100 mg
Injection – 5 mg in 10 ml
Syrup – 25 mg in 5 ml

Actions and uses
Atenolol is a cardioselective beta-adrenoreceptor blocking drug and the section on Beta-blockers (p. 51) should be consulted for a full account of its actions.

Dosage
- Atenolol is particularly long acting. Single daily doses of 100–200 mg in adults are usually adequate.
- By injection in cardiac dysrhythmias, 2.5 mg by slow intravenous injection (over 2½ minutes) repeated after 5 minute intervals to a maximum total dose of 10 mg.

Nursing implications
- See the section on Beta-blockers.
- Atenolol is a particularly useful drug in patients who have experienced central nervous system side effects from other

beta-blockers such as nightmares and hallucinations, since very little is able to enter the CNS across the blood–brain barrier.

Storage
Atenolol tablets and injection are stored at room temperature.

ATORVASTATIN (Lipitor)

Presentation
Tablets – 10 mg, 20 mg and 40 mg

Actions and uses
This is a new member of the statin group of lipid-lowering drugs used in the treatment of conditions associated with familial hypercholesterolaemia or in the secondary prevention of coronary heart disease (CHD). Early evidence suggests that it may be very potent with respect to other statins and that it may, in addition, reduce levels of triglycerides (which appear to be an independent risk factor for CHD).

Dosage
Adults only: the starting dose is 10 mg which should be increased gradually (every 4 weeks) until optimum dosage (up to 80 mg) is achieved. It is important to titrate dose against the response, i.e. the target cholesterol level, and to ensure that this is in fact achieved.

Nursing implications
- Assisting patients to comply with dietary advice is an important aspect of the nurse's role.
- It is important that pharmacological intervention is reserved for patients who do not respond to low fat and reducing diets or who have very high lipid levels.
- A baseline lipid profile should be obtained in order to evaluate the effectiveness of pharmacological intervention.

A

- Gastrointestinal upsets, headaches, myalgia and feelings of tiredness and sleep disturbances are the most commonly reported side effects of treatment with lipid-lowering drugs of this type.
- The potential for liver dysfunction should be noted and liver function tests carried out periodically.
- Drugs of this type should generally be avoided in pregnancy (or pregnancy avoided if on therapy) since their effects on fetal development and the course of pregnancy are unclear.
- Statins may interact with other drugs administered concomitantly, in particular warfarin (increased risk of bleeding), digoxin (increased risk of concentration-dependent toxicity) and the oral contraceptives (levels of oestrogen increased in line with high oestrogen-containing oral contraceptives).

Storage

Atorvastatin tablets are stored at room temperature.

ATRACURIUM (Tracrium)

Presentation

Injection – 25 mg in 2.5 ml; 50 mg in 5 ml; 250 mg in 25 ml

Actions and uses

Atracurium is a muscle relaxant of the non-depolarizing type. Thus it reversibly paralyses skeletal muscle by competitive inhibition of acetylcholine, the transmitter substance released at the junction of the (motor) nerve and muscle fibre (motor endplate receptor).

Drugs of this type are used to produce muscle relaxation during surgical anaesthesia.

Dosage

Adults and children: initially 300–600 microgram/kg followed by 100–200 microgram/kg as required by bolus intravenous injection. May also be administered by intravenous infusion at a rate of 5–10 microgram/kg/min (300–600 microgram/kg/h).

Nursing implications
- All patients must have their respiration assisted or controlled.
- Muscle relaxants of this type are also used to produce paralysis in patients on assisted ventilation in ICUs.
- Overdosage with muscle relaxant drugs of this type may result in paralysis of the respiratory muscles. If this occurs, an anticholinesterase such as neostigmine (which potentiates acetylcholine by blocking its inactivation) must be administered.

Storage

Atracurium injection is stored in a refrigerator and protected from light.

ATROPINE

Atropine is the main component of the belladonna alkaloids, a family of natural substances, found notably in the deadly nightshade plant. Hyoscine (scopolamine) is chemically closely related to atropine and the same considerations apply to both drugs in clinical practice. Atropine is generally used in the form of atropine sulphate and hyoscine as hyoscine hydrobromide.

Presentation

Injection – 600 microgram in 1 ml; 500 microgram in 5 ml; 1 mg and 3 mg (1000 and 3000 microgram) in 10 ml
Eye drops – 0.5% and 1%

Actions and uses

Atropine blocks the actions of the neurotransmitter acetylcholine at nerve endings (muscarinic sites) in the parasympathetic nervous system. This action is often referred to as 'anticholinergic' or, more accurately, 'antimuscarinic' which denotes the precise site of acetylcholine blockade. Atropine has several uses in clinical practice.

- It increases heart rate by blocking the restraining effects of the vagus nerve on the sinus node and for this reason is used in the treatment of sinus bradycardia, especially if complicated by hypotension following myocardial infarction. It may also be administered in asystolic cardiac arrest unresponsive to DC shock therapy.
- It reduces bronchial and salivary secretions and is used in preoperative medication to inhibit excess of these secretions in response to intubation and some inhalation anaesthetics.
- In the eye, atropine dilates the pupil and causes prolonged paralysis of the ciliary muscle, i.e. it is a mydriatic and long-acting cycloplegic and is used for refraction procedures and in the treatment of iridocyclitis. Homatropine may also be used for this indication.
- It reduces gut motility and may be used as a gastrointestinal antispasmodic (gastrointestinal sedative) in irritable bowel syndrome and diverticular disease, though hyoscine and other synthetic antimuscarinic drugs are more often used. Atropine is also combined with diphenoxylate in the antidiarrhoeal preparation Lomotil.
- It reduces gastric acid secretion and may be used to relieve dyspeptic symptoms, usually in antacids sold over the counter which contain atropine in the form of belladonna extract. However, antimuscarinics are now rarely used to treat peptic ulcer.
- Atropine is often given at the same time as a cholinesterase inhibitor, e.g. neostigmine, when it is used to reverse the effects of certain muscle relaxant drugs administered during surgery. Atropine prevents bradycardia and excessive salivation which might otherwise occur in response to the anticholinesterase agent.
- For similar reasons to the above, atropine is administered in emergencies associated with organophosphorus poisoning. These agents are commonly used as pesticides in agriculture and are potent and irreversible inhibitors of acetylcholinesterase. If swallowed, inhaled or absorbed in quantity through the skin, widespread and often fatal overstimulation of the parasympathetic nervous system results. Organophosphorus agents also form the main group of chemical (non-biological) warfare nerve gases.

Dosage

Cardiac arrhythmias.

- Sinus bradycardia: 300 microgram repeated if required.
- Asystolic cardiac arrest: single dose of 3 mg by slow intravenous injection (or 6–9 mg via the ET tube).

Preoperative medication.

- Adults: 300–600 microgram, 30 minutes to 1 hour before induction anaesthesia. Usually by intramuscular injection.
- Children: 20 microgram/kg as above.

Ophthalmology: single drop 1 hour before refraction. Used daily in uveitis. Control of side effects to neostigmine when used to reverse the effects of muscle relaxant drugs in surgery: 600 microgram (0.6 mg) to 1.2 mg by intravenous injection at the same time that neostigmine is administered. Organophosphorus poisoning: 2 mg by intravenous (if severe poisoning) or intramuscular (less severe poisoning) injection, repeated until the skin becomes flushed and dry, the pupils dilated and tachycardia occurs.

Nursing implications
- The side effects of atropine can be summed up as representing parasympathetic underactivity or resultant unrestrained sympathetic activity.
- This includes typically dry mouth, flushing, dry skin, swallowing difficulty due to reduced oesophageal motility, tachycardia and palpitations, dilatation of the pupil and loss of accommodation, raised

A

intraocular pressure, urinary retention and constipation.
- It follows that the elderly, in particular, may be vulnerable to the above effects. Caution is warranted in patients with dysphagia, reflux oesophagitis, myocardial insufficiency, glaucoma, lower GI obstruction and prostatic hypertrophy.

Storage
Preparations containing atropine are stored at room temperature.

AURANOFIN (Ridaura)

Presentation
Tablets – 3 mg

Actions and uses
Auranofin is a gold salt used in the treatment of active rheumatoid arthritis which is progressive and unresponsive to other first-line treatments. It is one of a number of agents which collectively are termed 'disease modifying' although its precise mechanism of action is unknown (its antirheumatic action was discovered by accident). Gold salts inhibit production of the inflammatory mediator prostaglandins but they also bind to products of the immune response such as immunoglobulins and complement and in doing so may modify the autoimmune process which underlies rheumatoid arthritis.

Dosage
Adults only: initially, 3 mg twice daily or 6 mg as a single daily dose is given for up to 6 months and the response is then assessed. Thereafter, the dose may be increased to 3 mg three times daily but treatment should be discontinued if there is no response within a further 3 months.

Nursing implications
- In order that good compliance is maintained during the early treatment period, patients should be made aware that

there may be a delay of 1–2 months before a response is achieved.
- Diarrhoea, nausea and abdominal pain are common. The incidence of diarrhoea may be reduced by combined use of dietary fibre supplement (e.g. bran) which adds bulk to the stool.
- Adverse effects which must be reported immediately include oral ulceration (a possible sign of haematological toxicity), altered (metallic) taste sensation, bleeding, skin reactions, peripheral neuritis, breathlessness, alopecia and jaundice.
- Gold salts are poorly tolerated by many patients and some adverse reactions are particularly severe. It is estimated that as many as 5% will experience a severe reaction so that close support and careful monitoring of the early indication of side effects are therefore essential.
- Regular blood counts are recommended.
- Contraindications to auranofin include existing liver and kidney impairment, exfoliative dermatitis, systemic lupus erythematosus, a history of blood disorders suggestive of bone marrow aplasia, pulmonary fibrosis and enterocolitis.
- Auranofin must not be administered during pregnancy.

Storage
Auranofin tablets are stored at room temperature.

AZAPROPAZONE (Rheumox)

Presentation
Capsules – 300 mg
Tablets – 600 mg

Actions and uses
See the section on Non-steroidal Antiinflammatory Analgesic Drugs (NSAIDs) (p. 250). This drug is generally reserved for the treatment of acute gout.

Dosage

The initial adult dose is 1200 mg daily taken in 2–4 divided doses. Once adequate clinical effect has been obtained, the dose is reduced to the minimum that will continue to keep the patient comfortable.

Nursing implications

- See the section on Non-steroidal Antiinflammatory Analgesic Drugs (NSAIDs) (p. 250).
- Azapropazone is especially likely to interact with warfarin, so increasing the possibility of haemorrhage. Reduced daily doses of warfarin may therefore be required if azapropazone is commenced in an anticoagulated patient and close monitoring of the prothrombin time is essential for the first 48 hours.

Storage

Azapropazone tablets and capsules are stored at room temperature.

AZATADINE (Optimine)

Presentation

Tablets – 1 mg
Syrup – 0.5 mg in 5 ml

Actions and uses

Azatadine is an antihistamine. The actions and uses of antihistamines in general are described on p. 33. Azatadine is used specifically:

- to suppress generalized minor allergic responses to allergens such as foodstuffs and drugs
- to suppress local allergic reactions, i.e. inflammatory skin responses to insect stings and bites, contact allergens and urticaria
- orally for other allergic conditions, e.g. hay fever and allergic rhinitis.

Dosage

Adults: 1–2 mg twice daily.
Children: 1–6 years, 0.25 mg twice daily, 6–12 years, 0.5–1 mg twice daily.

Nursing implications

- See the section on Antihistamines (p. 33).

Storage

Azatadine tablets and liquid are stored at room temperature and protected from light.

AZATHIOPRINE (Imuran)

Presentation

Tablets – 25 mg, 50 mg
Injection – vials containing 50 mg

Actions and uses

Azathioprine is the precursor of an immunosuppressant drug, 6-mercaptopurine, to which it is slowly converted after absorption. It has the following actions.

- It suppresses the immune response after organ or tissue transplantation and therefore prevents tissue rejection and enhances the survival and function of transplanted organs.
- It is also used in a number of other diseases where it appears to alter the disease process, producing an improvement in symptoms. Examples of such diseases are rheumatoid arthritis, systemic lupus erythematosus and Crohn's disease.

Dosage

- For immunosuppression after organ transplantation: an initial dose 5 mg/kg is followed by a maintenance dose 1–4 mg/kg body weight daily (average 2.4 mg/kg) in divided doses.
- For the treatment of the other diseases mentioned above: it is usually given in a dose range of 1–2.5 mg/kg.
- It may be given by intravenous injection at the above doses for short periods when oral treatment is unsuitable.
- The combination of azathioprine with a corticosteroid drug usually permits the use of lower doses of both drugs while maintaining their clinical effect.

Nursing implications

- Azathioprine commonly causes gastrointestinal upsets including anorexia, nausea, vomiting and diarrhoea.

- Regular monitoring of full blood count is required while patients are undergoing treatment with azathioprine.
- It depresses the bone marrow and seems particularly to affect white cell function, leading to an increased risk of infection. Patients suffering from acute infection should therefore not be given the drug or very closely monitored. They should be made aware of the symptoms of bone marrow suppression, e.g. unexpected bruising or bleeding and the hazards of exposure to infection.
- Infections by bacteria, fungi, protozoa and viruses which do not normally occur in healthy adults may occur in patients on this drug.
- It should be used with caution in patients who have existing liver disease; cases of hepatitis and biliary stasis have been reported. Despite this, it is worth noting that it is actually used in the treatment of active chronic hepatitis.
- The drug has been shown to cause fetal abnormality if taken either during pregnancy or by the father prior to conception. It is important therefore to encourage patients to take adequate contraceptive measures.
- Serious toxicity is likely to occur if azathioprine accumulates in the body. This will occur in two instances:
  - in patients with reduced renal function
  - in patients who are also taking allopurinol which inhibits the body's capacity to metabolize azathioprine. In such cases the dose of azathioprine should be substantially reduced.
- Injection solutions are prepared by adding not less than 5 ml water to each 50 mg vial.
- Solutions are alkaline and very irritant to the venous tract. They should be injected slowly, preferably via the drip tubing of a running 5% dextrose or 0.9% sodium chloride infusion. Any unused solution should be discarded immediately.

Storage
Azathioprine tablets and injection are stored at room temperature.

AZELASTINE (Rhinoplast)

Presentation
Metered dose nasal spray – 0.1%

Actions and uses
Azelastine is an antihistamine. The actions and uses of this group are described on p. 33. Azelastine is used specifically as a local nasal decongestant in the treatment of perennial and seasonal allergic rhinitis.

Dosage
Adults only: one metered dose sprayed into each nostril twice daily.

Nursing implications
- Azelastine administered locally may produce mild irritation to the nasal mucosa and taste disturbance but is otherwise well tolerated.
- Since it is intended for local use only, systemic toxicity is most unlikely.

Storage
Azelastine metered dose aerosol may be stored at room temperature. As with all pressurized devices, it must not be incinerated when discarded.

AZITHROMYCIN (Zithromax)

Presentation
Capsules – 250 mg
Suspension – 200 mg in 5 ml

Actions and uses
Azithromycin is an antibiotic of the erythromycin group which has a notably long action (once daily dosing is permissible) and good tissue penetration. It is somewhat less active

than erythromycin against Gram-positive bacteria but has enhanced activity against certain Gram-negative organisms. Azithromycin is indicated for the treatment of infections of the upper and lower respiratory tract, skin and soft tissues, otitis media and genital infections due to *Chlamydia trachomatis*.

Dosage
Adults: usually a short course (e.g. 3 days) of 500 mg once daily. In genital chlamydial infections, as a single dose of 1 g.
Children: up to 15 kg body weight, 10 mg/kg once daily for 3 days; 15–25 kg body weight, 200 mg once daily for 3 days; 25–35 kg body weight, 300 mg once daily for 3 days; 35–45 kg body weight, 400 mg once daily for 3 days.

Nursing implications
- Azithromycin causes notably fewer gastrointestinal upsets (abdominal pain, diarrhoea, etc.) than does erythromycin.
- Allergic reactions including skin rashes, angiooedema and even anaphylaxis are, however, possible. Caution is therefore advised if used in patients known to be allergic to erythromycin.
- Other uncommon but potentially severe adverse effects include hearing loss or disturbance (tinnitus) and liver impairment.
- Azithromycin should be used with caution in those with existing liver and kidney impairment and avoided in the presence of severe liver disease, pregnancy and breastfeeding.

Storage
Azithromycin capsules and powder for suspension are stored at room temperature.

AZLOCILLIN (Securopen)

Presentation
Injection – 1 g, 2 g and 5 g vials

Actions and uses
Azlocillin is a member of the penicillin group of antibiotics. It has a much wider spectrum of activity than the parent drug, benzylpenicillin. Its indications are for the treatment of bacterial infection in any tissue of the body when the organism has been shown to be sensitive to it. It is of particular interest that this drug is useful in the treatment of serious infections due to Pseudomonas species which are frequently resistant to other antibacterial drugs.

Dosage
Adults: 2–5 g every 8 hours according to the severity of infection.
Premature infants and children under 3 kg: 50 mg/kg body weight every 12 hours; under 3 months: 0.15–0.25 g every 8 hours; 3 months to 1 year: 0.25–0.5 g every 8 hours; 1–2 years: 0.5 g every 8 hours; 2–6 years: 0.5–1 g every 8 hours; 6 years and over: 1–3 g every 8 hours.

Nursing implications
- Like other beta-lactam (penicillin or cephalosporin) drugs, cross-reactive hypersensitivity may arise.
- Doses below 2 g are administered by intravenous bolus injection. Higher doses should be given by rapid intravenous infusion over 20–30 minutes. Solutions for injection should be prepared in a concentration of 10% in water for injections.

Storage
- Azlocillin vials are stored at room temperature.
- A 10% solution for injection should be prepared immediately before use and any remaining solution discarded.

AZTREONAM (Azactam)

Presentation
Injection – 500 mg, 1 g and 2 g vial

Actions and uses
Aztreonam is a monocyclic beta-lactam antibiotic which in effect

A

means that, while it shares some features in common with the penicillins and cephalosporins, it also has important structural differences. For this reason it can be safely used as an alternative to penicillins and cephalosporins for patients who are allergic to these drugs but who nevertheless require a drug of that type. The antibiotic spectrum of aztreonam is, however, restricted to the Gram-negative organisms, *E. coli*, Klebsiella spp. and occasionally Pseudomonas, *Proteus mirabilis, Serratia marcescens* and *Neisseria gonorrhoeae*: it is also effective in the treatment of ampicillin-resistant *Haemophilus influenzae* infections. Typical infections which may respond to aztreonam include the infections of the lower urinary and respiratory tracts, bacteraemia, septicaemia, venereal disease, skin and soft tissues, intraabdominal and gynaecological infections.

Dosage

Adults: usually 4 g daily in 3–4 divided doses but up to 8 g daily may be given.

Nursing implications

- Intramuscular injections may be given up to total doses of 1 g, above which the intravenous route is recommended.
- For intramuscular injection each 500 mg is prepared by the addition of 1.5 ml water for injections or sodium chloride 0.9% injection. The dose is administered into deep, large muscle, e.g. lateral thigh.
- For bolus intravenous injection add 6–10 ml water for injection to each 1 g or 2 g vial and administer slowly over 3–5 minutes.
- Intravenous infusions are given over 20–60 minutes as a 2% solution. If dilution is required, this may be administered in standard sodium chloride or glucose solutions or mixtures thereof.
- The common side effects of aztreonam are similar to those reported with the penicillins, e.g. allergic skin reactions, local reactions or pain at the injection site and gastrointestinal upsets. Also blood disorders and jaundice have been reported.
- The clotting time should be closely monitored in patients also treated with warfarin.
- The dose of aztreonam should be halved for patients with moderate renal failure (creatinine clearance 10–30 ml/min) and reduced to one-quarter for those with severe renal failure (<10 ml/min).
- Aztreonam should be avoided in pregnancy and breastfeeding.

Storage

- Aztreonam injection is stored at room temperature.
- Reconstituted solution remains stable if stored in a refrigerator for up to 24 hours.

B

BACAMPICILLIN (Ambaxin)

Presentation
Tablets – 400 mg

Actions and uses
Bacampicillin is an ampicillin ester, i.e. a chemical form which is well absorbed, so producing rapid high blood levels of ampicillin to which it is subsequently converted. Bacampicillin is used in the treatment of respiratory tract infections, skin and soft tissue infection and UTI but its major use is as a single large dose in the treatment of gonorrhoea when the high levels of ampicillin which result are especially advantageous.

Dosage
Adults.

- General use: 400–800 mg two or three times daily.
- Gonorrhoea: 1.6 g (with probenecid 1 g) as a single dose.

Children over 5 years: 200 mg three times daily.

> **Nursing implications**
> - Since it is a precursor of Ampicillin, the section on that drug (p. 28) should be consulted.

Storage
Bacampicillin tablets are stored at room temperature.

BACLOFEN (Lioresal)

Presentation
Tablets – 10 mg
Liquid – 5 mg in 5 ml

Actions and uses
Baclofen is used in the treatment of chronic severe spasticity of voluntary muscle. Spasticity is a disorder associated with increased muscle tone but loss of muscle power as a result of damage to cortico-motor neurone pathways in the brain and spinal cord. Baclofen reduces spasticity and flexor spasms by enhancing the activity of an inhibitory presynaptic neurotransmitter, gamma-aminobutyric acid (GABA), in the spinal cord and by its depressant effect in the CNS.

Examples of conditions in which a spastic state may develop include cerebral palsy, post-meningitis and stroke, multiple sclerosis and spinal injury.

Dosage
Adults: initially, 5 mg three times a day increased gradually (e.g. at 3-day intervals) by 5 mg three times a day until a response is obtained. Up to 100 mg daily may be required. Children: over 10 years, 0.75–2 mg/kg/day (maximum 2.5 mg/kg/day) or 2.5 mg four times daily increased gradually to a maintenance dose of 10–20 mg daily (1–2 years), 20–30 mg (2–6 years) or 30–60 mg (6–10 years).

> **Nursing implications**
> - The list of possible side effects with this drug is extensive and is the reason for careful dosage adjustment initially. Patients may be tempted to discontinue therapy and must be warned against doing so abruptly.
> - Baclofen is a CNS depressant and frequently causes sedation or drowsiness. Patients may also complain of nausea and light-headedness.
> - Other CNS side effects include ataxia, dizziness, confusion,

B

headaches, hallucinations, euphoria, depression, insomnia, tremors and (with very high doses) convulsions. Paraesthesia, muscle pain and weakness may develop.
- Other side effects include visual, gastrointestinal and urinary disturbances, sweating, skin rashes and altered liver function. Even a paradoxical increase in spasticity may occur rarely.
- The elderly patient may be particularly susceptible to the above range of side effects. Clearly, baclofen must also be used with caution in those with a history of epilepsy, stroke and psychiatric disturbance. Dosage adjustment may be required for patients with liver and/or kidney impairment.
- Baclofen is contraindicated in patients with active peptic ulcer disease.

Storage
Baclofen tablets and liquid are stored at room temperature.

BECLOMETHASONE (Becotide, Propaderm, Beconase)

Presentation
Inhalation, metered dose aerosol – 50, 100 and 250 microgram per dose
Intranasal, metered dose aqueous – 50 microgram per dose
'Rotacaps' – 100, 200 and 400 microgram
Cream/ointment – 0.025%

Actions and uses
Beclomethasone is a corticosteroid used either for application to the skin or by inhalation. See the section on Corticosteroids (p. 107) for an account of the action of this important class. Beclomethasone is:

- administered to the skin for treatment of inflammatory conditions such as psoriasis, eczema and dermatitis
- given by inhalation in asthma

- instilled intranasally in the management of allergic rhinitis and hay fever.

Dosage
Skin: apply sparingly twice daily.
Inhalation: 100–500 microgram twice daily. Four times daily inhalation may be necessary in acute exacerbations. Children usually receive half the adult dose but should not be denied the maximum daily dose required by inhalation to control brittle asthma. Intranasal use (adults and children): two applications (two metered doses or 100 microgram) into each nostril twice daily.

Nursing implications
See the section on Corticosteroids (p. 107).

Storage
- Preparations containing beclomethasone may be stored at room temperature.
- In common with other pressurized containers, metered aerosols and nasal sprays should not be punctured or incinerated after use.
- If necessary, beclomethasone cream may be diluted with cetomacrogol cream, Formula A, or the ointment with white soft paraffin.

BENDROFLUAZIDE

Presentation
Tablets – 2.5 mg, 5 mg

Actions and uses
See the section on Thiazide and Related Diuretics (p. 357).

Dosage
Adults: the daily adult dose range is 2.5–10 mg which may be taken as a single morning dose since the duration of action of bendrofluazide is approximately 24 hours.
Children.

- Up to 5 years: 1.25 mg.
- 5 years plus: 2.5 mg.

> **Nursing implications**
> See the section on Thiazide and
> Related Diuretics (p. 357).

Storage
Bendrofluazide tablets are stored at
room temperature.

BENORYLATE (Benoral)

Presentation
Tablets – 750 mg
Suspension – 4 g in 10 ml
Sachet – 2 g powder

Actions and uses
Benorylate is converted in the
blood to aspirin and paracetamol.
It is used in the treatment of pain
but mainly that associated with
acute or chronic inflammation. As a
product of aspirin and paracetamol,
its actions and uses are similar to
either or both. However, it may
be tried for patients unable
to tolerate aspirin due to its
gastric irritant effect.

Dosage
Adults: average dosage is 1.5 g
(two tablets) three times a day or
4 g (10 ml suspension) twice
daily.

> **Nursing implications**
> Since it is converted to aspirin, this
> drug is not recommended for use in
> children. The nursing implications
> notes for Aspirin (p. 35) are also
> applicable.

Storage
Benorylate tablets and suspension may
be stored at room temperature.

BENZHEXOL (Artane)

Presentation
Tablets – 2 mg and 5 mg

Actions and uses
Benzhexol has a number of actions
known as 'anticholinergic' since it
blocks the action of the stimulant
neurotransmitter acetylcholine at sites
on skeletal muscle. It therefore has the
potential to relax muscle and abolish
rigidity and tremor. This makes it
useful for the treatment of Parkinson's
disease. It is also used in schizophrenic
patients treated with phenothiazine
tranquillizers who may develop
muscular rigidity (pseudoparkinsonism)
as a side effect of therapy.

Dosage
Adults only: 5–15 mg daily in three
divided doses.

> **Nursing implications**
> - The drug's anticholinergic
>   actions produce dry mouth,
>   blurred vision, constipation and
>   urinary retention.
> - Further common adverse effects
>   include dizziness,
>   nervousness and nausea.
> - Mental confusion and
>   agitation are less common
>   problems.
> - The drug should be used with
>   caution in patients with:
>   – glaucoma
>   – gastrointestinal obstruction
>   – symptomatic prostatism.

Storage
Benzhexol tablets are stored at room
temperature.

BENZODIAZEPINES

Presentation
See individual drugs.

Actions and uses
Benzodiazepines are sedative drugs.
Some, however, have a specific action
on an area of the brain known as
the limbic system, thought to be
concerned with the control of
emotion. They are therefore used in
the symptomatic treatment of anxiety,
including situational (but not
psychotic) anxiety. The advantage
that benzodiazepines have over
other general sedative drugs is their
lack of respiratory depression, in
particular following overdosage. As
well as their selective sedative action,

B

certain drugs in this group have other uses.

- Nitrazepam, flunitrazepam, lormetazepam and temazepam have marked sedative effects and may be taken at night to induce sleep.
- Clobazam and clonazepam have a specific anticonvulsant action and are taken orally in the treatment of epilepsy.
- Chlordiazepoxide has a specific indication for the control of delirium tremens in alcoholic patients.
- Diazepam is particularly useful for intramuscular or intravenous administration as it provides sufficient sedation to relieve either acute anxiety or to allow minor practical procedures such as dental surgery or endoscopy. Diazepam is also useful in the treatment of status epilepticus and tetanus when it may be given by the intramuscular or intravenous route.

Dosage

See individual drugs.

Nursing implications

- When used in the treatment of anxiety there may be a degree of sedation occasionally leading to daytime drowsiness and accompanied by incoordination and staggering gait (ataxia). If troublesome, it may be necessary to review dosage and/or consider a less sedative alternative.
- The above effect is seen particularly when alcohol is taken in addition to a benzodiazepine. Patients must therefore be encouraged not to consume alcohol while taking these drugs and in addition they should be warned about the potential dangers of excess sedation when driving or operating machinery.
- Benzodiazepines, when given at night as hypnotics, may produce 'hangover' effects

lasting into the following day. These include symptoms of drowsiness, lethargy and headache and may, especially in elderly patients when high dosage has been given, cause frank confusion. Patients themselves may not notice effects of oversedation and nurses can play an important role in their detection.

- Occasionally when these drugs are given an unusual or paradoxical reaction may occur, especially in the very young and elderly. Patients become agitated, excited and may even experience hallucinations.
- Benzodiazepines, even when taken in massive overdosage, rarely produce profound neurological depression. When given intravenously for short-term sedation, they may, however, cause respiratory depression and should only be given by this route when facilities for resuscitation are available.
- These drugs are not recommended for regular use in pregnancy.
- Nursing mothers should be warned that if they take benzodiazepines while breastfeeding they will be excreted in their milk and may lead to marked drowsiness in the suckling infant.
- Side effects include gastrointestinal upset, blurred vision, dry mouth and headache.
- Benzodiazepine dependence and addiction is a major problem with long-term treatment which has become acknowledged over the past 20 years or more. This has, at least in part, resulted from overuse, often inappropriately for assumed anxiety. Benzodiazepine dependence is now widespread and occurs in patients who are not otherwise considered to be regular drug

abusers. Doctors are now requested to prescribe such drugs on a limited basis only (i.e. for 2–3 weeks). The symptoms of drug withdrawal are complex and may be difficult to interpret. They include anxiety, restlessness and agitation, sleep disturbances, hallucinations and even convulsions. Once detected, it is important that patients receive reassurance and support in attempting to 'wean off' the habit. This is often a prolonged and painstaking process and requires specialist psychiatric support for many.

Storage
See individual drugs.

BENZTROPINE (Cogentin)

Presentation
Tablets – 2 mg
Injection – 2 mg in 2 ml

Actions and uses
Benztropine has a number of actions known as 'anticholinergic' since it blocks the action of the stimulant neurotransmitter acetylcholine at sites on skeletal muscle. It therefore has the potential to relax muscle and abolish rigidity and tremor. Benztropine is used in the following situations where skeletal muscle rigidity and/or tremor is apparent.

- In Parkinson's disease.
- As an adjunct to treatment with the phenothiazine tranquillizers in schizophrenic patients who may develop muscular rigidity (pseudoparkinsonism) as a side effect of therapy.
- By injection for emergency treatment of acute dystonic reactions such as torticollis and oculogyric crises.

Dosage
For the treatment of parkinsonism: the adult dose is 1–6 mg per day as a single dose at bedtime. The dose may

alternatively be divided and given two or three times a day.
For the emergency treatment of acute dystonic reactions: 1–2 mg is given by intramuscular or intravenous injection.

Nursing implications
- The drug's anticholinergic actions produce dry mouth, blurred vision, constipation and urinary retention.
- Further common adverse effects include dizziness, nervousness and nausea.
- Mental confusion and agitation are less common problems.
- The drug should be used with caution in patients with:
  - glaucoma
  - gastrointestinal obstruction
  - symptomatic prostatism.

Storage
- Benztropine tablets and injection are stored at room temperature.
- Solution for injection should be protected from light.

BENZYLPENICILLIN (Crystapen G)

Also referred to as penicillin G available as the sodium salt.

Presentation
Injection – 600 mg (1 mega unit) powder in vial

Actions and uses
Benzylpenicillin was the first of the penicillin group of antibiotics. It has a mainly bactericidal action, i.e. it kills bacteria, by interference with the synthesis of the cell wall causing bacterial lysis. Benzylpenicillin has a notably narrow antibacterial spectrum restricted to streptococci, meningococci and gonococci. It has little or no anti-staphylococcal activity nor is it active against common Gram-negative pathogens. It has the following clinical uses.

B

- In the treatment of streptococcal and meningococcal infection including bacterial endocarditis related to the Viridans group and meningitis.
- The treatment of venereal disease, both syphilis and gonorrhoea.
- In the treatment of gonococcal infection of the eye in the newborn (ophthalmia neonatorum). A special eye drop formulation is available, freshly prepared in the pharmacy.

Dosage

- Adults: usually 600–1200 mg every 6 hours by intramuscular or intravenous bolus injection or intravenous infusion. The precise dose depends upon the sensitivity of the organism in question.
- In serious infection (e.g. treatment of bacterial endocarditis), 1.2 g every 4 hours (total 7.2 g/day) or 2.4 g every 6 hours (total 9.6 g) is required.
- Children aged 1 month to 12 years: 25 mg/kg body weight every 6 hours.
- Children less than 1 month: 25 mg/kg body weight every 8 hours.
- Premature infants: 25 mg/kg body weight every 12 hours.
- Meningococcal meningitis in children aged 1 month to 12 years: 75 mg/kg body weight at least every 6 hours and preferably every 4 hours.
- Meningococcal meningitis in children less than 1 month: 50 mg/kg body weight every 8 hours.
- Meningococcal meningitis in premature infants: 50 mg/kg body weight every 12 hours.
- A single intramuscular or intravenous injection should be given by the general practitioner if meningococcal infection is suspected. Patients with meningitis become seriously ill within a few hours and prompt treatment is therefore essential prior to hospitalization. Recommended single dose for adults is 1.2 g, for children 600 mg and for infants 300 mg.
- Eye drops: regular (e.g. 2–4 hourly) administration required initially in ophthalmia neonatorum.

- Intrathecal route: rarely benzylpenicillin is given intrathecally for the treatment of bacterial meningitis. Injection of an excessive dose by this route is dangerous and in many centres it is now felt that intravenous dosage is quite adequate. Maximum doses recommended are as follows.
  - Adults: 6 mg dissolved in 10 ml of sodium chloride or 10 ml of the patient's CSF. The usual daily dose is 6 mg but on occasions up to 12 mg may be used.
  - For infants and children: 0.1 mg/kg body weight is suitable. The concentration of penicillin in the injection should not exceed 0.6 mg/ml.
- Intraocular: in certain eye infections 300–600 mg may be given by subconjunctival injection.
- By the intravenous route at least 1 minute should be taken for each 300 mg injected.

Nursing implications

- Penicillins are most noted for the production of adverse effects in patients who are hypersensitive to the drug group. The effects produced may range from skin rash and urticaria to anaphylactic shock. **Patients with a history of penicillin allergy should never be given penicillin under any circumstance by any route.**
- As allergy to penicillin can be dangerous, the nurse plays an important role in the management of these patients by ensuring that their allergy, once identified, is duly recorded and brought to the attention of medical staff.
- The oral absorption of benzylpenicillin is so poor that it is now never used by this route. Penicillin V (phenoxymethylpenicillin) is preferred.
- Very high doses of benzylpenicillin have rarely been associated with haemolytic anaemia and convulsions.

Storage

- Preparations containing benzylpenicillin are stored at room temperature.
- Once prepared, solutions should be used immediately or within 6 hours if stored in a refrigerator.
- Eye drops, once prepared, should similarly be stored in a refrigerator and renewed daily or every 48 hours at most.

BETA-BLOCKERS (Beta-adrenoceptor blocking drugs)

Presentation

See individual drugs.

Actions and uses
Receptors of the autonomic sympathetic nervous system

The sympathetic nervous system is activated at two distinct receptor subtypes, termed alpha- and beta-adrenoceptors. The latter are further subdivided into beta-1 receptors and beta-2 receptors.

Relative effects of beta receptors

When stimulated, beta-1 receptors produce an increase in heart rate and cardiac output while beta-2 receptors cause dilatation of the small airways in the lung and arteriolar dilatation in the blood supply to skeletal muscle and the peripheries.

Beta-blockers antagonize these various effects. They therefore produce a reduction in heart rate and cardiac output and may potentially cause bronchoconstriction and peripheral vasoconstriction.

Implications of cardioselectivity

Individual beta-blockers may be distinguished on the basis of relative selectivity for beta-1 over beta-2 receptors. While all beta-blockers stimulate both types to a greater or lesser extent, some drugs (termed cardioselective) exert their effects mainly on the heart and are less likely to cause bronchoconstriction or impaired peripheral vascular perfusion.

Indications for beta-blockers

- Management of essential hypertension. A beta-blocker is frequently used as first-line treatment in mainly younger patients, either alone or in combination with a diuretic. This is especially useful for patients with co-existing coronary heart disease. The mechanism of action is unclear. It seems that beta-blockers in some way bring about an adaptive change which results in maintenance of blood pressure within normal limits.
- Prevention of angina pectoris in which beta-blockers reduce heart work and hence oxygen demand. They protect the ischaemic myocardium from the effects of overstimulation and are especially useful for patients who have a high sympathetic drive.
- Cardiac dysrhythmias including supraventricular and ventricular tachyarrhythmias. This action, together with protection of the ischaemic myocardium from sympathetic overstimulation, is thought to underlie the benefits of beta-blockers in acute myocardial infarction and subsequent prevention of reinfarction and sudden death.
- Symptomatic hyperthyroidism in which overstimulation by the sympathetic nervous system (tachycardia, tremor, sweating, etc.) is apparent.
- Situational anxiety for reasons above, i.e. in which the peripheral manifestations of anxiety (tachycardia, tremor, sweating, etc.) are blocked, so allowing the subject to cope with their stressful circumstances.
- Prevention of migraine by an unknown mechanism but following the observation that migraine sufferers receiving beta-blockers for other indications had fewer and less severe attacks of migraine than patients not treated with these drugs.
- Treatment of glaucoma in which beta-blockers block the production of aqueous humour, so leading to a reduction in intraocular pressure.

Other specialist uses for beta-blockers exist but will rarely be encountered in practice.

B

Dosage
See individual drugs.

Nursing implications
- Just as many of the beneficial effects of beta-blockers can be explained by their action at beta receptors, so too can their common side effects be predicted.
- Excessive reduction in cardiac output can predispose some patients to heart failure. This arises in those who have poor cardiac function and who rely especially on a high sympathetic drive in order to maintain cardiac output. Regular monitoring for excessive bradycardia (pulse <50 beats/min) can identify those most at risk.
- Beta-blockers should be used with caution or avoided in those with uncompensated heart failure or heart block.
- As mentioned above, beta-blockade within the airways of the lung can lead to wheeze and bronchospasm. Thus patients with chronic obstructive pulmonary disease (chronic bronchitis, emphysema) may be severely compromised even by cardioselective beta-blockers. **In patients with asthma the use of beta-blockers is absolutely contraindicated**; deaths from bronchospasm have been frequently reported even when these drugs have been used topically in the eye.
- Patients should be informed that when beta-blocker therapy is commenced there may be a sensation of coldness in the fingers and toes and tiredness as a result of reduced cardiac output. These initial side effects will diminish and become much less problematic as treatment continues.
- If necessary, a cardioselective beta-blocker should be chosen if the patient already has established peripheral vascular disease or poor peripheral circulation. Cardioselective drugs are less likely than non-selective beta-blockers to exacerbate vascular insufficiency though they are not themselves devoid of such an effect.
- Many diabetics recognize the early symptoms of a hypoglycaemic attack (i.e. sweating, tremor and tachycardia) and can act to prevent its development. However, if diabetics are given beta-blockers these early symptoms may not be apparent and more severe hypoglycaemia might ensue. Thus beta-blockers must be used with caution in diabetic patients. There is some evidence that cardioselective beta-blockers are less likely to have this effect and they are therefore generally preferred.
- Common gastrointestinal side effects include nausea, vomiting and diarrhoea which may be reduced if the drug is taken just before meals.
- Central nervous system effects include dizziness, drowsiness, lassitude, depression, insomnia, nightmares and hallucinations. Such effects are more likely to be seen when lipid-soluble beta-blockers such as propranolol are used and it is worth noting that atenolol is one of the least lipid-soluble beta-blockers.
- Other side effects include skin rashes, pruritus and flushing.
- It is important that the nurse remembers that beta-blockers will by definition produce a slow pulse and pulse rates below 50 per minute are not

an indication to stop the drug unless symptoms suggest heart failure is present. A useful point to note is that pulse rates of less than 50 per minute are often acceptable as long as they can be shown to rise after exercise.

Storage
See individual drugs.

BETAHISTINE (Serc)

Presentation
Tablets – 8 mg, 16 mg

Actions and uses
Betahistine is a derivative of histamine which acts on the inner ear as a vestibular and labyrinthine sedative. In clinical practice it is used in the treatment of vertigo and the symptoms of vertigo, tinnitus, hearing loss and nausea due to Menière's disease.

Dosage
Adults: 8–16 mg three times daily.

Nursing implications
- Gastrointestinal upsets occur in some patients treated with betahistine.
- Since the drug is a histamine derivative it may stimulate gastric acid secretion and predispose to bronchospasm. Betahistine should therefore be used with caution or avoided in patients with active peptic ulcer disease, oesophagitis and asthma.
- Caution should be used during pregnancy and breastfeeding

Storage
Betahistine tablets are stored at room temperature.

BETAMETHASONE (Betnelan, Betnesol, Betnovate)

Presentation
Tablets – 0.5 mg (plain and soluble)
Injection – 4 mg in 1 ml
Ointment, cream, lotion and scalp application – 0.1%
Ready-diluted ointment – 0.025%
Rectal ointment – 0.05% (includes local anaesthetic)
Eye, ear and nose drops – 0.1%
Eye ointment – 0.1%

Actions and uses
Betamethasone is a potent member of the corticosteroid group used widely by the topical and systemic routes. See the section on Corticosteroids (p. 107) for a full account of the actions and uses of these important drugs.

When used systemically, betamethasone is approximately seven times more potent than prednisolone and 25–30 times more potent than hydrocortisone on a mg-for-mg basis.

Dosage
Doses vary considerably with the nature and severity of the illness being treated and it is not therefore appropriate to quote specific instances.

Nursing implications
- See the section on Corticosteroids (p. 107).
- Intravenous injections are given slowly over 30 seconds to 1 minute.
- Perineal itching or burning discomfort may develop during or soon after injection. A few patients also complain of chills, headaches and flushing. These effects are a form of hypersensitivity which are very short-lived.
- If given by intravenous infusion, first dilute in 50–100 ml sodium chloride 0.9% or glucose 5% injection.

B

B

Storage
- Preparations containing betamethasone may be stored at room temperature.
- The injection solution should be protected from light.

BETAXOLOL (Betoptic, Kerlone)

Presentation
Tablets – 20 mg
Eye drops – 0.5%

Actions and uses
Betaxolol is a cardioselective Beta-blocker, the actions of which are discussed on p. 51. It has two uses in clinical practice.

- As an antihypertensive agent.
- In the treatment of glaucoma (ocular hypertension).

Dosage
Hypertension: 10–20 mg daily as single dose.
Glaucoma: 1 drop instilled in the eye twice daily.

Nursing implications
- Systemic absorption may follow topical application; therefore side effects associated with the use of Beta-blockers (p. 51) may occur.
- Application of betaxolol to the eye may cause local irritation or discomfort.

Storage
- Betaxolol tablets and eye drops are stored at room temperature.
- Eye drops, once opened, have a relatively short life due to the risk of bacterial contamination during use. Normally eye drops of any kind should not be used after 1 week for a hospitalized patient or after 4 weeks for others.

BEZAFIBRATE (Bezalip)

Presentation
Tablets – 200 mg, 400 mg (slow release)

Actions and uses
This drug is a member of the fibrate group of lipid-lowering drugs. The exact mechanism of action of these agents is unknown: they reduce both triglyceride and low-density lipoprotein (LDL-cholesterol) levels, so favourably influencing the LDL to HDL cholesterol profile. Bezafibrate is used in the treatment of certain of the familial hyperlipidaemias and hyperlipidaemias associated with coronary risk in patients who fail on diet alone. It is occasionally necessary to combine therapy with other types of lipid-lowering drugs.

Dosage
Adults only: 200 mg three times daily or 400 mg slow-release tablet once daily at night or in the morning.

Nursing implications
- Dosages are best taken with or immediately after meals.
- Skin rashes and muscle pain may occur, especially in patients with impaired kidney function, and treatment should be avoided if this is severe.
- All drugs of the fibrate group enhance warfarin and may produce bleeding in patients already receiving anticoagulant therapy. Close monitoring of prothrombin time is especially important in this group.
- This drug is contraindicated in pregnancy and breastfeeding.
- Other side effects include urticaria, nausea, dizziness, gastric pain, hair loss.

Storage
Bezafibrate tablets are stored at room temperature.

BICALUTAMIDE (Casodex)

Presentation
Tablet – 50 mg

Actions and uses
Bicalutamide is an antiandrogen used in conjunction with surgical castration

or 'medical' castration with the gonadorelin (LHRH) analogues in the treatment of advanced prostatic cancer. It effectively denies access of androgen to the tumour and, in particular, reduces the tumour flare which often accompanies the early treatment of prostatic cancer with LHRH analogues.

Dosage

Single daily dose 50 mg commencing 3 days before starting therapy with a LHRH analogue or at the same time as surgery.

Nursing implications
- Relatively common side effects include anorexia, dyspepsia, dry mouth, constipation, skin rashes, sleep disturbances and weight gain.
- Chest pain, abdominal pain, hyperglycaemia and peripheral oedema may be experienced.
- The antiandrogenic effect is associated with hot flushes, itching, breast tenderness, weakness and decreased libido.
- Liver function should be monitored during treatment as liver impairment with cholestasis and jaundice has been reported.

Storage

Bicalutamide tablets are stored at room temperature.

BISACODYL (Dulco-Lax)

Presentation

Tablets – 5 mg
Suppositories – 5 mg and 10 mg

Actions and uses

Bisacodyl is a stimulant laxative, i.e. it promotes peristalsis in the colon and rectum and hence bowel clearance. It is used for the short-term treatment of constipation in which a stimulant laxative is required or administered regularly in conjunction with

regular opioid treatment of chronic pain.

Dosage

Adults: 10 mg orally at night or one 10 mg suppository inserted each morning.
Children: one 5 mg suppository inserted each morning.

Nursing implications
- Patient education, including encouraging mobility and a high-fibre diet, may avoid the need for stimulant laxatives such as bisacodyl.
- Bisacodyl increases intestinal mobility and may irritate the gut wall, leading to abdominal cramps. It should be avoided where intestinal obstruction is suspected.
- Stimulant laxatives, if continued inappropriately, can lead to poor bowel function and chronic constipation. The exceptions occur in elderly patients who have poor bowel tone (often as a result of overuse of stimulant laxatives in the past), are unable to take a high-residue diet and are relatively inactive and where long-term pain control is associated with drug-induced constipation.

Storage

Preparations containing bisacodyl are stored at room temperature.

BISOPROLOL (Emcor, Monocor)

Presentation

Tablets – 5 mg, 10 mg

Actions and uses

Bisoprolol is a beta-blocker which is reported to have a degree of cardioselectivity far in excess of other so-called cardioselective beta-blockers. With this in mind, the reader is referred to the general account of Beta-blockers on p. 51. In practice, bisoprolol is used in the treatment of hypertension and angina pectoris.

Dosage

Bisoprolol has a long duration of action and is required to be taken only once daily. The usual dose is in the range 5–20 mg irrespective of indication.

Nursing implications

- See the section under Beta-blockers (p. 51).
- Although a very high degree of cardioselectivity is claimed for bisoprolol, it should nonetheless be used with caution in patients with asthma and severe chronic obstructive airways disease.

Storage

Bisoprolol tablets are stored at room temperature.

BLEOMYCIN

Presentation

Injection – ampoules containing 5 and 15 mg

Actions and uses

Bleomycin is a cytotoxic drug derived from a family of antibiotics which have been found to have this action. Its action, though complex, results in scission (cutting) of the DNA strand formed during cell replication and subsequent growth. Bleomycin is used in treatment of the following.

- Squamous cell carcinomas, i.e. in the mouth, nose, throat and oesophagus.
- Hodgkin's disease and other lymphomas.
- Testicular teratoma.
- Bleomycin has also been used in melanoma and carcinoma of the thyroid, lung and bladder.
- It has a special use by the intracavitary route in treating malignant effusions (e.g. affecting the lung and abdomen).

Dosage

- Route of administration: bleomycin may be used alone but is usually given in combination with other cytotoxic drugs. It may be administered by various routes including intramuscular, intravenous, intraarterial, intrapleural or intraperitoneal injection. It has also been injected directly into tumours.
- Adult doses vary widely according to the age of the patient, the route used and the type of tumour being treated. Doses for children are calculated upon body surface area.
- By intracavitary injection, usually 60 mg (but up to 100 mg) dissolved in 100 ml sodium chloride 0.9% injection.

Nursing implications

- Bleomycin, in contrast to most other cytotoxics, has little or no harmful effect on the bone marrow.
- Gastrointestinal side effects such as anorexia, nausea and vomiting and stomatitis are relatively common. Therefore the nurse must encourage adequate fluid and dietary intake and regular oral hygiene.
- Bleomycin is irritant and local reactions, including thrombophlebitis, may occur. If given by the intravenous route it is preferably given by slow (30 minutes to 1 hour) infusion.
- Intravenous infusions (rather than bolus IV injections) are less likely to be associated with serious pulmonary reactions to bleomycin.
- Pretreatment with corticosteroids (e.g. dexamethasone 16 mg by IV injection) reduces the likelihood of systemic reactions (e.g. rigors, chills, fever, flushing) to IV bleomycin.

- Most patients develop skin lesions after receiving full courses. These skin lesions include hyperkeratosis, impaired nail formation, redness and peeling of the skin and alopecia. Nurses should be aware of the implications of patients' altered body image as a result of these effects.
- Interstitial pneumonia may develop during treatment and if the drug is continued fatal pulmonary fibrosis may result. This effect limits the total dose that can be given to any one patient.
- If patients are known to have impaired renal function, reduced dosages should be used.
- When bleomycin is to be given by the intramuscular route, it may be prepared using 1% lignocaine solution in order to limit local pain on injection.
- Nurses should be aware of the risks posed by cytotoxic drugs. Some are irritant to the skin and mucous surfaces and care must be exercised when handling them. In particular, spillage or contamination of personnel or the environment must be avoided. If cytotoxic drugs are handled regularly, it is theoretically possible that repeated skin contact or inhalation may produce systemic toxic effects in nurses who have developed hypersensitivity to them. Most hospitals now operate a centralized (pharmacy-organized) additive service. While this reduces the risk of exposure to cytotoxic drugs, it is essential that nurses recognize and understand the local policy on their safe handling and disposal. The Health and Safety Executive has decreed that such a policy should be in place wherever cytotoxic drugs are administered. These should be adapted, wherever possible, to care of patients in the community.

B

Storage

- Bleomycin injection is stored at room temperature.
- It is stable for up to 3 years and an expiry date is printed on the label of individual ampoules.
- Any solution remaining after injection should be immediately discarded.
- The recommended diluent is 0.9% sodium chloride.
- Bleomycin solutions should not be mixed with other drugs, except where lignocaine is added for intramuscular injection.

BROMOCRIPTINE (Parlodel)

Presentation

Tablets – 1 mg, 2.5 mg
Capsules – 5 mg, 10 mg

Actions and uses

Bromocriptine inhibits the release of prolactin and growth hormone, normally produced in the pituitary gland which lies within the brain. It is used in clinical practice in a number of situations.

- Treatment of acromegaly: a disease caused by excess secretion of growth hormone, usually by a tumour of the pituitary. Acromegaly is associated with excessive growth of the facial bones and the hands and feet with accompanied headache, sweating, hypertension, heart and chest disease.
- Inhibition of puerperal lactation stimulated by prolactin secretion.
- Treatment of infertility in females when this is found to be associated with an excess production of prolactin.
- Treatment of galactorrhoea (production of milk by the breast) when this is shown to be due to an excess production of prolactin.
- Bromocriptine is also dopaminergic, i.e. it exerts a stimulant action on

B

receptor sites in the brain which normally respond to the neurotransmitter substance dopamine. As a result, it is used in the treatment of Parkinson's disease thought to be due to dopamine lack and arising in a specific area of the brain (the extrapyramidal system) which coordinates movement. Bromocriptine produces benefit in symptoms associated with Parkinson's disease characterized by increased mobility and loss of rigidity and tremor.

Dosage

For the treatment of acromegaly: dosage is adjusted according to response, monitored both clinically and by measuring blood levels of growth hormone. It is worth noting that acromegalics require fairly high doses for effective treatment.

For the inhibition of puerperal lactation: 2.5 mg twice daily.

For the treatment of infertility: initially 2.5 mg once or twice a day is given and the dose is gradually increased until menstruation or pregnancy is achieved.

For the treatment of galactorrhoea: initially 2.5 mg once or twice a day with gradual increments until galactorrhoea ceases.

In the treatment of Parkinson's disease (usually in conjunction with levodopa): a daily dose ranging from 10 to 100 mg may be used depending upon the balance between patient response and the occurrence of unwanted side effects. Daily doses are achieved by the use of gradual dosage increments following an initial low dose until the optimum is reached in the individual.

Nursing implications

- Gastrointestinal upset, including severe nausea, is perhaps the major side effect of bromocriptine. It can be minimized by commencing with a very low initial dose which is gradually built up to the lowest effective

maintenance dose thereafter; for example, by starting therapy on a once-daily basis at night then increasing as necessary.
- Other side effects include postural hypotension, dizziness, headache, vomiting and constipation.
- Less commonly, drowsiness, confusion, agitation, hallucination, dyskinesia, dry mouth and leg cramps.
- Note that side effects are considerably more likely to occur with high doses such as those used in the treatment of Parkinson's disease.

Storage

Bromocriptine tablets and capsules are stored at room temperature.

BUDESONIDE (Entocort, Pulmicort, Rhinocort)

Presentation

Tablet – 3 mg (controlled release/enteric coated)
Pressurized metered dose inhaler – 50 and 200 microgram per dose
Dry powder Turbohaler – 100, 200 and 400 microgram per dose
Nebulizer solution – 500 and 1000 microgram (1 mg) in 2 ml 'Respules'
Nasal spray – 100 microgram aqueous pumped dose

Actions and uses

Budesonide is a corticosteroid for local use including oral treatment of inflammatory bowel disease. The actions of Corticosteroids are summarized on p. 107.

In practice, budesonide is used in the treatment of the following chronic inflammatory (autoimmune) conditions.

- Prevention of asthma, by inhalation.
- Prevention of seasonal (allergic) rhinitis, by nasal instillation.
- Suppression of ileocaecal Crohn's disease, using positioned-release tablets.

Dosage

Asthma: regular twice-daily (morning and night) inhalation in doses ranging from 50 to 400 microgram. The optimum dose is that which enables good control of chronic asthma and reduces the need for regular or frequent use of bronchodilator inhalers (e.g. salbutamol, terbutaline). In acute or severe chronic asthma: respirator solution may be nebulized, e.g. 0.5–2 mg twice daily or up to four times daily according to response. Seasonal and perennial rhinitis: 1–2 applications into each nostril twice daily.
Crohn's disease: 9 mg positioned-release, enteric-coated tablets usually taken once daily in the morning, e.g. before breakfast.

Nursing implications
- See the section on Corticosteroids (p. 107).
- It should be noted that overuse of the above products may result in systemic steroid effects but in practice only local problems are encountered.

Storage
- Budesonide preparations are stored at room temperature.
- Pressurized inhaler devices must not be incinerated, even when apparently empty.
- 'Respule'ampoules are **not for injection**.

BUMETANIDE (Burinex)

Presentation

Tablets – 1 mg, 5 mg
Injection – 1 mg in 4 ml, 6.25 mg in 25 ml

Actions and uses

Bumetanide is a rapid-acting, short-duration diuretic of the 'loop' acting type, so-called because their site of action is in the loop of Henle. Such diuretics interfere with sodium and water reabsorption which is the major mechanism for concentration of urine within the kidney tubule. As a result, a relatively large volume of dilute urine is produced within 30 minutes of oral dosing and for up to 4 hours thereafter.

Bumetanide is therefore used in the treatment of oedema and, in particular, heart failure. In acute left ventricular failure, it contributes a useful lowering of pulmonary arterial pressure and cardiac preload (by dilatation of the pulmonary and venous capacitance vessels), so reducing pulmonary oedema and acute breathlessness.

Frusemide is the most widely used of the loop diuretics since it is effective and very inexpensive. Bumetanide is, however, more reliably absorbed from the gastrointestinal tract and may be preferred for some patients in whom frusemide is relatively ineffective.

Dosage
- Bumetanide is 40 times more potent than frusemide, i.e. 1 mg bumetanide produces the same effect as 40 mg of frusemide. Recommended doses are therefore 1/40th of those discussed under frusemide, i.e. 1–2 mg daily.
- Much higher doses are used in acute renal failure.

Nursing implications
- In common with other diuretic drugs, it is essential that overuse does not result in salt and water depletion.
- Monitoring of serum sodium, potassium and blood urea is therefore warranted.
- In particular, hypokalaemia may predispose patients to serious cardiac arrhythmias, particularly if concurrently treated with digoxin.
- Very high dosage may be associated with hearing impairment and renal dysfunction
- Patients should be made aware of increased diuresis which occurs approximately 30 minutes after taking bumetanide.

B

Storage
- Bumetanide tablets and injection are stored at room temperature.
- The injection solution is sensitive to light and is therefore packed in amber-coloured ampoules.

BUPIVACAINE (Marcain)

Presentation
Injection – 0.25% and 0.5% (plain and with adrenaline)

Actions and uses
This potent local anaesthetic drug has a much longer duration of action than lignocaine. It is used in minor surgical and obstetric procedures to produce extradural block, digital block, nerve plexus block and pudendal block.

Dosage
Individual doses vary considerably with the type of procedure and the patient response. It is recommended that the maximum dosage in any 4-hour period should be 2 mg/kg body weight.

Nursing implications
- The onset of action is rapid (within a few minutes) and lasts for several hours, depending upon dosage and route of administration.
- Bupivacaine is well tolerated except in a few patients who are allergic to this and other local anaesthetics.

Storage
Bupivacaine injection is stored at room temperature but protected from light.

BUPRENORPHINE (Temgesic)

Presentation
Injection – 300 microgram (0.3 mg) in 1 ml
Tablets, sublingual – 200 microgram (0.2 mg) and 400 microgram (0.4 mg)

Actions and uses
This narcotic (opioid) drug has a moderate to potent analgesic action of relatively long duration. It is used for the treatment of conditions associated with moderate to severe pain but in practice it has been largely overused to the extent of abuse. As a result, buprenorphine is now subject to the legal requirements of the Controlled Drugs.

Dosage
Adults: 300–600 microgram (0.3–0.6 mg) every 6–8 hours by intramuscular or slow intravenous injection or 200–400 microgram (0.2–0.4 mg) by the sublingual route.
Children over 6 months: 3–9 microgram (0.3–0.9 mg)/kg body weight 6–8 hourly by slow intravenous or intramuscular route or 100–300 microgram (0.1–0.3 mg) may be given to children >16 kg every 6–8 hours.

Nursing implications
- The problem of addiction with continued use of this drug is now firmly established. This has arisen in the past as a result of persevering with treatment using increasing dosage in patients who actually required more effective pain control with more potent analgesics such as morphine and diamorphine.
- Buprenorphine is now therefore subject to the legal restrictions placed on other Controlled Drugs.
- Nausea and occasionally vomiting are relatively frequent side effects.
- Others include constipation and urinary hesitancy.
- There is a risk of prolonged sedation and respiratory depression with excessive dosage and treatment with repeated doses of the opioid antagonist naloxone may be required.

Storage

- Buprenorphine preparations must be stored in the Controlled Drug cupboard.
- Tablets and injection solution must be protected from light.

BUSERELIN (Suprecur, Suprefact)

Presentation

Injection – 5.5 mg in 5.5 ml
Nasal spray – 100 and
150 microgram/dose

Actions and uses

Buserelin is a chemical analogue of the hypothalamic hormone gonadotrophin-releasing hormone (GnRH), also known as LHRH (luteinizing hormone-releasing hormone) or gonadorelin. It acts by downregulating the release of pituitary gonadotrophins (it induces a desensitization to gonadotrophin release) with consequent suppression of pituitary gonadal function. Buserelin has three main uses.

- It is used in the treatment of advanced prostatic cancer (stages C or D) when suppression of testosterone is required (such tumours are testosterone dependent): its action has been described as equivalent to 'medical castration'.
- It inhibits ovarian secretion of sex steroids and it is used therefore in the treatment of endometriosis.
- It is used at specialist fertility clinics to desensitize the pituitary and so facilitate induction of ovulation by administered gonadotrophins.

Dosage

Prostatic cancer: at the start of therapy a series of subcutaneous injections, the usual dose is 500 microgram, is given 8-hourly for 1 week. This is followed by intranasal maintenance therapy with one application (100 microgram) into each nostril six times daily.
Endometriosis: one application (150 microgram) is sprayed into each nostril three times daily commencing on the first or second day of menstruation and continued for a maximum treatment duration of 6 months.

Anovulatory infertility: one application (150 microgram) is sprayed into each nostril four times daily commencing in early follicular phase (day 1) or, provided pregnancy is first excluded, in mid-luteal phase (day 21) and continued until suppression of pituitary function is achieved (usually after 2–3 weeks).

Nursing implications

- The effectiveness of treatment is highly dependent upon good patient compliance and patients require careful instruction in the use of maintenance therapy. For example, in prostatic cancer six daily doses are administered as follows: dose 1 (before breakfast), dose 2 (after breakfast), doses 3 and 4 (before and after the mid-day meal), doses 5 and 6 (before and after the evening meal).
- Since in prostatic cancer buserelin affects only testosterone-dependent tumours it should not be used if orchidectomy has been carried out. Also, failure to obtain a response (measured by falling testosterone levels) within 6 weeks on full doses indicates the presence of an insensitive tumour and buserelin therapy should be stopped.
- A high proportion of patients experience an initial flare-up in their condition associated with a transient rise in testosterone levels, accompanied by increased bone pain, at the start of therapy. To offset this, an antiandrogen may be administered concurrently, starting a few days before buserelin therapy and continued for about 3 weeks thereafter.
- Buserelin must not be used during pregnancy, breastfeeding or in patients with undiagnosed vaginal bleeding.

B

- Common side effects include hot flushing, loss of potency and libido, breast swelling and tenderness. Occasionally patients may complain of nasal irritation while on maintenance therapy.

Storage
- Buserelin injection and nasal spray are stored at room temperature.
- Nasal spray, once started, is used for 7 days and then discarded and replaced.

BUSPIRONE (Buspar)

Presentation
Tablets – 5 mg, 10 mg

Actions and uses
Buspirone is an anxiolytic and antidepressant which appears to combine the effects of the benzodiazepines and tricyclic and related antidepressants though its precise mechanism of action is unknown. It is used in the treatment of anxiety, particularly that in which depression is an associated finding.

Dosage
Adults: usually 5 mg taken 2–3 times daily but up to a maximum dose of 45 mg daily may be required.

Nursing implications
- Side effects commonly experienced during the early period of treatment include nausea, headache, dizziness or light-headedness and irritability.
- Tachycardia, palpitations, sweating, confusion and fatigue are also reported.

Storage
Buspirone tablets are stored at room temperature.

BUSULPHAN (Myleran)

Presentation
Tablets – 0.5 mg, 2 mg

Actions and uses
Busulphan is a cytotoxic drug which is converted in the body to a highly reactive product which in turn binds irreversibly to substances in cells which are essential for cell growth and division. The process of growth and division is therefore blocked by this action. Rapidly dividing cells such as tumour cells and cells of the bone marrow are more likely to be affected by this drug than slowly dividing cells.

In practice busulphan has the following uses.

- In the treatment of chronic myeloid/granulocytic leukaemia.
- In the treatment of primary polycythaemia.

Dosage
The average adult dose is 2–4 mg daily taken for a period of 6 months when an optimum response is usually achieved. If treatment is stopped at this stage relapse often occurs 6–18 months later. Patients are therefore usually continued on maintenance doses ranging from 0.5 to 3 mg per day. With maintenance therapy the disease may be controlled for longer periods of time, i.e. 2 years or more. This regime is not used in the treatment of children.

Nursing implications
- Excessive bone marrow depression may occur and thrombocytopenia with resultant haemorrhage is particularly common. Anaemia and opportunistic infection due to suppression of white cell production may also occur.
- If patients are given this drug for several years, pulmonary fibrosis may develop. This usually presents as progressive breathlessness on exertion or may be detected on routine

X-ray examination. If it is noticed at an early stage and treatment is stopped, a course of steroid therapy may reverse the process. If the effect is not recognized, progressive irreversible fibrosis with respiratory failure will follow. It is important therefore that patients on this treatment be observed for development of such symptoms.

- Other side effects include skin pigmentation, which may be extensive and especially affects light-exposed areas, pressure areas, skin creases, axillae and nipples.
- Amenorrhoea, testicular atrophy and gynaecomastia may also occur.
- Adrenal gland insufficiency (Addison's disease) has been reported as a rare complication of this treatment.
- Nurses should be aware of the risks posed by cytotoxic drugs. Some are irritant to the skin and mucous surfaces and care must be exercised when handling them. In particular, spillage or contamination of personnel or the environment must be avoided. If cytotoxic drugs are handled regularly, it is theoretically possible that repeated skin contact or inhalation may produce systemic toxic effects in nurses who have developed hypersensitivity to them. Most hospitals now operate a centralized (pharmacy-organized) additive service. While this reduces the risk of exposure to cytotoxic drugs, it is essential that nurses recognize and understand the local policy on their safe handling and disposal. The Health and Safety Executive has decreed that such a policy should be in place wherever cytotoxic drugs are administered. These should be adapted, wherever possible, to care of patients in the community.

Storage

Busulphan tablets are stored at room temperature.

C

CABERGOLINE (Dostinex)

Presentation
Tablet – 0.5 mg (500 microgram)

Actions and uses
Cabergoline is a centrally acting dopamine agonist, i.e. it stimulates receptors in the brain which are normally under the influence of the dopamine neurotransmitter. In this respect its actions and uses are identical to those of bromocriptine (p. 57). However, it is longer acting than bromocriptine and does not appear to be associated with the same wide-ranging side effects. In practice, cabergoline is used for the following indications.

- Inhibition or suppression of lactation.
- Infertility associated with hyperprolactinaemia.

Dosage
Inhibition or suppression of lactation: initially 1 mg (1000 microgram) on the first day post partum then 0.25 mg (250 microgram) every 12 hours for 2 days thereafter.
Infertility associated with hyperprolactinaemia: 0.5 mg (500 microgram) on one day each week (or half this dose taken on two days in the week) increased gradually (i.e. by 0.5 mg/week at monthly intervals) as required to a maximum weekly dose of 4.5 mg (4500 microgram or nine tablets).

Nursing implications
- Although related to bromocriptine (p. 57), the side effect profile of cabergoline is possibly much less severe. Close monitoring of patients and the need to document observed (suspected) toxicity are still important.
- Reported side effects include gastrointestinal discomfort, nausea and vomiting, bleeding, syncope, weakness and hot flushes.
- It is important to exclude pregnancy before starting treatment in patients with hyperprolactinaemic infertility. Treatment should be discontinued immediately if pregnancy occurs.
- In some patients, hypotension may be a problem, usually in the early treatment period. If affected, patients should be warned to avoid driving or operating machinery at this time.

Storage
Cabergoline tablets are stored at room temperature.

CALCIFEROL

Presentation
Present in various prescription and over-the-counter products in a range of strengths. Often available in combination with mineral calcium and other fat- and water-soluble vitamins.

Actions and uses
Calciferol is a mixture of ergocalciferol and cholecalciferol which are respectively vitamin D2 and D3. Vitamin D compounds are essential for proper bone development.

A deficiency in children causes rickets, characterized by stunted growth and a 'bowing' of the limbs as a result of failure of bone mineralization. In adults the deficiency also results in defective bone mineralization, leading to a condition known as osteomalacia.

- Vitamin D supplements containing low doses of calciferol are taken if there is a relative lack of vitamin D in the diet.
- Higher doses are required in chronic liver disease or other situations in which intestinal malabsorption of the vitamin occurs.

Dosage

- Dosage varies widely depending upon the need to prevent or treat established vitamin D deficiency. Specialist advice from dieticians or those with experience in treating rickets and osteomalacia should be sought
- In malnourished patients, a single injection of calciferol 300 000 unit every 6 months or 600 000 unit once a year by deep IM injection will often suffice in preventing long-term deficiency and bone mineralization defect.

Nursing implications

- Overzealous use of vitamin D (which is fat soluble and therefore likely to accumulate in the body) can lead to excessive absorption of calcium. It is important to check plasma calcium levels, especially in those who develop nausea and vomiting, in order to avoid serious hypercalcaemia.
- Note that vitamin D enters breast milk in large amounts and excessive amounts ingested by nursing mothers can cause hypercalcaemia in the suckling infant.
- Patients with chronic renal failure may not adequately convert calciferol into its active form (a process which takes place within the kidney). As a result, vitamin D treatment for renal osteodystrophy requires

administration of active forms of the vitamin (e.g. alfacalcidol or calcitriol).
- Symptoms of overdosage (usually due to excessive ingestion of supplements) include anorexia, nausea, vomiting, diarrhoea, tiredness, sweating, polyuria, thirst, headache and vertigo. This is in fact a result of raised plasma concentrations of calcium and phosphate.

Storage

- Check storage requirements for individual preparations.
- Calciferol injection is stored at room temperature and protected from light. If necessary, it can be diluted using arachis oil or olive oil.

CALCIPOTRIOL (Dovonex)

Presentation

Ointment – 50 microgram per 1 g
Cream – 50 microgram per 1 g
Scalp solution – 50 microgram/ml

Actions and uses

Calcipotriol is a chemical derivative of vitamin D which has been shown to reduce plaque formation in psoriasis. It is used in mild to moderate psoriasis affecting up to 40% of the body skin area.

Dosage

- Ointment or cream is applied to the affected area twice daily.
- Apply to scalp twice daily to treat scalp psoriasis.

Nursing implications

- It is recommended that application to the body be restricted to 100 g weekly and that application to the face be avoided.
- Similarly, a maximum recommended weekly dose to the scalp is 5 mg or 100 ml scalp solution.

C

- Since it is a vitamin D analogue, calcipotriol should not be used in patients with hypercalcaemia.
- The effects of large quantities of topical vitamin D in pregnancy and lactation are unknown and calcipotriol should therefore be avoided in these situations.
- A degree of irritation is reported which may be more marked when applied to the face. Perioral lesions in particular may occur.
- Hands should be washed thoroughly after application.

Storage
Calcipotriol preparations are stored at room temperature.

CALCITONIN (Calcitare)

Presentation
Injection – 160 units

Actions and uses
A form of calcitonin derived from pig (porcine) thyroid tissue. In this form it is more immunogenic than salmon calcitonin (salcatonin) which is therefore generally preferred.

Calcitonin is a hormone secreted by the thyroid and parathyroid glands which regulates bone turnover. It does so by lowering plasma calcium and phosphate levels and by antagonizing the actions of parathyroid hormone on bone. In particular, calcitonin:

- inhibits the activity of bone cells called osteoclasts which continuously digest bone tissue, releasing free calcium and phosphate
- promotes the renal excretion of calcium and phosphate
- inhibits the activation of vitamin D and hence calcium absorption from the gut.

It is used in conditions associated with rapid bone turnover including Paget's disease (to relieve pain and neutrological complications), postmenopausal osteoporosis, hypercalcaemia of malignancy and for pain relief in metastatic disease of the bone.

Dosage
Administration is usually by subcutaneous (occasionally intramuscular) injection.

- Paget's disease in adults: range from 80 unit on alternate days to 160 unit daily as a single dose or in 2–3 divided doses.
- Hypercalcaemia: based on 4 unit/kg and increased according to response.

Nursing implications
- As described above, calcitonin is to some extent immunogenic and injections may be poorly tolerated by some patients in whom it causes nausea, vomiting, flushing, diarrhoea, tingling sensation and skin rashes. Inflammatory reactions may occur at the injection site.
- Anaphylaxis has occurred.
- As a result of the above, patients may be assessed for likely allergy by prior skin prick or scratch testing.
- If used to arrest the rate of bone turnover in osteoporotic women, it is important that supplementary calcium and vitamin D be given also.
- The use of calcitonin should be avoided in pregnancy and lactation.

Storage
- Porcine calcitonin is supplied as a dry powder which must be reconstituted with a special gelatin diluent with which it is provided.
- Dry powder ampoules are stored at room temperature but solution, once prepared, should be used within 24 hours. If refrigerated, however, solutions can be stored for up to 7 days.

CALCITRIOL (Calcijex, Rocaltrol)

Presentation
Capsules – 0.25 microgram and 0.5 microgram
Injection – 1 and 2 microgram in 1 ml

Actions and uses

Calcitriol is 1,25-dihydroxy vitamin D which is the end-stage of calciferol metabolism (first via the kidney then the liver) to the final active form of the vitamin. The actions of vitamin D are described for Calciferol (p. 64).

In practice, calcitriol is used to correct calcium and phosphate metabolism in situations in which the conversion of calciferol is impaired.

- In the treatment of renal osteo-dystrophy associated with severe renal impairment.
- In the treatment of hypocalcaemia in patients undergoing dialysis for chronic renal failure.
- Calcitriol is also occasionally used in the treatment of postmenopausal osteoporosis.

Dosage

For the treatment of renal osteodystro-phy in adults: initially 0.25 microgram daily or on alternate days increased, as required, by doses of 0.25 microgram at 2–4 weekly intervals. Usually a dose of 0.5–1.0 microgram/day is required.

In conjunction with renal dialysis: ini-tially 0.5 microgram on alternate days by IV injection at the finish of dialysis increased, as required, by 250–500 microgram at 2–4 weekly intervals to a maximum of 9 microgram per week in total.

In postmenopausal osteoporosis: twice-daily dosing with 0.25 micro-gram according to the biochemical response.

Nursing implications

- Side effects of note are associ-ated with overuse of this drug which is the active form of vitamin D. See under Calciferol (p. 64).
- Although very active, the effects of calcitriol are short-lived so that toxicity, when it arises, is resolved within 1–2 days.

Storage

Preparations containing calcitriol are stored at room temperature and protected from light.

CALCIUM ANTAGONISTS

Presentation

See individual drugs.

Actions and uses

The calcium antagonists are a group of drugs which act on vascular smooth muscle and, to a lesser extent, the conducting cells of the heart. They block the flow of calcium (flux) into the cell via a calcium ion channel (Ca++) and so inhibit tissue activation. For this reason drugs of this type are often also referred to as calcium channel blockers.

Calcium antagonists are used in the following indications.

- Hypertension in which they produce arterial vasodilatation and hence reduction of peripheral vascular resistance. Calcium antagonists are frequently used in addition to drugs of the beta-blocker and thiazide diuretic groups.
- Angina pectoris (often in unstable or vasoplastic angina) in which they increase coronary artery flow and reduce the risk of coronary arterial spasm. To a lesser extent they also reduce heart work by dampening myocardial contractility.
- Individual members of the group have other specific indications described under specific calcium antagonists.

Dosage

See individual drugs.

Nursing implications

- As vasodilators, the calcium antagonists produce frequent flushing and occasional headache and dizziness. This is readily predictable and worth discussing with the patient at the outset. Patients may be reassured, however, that tolerance to these effects quickly follows and they become much less troublesome within a few weeks of commencing treatment.

C

- A common effect of certain of these drugs is the development of oedema of the foot and ankle (pedal oedema). It is important to note that this does not reflect heart or kidney failure but is rather an expected consequence of their action on the blood vessel wall, namely leakage of fluid into the surrounding tissues. The lower extremities are most affected as a result of gravitational influence and elevation of the feet brings some benefit. Pedal oedema can be found, if actively sought, in over one-third of patients but is rarely sufficently severe to warrant discontinuation of treatment.
- Calcium antagonists reduce myocardial contractility and should be used with caution in patients with cardiac conduction defects, including bradycardia and heart block. This is especially important when used with other drugs which reduce contractility including the beta-blockers and antiarrhythmics (with the exception of digoxin). Severe bradycardia and uncompensated heart failure are relative contraindications.
- Other side effects include gastrointestinal upsets, including abdominal pain and constipation, and skin rashes.
- Drugs of this group should be avoided in pregnancy since animal investigations suggest possible teratogenicity. If taken late in pregnancy they may inhibit uterine activity.

Storage
See individual drugs.

CAPTOPRIL (Acepril, Capoten)

Presentation
Tablets – 12.5 mg, 25 mg, 50 mg

Actions and uses
Captopril is an angiotensin-converting enzyme inhibitor. See the section on ACE Inhibitors (p. 4) for an account of the actions of this drug. In clinical practice, it is used in heart failure, hypertension and following myocardial infarction. In addition, its role in the prevention of diabetic nephropathy (microalbuminuria >30 mg/day) is becoming accepted in insulin-dependent diabetics, in particular.

Dosage
Heart failure: 6.25–12.5 mg twice daily increased up to 50 mg three times per day.
Hypertension: usual dose is 6.25–12.5 mg twice daily.
Diabetic nephropathy: 25 mg three or four times daily.

Nursing implications
- See section on ACE Inhibitors (p. 4).
- Captopril, in particular, is associated with (potentially severe) hypersensitivity reactions, especially when high dosage is used.

Storage
Captopril tablets are stored at room temperature.

CARBAMAZEPINE (Tegretol)

Presentation
Tablets – 100 mg, 200 mg and 400 mg
Chewable tablets – 100 mg, 200 mg
Controlled-release tablets – 200 mg, 400 mg
Liquid – 100 mg in 5 ml
Suppositories – 125 mg, 250 mg

Actions and uses
Carbamazepine is a centrally acting drug which, as a result of stabilization of nerve activity, has four main uses in clinical practice.

- It is an anticonvulsant and a treatment of choice in all forms of epilepsy with the exception of absence seizures.
- It is an effective analgesic for the treatment of pain associated with trigeminal neuralgia.
- Prophylaxis of manic-depressive psychosis unresponsive to treatment with lithium.

- Finally, it has become recognized that carbamazepine causes water retention, probably by blocking free water clearance by the kidney. This is thought to result from a reduction in the sensitivity of the kidney tubules to the effect of vasopressin (antidiuretic hormone or ADH). As a result, carbamazepine is used in the treatment of nephrogenic and partial pituitary diabetes insipidus.

Dosage

Epilepsy in adults: a gradually increasing dosage regime is used which is adjusted to suit the needs of the individual patient. For example: adults: initially 100–200 mg once or twice daily followed by a slow increase until the best response is obtained. This usually occurs when the patient is receiving 800–1200 mg in total per day but in some instances 1600 mg daily may be necessary.

Rectally: using the oral dose as a guide with 125 mg and 250 mg rectally corresponding to 100 mg and 200 mg orally respectively (i.e. an increase in dose of 25% to account for slightly poorer absorption from the rectum).

Epilepsy in children: less than 1 year, 100–200 mg/day given in divided doses; 1–5 years, 200–400 mg per day given in divided doses; 5–10 years, 400–600 mg per day in divided doses; 10–15 years, 600–1000 mg per day given in divided doses.

The above are maintenance doses. Initial doses should be considerably smaller.

For the treatment of trigeminal neuralgia: the individual dosage requirements of carbamazepine vary considerably depending on age and weight of the patient. An initial dose of 100 mg per day is recommended. Under normal circumstances, 200 mg 3–4 times daily is sufficient to maintain a pain-free state but in rare instances a total dose of 1600 mg per day may be necessary.

Manic-depressive psychosis: in adults and children, initially 400 mg daily in divided doses increased gradually as required to a maximum dose of 1.6 g/day. In practice, 400–600 mg daily is sufficient for most patients.

Nephrogenic diabetes insipidus: 200 mg taken once or twice daily.

Nursing implications

- Drowsiness and dizziness are common at the start of treatment, especially if the initial dose is high or is subsequently increased too quickly.
- Dry mouth, diarrhoea, nausea and vomiting are common side effects.
- Unusual side effects include skin rash, light-sensitive dermatitis, jaundice, leucopenia and aplastic anaemia.
- Suppositories are generally used to cover periods when the oral route is unavailable, e.g. due to severe nausea and vomiting or in the perioperative period.
- Rectal carbamazepine is reported occasionally to produce local irritation.
- Carbamazepine is a potent inducer of the liver microsomal enzyme system and as such it may increase the rate of metabolism of other drugs taken concurrently. Interactions of this type occur with the following drugs which are extensively metabolized by the liver: corticosteroids, cyclosporin, other anticonvulsants, theophylline, thyroxine and warfarin. It may be necessary to review the dosage of such drugs to avoid a loss of effect if one is already being prescribed for a patient commenced on carbamazepine.
- As carbamazepine is associated with an increased risk of teratogenicity, women treated with this drug who are contemplating pregnancy should seek medical advice.

Storage

Carbamazepine preparations are stored at room temperature.

CARBIMAZOLE (Neomercazole)

Presentation

Tablets – 5 mg, 20 mg

C

Actions and uses

Carbimazole inhibits the production of thyroxine by the thyroid gland. This action is shared by its active metabolite, methimazole. Both are therefore termed antithyroid drugs and are used in the treatment of thyrotoxicosis. They may be used on their own for prolonged periods in the treatment of this disease or they may be given for a short period only in thyrotoxic patients prior to surgery.

Dosage

Adults: a high dose is used initially in order to render the patient euthyroid (i.e. to produce a normal thyroid function). For example, 20–60 mg daily for the first month after which the dose is gradually reduced to maintain the patient in a clinically and biochemically euthyroid state. The total amount daily is usually taken in three divided doses. Children: an average daily dose for children is 5 mg three times per day initially, reducing to doses as determined by the clinical and biochemical state of the patient.

Nursing implications

- A rare but important adverse effect of this drug is the production of bone marrow depression affecting white cell function, in particular, and leading to an increased risk of infection. This usually manifests as throat infection and patients should be warned to report sore throat immediately, whereupon treatment should be stopped pending the results of WBC tests.
- Other side effects include nausea, headache, arthralgia, gastrointestinal upset, skin rash and hair loss.
- If carbimazole is given to a pregnant patient adverse effects on thyroid function of the developing fetus may occur. It is therefore important to achieve the minimum effective dose in pregnancy.
- As the drug is actively secreted in breast milk, mothers receiving this drug should be advised not to breastfeed.

Storage

Carbimazole tablets are stored at room temperature.

CARBOPLATIN (Paraplatin)

Presentation

Injection – 50 mg in 5 ml, 150 mg in 15 ml, 450 mg in 45 ml

Actions and uses

Carboplatin is a platinum-containing cytotoxic drug which is similar to cisplatin. It appears to interfere with cellular reproduction and since tumour cells reproduce at a rapid rate they are particularly sensitive to its effects. It is mainly used in the treatment of advanced ovarian carcinoma and small cell carcinoma of the lung.

Dosage

This is largely determined by specific indication and current schedules which are subject to change in line with existing knowledge. Current schedules should be consulted for up-to-date details of dosage and route of administration. Doses in the region of 400 mg/m^2 body surface area have been used.

Nursing implications

- Carboplatin is generally better tolerated and, overall, it is less toxic than is cisplatin. Nevertheless the toxic potential of both drugs is somewhat similar.
- Carboplatin produces less nausea and vomiting than does cisplatin but this effect arises in almost all patients treated with cisplatin.
- Nephrotoxicity, neurotoxicity and ototoxicity are also much less likely to occur. The exception is bone marrow toxicity (myelosuppression) which is more common in patients treated with carboplatin who must be closely monitored as a result. This makes patient education regarding control of infection and enhanced bleeding tendency an

important aspect of the nurse's role.

- Nurses should be aware of the risks posed by cytotoxic drugs. Some are irritant to the skin and mucous surfaces and care must be exercised when handling them. In particular, spillage or contamination of personnel or the environment must be avoided. If cytotoxic drugs are handled regularly, it is theoretically possible that repeated skin contact or inhalation may produce systemic toxic effects in nurses who have developed hypersensitivity to them. Most hospitals now operate a centralized (pharmacy-organized) additive service. While this reduces the risk of exposure to cytotoxic drugs, it is essential that nurses recognize and understand the local policy on their safe handling and disposal. The Health and Safety Executive has decreed that such a policy should be in place wherever cytotoxic drugs are administered. These should be adapted, wherever possible, to care of patients in the community.

Storage

Carboplatin injection is stored at room temperature. Infusions are prepared in glucose 5% or sodium chloride 0.9% injection diluted to concentrations as low as 0.5 mg in 1 ml.

CARBOPROST (Hemabate)

Presentation

Injection – 250 microgram in 1 ml

Actions and uses

Carboprost is a prostaglandin derivative used to treat postpartum haemorrhage which is unresponsive to first line treatment with ergotamine and oxytocin.

Dosage

250 microgram by deep intramuscular injection repeated as required at intervals as short as 15 minutes and up to 90 minutes. A maximum of 12 mg (48 doses) may be given.

Nursing implications

- Carboprost injection may produce nausea, vomiting, diarrhoea, flushing and bronchospasm. Other adverse effects include a raised blood pressure, pulmonary oedema, chills and sweating, dizziness and erythema. There may also be a local reaction at the injection site.
- It must be avoided in acute pelvic inflammatory disease and cardiac, pulmonary and hepatic disease. Caution is necessary in patients with a history of glaucoma, asthma, hypertension, anaemia, jaundice, diabetes, epilepsy and uterine scars since excessive dosage may cause uterine rupture.

Storage

This drug has a 3-year shelf life when stored in a refrigerator.

CARMUSTINE (BiCNU)

Presentation

Injection – 100 mg (plus ethanol diluent 3 ml)

Actions and uses

Carmustine is a cytotoxic drug of the nitrogen mustard group which arrests cell proliferation and growth by a chemical binding (alkylation) action on DNA and other cellular substances which are essential for cell division to proceed. Its main use is in the treatment of myeloma, lymphoma and brain tumours.

Dosage

This is largely determined by specific indication and current schedules which are subject to change in line with existing knowledge. Current schedules should be consulted for up-to-date details of dosage and route of administration. Courses of 200 mg/m^2, either as a single dose or a series of daily doses, have been used and repeated several weeks later.

C

Nursing implications
- Delayed myelotoxicity is the most common, and serious, adverse effect of this drug. Anaemia, leucopenia and, in particular, thrombocytopenia may develop up to 6 weeks after the drug has been administered and is dose related. This makes patient education regarding control of infection and enhanced bleeding tendency an important aspect of the nurse's role.
- Carmustine causes frequent nausea and vomiting within 2 hours of dosing and lasting for about 4–6 hours.
- Adverse effects are also reported on the liver (raised liver enzymes), lung (pulmonary infiltration/fibrosis) and kidney (renal failure).
- Carmustine causes a burning irritation at the injection site and extravasation must be avoided. If administered too rapidly, there may be intense flushing lasting for several hours.
- Nurses should be aware of the risks posed by cytotoxic drugs. Some are irritant to the skin and mucous surfaces and care must be exercised when handling them. In particular, spillage or contamination of personnel or the environment must be avoided. If cytotoxic drugs are handled regularly, it is theoretically possible that repeated skin contact or inhalation may produce systemic toxic effects in nurses who have developed hypersensitivity to them. Most hospitals now operate a centralized (pharmacy-organized) additive service. While this reduces the risk of exposure to cytotoxic drugs, it is essential that nurses recognize and understand the local policy on their safe handling and disposal. The Health and Safety Executive has decreed that such a policy should be in place wherever cytotoxic drugs are administered. These should be adapted, wherever possible, to the care of patients in the community.
- The infusion, once prepared, may be stored under refrigeration for 48 hours before use. It must be protected from light and rapidly degrades at room temperature.

Storage
- Carmustine injection must be stored in a refrigerator. It is reconstituted using the ethanol diluent supplied and further diluted in 500 ml glucose 5% or sodium chloride 0.9% injection.

CARTEOLOL (Teoptic)

Presentation
Eye drops – 1% and 2%

Actions and uses
Carteolol is a beta-adrenoceptor antagonist with the actions of other drugs described in the section on Beta-blockers (p. 51). In practice, however, carteolol is only used in the form of eye drops for the treatment of ocular hypertension and chronic open angle glaucoma. Topical beta-blockers lower raised intraocular pressure by an unknown mechanism associated with a reduction in aqueous humour production.

Dosage
Glaucoma: one drop is instilled in the affected eye twice daily, therapy being initiated with 1% strength drops and increased in time as necessary.

Nursing implications
- Despite the fact that this drug is administered externally, sufficient may be absorbed from the cornea to produce systemic side effects in susceptible patients (see Beta-blockers, p. 51).
- Thus patients with obstructive airways disease (particularly asthmatics) and those with

uncontrolled heart failure should not be treated with beta-blocker eye drops.

- Other patients in whom carteolol must be used with caution include those with sinus bradycardia and second- or third-degree heart block.
- Carteolol eye drops may cause stinging of the eye on application and should be avoided if the patient uses soft contact lenses.

Storage

- Carteolol eye drops are stored at room temperature.
- They have a relatively short life during use when a risk of bacterial contamination after opening exists and normally eye drops of any kind should not be used after 1 week for a hospitalized patient or after 4 weeks for others.

CARVEDILOL (Eucardic)

Presentation

Tablets – 12.5 mg, 25 mg

Actions and uses

Carvedilol is a beta-adrenoceptor antagonist with the actions of other drugs described in the section on Beta-blockers (p. 51). This drug, however, has a dual action in the sympathetic nervous system in that it also blocks noradrenaline and adrenaline at alpha sites, notably in the peripheral vasculature. Thus it produces arteriolar vasodilatation which may contribute to the blood pressure lowering effect and reduce the degree of vasoconstriction which is a problem for patients with peripheral vascular disease treated with beta-blockers.

Carvedilol is used mainly in the treatment of heart failure.

Dosage

Adults: initially 12.5 mg once daily, increased as necessary to 25 mg once daily, then to a maximum of 50 mg daily given in 1–2 doses.

Nursing implications

- The nursing implications described for the Beta-blockers (p. 51) also apply to this drug.
- Although less likely than other beta-blockers to compromise blood flow in patients with peripheral vascular disease, carvedilol does not eliminate the problems associated with vascular insufficiency.

Storage

Carvedilol tablets are stored at room temperature.

CEFACLOR (Distaclor)

Presentation

Capsules – 500 mg
Tablets – 375 mg (sustained release)
Syrup – 125 mg in 5 ml, 250 mg in 5 ml

Actions and uses

This drug is a member of the cephalosporin group of antibiotics which, like penicillins, kill dividing bacteria by preventing formation of an intact cell wall, leading to bacterial lysis. In practice, cefaclor is used in the treatment of infections of the respiratory tract (including otitis media), urinary tract, skin and soft tissue. Its spectrum includes most common Gram-positive and Gram-negative pathogens and, in particular, it is uniformly active against *Haemophilus influenzae*.

Dosage

Adults: usually 250–500 mg 8-hourly but up to 1 g 6-hourly may be given in severe infection. Alternatively, 375–750 mg twice daily using sustained-release tablets.
Children <1 year, 62.5 mg 8-hourly: 1–5 years, 125 mg 8-hourly: >5 years, 250 mg 8-hourly.

Nursing implications

- As with the penicillins, the only side effects of note arise in patients who prove to be allergic to drugs of the cephalosporin group.

- A careful history to exclude previous hypersensitivity reactions to drugs of this type (usually manifesting as generalized skin rashes, angiooedema and anaphylaxis) is therefore necessary.
- Note that a proportion of patients with established penicillin allergy (around 10%) will develop cross-hypersensitivity to drugs of the cephalosporin group. Careful monitoring of such patients is therefore recommended.
- In common with other broad-spectrum antibiotics, gastrointestinal upset, including diarrhoea, may arise as a consequence of altered bowel flora.

Storage

- Cefaclor preparations are stored at room temperature.
- Once prepared, the syrup should be stored in a refrigerator and used within 14 days.

CEFADROXIL (Baxan)

Presentation

Capsules – 500 mg
Suspension – 125 mg in 5 ml, 250 mg in 5 ml, 500 mg in 5 ml

Actions and uses

This drug is a member of the cephalosporin group of antibiotics which, like penicillins, kill dividing bacteria by preventing formation of an intact cell wall, leading to bacterial lysis. In practice, cefadroxil is used in the treatment of infections of the respiratory tract (including otitis media), urinary tract, skin and soft tissue. Its spectrum includes most common Gram-positive and Gram-negative pathogens. The relatively long half-life of cefadroxil permits twice daily, instead of three or four times daily, dosage.

Dosage

Adults: 1 g twice daily (or once daily for urinary tract infection).
Children <1 year, 25 mg/kg body weight in total daily in two divided doses; 1–6 years, 125–250 mg twice daily; over 6 years, 250–500 mg twice daily.

Nursing implications

- As with the penicillins, the only side effects of note arise in patients who prove to be allergic to drugs of the cephalosporin group.
- A careful history to exclude previous hypersensitivity reactions to drugs of this type (usually manifesting as generalized skin rashes, angiooedema and anaphylaxis) is therefore necessary.
- Note that a proportion of patients with established penicillin allergy (around 10%) will develop cross-hypersensitivity to drugs of the cephalosporin group. Careful monitoring of such patients is therefore recommended.
- In common with other broad-spectrum antibiotics, gastrointestinal upset, including diarrhoea, may arise as a consequence of altered bowel flora.

Storage

- Cefadroxil preparations are stored at room temperature.
- Once prepared, the suspension is stable if stored at room temperature for 7 days (or 14 days if refrigerated).

CEFAMANDOLE (Kefadol)

Presentation

Injection – 1 g dry powder vial

Actions and uses

This drug is a member of the cephalosporin group of antibiotics which, like penicillins, kill dividing bacteria by preventing formation of an intact cell wall, leading to bacterial lysis. In practice, cefamadole is effective against most common Gram-positive and Gram-negative pathogens including several which have acquired resistance to drugs of the penicillin/cephalosporin group through production of a beta-lactamase enzyme which destroys such antibiotics. It is used in the treatment of infections of the respiratory tract, skin and soft tissue when it has notable activity against beta-lactamase producing strains of *Staphylococcus aureus* and *Haemophilus influenzae*.

Dosage

Adults: range 500 mg–2 g, 4–8 hourly by the IV or deep IM route. Low doses (e.g. 500 mg) only should be given by IM or slow bolus IV injection (over 3–5 minutes). Higher doses preferably by IV infusion over 30 minutes to 1 hour in 100 ml sodium chloride 0.9% or glucose 5% injection or glucose/saline mixtures.

Children: range is 50–100 mg/kg body weight (up to 150 mg/kg in life-threatening infection) daily in 4–8 hourly dosage, as above.

Nursing implications

- As with the penicillins, allergy to drugs of the cephalosporin group is a particular problem.
- A careful history to exclude previous hypersensitivity reactions to drugs of this type (usually manifesting as generalized skin rashes, angiooedema and anaphylaxis) is therefore necessary.
- Note that a proportion of patients with established penicillin allergy (around 10%) will develop cross-hypersensitivity to drugs of the cephalosporin group. Careful monitoring of such patients is therefore recommended.
- In common with other broad-spectrum antibiotics, gastro-intestinal upset, including diarrhoea, may arise as a consequence of altered bowel flora. Sustained and bloody diarrhoea may be indicative of colitis and should be immediately brought to the attention of medical staff.

- Pain and discomfort at the injection site is relatively common; hence the need for slow administration. Also, care must be taken to avoid extravasation.
- During prolonged therapy it is advisable to monitor liver function and carry out full blood counts.
- The effects of injectable cephalosporins are synergistic with those of the aminoglycoside group (e.g. gentamicin) and combination therapy is often used to extend the spectrum of activity of both drugs. **However, drugs of this type should never be mixed together during administration since they are chemically incompatible.**

Storage

- Cefamandole injection vials are stored at room temperature.
- After reconstitution, vials should be stored in a refrigerator and must be discarded if unused within 96 hours.
- Prolonged storage at room temperature will generate carbon dioxide gas and create increased pressure within the vial.

CEFIXIME (Suprax)

Presentation

Tablets – 200 mg
Suspension – 100 mg in 5 ml

Actions and uses

This drug is a member of the cephalosporin group of antibiotics which, like penicillins, kill dividing bacteria by preventing formation of an intact cell wall, leading to bacterial lysis. In practice, cefixime's use is restricted to the treatment of infections of the respiratory tract (including otitis media) and urinary tract. Its spectrum includes most common Gram-positive and Gram-negative pathogens. The relatively long half-life of cefixime allows for simple once-daily dosage.

C

Dosage
Adults: 200–400 mg once daily.
Children <1 year, 75 mg/kg body
weight once daily; 1–5 years, 100 mg
once daily; over 5 years, 200 mg once
daily.

Nursing implications
- As with the penicillins, the only
  side effects of note arise in
  patients who prove to be
  allergic to drugs of the
  cephalosporin group.
- A careful history to exclude
  previous hypersensitivity
  reactions to drugs of this type
  (usually manifesting as generalized skin rashes, angiooedema
  and anaphylaxis) is therefore
  necessary.
- Note that a proportion of
  patients with established
  penicillin allergy (around 10%)
  will develop cross-hypersensitivity
  to drugs of the cephalosporin
  group. Careful monitoring of
  such patients is therefore
  recommended.
- In common with other
  broad-spectrum antibiotics,
  gastrointestinal upset, including
  diarrhoea, may arise as a consequence of altered bowel flora.

Storage
- Cefixime preparations are stored at
  room temperature.
- Once prepared, the suspension is
  stable if stored at room temperature for 7 days (or 14 days if
  refrigerated).

CEFODIZIME (Timecef)

Presentation
Injection – 1 g dry powder vial

Actions and uses
This drug is a member of the
cephalosporin group of antibiotics
which, like penicillins, kill dividing
bacteria by preventing formation of
an intact cell wall, leading to bacterial
lysis. In practice, cefodizime has a
broad antibacterial spectrum but is less
active than other injectable
cephalosporins against certain Gram-
positive organisms, most notably
Staphylococcus aureus. On the other
hand it has excellent activity against
common Gram-negative pathogens.
   It is used in the treatment of infections of the lower respiratory tract and
occasionally of the urinary tract.

Dosage
Adults only: usually 2 g daily in two
divided doses or single dose in the
treatment of urinary tract infections.
It may be given by the deep IM
route but doses >1 g should be
administered by slow bolus IV injection
(over 3–5 minutes) or preferably by IV
infusion over 30 minutes to 1 hour in
100 ml sodium chloride 0.9% or
glucose 5% injection or glucose/saline
mixtures.

Nursing implications
- As with the penicillins, allergy to
  drugs of the cephalosporin
  group is a particular problem.
- A careful history to exclude
  previous hypersensitivity
  reactions to drugs of this type
  (usually manifesting as
  generalized skin rashes,
  angiooedema and anaphylaxis)
  is therefore necessary.
- Note that a proportion of
  patients with established penicillin allergy (around 10%) will
  develop cross-hypersensitivity to
  drugs of the cephalosporin
  group. Careful monitoring of
  such patients is therefore
  recommended.
- In common with other
  broad-spectrum antibiotics,
  gastrointestinal upset, including
  diarrhoea, may arise as a consequence of altered bowel flora.
  Sustained and bloody diarrhoea
  may be indicative of colitis and
  should be immediately brought
  to the attention of medical staff.
- Pain and discomfort at the injection site are relatively common,
  hence the need for slow administration. Also, care must be
  taken to avoid extravasation.
- During prolonged therapy it
  is advisable to monitor liver

C

function and carry out full blood counts.

- The effects of injectable cephalosporins are synergistic with those of the aminoglycoside group (e.g. gentamicin) and combination therapy is often used to extend the spectrum of activity of both drugs. **However, drugs of this type should never be mixed together during administration since they are chemically incompatible.**

Storage

- Cefodizime injection vials are stored at room temperature.
- After reconstitution, vials should be stored in a refrigerator and must be discarded if unused within 96 hours.
- Prolonged storage at room temperature will generate carbon dioxide gas and create increased pressure within the vial.

CEFOTAXIME (Claforan)

Presentation

Injection – 500 mg, 1 g and 2 g dry powder vials

Actions and uses

This drug is a member of the cephalosporin group of antibiotics which, like penicillins, kill dividing bacteria by preventing formation of an intact cell wall, leading to bacterial lysis. In practice, cefotaxime has a broad antibacterial spectrum which includes many common Gram-positive and Gram-negative pathogens.

It is used in the treatment of septicaemia and infections of the respiratory tract, skin and soft tissue and notably in meningitis (especially in neonates for whom various other modern antibiotics are contraindicated). It is occasionally of use in treating infections of the urinary tract.

Dosage

Adults: usually 1–2 g 8-hourly but up to 12 g per day may be required in life-threatening infections. Twice-daily dosage of 1 g IM is sufficient in urinary tract infection and a single IM dose is used in the treatment of gonorrhoea. Higher doses are given preferably by IV infusion over 30 minutes to 1 hour in 100 ml sodium chloride 0.9% or glucose 5% injection or glucose/saline mixtures.

Children: 100–150 mg/kg body weight (up to 200 mg/kg in life-threatening infection) daily in 2–4 divided doses, as above.

Neonates: in severe infections 150 mg/kg daily (but up to 200 mg/kg in meningitis) administered in 2–4 divided doses.

Nursing implications

- As with the penicillins, allergy to drugs of the cephalosporin group is a particular problem.
- A careful history to exclude previous hypersensitivity reactions to drugs of this type (usually manifesting as generalized skin rashes, angiooedema and anaphylaxis) is therefore necessary.
- Note that a proportion of patients with established penicillin allergy (around 10%) will develop cross-hypersensitivity to drugs of the cephalosporin group. Careful monitoring of such patients is therefore recommended.
- In common with other broad-spectrum antibiotics, gastro-intestinal upset, including diarrhoea, may arise as a consequence of altered bowel flora. Sustained and bloody diarrhoea may be indicative of colitis and should be immediately brought to the attention of medical staff.
- Pain and discomfort at the injection site are relatively common, hence the need for slow administration. Also, care must be taken to avoid extravasation.
- During prolonged therapy it is advisable to monitor liver function and carry out full blood counts.
- The effects of injectable cephalosporins are synergistic with those of the aminoglycoside group (e.g. gentamicin) and

C

combination therapy is often used to extend the spectrum of activity of both drugs. **However, drugs of this type should never be mixed together during administration since they are chemically incompatible.**

Storage

- Cefotaxime injection vials are stored at room temperature.
- After reconstitution, intramuscular and intravenous injections should be administered immediately and any drug remaining should be discarded. Solutions for infusion should be discarded after 24 hours.

CEFOXITIN (Mefoxin)

Presentation

Injection – 1 g and 2 g vials

Actions and uses

Although more correctly described as a 'cephamycin', this drug is effectively a member of the cephalosporin group of antibiotics. Cephalosporins, like penicillins, kill dividing bacteria by preventing formation of an intact cell wall, leading to bacterial lysis. Cefoxitin has a broad antibacterial spectrum which includes many common Gram-positive and Gram-negative pathogens and it may be used in the treatment of septicaemia and infections of the respiratory tract, skin and soft tissue infection. In practice, however, it has a special role in prevention and treatment of peritonitis because of its excellent activity against organisms of the bowel flora, notably the anaerobe *Bacteroides fragilis*. It is therefore also indicated for infections in gynaecological surgery in which bowel organisms may be implicated.

Dosage

Adults: usually 1–2 g every 6–8 hours but up to 12 g per day may be required in life-threatening infections. Doses of 1 g may be given by the IM route but more often it is administered by slow IV bolus injection or preferably by IV infusion over 30 minutes to 1 hour in 100 ml sodium chloride 0.9% or glucose 5% injection or glucose/saline mixtures.
Children: age <1 week, 40 mg/kg 12-hourly: 1 week to 1 month, 40 mg/kg 8-hourly: >1 month, 40 mg/kg 6–8 hourly.
Prophylaxis in gastrointestinal and gynaecological surgery: single 2 g dose 1–2 hours before surgery or on clamping (in gynaecological procedures).

Nursing implications

- As with the penicillins, allergy to drugs of the cephalosporin group is a particular problem.
- A careful history to exclude previous hypersensitivity reactions to drugs of this type (usually manifesting as generalized skin rashes, angiooedema and anaphylaxis) is therefore necessary.
- Note that a proportion of patients with established penicillin allergy (around 10%) will develop cross-hypersensitivity to drugs of the cephalosporin group. Careful monitoring of such patients is therefore recommended.
- In common with other broad-spectrum antibiotics, gastrointestinal upset, including diarrhoea, may arise as a consequence of altered bowel flora. Sustained and bloody diarrhoea may be indicative of colitis and should be immediately brought to the attention of medical staff.
- Pain and discomfort at the injection site are relatively common, hence the need for slow administration. Also, care must be taken to avoid extravasation.
- During prolonged therapy it is advisable to monitor liver function and carry out full blood counts.
- The effects of injectable cephalosporins are synergistic with those of the aminoglycoside group (e.g. gentamicin) and combination therapy is often used to extend the spectrum of activity of both drugs.

> However, drugs of this type should never be mixed together during administration since they are chemically incompatible.

Children (IV route only): age <2 months, 30 mg/kg 12-hourly: >2 months, 30 mg/kg 8-hourly or 50 mg/kg 12-hourly or 8-hourly in life-threatening infections.
Cystic fibrosis (adults and children): 50 mg/kg 8-hourly by IV injection.

C

Storage
- Cefoxitin injection vials are stored in a refrigerator.
- Reconstituted solutions for injection (prepared aseptically) must be used within 24 hours if kept at room temperature or 1 week if refrigerated.

CEFTAZIDIME (Fortum)

Presentation
Injection – 250 mg, 500 mg, 1 g, 2 g and 3 g dry powder vials

Actions and uses
This drug is a member of the cephalosporin group of antibiotics which, like penicillins, kill dividing bacteria by preventing formation of an intact cell wall, leading to bacterial lysis. In practice, ceftazidime has a broad antibacterial spectrum which includes many common Gram-positive and Gram-negative pathogens.

It is used in the treatment of septicaemia (especially in neutropenic/immunocompromised patients) and infections of the respiratory tract, skin and soft tissue, bone and joint and the gastrointestinal tract. It has notable activity against *Pseudomonas aeruginosa* and it may be reserved as second-line back-up for infections associated with this important pathogen. In this respect, ceftazidime has a particular role in the treatment of recurrent chest infections in cystic fibrosis.

Dosage
Adults: usually 1 g every 8 hours or 2 g every 8–12 hours depending upon severity of infection. Doses of 1 g may be given by the IM route but more often it is administered by slow IV bolus injection or preferably by IV infusion over 30 minutes to 1 hour in 100 ml sodium chloride 0.9% or glucose 5% injection or glucose/saline mixtures.

Nursing implications
- As with the penicillins, allergy to drugs of the cephalosporin group is a particular problem.
- A careful history to exclude previous hypersensitivity reactions to drugs of this type (usually manifesting as generalized skin rashes, angiooedema and anaphylaxis) is therefore necessary.
- Note that a proportion of patients with established penicillin allergy (around 10%) will develop cross-hypersensitivity to drugs of the cephalosporin group. Careful monitoring of such patients is therefore recommended.
- In common with other broad-spectrum antibiotics, gastrointestinal upset, including diarrhoea, may arise as a consequence of altered bowel flora. Sustained and bloody diarrhoea may be indicative of colitis and should be immediately brought to the attention of medical staff.
- Pain and discomfort at the injection site are relatively common, hence the need for slow administration. Also, care must be taken to avoid extravasation.
- During prolonged therapy it is advisable to monitor liver function and carry out full blood counts.
- The effects of injectable cephalosporins are synergistic with those of the aminoglycoside group (e.g. gentamicin) and combination therapy is often used to extend the spectrum of activity of both drugs. **However, drugs of this type should never be mixed together during administration since they are chemically incompatible.**

C

Storage

- Ceftazidime injection vials are stored at room temperature.
- Carbon dioxide gas is formed during the mixing of ceftazidime injection, creating an increase in the internal pressure of the vial.
- Prepared solutions for injection may be stored for up to 18 hours at room temperature if not immediately used but are preferably administered within 6 hours of preparation.

CEFTRIAXONE (Rocephin)

Presentation

Injection – 250 mg, 1 g, 2 g vials

Actions and uses

This drug is a member of the cephalosporin group of antibiotics which, like penicillins, kill dividing bacteria by preventing formation of an intact cell wall, leading to bacterial lysis. Of particular interest is its very long half-life compared to other cephalosporins which enables it to be used in a single daily dosage regimen. Although it has a broad spectrum, ceftriaxone has notable anti-staphylococcal activity which reflects its use in the treatment of infections of skin and soft tissue, bone, lower respiratory tract and septicaemia, and for surgical prophylaxis to prevent postoperative wound infections. It is also of particular value in treating meningitis in adults and children (but not neonates) and in gonorrhoea but it has little useful activity in pseudomonal infections.

Finally, ceftriaxone has a special use in the treatment of close ('kissing') contacts of patients with meningitis infection.

Dosage

Adults: by intravenous infusion in 50–100 ml sodium chloride 0.9% or glucose 5% over 30 minutes, usually 2 g administered once daily but this is doubled in severe or life-threatening infections such as meningitis. Very high doses may be split and administered 12-hourly to reduce the occurrence of high peak concentrations.

Single doses of 250 mg IM are effective in uncomplicated gonorrhoea.

For surgical prophylaxis a single dose of 1 g is administered by the intravenous route at induction of anaesthesia.

Children (>6 weeks only): 20–50 mg/kg body weight daily as above up to 80 mg/kg in severe infections, e.g. meningitis.

Nursing implications

- As with the penicillins, allergy to drugs of the cephalosporin group is a particular problem.
- A careful history to exclude previous hypersensitivity reactions to drugs of this type (usually manifesting as generalized skin rashes, angiooedema and anaphylaxis) is therefore necessary.
- Note that a proportion of patients with established penicillin allergy (around 10%) will develop cross-hypersensitivity to drugs of the cephalosporin group. Careful monitoring of such patients is therefore recommended.
- In common with other broad-spectrum antibiotics, gastrointestinal upset, including diarrhoea, may arise as a consequence of altered bowel flora. Sustained and bloody diarrhoea may be indicative of colitis and should be immediately brought to the attention of medical staff.
- Pain and discomfort at the injection site are relatively common, hence the need for slow administration. Also, care must be taken to avoid extravasation.
- During prolonged therapy it is advisable to monitor liver function and carry out full blood counts.
- The effects of injectable cephalosporins are synergistic with those of the aminoglycoside group (e.g. gentamicin) and combination therapy is often used to extend the spectrum of activity of both drugs.

> However, drugs of this type should never be mixed together during administration since they are chemically incompatible.

Storage
- Ceftriaxone injection vials are stored at room temperature.
- Do not mix with calcium-containing salts.

CEFUROXIME (Zinacef, Zinnat)

Presentation
Tablets – 125 mg and 250 mg
Oral suspension – 125 mg in 5 ml
Oral granules – 125 mg per sachet
Injection – 250 mg, 750 mg, 1.5 g

Actions and uses
This drug is a member of the cephalosporin group of antibiotics which, like penicillins, kill dividing bacteria by preventing formation of an intact cell wall, leading to bacterial lysis. Although it has a broad spectrum of activity, cefuroxime is particularly useful for the treatment of infections due to *Haemophilus influenzae* and *Neisseria gonorrhoeae* which effectively means that it is useful in the treatment of respiratory tract infections, gonorrhoea, skin and soft tissue infection. In addition, cefuroxime by the IV route is a drug of choice for prophylaxis of abdominal surgery.

Dosage
Adults: range is 750 mg to 1.5 g three times daily by intramuscular or intravenous bolus injection or rapid intravenous infusion over 30 minutes. The intravenous infusion may be given in most common infusion fluids.
An oral dose of 250 mg (as axetil) two, three or four times daily may be used in the treatment of infections due to sensitive organisms.
Children: intravenous dose varies from 30 to 60 mg/kg body weight in 3–4 divided doses depending upon specific indication.
Neonates: dose is 25–50 mg/kg body weight 8- or 12-hourly.

Nursing implications
- As with the penicillins, allergy to drugs of the cephalosporin group is a particular problem.
- A careful history to exclude previous hypersensitivity reactions to drugs of this type (usually manifesting as generalized skin rashes, angiooedema and anaphylaxis) is therefore necessary.
- Note that a proportion of patients with established penicillin allergy (around 10%) will develop cross-hypersensitivity to drugs of the cephalosporin group. Careful monitoring of such patients is therefore recommended.
- In common with other broad-spectrum antibiotics, gastrointestinal upset, including diarrhoea, may arise as a consequence of altered bowel flora. Sustained and bloody diarrhoea may be indicative of colitis and should be immediately brought to the attention of medical staff.
- Pain and discomfort at the injection site are relatively common, hence the need for slow administration. Also, care must be taken to avoid extravasation.
- The effects of injectable cephalosporins are synergistic with those of the aminoglycoside group (e.g. gentamicin) and combination therapy is often used to extend the spectrum of activity of both drugs. However, drugs of this type should never be mixed together during administration since they are chemically incompatible.

Storage
- Cefuroxime in injectable form should be stored at room temperature and protected from light.
- After reconstitution solutions may be kept for 4 hours at room temperature or 24 hours if refrigerated.

C

CELIPROLOL (Celectol)

Presentation
Tablets – 200 mg, 400 mg

Actions and uses
Celiprolol is a beta-adrenoceptor blocking drug and the section under Beta-blockers (p. 51) should be consulted for a general account of these compounds. However, celiprolol is notably different from other beta-blockers in that it is a potent beta-2 partial antagonist (i.e. it stimulates rather than blocks the effects of sympathetic stimulation at this site) and it possesses additional vasodilator activity. Thus celiprolol is particularly useful in the treatment of hypertension and for patients with peripheral vascular insufficiency which is aggravated by therapy with other beta-blockers. Celiprolol is also less likely to interfere with lipid profile and, indeed, it may have a beneficial effect on the blood lipid pattern, so improving this recognized risk factor for coronary heart disease.

Dosage
Adults: 200–400 mg once daily in the morning.

Nursing implications
- As for Beta-blockers (p. 51).
- Although celiprolol has pronounced beta-2 stimulant properties its use is contraindicated in asthma, despite an early report that it improved airways performance in a small group of asthmatics.

Storage
Celiprolol tablets are stored at room temperature.

CEPHALEXIN (Ceporex, Keflex)

Presentation
Tablets – 250 mg, 500 mg and 1 g
Capsules – 250 mg, 500 mg
Syrup – 125 mg in 5 ml, 250 mg in 5 ml, 500 mg in 5 ml

Actions and uses
This drug is a member of the cephalosporin group of antibiotics which, like penicillins, kill dividing bacteria by preventing formation of an intact cell wall, leading to bacterial lysis. In practice, cephalexin is used in the treatment of infections of the respiratory tract (including otitis media), the urinary tract, skin and soft tissue. Its spectrum includes most common Gram-positive and Gram-negative pathogens.

Dosage
Adults: 1–2 g daily in 2–4 divided doses.
Children: <3 months, 62.5–125 mg twice daily: 3 months to 2 years, 125–250 mg twice daily: 2–7 years, 250–500 mg twice daily: 7–12 years, 500 mg to 1 g twice daily.

Nursing implications
- As with the penicillins, the only side effects of note arise in patients who prove to be allergic to drugs of the cephalosporin group.
- A careful history to exclude previous hypersensitivity reactions to drugs of this type (usually manifesting as generalized skin rashes, angiooedema and anaphylaxis) is therefore necessary.
- Note that a proportion of patients with established penicillin allergy (around 10%) will develop cross-hypersensitivity to drugs of the cephalosporin group. Careful monitoring of such patients is therefore recommended.
- In common with other broad-spectrum antibiotics, gastrointestinal upset, including diarrhoea, may arise as a consequence of altered bowel flora.

Storage
- Cephalexin preparations are stored at room temperature.
- The syrup should be used within 10 days of preparation.

CEPHAZOLIN (Kefzol)

Presentation
Injection – 500 mg and 1 g vials

Actions and uses
This drug is a member of the cephalosporin group of antibiotics which, like penicillins, kill dividing bacteria by preventing formation of an intact cell wall, leading to bacterial lysis. In practice, cephazolin is used in the treatment of infections of the respiratory tract, the urinary tract, skin and soft tissue. Its spectrum includes most common Gram-positive and Gram-negative pathogens.

Dosage
- Cephazolin is given by IM or IV bolus injections or IV infusions in 50–100 ml sodium chloride or glucose 5% over 30 minutes.
- Adult dosage ranges from 500 mg twice daily to 1 g 3–4 times daily depending upon the nature and severity of infection.
- Children's doses are in the range 25–50 mg/kg body weight daily in 3–4 divided doses.

Nursing implications
- As with the penicillins, the only side effects of note arise in patients who prove to be allergic to drugs of the cephalosporin group.
- A careful history to exclude previous hypersensitivity reactions to drugs of this type (usually manifesting as generalized skin rashes, angiooedema and anaphylaxis) is therefore necessary.
- Note that a proportion of patients with established penicillin allergy (around 10%) will develop cross-hypersensitivity to drugs of the cephalosporin group. Careful monitoring of such patients is therefore recommended.
- In common with other broad-spectrum antibiotics, gastrointestinal upset, including diarrhoea, may arise as a consequence of altered bowel flora.

Storage
- The drug may be stored at room temperature.
- This drug should not be mixed with other antibiotics in the same syringe or infusion fluid.

CEPHRADINE (Velosef)

Presentation
Capsules – 250 mg, 500 mg
Syrup – 250 mg in 5 ml
Injection – 500 mg and 1 g powder in vial

Actions and uses
This drug is a member of the cephalosporin group of antibiotics which, like penicillins, kill dividing bacteria by preventing formation of an intact cell wall, leading to bacterial lysis. In practice, cephradine is used in the treatment of infections of the respiratory tract, the urinary tract, skin, soft tissue and bone and joint. Its spectrum includes most common Gram-positive and Gram-negative pathogens.

Dosage
Adult dosage varies from 1–2 g twice daily to 500 mg to 1 g four times daily by any route. Injections are administered by the IM or IV (bolus or infusion) route.
Children's doses are based on 50–100 mg/kg body weight per day given in 2–4 divided doses orally or by the parenteral route.

Nursing implications
- As with the penicillins, the only side effects of note arise in patients who prove to be allergic to drugs of the cephalosporin group.
- A careful history to exclude previous hypersensitivity reactions to drugs of this type (usually manifesting as generalized skin rashes, angiooedema and anaphylaxis) is therefore necessary.
- Note that a proportion of patients with established penicillin allergy (around 10%)

will develop cross-hypersensitivity to drugs of the cephalosporin group. Careful monitoring of such patients is therefore recommended.
In common with other broad-spectrum antibiotics, gastrointestinal upset, including diarrhoea, may arise as a consequence of altered bowel flora.

Storage
- Cephradine preparations are stored at room temperature.
- Syrup should be used within 7 days if kept at room temperature or 14 days if refrigerated following reconstitution.

CETIRIZINE (Zirtek)

Presentation
Tablets – 10 mg
Oral solution – 5 mg in 5 ml

Actions and uses
Cetirizine is a non-sedative, long-acting antihistaminic used in the treatment of perennial and seasonal rhinitis and in urticaria. The section on Antihistamines (p. 33) should be consulted for a full account of the actions and uses of this group.

Dosage
Adults: standard dose is 10 mg once daily.
Children 2–6 years, 5 mg once daily; >6 years, use adult dose.

Nursing implications
- See the section on Antihistamines (p. 33).
- Note that cetirizine is a non-sedative drug.

Storage
- Cetirizine tablets and oral liquid are stored at room temperature.
- Protect liquid preparation from direct light.

CHENODEOXYCHOLIC ACID (Chendol, Chenofalk)

Presentation
Capsules – 125 mg, 250 mg

Actions and uses
This is a naturally occurring bile acid which, after oral administration, increases the bile acid pool and thus the amount of dissolved cholesterol and phospholipid. In addition, it is likely that the output of cholesterol secreted into the bile is reduced. The net result is to prevent the precipitation of cholesterol from solution and therefore the formation of cholesterol gallstones; existing cholesterol stones will gradually dissolve, possibly avoiding the need for surgical removal.

Dosage
Adults only: usually 10–15 mg/kg body weight daily in divided doses or as a single dose at bedtime. Treatment courses are determined by the size of stones, e.g. a few months for small gallstones with as long as 2 years for large stones.

Nursing implications
- It is important to note that chenodeoxycholic acid therapy is not a suitable treatment for all patients with gallstones and that the nature and size of the stones are important. Those for whom treatment is unsuitable are:
  - patients with radioopaque stones
  - those with non-functioning gallbladders
  - pregnant patients or female patients contemplating pregnancy
  - patients with chronic liver disease or inflammatory bowel disease.
- The only side effects of treatment are diarrhoea and pruritus, which commonly occur. The incidence of diarrhoea is reduced following a dosage reduction.

- Abnormal liver function tests and liver damage have occurred during administration of this drug.

Storage
Chenodeoxycholic acid capsules are stored at room temperature in well-sealed containers.

CHLORAL HYDRATE (Noctec)

Presentation
Capsules – 500 mg
Mixture – 500 mg in 5 ml
Paediatric elixir – 200 mg in 5 ml

Actions and uses
Chloral hydrate is a general central nervous system depressant. It has been in clinical use for many years and has maintained its popularity as a sleep-inducing agent despite the development of many newer hypnotic drugs during this period. In particular, the drug has found widespread popularity in young and elderly patients who generally tolerate it well. The sedative action of chloral hydrate is partly due to trichloroethanol, a metabolite to which it is converted in the body.

Dosage
Adults: 500 mg–2 g taken on retiring.
Children: 30–50 mg/kg body weight as a single dose up to a maximum of 1 g.

Nursing implications
- Chloral hydrate administration may be associated with a degree of nausea and gastrointestinal discomfort and patients should be advised to take their dosages well diluted with water, fruit juices or beverages to minimize the irritant effect on the gut mucosa.
- Skin rashes occasionally occur and contact of liquid chloral hydrate with skin can produce skin irritation; if this occurs the area of contact should be thoroughly washed.

- Chloral hydrate capsules must never be bitten since they contain concentrated liquid drug which can produce severe irritation if liberated in the mouth.
- Despite its irritant effect, chloral hydrate is generally well tolerated. In patients who suffer troublesome gastrointestinal upsets, a more palatable alternative is triclofos.

Storage
- Chloral hydrate capsules and mixtures are stored at room temperature.
- Once diluted, liquid doses must be taken immediately.
- Mixtures are relatively unstable and have to be freshly prepared for each prescription: these should not be kept by patients for longer than 2 weeks from time of issue.

CHLORAMBUCIL (Leukeran)

Presentation
Tablets – 2 mg, 5 mg

Actions and uses
Chlorambucil is a cytotoxic drug of the nitrogen mustard group which damages cells by irreversibly binding important constituents necessary for cellular growth and reproduction. The drug has been shown in practice to be particularly active against lymphoid tissues and appears to destroy not only proliferating cells but also mature circulating lymphocytes. This makes it particularly useful in the treatment of lymphoproliferative disorders. Its main uses are as follows.

- Lymphoproliferative disorders such as chronic lymphatic leukaemia and the lymphomas.
- It is the drug of choice for the rare condition of Waldenstrom's microglobulinaemia.
- It has been used in the treatment of carcinoma of the breast, lung and ovary.
- It has an immunosuppressant action and may be used in the

management of some autoimmune diseases such as rheumatoid arthritis and systemic lupus erythematosus. It is worth noting that it is used only in severe cases of rheumatoid arthritis which have proved rapidly progressive and resistant to treatment with alternative regimes.

Dosage

See current dosage schedules since these are subject to frequent revision in line with developments in the field of cancer chemotherapy. Immunosuppressive dosage is in the range 100–300 microgram/kg per day.

Nursing implications

- Chlorambucil exerts a depressant effect on the bone marrow and may cause leucopenia, thrombocytopenia and anaemia. Patients may therefore suffer from severe, occasionally life-threatening, infection or may develop serious haemorrhage. In addition, long-term treatment may lead to irreversible bone marrow damage, resulting in aplastic anaemia.
- Nausea and vomiting are common at higher dosages.
- Skin rash, alopecia and liver damage are occasional complications.
- As the drug affects dividing cells it reduces sperm formation and may affect the growing fetus. It is therefore essential that effective contraception is used to avoid pregnancy during treatment.
- Nurses should be aware of the risks posed by cytotoxic drugs. Some are irritant to the skin and mucous surfaces and care must be exercised when handling them. In particular, spillage or contamination of personnel or the environment must be avoided. If cytotoxic drugs are handled regularly, it is theoretically possible that repeated skin contact or inhalation may produce systemic toxic effects in nurses who have developed

hypersensitivity to them. Most hospitals now operate a centralized (pharmacy-organized) additive service. While this reduces the risk of exposure to cytotoxic drugs, it is essential that nurses recognize and understand the local policy on their safe handling and disposal. The Health and Safety Executive has decreed that such a policy should be in place wherever cytotoxic drugs are administered. These should be adapted, wherever possible, to care of patients in the community.

Storage

Chlorambucil tablets are stored in the refrigerator.

CHLORAMPHENICOL (Chloromycetin)

Presentation

Capsules – 250 mg
Injection – 1 g and 1.2 g vials
Eye ointment – 1%
Eye drops – 0.5%
Ear drops – 5%

Actions and uses

Chloramphenicol is an antibiotic which has a bacteriostatic action. It blocks protein synthesis, so inhibiting bacterial growth and replication but, although very effective, its use in practice is limited by potentially severe toxicity. Chloramphenicol is therefore reserved for the following infections.

- Treatment of typhoid fever.
- Treatment of septicaemia, epiglotitis and meningitis due to *Haemophilus influenzae* infection.
- Topical applications of the drug are not associated with its more serious side effects and are used widely for the treatment of infections of the eye and external ear.

Dosage

Oral/intravenous for adults and children: based on 12.5–25 mg four times a day with highest doses used short term in life-threatening infections.

Infants: 2 weeks–1 year, 12.5 mg/kg 6-hourly; <2 weeks, 6.25 mg/kg 6-hourly.
Eye drops 0.5% or eye ointment 1%: a small quantity of ointment or two drops in the affected eye every 1–3 hours until the eye has been free of visible signs of infection for 48 hours. Ear drops: 1–3 drops every 3–4 hours is recommended.

Nursing implications
- The reason that this highly effective antibiotic is now recommended for restricted use only is that it has a number of serious and potentially fatal side effects. It may depress bone marrow function and regular blood monitoring is essential since potentially serious abnormalities will reverse if treatment is stopped early. However, an irreversible aplastic anaemia with depression of formation of all types of blood cells may develop. This can occur suddenly and lead to anaemia and the risk of severe haemorrhage and infection. Although this effect is more common when the drug is used in high dosage and for prolonged periods, the fact that it is irreversible and commonly fatal makes it a strong contraindication to the general use of chloramphenicol in the treatment of mild infection.
- A specific toxic effect known as 'grey baby syndrome' may occur in the very young who cannot metabolize chloramphenicol in the same way that adults and older children can. Therefore high dosage (similar to that for adults and older children) can result in excessive concentrations of chloramphenicol in the blood. This leads to circulatory collapse with shock, respiratory difficulty, cyanosis, vomiting, refusal to suckle and passage of loose green stools. If this syndrome is not recognized early, it may be rapidly fatal.

- Other side effects include nausea, vomiting, an unpleasant taste in the mouth, abdominal pain, diarrhoea and, very rarely, optic neuritis.
- Injections are given by slow IV bolus via the tubing of a running IV infusion or over 30 minutes in 50 ml sodium chloride 0.9% or glucose 5% injection.

Storage
- Chloramphenicol capsules and injection are stored at room temperature.
- Eye and ear drops are preferably stored in a refrigerator when not in use.

CHLORDIAZEPOXIDE (Librium)

Presentation
Tablets – 5 mg, 10 mg, 25 mg
Capsules – 5 mg, 10 mg

Actions and uses
Chlordiazepoxide is a member of the Benzodiazepine group: see p. 47 for a full account of the actions of these drugs. Chlordiazepoxide is used mainly in the treatment of anxiety but it has also proved to be particularly useful in the control of symptoms associated with acute withdrawal of alcohol in chronic alcoholism (delirium tremens).

Dosage
Treatment of anxiety: adults receive a total of up to 30 mg daily in divided doses. Up to 100 mg may be required to control symptoms of acute alcohol withdrawal.

Nursing implications
See the section on Benzodiazepines (p. 47).

Storage
Chlordiazepoxide tablets and capsules are stored at room temperature.

CHLORMETHIAZOLE (Heminevrin)

Presentation
Capsules – 192 mg

C

Syrup – 250 mg in 5 ml (as edisylate)
Injection – 0.8% solution for
intravenous infusion

Actions and uses

Chlormethiazole is a central nervous
system depressant which has several
uses in clinical practice.

- It is a general sedative and hypnotic
  drug which alleviates acute restlessness and anxiety and induces sleep.
- It possesses anticonvulsant activity
  and is administered by intravenous
  infusion in acute convulsive states,
  e.g. status epilepticus, preeclampsia.

Dosage

Sedation: adult dose is 1 capsule
(or 5 ml syrup) taken three times daily.
Insomnia: adult dose is 2 capsules
(or 10 ml syrup) at bedtime.
By intravenous infusion (adults): dose
range is 40–120 mg (5–15 ml)/min of
0.8% chlormethiazole infusion up to a
maximum total dose of 800 mg
(500 ml). This may be continued at a
maintenance rate but the anaes-
thetist's supervision is recommended.

Nursing implications

- It is important that the apparent
  difference in the strengths of
  chlormethiazole capsules and
  syrup is understood since confusion when substituting one
  dosage form for another can
  lead to over- or underdosage.
  Capsules contain 192 mg
  chlormethiazole (base) while the
  syrup contains 250 mg chlormethiazole edisylate/5 ml. The
  difference in weight is due to
  the inactive edisylate group and
  is irrelevant to the clinical effect.
  Therefore when substituting
  capsules for syrup, or vice versa,
  one capsule is equivalent to 5 ml
  syrup.
- Chlormethiazole frequently
  causes nasal congestion and,
  occasionally, conjunctival irritation about 15–30 minutes after
  a dose is administered. If these
  effects are severe or prevent
  sleep, alternative treatment may
  be necessary.

- A less common, but equally
  important, side effect is
  headache which may prove
  severe.
- Chlormethiazole is often used
  as a hypnotic in elderly subjects
  because it is generally well tolerated and is short acting.
  However, it should be stressed
  that occasionally a prolonged
  'hangover' effect lasting into
  the following day is noted
  which can impair mobility and
  awareness in elderly patients.
- Intravenous administration may
  produce a fall in blood pressure
  and depression of respiration,
  particularly if given too quickly,
  and it may be necessary to
  monitor patients accordingly.
- Irritation at the intravenous site
  is associated with superficial
  thrombophlebitis.
- Since chlormethiazole is a
  depressant of the central
  nervous system, concurrent use
  of other CNS depressant drugs
  (including alcohol) will produce
  excessive sedation.

Storage

- Chlormethiazole capsules and
  syrup are stored at room
  temperature.
- Solution for intravenous infusion
  should, however, be stored in a
  refrigerator.

CHLOROQUINE
(Nivaquine, Avloclor)

Presentation

Tablets – 200 mg (as sulphate), 250 mg
(as phosphate)
Syrup – 50 mg in 5 ml

Actions and uses

Chloroquine was originally developed
for use in the treatment of malaria
(it is related to quinine) but has
also proved to be effective as a
'disease-modifying' drug in the
treatment of connective tissue
disease, including rheumatoid
arthritis.

Dosage

Prevention of malaria in travellers abroad: adults, 300–600 mg taken once weekly during exposure to risk and for 4–6 weeks thereafter. Children receive weekly doses based on 5 mg/kg body weight as above. Rheumatoid arthritis in adults: control of symptoms is achieved by treatment for 2–3 months with doses of between 75 and 300 mg of chloroquine base daily. Discoid lupus erythematosus: usually 150 mg of chloroquine base is taken two or three times daily, reducing to a maintenance dose of 150 mg or less per day.

Nursing implications

- Chloroquine is generally well tolerated when used in doses for suppression of malaria.
- Higher, prolonged doses given for the treatment of rheumatoid arthritis and lupus erythematosus are associated with side effects, the early detection of which is very important.
- Pruritus, gastrointestinal disturbances and headache are relatively common.
- Rarely the bone marrow may be suppressed, inducing blood dyscrasias such as agranulocytosis, thrombocytopenia and neutropenia. Other rare side effects include altered skin pigmentation and muscle weakness.
- The major problem with prolonged or high-dose treatment with chloroquine is damage to the retina which may result in permanent visual impairment. Patients should be regularly assessed by measurement of visual acuity and treatment stopped if visual impairment occurs.
- Chloroquine should be used with caution in patients with liver disease, psoriasis, gastrointestinal, neurological or blood disorders.

Storage

- Chloroquine tablets and oral liquid are stored at room temperature.

- The syrup must be protected from light.

CHLOROTHIAZIDE (Saluric)

Presentation

Tablets – 500 mg

Actions and uses

Chlorothiazide is one of the Thiazide and Related Diuretics, an account of which is given on p. 357.

Dosage

Adults: 125 mg to 1 g (1000 mg) daily. The duration of action is approximately 12 hours.
Children up to 1 year, 125 mg; 1–7 years, 250 mg; 7 years plus, 500 mg. The above doses are taken once daily.

Nursing implications

See the section on Thiazide and Related Diuretics.

Storage

Chlorothiazide tablets are stored at room temperature.

CHLORPHENIRAMINE (Piriton)

Presentation

Tablets – 4 mg
Syrup – 2 mg in 5 ml
Injection – 10 mg in 1 ml

Actions and uses

Chlorpheniramine is a traditional antihistamine still widely used despite the introduction of newer, longer-acting and less sedative drugs. The actions and uses of the Antihistamines are described on p. 33.

In practice, chlorpheniramine is used as follows.

- To suppress generalized minor allergic reactions to allergens such as foodstuffs and drugs.
- To suppress local allergic reactions, i.e. inflammatory skin responses to insect stings and bites, contact allergens and urticaria.
- In the control of symptoms associated with hay fever and allergic rhinitis.

Dosage

Adults orally: 4 mg three to four times daily.

Adults, in acute control of allergy by intravenous, intramuscular or subcutaneous injection: 10–20 mg repeated as required up to 40 mg/day. Children: <1 year, 1 mg (2.5 ml syrup) twice daily; 1–5 years, 1–2 mg (2.5–5 ml syrup) three times daily; 6–12 years, 2–4 mg three times daily.

Nursing implications
See the section on Antihistamines (p. 33).

Storage

Chlorpheniramine preparations are stored at room temperature but protected from light.

CHLORPROMAZINE (Largactil)

Presentation

Tablets – 10 mg, 25 mg, 50 mg, 100 mg
Syrup – 25 mg in 5 ml
Suspension – 100 mg in 5 ml
Injection – 50 mg in 2 ml

Actions and uses

Chlorpromazine is an original member of the Phenothiazine class with the actions and uses associated with this extensive range of drugs (see p. 281). In addition to its role as a major tranquillizer, used in the control of psychoses and severe anxiety/agitation, its less common uses include the following.

- Control of intractable hiccoughs.
- To induce hypothermia.
- In obstetric practice for the treatment of preeclampsia and eclampsia.

Dosage

Adult dosage varies widely. The following regimes are suggested.

- Oral: 25 mg three times is an average dose, although in some cases total dosage may be increased up to 1 g per day, if necessary.
- Intramuscularly: 25–50 mg is administered and repeated at 6–8 hourly intervals as required.

- Intravenously: the drug should be diluted with at least 10 times its own volume of sodium chloride 0.9% and given extremely slowly (over at least 30 minutes). Administration by this route is rarely necessary and should only be carried out under the supervision of senior medical staff.
- Children <5 years, 5–10 mg three times daily; >5 years one-third to one-half of the adult dosage is suggested.

Nursing implications
See the section on the Phenothiazines (p. 281).

Storage

- Preparations containing chlorpromazine are stored at room temperature.
- It is important that syrup, suspension and injection ampoules are protected from light.
- The injection may develop a pink or yellow discolouration, in which case it should be discarded.

CHLORPROPAMIDE (Diabinese)

Presentation

Tablets – 100 mg, 250 mg

Actions and uses

Chlorpropamide is a member of the Sulphonylurea group of oral hypoglycaemic drugs. It is used in the treatment of non-insulin dependent diabetes mellitus but due to problems related to its very long action (i.e. prolonged periods of hypoglycaemia) it is now rarely commenced in newly diagnosed diabetic patients.

Dosage

Adults: usually late-onset diabetes, range 50–500 mg as a single morning dose as required to control blood glucose or, more often, to prevent ketonuria.

Nursing implications
- See the section on glibenclamide (p. 160).

- Note the very long action of chlorpropamide, the relatively frequent occurrence of hypoglycaemia and its waning popularity as a result.

Storage
Chlorpropamide tablets are stored at room temperature and protected from light.

CHLORTHALIDONE (Hygroton)

Presentation
Tablets – 50 mg

Actions and uses
This drug is one of the Thiazide and Related Diuretics, the actions and uses of which are described on p. 357. Chlorthalidone is notable for its prolonged diuretic action of up to 48 hours in duration.

Dosage
The usual adult dose range is 50–100 mg daily or on alternate days.

Nursing implications
The nursing implications for the Thiazide and Related Diuretics (p. 357) apply to this drug.

Storage
Chlorthalidone tablets are stored at room temperature.

CHOLESTYRAMINE (Questran)

Presentation
Sachets – 4 g (orange flavoured including sugar-free)

Actions and uses
Cholestyramine is an ion exchange resin which is active in the gastrointestinal tract. It binds bile acids by a physicochemical action with the following results.

- It increases faecal excretion of bile acids, so increasing the liver conversion of cholesterol to new bile acids with consequent fall in low-density lipoprotein level. It is thus used in conjunction with dietary measures to treat hypercholesterolaemia.
- It relieves pruritus associated with elevated plasma bile acid levels in patients with cholestatic jaundice.
- It reduces diarrhoea associated with the presence of free bile acids in the gut, particularly in Crohn's disease, diabetic neuropathy or after ileal resection, vagotomy and other gastrointestinal surgery or radiotherapy.

Dosage
Treatment of hypercholesterolaemia: usual dose is 3–6 sachets (12–24 g) daily, taken as a single or in up to four divided doses. Maximum dose up to 36 g per day.

- Treatment of pruritus: 1 or 2 sachets (4–8 g) daily.
- Treatment of diarrhoea: dose as for treatment of hypercholesterolaemia.

Nursing implications
- Cholestyramine is particularly unpleasant for many patients to consume. This may be alleviated by encouraging patients to mix it with water, fruit juice, soup or soft fruit.
- It is important to note that cholestyramine may also bind and inactivate other drugs in the gastrointestinal tract and it is advisable to take other medication 30 minutes to 1 hour before cholestyramine dosing.
- Since it interferes with fat absorption, cholestyramine may reduce the absorption of the fat-soluble vitamins A, D and K. When such vitamin deficiency is identified, parenteral vitamin supplementation may be required.
- The most frequent side effects associated with treatment are gastrointestinal upsets and constipation. As cholestyramine is not absorbed, systemic toxicity does not occur.

Storage
Cholestyramine sachets are stored at room temperature.

CILAZAPRIL (Vascace)

Presentation
Tablets – 0.25 mg, 0.5 mg, 1 mg, 2.5 mg, 5 mg

Actions and uses
Cilazapril is an angiotensin-converting enzyme inhibitor. See the section on ACE Inhibitors (p. 4) for an account of the actions of this drug. In clinical practice, it is used in the treatment of heart failure and essential and renovascular hypertension.

Dosage
Heart failure: 0.5 mg initially, increased gradually to maintenance dose up to 5 mg once daily.
Hypertension: 0.5 mg (0.25 mg if renovascular hypertension) initially, increased gradually to the usual maintenance dose of 1.0–2.5 mg once daily.

Nursing implications
See section on ACE Inhibitors (p. 4).

Storage
Cilazapril tablets are stored at room temperature.

CIMETIDINE (Tagamet, Dyspamet)

Presentation
Tablets – 200 mg, 400 mg, 800 mg
Syrup – 200 mg in 5 ml
Injection – 200 mg in 2 ml, 400 mg in 100 ml

Actions and uses
Cimetidine is one of the Histamine H2-Receptor Antagonists, the actions and uses of which are described on p. 169.

Dosage
- Adults (oral treatment): 400 mg twice daily or 800 mg at night but up to 1000–1600 mg in 4–5 divided doses may be necessary. For maintenance therapy, a single bedtime dose is often used since overnight acid suppression appears to be important in determining ulcer relapse rates.
- Note that much lower doses (e.g. half the above) may be taken by patients buying cimetidine over the counter for ulcer and non-ulcer dyspepsia.
- Adults (injection therapy in active bleeding): intravenous doses of 200 mg are given slowly over several minutes and repeated at intervals of 4–6 hours. Alternatively, 400 mg may be administered over 15–30 minutes by rapid IV infusion or by continuous intravenous infusion (dose 50–100 mg/h) to a total dose 2.4 g daily.
- Intramuscular use may be substituted for oral treatment when necessary.
- Children >1 year: dose is based on 25–30 mg/day in divided doses as for adults.

Nursing implications
- See Histamine H2-Receptor Antagonists (p. 169) for a full account.
- Note that cimetidine is a potent inhibitor of the liver metabolism of many drugs. Thus it reduces the metabolism of warfarin, theophylline, anticonvulsants and antidepressants. When commenced in any patient already receiving drug therapy, a careful check of such interactions is warranted in order to prevent the development of sudden and unexpected toxicity. Seek advice from the pharmacy if in doubt. Note that the elderly and those on multiple drug treatment are most at risk from such interactions.
- Cimetidine is also available over the counter in chemists' shops. Patients who regularly self-medicate may be better advised to seek medical advice concerning their chronic dyspepsia.

Storage
- Cimetidine preparations are stored at room temperature.
- Syrup and injection solutions must be protected from light during storage.

CINNARIZINE (Stugeron)

Presentation
Tablets – 15 mg
Capsules – 75 mg

Actions and uses
Cinnarizine is an antihistamine and calcium channel blocker which, in practice, is used for its effects both as a labyrinthine sedative and peripheral vasodilator. It is used in the management of the following disorders.

- In the treatment of nausea and vomiting, particularly motion sickness.
- In the treatment of vertigo and the symptoms of vertigo and nausea due to Menière's disease.
- To improve blood flow in peripheral vascular disease.

Dosage
Nausea/vomiting and Menière's disease: adults, 30 mg initially, then 15–30 mg 8-hourly. Children: half the adult dose.
As a vasodilator (adults only): 75 mg 8-hourly.

Nursing implications
The nursing implications of this drug are the same as those described for Antihistamines (p. 33).

Storage
Cinnarazine preparations are stored at room temperature.

CIPROFIBRATE (Modalim)

Presentation
Tablets – 100 mg

Actions and uses
This drug is a member of the fibrate group of lipid-lowering drugs. The exact mechanism of action of these agents is unknown: they reduce both triglyceride and low-density lipoprotein (LDL-cholesterol) levels, so favourably influencing the LDL to HDL cholesterol profile. Ciprofibrate is used in the treatment of certain of the familial hyperlipidaemias and hyperlipidaemias associated with coronary risk in patients who fail on diet alone. It is occasionally necessary to combine therapy with other types of lipid-lowering drugs.

Dosage
Adults only: 100 mg once daily

Nursing implications
- Dosages are best taken with or immediately after meals.
- Skin rashes and muscle pain may occur, especially in patients with impaired kidney function, and treatment should be avoided if this is severe.
- All drugs of the fibrate group enhance warfarin and may produce bleeding in patients already receiving anticoagulant therapy. Close monitoring of prothrombin time is especially important in this group.

Storage
Ciprofibrate tablets are stored at room temperature.

CIPROFLOXACIN (Ciproxin)

Presentation
Tablets – 250 mg
Injection – 100 mg in 50 ml, 200 mg in 100 ml, 400 mg in 200 ml

Actions and uses
Ciprofloxacin is the forerunner of a series of antibiotics, collectively called the aminoquinolones, which have a broad spectrum of activity against Gram-positive and Gram-negative bacteria. Ciprofloxacin is notable as the first truly effective oral drug for the treatment of infections due to *Pseudomonas aeruginosa*. The major roles for ciprofloxacin are in the following settings.

- Empirical therapy of bacteraemia/septicaemia in seriously ill patients when the responsible pathogen cannot be readily identified.
- Respiratory infections, particularly those associated with bronchiectasis and cystic fibrosis, in which

C

Pseudomonas aeruginosa is frequently implicated.

- Urinary tract infections where resistance to standard drugs has been demonstrated and including that due to Pseudomonas.
- Skin and soft tissue infections as a result of its antistaphylococcal activity.
- Infections of bone and joint tissues for the reasons described above.
- Infective diarrhoeas due to its excellent activity against Salmonella, Shigella, Campylobacter.
- Sexually transmitted disease (e.g. gonococcal infection).

Dosage
- Adults: treatment of sensitive organisms (e.g. in urinary tract infection), 250 mg twice daily orally.
- Adults: treatment of skin and soft tissue infection, 500 mg twice daily orally.
- Adults: chest infection unresponsive to first-line therapy, 750 mg twice daily orally.
- Adults: acute treatment of severe infection, 400 mg by intravenous infusion undiluted over 30 minutes to 1 hour. Usually twice daily but 8-hourly in life-threatening infections.
- Children: if considered necessary, 7.5 mg/kg twice daily orally or 5 mg/kg twice daily by IV infusion.
- In children with cystic fibrosis, up to 40 mg/kg orally per day has been administered in severe respiratory infection.
- Gonococcal infection: 250–500 mg single dose.

Nursing implications
- Commonly reported side effects include gastrointestinal upsets (nausea, abdominal pain, diarrhoea) and dizziness and/or drowsiness.
- Ciprofloxacin is a contact irritant and intravenous injection may be associated with redness of the injection site and phlebitis.
- Ciprofloxacin is potentially neuro-toxic and patients with a history of convulsions must be closely monitored during treatment.

- Serum levels of theophylline may be sharply elevated by ciprofloxacin so that an appropriate dosage reduction in theophylline is warranted.
- Similarly, ciprofloxacin inhibits the liver metabolism of warfarin and may increase the risk of bleeding if commenced in an already anticoagulated patient. It is essential therefore to monitor clotting function very closely.
- Crystalluria (precipitation of insoluble ciprofloxacin in the urinary tract) may occur unless patients are well hydrated. Also excessive alkalinization of the urine should be avoided, e.g. ingestion of sodium bicarbonate and other antacids.
- The safety of ciprofloxacin in children is uncertain. Evidence from experimental animal studies indicates possible association with arthropathy in weight-bearing joints and there is concern that growing joints may be adversely affected as a result.

Storage
- Ciprofloxacin tablets and injections are stored at room temperature.
- The injection solution must be protected from light during storage. It is compatible with sodium chloride, glucose and fructose solutions but such dilutions should be administered within 24 hours of preparation.

CISAPRIDE (Alimix, Prepulsid)

Presentation
Tablets – 10 mg
Suspension – 5 mg in 5 ml

Actions and uses
This drug is often described as a gastrointestinal prokinetic because it stimulates gut motility throughout the gastrointestinal tract, from mouth to anus. The precise mechanism of action is not clearly understood. Although cisapride is chemically related to domperidone and metoclopramide, it

appears to have a unique action which is related, at least in part, to facilitation of the release or subsequent action of the neurotransmitter substance acetylcholine in the gastrointestinal tract. Cisapride has several uses in practice.

- It stimulates oesophageal transit and is therefore used in disorders associated with reduced oesophageal motility.
- It stimulates upper gastrointestinal motility and so increases gastric emptying and is used in the treatment of reflux oesophagitis, gastric stasis and non-ulcer dyspepsia.
- Its action in the upper gastrointestinal tract, together with a possible inhibitory action on the chemoreceptor trigger zone, make it a useful antiemetic.
- Its stimulant action in the colon has led to its use as a laxative.

Dosage
Adults: 10 mg taken two, three or four times a day. A single bedtime dose of 20 mg may be used to treat heartburn. Children (including neonates) with gastrooesophageal reflux disorders: 0.1–0.3 mg/kg three times daily.

Nursing implications
- This drug is generally well tolerated but a few problems related to an unwanted increase in gut motility may arise. These include diarrhoea, abdominal cramps and stomach rumbling.
- Cisapride should be avoided in those with gastrointestinal obstruction or perforation. It is also contraindicated in pregnancy.
- Since cisapride increases the rate of gastric emptying it may increase the rate of absorption and so enhance the action of other drugs. It has so far been shown to potentiate the action of warfarin and close monitoring of anticoagulant control is advised.

Storage
Cisapride tablets and suspension are stored at room temperature.

CISPLATIN (Neoplatin)

Presentation
Injection – 10 mg, 50 mg, 100 mg vials

Actions and uses
Cisplatin is a platinum-containing cytotoxic drug similar to carboplatin. It appears to interfere with cellular reproduction and since tumour cells reproduce at a rapid rate, they are particularly sensitive to its effects. It is mainly used in the treatment of advanced ovarian carcinoma and testicular teratoma.

Dosage
This is largely determined by specific indication and current schedules which are subject to change in line with existing knowledge.

- When used as a sole antitumour agent, the recommended dose for adults and children has been in the range 50–75 mg/m^2 body surface area as a single intravenous infusion every 3–4 weeks.
- An alternative regime is to give 15–20 mg/m^2 by intravenous infusion daily for 5 days every 3–4 weeks.
- When used in combination with other cytotoxic drugs, lower doses may be given.

Nursing implications
- Cisplatin is particularly toxic to the kidney and a progressive fall in renal function may occur. As this is dose related, laboratory testing should confirm that renal function has returned to normal before repeat courses are given. Regular 24-hour urine collections for creatinine clearance should be obtained.
- Almost all patients treated with this drug suffer from anorexia, nausea and vomiting.
- Bone marrow suppression may occur, leading to anaemia, haemorrhage due to thrombocytopenia and infection due to suppression of white blood cell function.

- Other adverse effects include tinnitus, hearing loss, peripheral neuropathy, abnormal liver function and abnormal cardiac function.
- Anaphylactic reaction characterized by facial oedema, wheezing, tachycardia and hypotension may occur within minutes of drug administration.
- In common with all cytotoxic drugs there are potential risks to normal fetal development if treatment is given during pregnancy.
- Nurses should be aware of the risks posed by cytotoxic drugs. Some are irritant to the skin and mucous surfaces and care must be exercised when handling them. In particular, spillage or contamination of personnel or the environment must be avoided. If cytotoxic drugs are handled regularly, it is theoretically possible that repeated skin contact or inhalation may produce systemic toxic effects in nurses who have developed hypersensitivity to them. Most hospitals now operate a centralized (pharmacy-organized) additive service. While this reduces the risk of exposure to cytotoxic drugs, it is essential that nurses recognize and understand the local policy on their safe handling and disposal. The Health and Safety Executive has decreed that such a policy should be in place wherever cytotoxic drugs are administered. These should be adapted, wherever possible, to care of patients in the community.

Storage
- Cisplatin vials are stored at room temperature.
- Vials are reconstituted with 10 ml or 50 ml of water for injection to provide a solution containing 1 mg in 1 ml.
- The drug is diluted in 2 litres of dextrose/saline mixture and infused over a 6–8 hour period.

- Prepared solutions are kept at room temperature and are stable for up to 24 hours.
- Refrigeration will produce precipitation from solution and is therefore not advised.

CITALOPRAM (Cipramil)

Presentation
Tablets – 20 mg

Actions and uses
Citalopram is one of the new range of antidepressant drugs. It is a selective inhibitor of serotonin reuptake into nerve endings in the brain. The actions and uses of this drug are described under Antidepressant Drugs (p. 31).

Dosage
Adults only: initially 20 mg once daily increasing as required to a maximum 60 mg once daily.
Note that elderly patients generally require lower doses.

Nursing implications
- Possible side effects include dry mouth, nausea, sweating and tremor.
- Must not be given with or within 14 days of monoamine oxidase inhibitors.
- Patient and carers should be advised that the full effect of the therapy may take several weeks.
- Care should be taken when driving or operating machinery.
- Also see Antidepressant Drugs (p. 31).

Storage
Citalopram tablets are stored at room temperature.

CLARITHROMYCIN (Klaricid)

Presentation
Tablets – 250 mg, 500 mg
Oral suspension – 125 mg in 5 ml
Injection – 500 mg vial

Actions and uses

Clarithromycin is an antibiotic of the erythromycin group which is, however, more active and longer acting than erythromycin and also reaches higher tissue concentrations. It is also claimed that gastrointestinal tolerance is improved with this drug. The antibacterial activity of clarithromycin is nevertheless similar to that of erythromycin, as are its indications. In particular, clarithromycin is used in the treatment of lower respiratory tract infections, skin and soft tissue infection and infections of the upper respiratory tract including acute otitis media.

Dosage

Adults: 250–500 mg twice daily for courses of 7–14 days depending upon the nature and severity of infection.
Children: up to 1 year (<8 kg), 7.5 mg/kg twice daily; 1–2 years (8–11 kg), 62.5 mg twice daily; 2–6 years (12–19 kg), 125 mg twice daily; 6–9 years (20–29 kg), 187.5 mg twice daily; older children, 250 mg twice daily.

Nursing implications

The nursing implications section for Erythromycin (p. 134) also applies to this drug with the additional comment that gastrointestinal upsets are less likely or less severe.

Storage

- Clarithromycin preparations are stored at room temperature and protected from light.
- To reconstitute injection, 10 ml water for injection is first added to the vial to produce a stock solution containing 50 mg in 1 ml. This stock solution can be stored at room temperature or under refrigeration for up to 24 hours.
- The required volume is then transferred to 250–500 ml sodium chloride or glucose injection and administered over 4–6 hours. Prepared infusions can be stored under refrigeration only but must be used within 24 hours.

CLEMASTINE (Tavegil)

Presentation

Tablets – 1 mg
Elixir – 0.5 mg (500 microgram) in 5 ml

Actions and uses

Clemastine is an antihistamine. See the section on Antihistamines (p. 33) for an account of the actions and uses of this drug. Clemastine is used in clinical practice for the following indications.

- To suppress generalized minor allergic responses to allergens such as foodstuffs and drugs.
- To suppress local allergic reactions, i.e. inflammatory skin responses to insect stings and bites, contact allergens, urticaria, etc.

Dosage

Adults: 1 mg twice daily.
Children: 1–3 years, 0.25–0.5 mg twice daily; 3–6 years, 0.5 mg twice daily; >6 years, 0.5–1 mg twice daily.

Nursing implications

The account under Antihistamines (p. 33) applies to this drug.

Storage

- Clemastine tablets and elixir are stored at room temperature.
- Elixir should be protected from light.

CLINDAMYCIN (Dalacin C, Dalacin T)

Presentation

Capsules – 75 mg, 150 mg
Syrup – 75 mg in 5 ml
Injection – 300 mg in 2 ml, 600 mg in 4 ml
Topical solution – 10 mg in 1 ml (30 ml roll-on application)
Vaginal cream – 2% (40 g tube plus applicators)

Actions and uses

Clindamycin is an antibiotic of the lincosamide group having a mainly bacteriostatic action in that it inhibits

C

further growth and multiplication of bacterial microorganisms in the body. It is effective in the treatment of infections due to Gram-positive cocci, including Pneumococcus and penicillin-resistant staphylococci and also anaerobic organisms. It is therefore used in the treatment of the following.

- Skin and soft tissue infections.
- Infections of bone and joint tissue, including osteomyelitis.
- Prophylaxis of bacterial endocarditis in 'at-risk' dental patients.
- Topically in the treatment of acne vulgaris when an infective component is involved.
- By local application in bacterial vaginosis.

Dosage
- Adults: orally 150–450 mg 6-hourly.
- Adults: injection 600–1200 mg 6-hourly. Usually by IV injection though doses up to 600 mg may be given by the IM route.
- Prophylaxis of endocarditis (adults): a single dose of 600 mg taken 1 hour before the dental procedure.
- Children: orally 3–6 mg/kg 6-hourly or 10 mg/kg 6-hourly by injection to a dose of 300 mg daily regardless of body weight in life-threatening infection.
- Children: prophylaxis of endocarditis, a single dose of 6 mg/kg as above.
- For treatment of acne, in adults and children: apply topical solution to the affected area twice daily for up to 12 weeks.
- In bacterial vaginosis, insert 5 g via applicator every night for 1 week.

Nursing implications
- Intramuscular injections should be made deeply into the gluteal muscles to prevent abscess formation.
- For intravenous injection: 600 mg should be diluted in 100 ml or more of 5% glucose or normal saline and given over a period of not less than 1 hour. Children's doses should be diluted appropriately.

- Gastrointestinal upsets are the only major side effects associated with clindamycin. If diarrhoea occurs in any patient the drug should be immediately stopped as a proportion of these patients may develop pseudomembranous enterocolitis. This serious condition arises as the result of the action of one or more endotoxins on the gut mucosa following release by the bowel organism *Clostridium difficile*.
- The drug must be given with caution to the newborn, during pregnancy or breastfeeding and to patients with preexisting kidney, liver, endocrine or metabolic disease.
- It is important to avoid contact with the eyes or mucous membranes when applying topical solutions.

Storage
- All preparations containing clindamycin are stored at room temperature.
- Avoid refrigeration.

CLOBAZAM (Frisium)

Presentation
Capsules – 10 mg

Actions and uses
Clobazam is one of the Benzodiazepines (see p. 47) which is used in the treatment of anxiety or as additional therapy in epilepsy.

Dosage
Anxiety in adults: 10 mg, 2–3 times daily or 20–30 mg, single dose at night.
Epilepsy in adults: 20–60 mg in divided doses as above.
Epilepsy in children >3 years: up to one-half the adult dose.

Nursing implications
See Benzodiazepines (p. 47).

Storage

- Clobazam capsules are stored at room temperature.
- Capsules should be protected from light.

CLOBETASOL (Dermovate)

Presentation

Cream – 0.05%
Ointment – 0.05%
(Also cream and ointment with neomycin plus nystatin)
Scalp application – 0.05%

Actions and uses

Clobetasol is a very potent topical corticosteroid which is used for the treatment of inflammatory skin conditions, e.g. psoriasis, eczema, dermatitis, etc.

Dosage

All preparations are applied sparingly once or twice daily to the affected area.

Nursing implications

See Corticosteroids, Topical for a full account of the nursing implications which apply to this drug.

Storage

All clobetasol preparations are stored at room temperature.

CLOBETASONE (Eumovate)

Presentation

Cream – 0.05%
Ointment – 0.05%

Actions and uses

Clobetasone (as butyrate) is a moderately potent topical corticosteroid which is used for the treatment of inflammatory skin conditions, e.g. psoriasis, eczema, dermatitis, etc.

Dosage

All preparations are applied sparingly from one to four times daily to the affected area.

Nursing implications

See Corticosteroids, Topical for a full account of the nursing implications which apply to this drug.

Storage

- Clobetasone butyrate preparations are stored at room temperature.
- Do not dilute, otherwise stability of the preparation may be adversely affected.

CLOMIPHENE (Clomid)

Presentation

Tablets – 50 mg

Actions and uses

During each menstrual cycle the growth of a follicle, ovulation and the development of the endometrium is stimulated by two pituitary hormones: luteinizing hormone (LH) and follicle-stimulating hormone (FSH). Late in the menstrual cycle, sufficient oestrogen is produced for these pituitary hormones to be inhibited and by this process a regular cycle of menstruation results. Clomiphene blocks the inhibitory action of oestrogens on the pituitary and therefore stimulates further production of pituitary hormones. This action is useful in the treatment of infertility when it has been shown that ovulation is not taking place, as the stimulation of pituitary hormones may induce ovulation.

Dosage

50 mg daily for 5 days with subsequent courses for up to six cycles until pregnancy occurs.

Nursing implications

- Because of its mechanism of action, clomiphene is likely to lead to the stimulation of the development of more than one ovum and multiple pregnancies may occur. This risk is usually explained to patients prior to commencing treatment.

C

- As clomiphene stimulates the ovaries and produces ovarian enlargement its administration is contraindicated should the patient be known to have an ovarian cyst.
- Common side effects include hot flushes and abdominal pain and distension.
- Less common side effects include blurring of vision, occular damage, fatigue, dizziness, headache, nausea, vomiting, breast tenderness, heavy periods, urinary frequency and, very rarely, loss of hair.
- Abnormalities in liver function have occurred when patients receive this drug.

Storage
- Clomiphene tablets are stored at room temperature.
- Tablets should be protected from moisture, light and excessive heat.

CLOMIPRAMINE (Anafranil)

Presentation
Capsules – 10 mg, 25 mg, 50 mg
Tablets – 75 mg, slow release
Syrup – 25 mg in 5 ml
Injection – 25 mg in 2 ml

Actions and uses
Clomipramine is a tricyclic antidepressant drug. Its actions and uses are described under Antidepressants (p. 31).

Dosage
- Orally: 30–150 mg daily in three divided doses.
- Up to 250 mg daily may be necessary.
- Alternatively the entire daily dose may be taken on retiring or as a single dose using 75 mg slow-release tablets.
- Where injections are necessary, e.g. for the treatment of uncooperative patients or at the beginning of therapy when a more rapid effect is required: 25 mg by intramuscular injection may be given up to six times daily.

Nursing implications
See Antidepressants (p. 31) for a full account.

Storage
- Preparations containing clomipramine are stored at room temperature.
- Solutions for injection and syrup must be protected from light.

CLONAZEPAM (Rivotril)

Presentation
Tablets – 0.5 mg, 2 mg
Injection – 1 mg in 1 ml

Actions and uses
Clonazepam is a member of the Benzodiazepine group (see p. 47). However, it has a marked anticonvulsant action and is used solely for this indication. It is indicated in the treatment of both myoclonic and generalized tonic-clonic seizures, but is potentially sedative and associated with tolerance.

Clonazepam is administered orally to prevent seizures and by slow intravenous injection for the treatment of status epilepticus.

Dosage
Adult oral dose: 4–8 mg daily in three or four divided doses.
Children: up to 1 year, 0.5–1 mg; 1–5 years, 1–3 mg; 5–12 years, 3–6 mg. The above are total daily dosages administered in three or four divided doses daily.
For the treatment of status epilepticus: slow intravenous injection is administered over a period of 30 seconds. More rapid injections produce hypotension and apnoea. Recommended doses are 1 mg for adults and 0.5 mg for infants and children.

Nursing implications
- See Benzodiazepines for nursing implications (p. 47).

- A particular problem with clonazepam is the occurrence of increased salivation and bronchial hypersecretion, resulting in drooling. It may prove troublesome in patients with obstructive airways disease.
- In common with anticonvulsant drug therapy in general, clonazepam should never be abruptly withdrawn but should be replaced with alternative medication after gradual reduction in dose.
- Care should be taken when performing skilled tasks, including driving, as drowsiness and coordination disturbances may occur with treatment.
- The effects of alcohol may be enhanced.

Storage
- Preparations containing clonazepam are stored at room temperature.
- Injection solution should be protected from light.
- The injection consists of dry powder in a vial with 1 ml of water for injection as solvent. It should be added immediately before use. If necessary the injection can be diluted in an intravenous infusion containing sodium chloride or glucose.
- Any injection not used immediately must be discarded.
- Intravenous infusions must be used within 12 hours.

CLONIDINE (Catapres, Dixarit)

Presentation
Tablets – 0.025, 0.1 and 0.3 mg (or 25, 100 and 300 microgram)
Capsules – 0.25 mg (250 microgram) sustained-release
Injection – 0.15 mg (150 mg) in 1 ml

Actions and uses
This drug blocks the outflow of sympathetic nerve stimulation from the brain, so reducing the response of peripheral arterioles to vasoconstrictor substances.

Small doses of clonidine have been found to be effective in the prophylaxis of migraine as well as in the treatment of vascular flushes in the menopause. Clonidine is, however, now rarely used in the treatment of hypertension in which more cardiovascular-specific drugs exist.

Dosage
For the prophylaxis of migraine and the treatment of menopausal flushing, a dose of 50–150 microgram per day is recommended.

Nursing implications
- The most important problem associated with clonidine occurs when used to treat hypertension. In such a circumstance, when discontinued abruptly, serious rebound hypertension may occur within 24 hours. Therefore the drug should never be stopped suddenly unless the patient is under constant medical supervision.
- Clonidine may worsen symptoms of depression and it is therefore contraindicated in depressed patients.
- Dry mouth, sedation and postural hypotension commonly occur during the early stages of treatment.
- Other reported side effects include bradycardia, headache, sleep disturbances, nausea, constipation and impotence in males.

Storage
Clonidine tablets and injection are stored at room temperature.

CLOTRIMAZOLE (Canesten)

Presentation
Cream – 1%
Powder – 1%
Topical spray – 1%
Pessaries – 100 mg, 200 mg and 500 mg
Ear drops – 1%
Vaginal cream – 1%, 2%, or 10% (single dose)

Actions and uses

This drug is an antifungal agent which interferes with the integrity of the fungal cell wall, so leading to intracellular leakage and hence cell death. It is indicated for the treatment of the following.

- Fungal skin infections due to dermatophytes, yeasts, moulds and other fungi including Trichophyton species, candida, ringworm (tinea) infections, athlete's foot, paronychia, pityriasis versicolor, erythrasma, intertrigo, fungal nappy rash, candida vulvitis and balanitis. It should be noted that the drug is not recommended as a sole treatment for pure trichomoniasis.
- Fungal otitis externa (otomycoses).

Dosage

Cream, powder or spray: to be thinly and evenly applied to the affected area two or three times daily and rubbed in gently. Treatment should be continued for at least 1 month or for at least 2 weeks after the disappearance of all signs of infection.
Pessaries: 200 mg should be inserted at night for three consecutive days. Alternatively 100 mg may be inserted daily for 6 days or a single 500 mg pessary inserted once.

Nursing implications
Rarely patients may experience local mild burning or irritation immediately after applying the preparation.

Storage

Preparations containing clotrimazole are stored at room temperature.

CLOXACILLIN (Orbenin)

Presentation

Capsules – 250 mg, 500 mg
Injection – vials containing 250 mg and 500 mg

Actions and uses

Cloxacillin is a member of the penicillin group of antibiotics. Its bactericidal action therefore results from its ability to prevent formation of an intact bacterial cell wall, thus leading to lysis of the growing bacterium. In practice, cloxacillin, like flucloxacillin, is used exclusively in the treatment of infections due to staphylococci since it is relatively unaffected by the beta-lactamase (drug-destroying) enzyme frequently secreted by this significant pathogen.

Its use therefore is usually restricted to infections of the respiratory tract and of skin and soft tissue frequently associated with *Staphylococcus aureus*.

Unlike some penicillins, cloxacillin is well absorbed after oral administration.

Dosage

Adults, orally: 500 mg four times a day; by intravenous or intramuscular injection, 250–500 mg 4–6-hourly.
Children: <2 years, one-quarter of the adult dose; 2 years or over, one-half of the adult dose.
Above doses may be doubled in severe infection though flucloxacillin is often preferred, especially by the oral route, due to its better absorption.

Nursing implications

- In common with other penicillins, it is important to determine the existence of penicillin allergy before administering cloxacillin.
- Note also that a proportion of patients who report allergy to drugs of the cephalosporin group will 'cross-react' with the penicillins.
- The only side effect of note, allergy excepted, is gastrointestinal upset with nausea, vomiting and diarrhoea.
- It is not necessary to instruct patients to take cloxacillin before meals since its absorption is relatively unaffected by the presence of food in the gut.

Storage

- Preparations containing cloxacillin are stored at room temperature.
- Once reconstituted, injection solutions must be used immediately.

Injections are prepared as follows:
- for intramuscular injection the vials should be diluted with 1.5–2 ml of water
- for intravenous injection: 1 g should be dissolved in 20 ml of water for injections and given either directly over 3–4 minutes or added to 0.9% sodium chloride, 5% glucose or glucose/saline mixtures and infused over 4–6 hours
- for intraarticular or intrapleural injection: the vials should be diluted with 5–10 ml water for injection.

CO-AMOXICLAV (Augmentin)

This drug is a combination of amoxycillin and clavulanic acid.

Presentation
Tablets – contain amoxycillin 250 mg and clavulanic acid 125 mg (Augmentin 375) including 'Dispersible tablets'; or amoxycillin 500 mg and clavulanic acid 125 mg (Augmentin 625)
Mixtures – contain: amoxycillin 125 mg and clavulanic acid 31 mg in 5 ml; amoxycillin 250 mg and clavulanic acid 62 mg in 5 ml; amoxycillin 400 mg and clavulanic acid 57 mg in 5 ml
Injections – contain: amoxycillin 500 mg and clavulanic acid 100 mg; or amoxycillin 1 g and clavulanic acid 200 mg

Actions and uses
This drug has the actions and uses of Amoxycillin (see p. 26). In addition, it contains clavulanic acid/clavulanate potassium which effectively broadens its spectrum of activity by blocking the inactivation of amoxycillin by penicillinase (beta-lactase) enzyme. Penicillinase effectively renders some microorganisms penicillin resistant so that such bacteria, normally unaffected by amoxycillin alone, may in fact be sensitive to co-amoxiclav. Good examples of this include amoxycillin-resistant strains of Staphylococcus and E. coli which are responsible for infections of the respiratory tract (including otitis media) and of the urinary tract. In practice, co-amoxiclav also has activity against important anaerobes (e.g. Bacteroides) and is used therefore as a good broad-spectrum agent in the treatment of abdominal sepsis and septicaemia. It is also a standard drug for prophylaxis in various surgical procedures.

Dosage
Doses may be calculated on the basis of the amoxycillin content and full prescribing instructions are given under Amoxycillin (p. 26).

Nursing implications
- The nursing implications already discussed for amoxycillin apply to this drug.
- The addition of clavulanic acid appears to increase the incidence of diarrhoea due to amoxycillin.
- Cholestatic jaundice is reported to occur in association with co-amoxiclav, to a much greater extent than with amoxycillin alone. Liver function tests should be monitored during prolonged therapy.

Storage
- Co-amoxiclav tablets, suspension and injections may be stored at room temperature.
- Injection solution should be used within 24 hours of preparation.
- Oral mixtures should be used within 1 week of preparation.

CODEINE PHOSPHATE

Presentation
Tablets – 15 mg, 30 mg and 60 mg
Linctus – 15 mg in 5 ml, 3 mg in 5 ml (paediatric)
Syrup – 25 mg in 5 ml

Actions and uses
Codeine phosphate is a member of the opioid group of analgesics, though it has relatively low potency which is limited within a narrow dosage range. It is also antitussive (i.e. it suppresses the cough reflex) and it slows gastrointestinal motility by a direct action on the

intestinal wall. It has the following uses.

- As a mild analgesic, usually in combination with aspirin (co-codaprin) or paracetamol (co-codamol), for use when aspirin or paracetamol alone is unable to control pain.
- As a cough suppressant in the treatment of persistent, often dry, cough.
- To treat diarrhoea associated with excessive gastrointestinal motility.

Dosage

For mild analgesia: in combination with aspirin or paracetamol, adults should receive two codeine compound tablets 4–6 hourly.

As an antidiarrhoeal: adults should receive 15–60 mg three or four times a day. Children: <1 year old, the drug is not recommended; 1–7 years, 1.25–2.5 ml of linctus (15 mg in 5 ml) three or four times a day.

As a cough suppressant: 2.5–10 ml of syrup or 5–10 ml of linctus, taken 3–4 times daily.

Nursing implications
- Although not normally associated with the severe problems encountered with more potent opioid drugs, codeine preparations are nonetheless a problem since they are widely prescribed or purchased over the counter in large quantities.
- Patients frequently become 'habituated' in that they may crave regular high dosage.
- The constipating action of codeine may be a problem when taken regularly other than for the treatment of diarrhoea.
- Elderly patients, in particular, may experience drowsiness and confusion, especially if preparations such as Tylex or Solpidol are taken since they contain high amounts of codeine per unit dose.

Storage
Codeine preparations are stored at room temperature.

COLCHICINE

Presentation
Tablets – 250 microgram, 500 microgram

Actions and uses
Colchicine interferes with the uptake of uric acid crystals by white cells present in gouty joints. The result of this is that inflammation is rapidly reduced and symptoms of pain are relieved. Its main use is in the treatment of acute gout but it is occasionally used as an alternative to the non-steroidal anti-inflammatory analgesics to prevent attacks of gout, especially during the introduction of allopurinol therapy.

Dosage
Adults: single course is used in acute gout. Initially 1000 microgram (1 mg) is given followed by subsequent doses of 500 microgram every 2 hours until relief of pain is obtained or vomiting or diarrhoea occur or a total dose of 10 mg has been reached. Such courses should not be repeated within 3 days. For prophylaxis, a dose of 250–500 microgram twice daily may be used.

Nursing implications
- Although very effective, use of colchicine is limited by the frequent occurrence of side effects such as nausea, abdominal pain and diarrhoea. Indeed, such side effects may necessitate withdrawal of treatment.
- High dosage may cause skin rashes and renal damage. Alopecia has followed prolonged use.
- It is recommended that colchicine be used with caution in elderly patients with heart disease and in patients with kidney or gastrointestinal disease.
- Fatalities have occurred after overdosage of colchicine with doses as low as 7 mg and therefore any patient accidentally or purposefully ingesting large amounts of this drug must be referred for immediate treatment.

Storage
- Colchicine tablets are stored at room temperature.
- Tablets should be protected from light.

CONTRACEPTIVES, ORAL

Numerous preparations are available which are listed in the British National Formulary. Oral contraceptives contain either a combination of oestrogen plus progestogen or progestogen alone. The oestrogen is usually ethinyloestradiol or mestranol. Progestogens include norethisterone, levonorgestrel, desogestrel or gestodene.

Actions and uses

Oral contraceptives act by the following mechanisms.

- Oestrogens inhibit the secretion of gonadotrophin-releasing hormone by the hypothalamus in the brain which in turn 'switches off' the pituitary release of substances known as gonadotrophins which stimulate ovulation. Oral contraceptives halt this action.
- Progestogens, on the other hand, do not necessarily inhibit ovulation (though they occasionally do) but, rather, make conception much less likely. They do so by affecting conditions within the endometrium (the lining of the uterus), making the implantation of an ovum less likely and therefore reducing the chances of successful pregnancy.
- The cervical mucus is made more viscous such that the motility of spermatozoa is impaired with greater difficulty in reaching the uterus and fertilizing the ovum.

Generally combined (oestrogens + progestogen) oral contraceptives are most effective. These two hormones may be combined for the purposes of contraception in two different ways.

1. The combination of both drugs may be started on the fifth day after the start of menstruation and continued for 20 days. No further drugs are taken until the fifth day of the next episode of bleeding.

2. Oestrogen only may be given for 15–21 days with progestogen (sometimes in variable but increasing dose) being added to the last 5–10 days of the 21-day course.

Dosage

For combination tablets: one tablet is taken daily for 21 days starting on the fifth day of menstruation. To assist patients who have difficulty remembering when to stop and start treatment, many contraceptives come in packs of 28 days, seven of these being dummy tablets.

Progestogen-only tablets are taken every day without a break during the cycle. Up to 1 mg oestrogen (around four times the standard dose) may be given twice for postcoital contraception using a combined preparation. The first dose is taken within 72 hours of intercourse then the follow-up dose 12 hours later.

Nursing implications
- It is recommended that the pill be avoided in certain groups (see product package insert for details). Generally contraindications include the following.
  - Women with cardiovascular disease including hypertension, previous stroke, angina pectoris, myocardial infarction or venous thrombosis.
  - Women with liver disease; however, some authorities believe that the contraceptive pill may be given to patients with liver disease if their liver function tests are normal.
  - Any patient who has or has in the past had breast cancer or cancer of gynaecological origin.
  - It is felt that patients who have or have had hypertension, facial nerve palsy or migraine may be at risk of cerebral thrombosis and therefore they should be discouraged from using the contraceptive pill.

- Women should be advised to wait for the first period to occur prior to commencing the contraceptive pill. During this time it is important to ensure that alternative precautions are taken.
- If a woman is breastfeeding, there is still a risk of pregnancy. There is very little risk to the suckling infant from the low doses of oestrogen and progestrogen in the contraceptive pill and therefore it is not contraindicated from the point of view of the infant. However, there may be a reduction in milk production after recommencing the pill and this may lead to failure of breastfeeding. A progestogen-only pill is therefore preferred.
- If a dose of combined preparation pill is missed, the dose may be taken for up to 12 hours after the usual dosage time. After 12 hours there is a definite risk of contraceptive failure and if 3 days or more have elapsed then the course should be completed, missing out the tablets which have been omitted, but alternative precautions to avoid pregnancy must be used.
- With the progestogen-only pill, missing a dose by even 3 hours or more may result in contraceptive failure and additional precautions are advised until at least 14 consecutive days treatment have again been taken.
- It is best to wait until at least one true period has occurred after stopping the pill before attempting to conceive. This allows calculation of dates and assessment of maturity and development of the fetus to be performed more accurately.
- If pregnancy occurs while the contraceptive pill is still being taken, there is a theoretical risk of damage to the fetus but in practice there is no evidence that any damage occurs.

- Provided no severe side effects occur and regular checks are made at visits to a general practitioner or family planning clinic, the pill may be continued for as long as the patient desires. More specific advice on this point should be sought from the patient's own general practitioner or family planning clinic.
- A combined preparation should be stopped 4 weeks prior to an operation. Progestogen-only pills may be continued. If surgery is necessary at short notice the doctor or surgeon involved should be informed that the patient is on the pill so that specific measures to limit the risk of thromboembolism can be taken.
- It is important to inform women that the bleeding which occurs is not actually a period but rather withdrawal bleeding during the pill-free period of time. Such episodes of bleeding will tend to occur regularly if the combined preparations are used. A beneficial effect is that bleeding may become lighter and pain encountered with periods may be diminished. If progestogen-only pills are used, irregularities in the menstrual cycle and therefore irregular bleeding may occur in the early months of treatment and occasionally periods may be missed altogether.
- A number of drugs including antibiotics (particularly rifampicin), barbiturates and anticonvulsants can reduce the effectiveness of low oestrogen-containing contraceptives especially. They do so by mechanisms including increased liver metabolism and diarrhoea with reduced gastrointestinal absorption as a result. They are, however, more likely to induce mid-cycle or breakthrough bleeding when alternative contraception measures should be used. Another option is to use a high (50 microgram)

oestrogen-containing pill but if in doubt, women should be advised to consult their doctor or family planning clinic.

- Side effects with the contraceptive pill are common and these may be divided into two major groups.
  1. Those arising just after the commencement of the contraceptive pill for the first time. These are largely due to the oestrogen and include nausea, vomiting, breast discomfort, fluid retention, depression, headache, lethargy, abdominal discomfort, vaginal discharge, cervical erosions and a syndrome of general irritability.
  2. Actual side effects include depression, altered sexual drive, jaundice, salt and water retention, hypertension, altered glucose tolerance, thrombophlebitis and thromboembolism.
- The results of many biochemical tests may be altered in patients taking the pill. In order to avert unnecessary worry for the patient and unnecessary use of health service resources, patients must be encouraged to inform medical staff at consultation that they are using the oral contraceptive.

Storage

All oral contraceptive preparations are blister packed and stored at room temperature.

CORTICOSTEROIDS

The corticosteroids include a large family of drugs having a wide range of uses in clinical practice.

Actions and uses

Corticosteroids are synthetic substances derived from hydrocortisone produced in the body by the cortex of the adrenal glands. They have effects described as 'glucocorticoid' or 'mineralocorticoid' based on their ability to respectively raise blood glucose or cause sodium retention.

- Glucocorticoid activity is responsible for the antiinflammatory/antiallergic or 'disease-modifying' action of the corticosteroids in numerous autoimmune conditions, which represents their major use. The list of potential indications for the glucocorticoids is almost limitless and includes the following:
  - rheumatoid arthritis and related connective tissue diseases (including systemic lupus erythematosus)
  - inflammatory bowel disease
  - other autoimmune conditions (e.g. nephrotic syndrome)
  - acute and chronic allergic and inflammatory states, e.g. asthma, dermatoses (including eczema and psoriasis)
  - local treatment of allergic rhinitis
  - topically for inflammatory conditions of the eye, ear and body cavities.
- Mineralocorticoid effects have little useful application – their tendency to cause salt and water retention and raise blood pressure is often seen as an unwanted side effect. It is also the reason why the parent drug, hydrocortisone, is rarely used (except in acute conditions) or in adrenal cortical replacement therapy.
- A major effect of the corticosteroids arises as a result of their ability to suppress blood-forming and lymphoid tissues so that they are routinely included in cytotoxic drug regimens for the treatment of leukaemias (especially acute lymphoblastic leukaemia in childhood) and lymphomas.

Corticosteroids are used both systemically and topically in the form of tablets, injections, ointments, creams, eye drops, enemas, suppositories, etc.

Dosage

The dosage range is potentially vast given the number of drugs available and the wide routes of administration. See individual corticosteroids.

C

Nursing implications

- Corticosteroids potentially have many side effects, especially if given systemically in high dose or for prolonged periods of time. By far the most important is suppression of the ability of the adrenal gland to produce hydrocortisone, especially when required in acute stressful conditions. Thus patients receiving steroids in prolonged (1–2 months or more) or high dosage (especially >30–40 mg/day) will usually exhibit significant 'adrenal suppression' which will compromise them in stressful situations such as infection or injury. Such an effect may be potentially severe or life threatening unless 'replacement' intravenous hydrocortisone is administered. It is essential, therefore, to note such risk in acutely ill patients or patients undergoing surgery so that remedial measures can be taken promptly. For example, the dose of steroid may need to be increased, at least twofold, to compensate for adrenal suppression.
- Patients who have been on steroids for prolonged periods frequently develop what is known as 'Cushingoid' symptoms, i.e. signs of steroid excess which include a characteristic 'moon face', obesity, purple striae and acne.
- Electrolyte disturbances associated with corticosteroid treatment include:
  - salt and water retention with hypertension
  - hypokalaemia with resultant muscle weakness
  - altered glucose metabolism with the possible precipitation of diabetes
  - altered calcium/phosphorus balance producing osteoporosis and a tendency towards bone fracture.
- Depression and psychosis are occasionally associated with steroid treatment.

- Gastric upset and occasionally peptic ulceration may arise as a result of reduced gastrointestinal mucosal protection associated with steroid treatment.
- Wound healing may be delayed significantly. This is especially important in patients who have to undergo an operation while on steroid treatment. Note also that Achilles tendon rupture is frequently encountered in long-term steroid users.
- Corneal ulceration and cataract formation may occur.
- There is an increased risk of infection by bacteria, viruses and fungi, such as oral candidiasis, when patients are treated with steroids.
- It is important to note that the above effects can occur with prolonged or high dosage of steroids administered by any route, **including topical application** to the skin.
- It is also extremely important to note that corticosteroids should not be given to patients who have active infection such as chickenpox, poliomyelitis, tuberculosis and infection due to herpes virus since they impair the body's natural immunity (i.e. are immunosuppressive).
- Similarly, disseminated (even fatal) infection may result if live vaccines are administered to immunosuppressed steroid users.

Storage
See individual steroid preparations.

CYCLIZINE (Valoid)

Presentation
Tablets – 50 mg
Injection – 50 mg in 1 ml
Note also the administration of cyclizine together with morphine in the Cyclimorph combination.

Actions and uses
Cyclizine is an Antihistamine (see p. 33 for a full account of this diverse

range of drugs). However, its major use is as an antiemetic in the treatment of nausea and vomiting, particularly due to motion sickness, neoplastic disease and co-administration of potent analgesia (e.g. morphine). The use of cyclizine in the management of emesis is related to its labyrinthine sedative action combined with its inhibitory effect on the chemoreceptor trigger zone (CTZ) within the brain which in turn stimulates the vomiting centre.

Dosage
Adults: orally, intramuscularly or intravenously: 50 mg 8-hourly or up to 150 mg over 24 hours by continuous intravenous or subcutaneous infusion.
Children: over 6 years require doses of up to 25 mg 8-hourly.

Nursing implications
- Patients should be advised that the performance of skilled tasks such as driving may be adversely affected by the sedative action of this drug and its ability to enhance the effects of alcohol.
- See under Antihistamines (p. 33).

Storage
- Cyclizine tablets and injection are stored at room temperature.
- Preparations should be protected from light.

CYCLOPENTHIAZIDE (Navidrex)

Presentation
Tablets – 0.5 mg (500 microgram)

Actions and uses
See the section on Thiazide and Related Diuretics (p. 357) of which cyclopenthiazide is a member.

Dosage
The daily adult range is 0.25–1 mg (250–1000 microgram), usually as a single daily dose. The duration of action is 12 hours plus.

Nursing implications
See under Thiazide and Related Diuretics (p. 357).

Storage
Cyclopenthiazide tablets are stored at room temperature.

CYCLOPHOSPHAMIDE (Endoxana)

Presentation
Tablets – 50 mg
Injection – 100 mg, 200 mg, 500 mg, 1000 mg (1 g)

Actions and uses
Cyclophosphamide is a member of the nitrogen mustard group of cytotoxic drugs. It is converted by the liver to a number of highly reactive metabolites which interfere with enzyme systems essential for growth and development of tumour cells. It also possesses immunosuppressive activity when used in low dosage. It has a wide range of uses which are as follows.

- In the treatment of Hodgkin's disease, lymphosarcoma, multiple myeloma, reticulum cell sarcoma, chronic lymphocytic leukaemia and ovarian carcinoma.
- In the treatment of carcinoma of the breast and lung.
- In non-malignant diseases including rheumatoid arthritis, systemic lupus erythematosus, nephrotic syndrome and other autoimmune conditions.

Dosage
As a cytotoxic drug, dosage depends on tumour type, the state of the patient and other factors including coincident administration of other cytotoxic drugs. Various regimens are used, the components of which do vary from time to time as knowledge of how best to apply cytotoxic chemotherapy develops.
As an immunosuppressant, daily oral doses of 1.5–3 mg/kg are commonly used.

Nursing implications
- Cyclophosphamide may be given orally or intravenously

C

(and occasionally into body cavities in the treatment of malignant effusions) but it is **unsuitable for intramuscular administration**.

- It is essential that all patients receiving this drug should maintain an adequate fluid intake. This reduces, by a dilutional effect, the incidence of haemorrhagic cystitis which results from an irritant effect on the bladder surface from various metabolites.
- Bone marrow suppression is a common side effect of cyclophosphamide. White blood cells are most often affected, leading to the risk of serious infection in some patients which may even prove life threatening.
- Gastrointestinal toxicity commonly presents as anorexia, nausea and vomiting.
- Alopecia is a common occurrence with risk increasing as higher (anticancer) doses of the drug are used. As it is a particularly distressing side effect, patients often require psychological support and reassurance that their hair will eventually return on cessation of treatment. Indeed, in some patients, the hair will reappear while they are still receiving treatment.
- Less common side effects include liver dysfunction, cardiac damage, skin and nail pigmentation, dizziness, diarrhoea, thyroid dysfunction and the syndrome of inappropriate secretion of antidiuretic hormone.
- Jaundice, colitis, mucosal ulceration, interstitial pulmonary fibrosis and adverse effects on the clotting mechanism are also occasionally noted.
- Cyclophosphamide enhances the effect of oral antidiabetic drugs of the sulphonylurea group and should therefore be used with caution in non-insulin dependent diabetics. Any diabetic receiving this drug should be carefully monitored as change in hypoglycaemic therapy may be necessary.
- Nurses should be aware of the risks posed by cytotoxic drugs. Some are irritant to the skin and mucous surfaces and care must be exercised when handling them. In particular, spillage or contamination of personnel or the environment must be avoided. If cytotoxic drugs are handled regularly, it is theoretically possible that repeated skin contact or inhalation may produce systemic toxic effects in nurses who have developed hypersensitivity to them. Most hospitals now operate a centralized (pharmacy-organized) additive service. While this reduces the risk of exposure to cytotoxic drugs, it is essential that nurses recognize and understand the local policy on their safe handling and disposal. The Health and Safety Executive has decreed that such a policy should be in place wherever cytotoxic drugs are administered. These should be adapted, wherever possible, to care of patients in the community.

Storage
- Cyclophosphamide tablets and vials for injection may be stored at room temperature.
- It is important to note that solutions prepared using water for injection should be used within 2 hours.

CYCLOSPORIN
(Neoral, Sandimmun)

Presentation
Capsules – 25 mg, 50 mg 100 mg
Injection – 50 mg in 1 ml, 250 mg in 5 ml
Oral solution – 100 mg in 1 ml

Actions and uses
Cyclosporin is an immunosuppressant drug used after organ transplantation (involving various donor organs) to reduce the likelihood of rejection and

graft-versus-host disease. It suppresses relevant T-lymphocytes which undergo a complex change during the development of the normal immune response. Cyclosporin is also used in the control of a variety of autoimmune diseases (e.g. psoriasis) as a steroid-sparing agent and an alternative to other first-line immunosuppressant drugs.

Dosage

Highly variable depending upon indication (transplantation or treatment of autoimmune disease), target blood level(s) and clinical response. Therefore, seek advice on optimum dosage, if in doubt.

Nursing implications

- Cyclosporin produces a series of side effects which are all dose related, including increased growth of body hair (hirsutism), tremor, kidney and liver impairment, gingival hypertrophy and gastrointestinal upsets.
- Close monitoring of liver and kidney function and of drug blood levels is essential in determining efficacy and toxicity.
- Intravenous infusion may be associated with hypersensitivity reactions (chills, fever, rigors, etc.) which are often associated with an 'inactive' constituent of the preparation. If severe, medical staff must be advised in order that intravenous therapy be reviewed.
- Cyclosporin given in combination with other drugs which carry a known risk of producing renal damage will increase the possibility of kidney dysfunction.
- Concurrent administration of many other drugs has been shown to increase blood levels of cyclosporin and hence the incidence of side effects. These include the antiarrhythmics, some antiinfectives, calcium antagonists, colchicine, danazol, oral contraceptives and hormone replacement therapy. If in doubt, seek advice from the pharmacy.

- In contrast to the above, drugs which may reduce cyclosporin blood levels and so increase the risk of tissue rejection include the following: barbiturates, some anticonvulsants and rifampicin.

Storage

- Preparations of cyclosporin are stored at room temperature.
- In particular, cyclosporin oral solution **must not be refrigerated** since precipitation of the drug will occur.
- Once opened, the oral solution should be discarded if unused after 2 months.

CYPROTERONE ACETATE (Androcur, Cyprostat, Dianette)

Presentation

Tablets – 50 mg
Capsules – 100 mg
Also combination of cyproterone acetate 2 mg with ethinyloestradiol 35 microgram in the Dianette formulation.

Actions and uses

Cyproterone acetate has an antiandrogenic action: it blocks the metabolic actions of testosterone, the male androgenic hormone. In clinical practice it has the following indications.

- It may be used to treat hirsutism in the female which is associated with androgen excess.
- It is also given to treat symptoms of sexual precocity and sexual deviation in the male.
- It reduces sebum secretion (normally stimulated by androgen) and is administered cyclically in combination with ethinyloestradiol (Dianette) in female acne unresponsive to oral antibiotic therapy.
- It is used in the treatment of symptomatic metastatic cancer of the prostate which is an androgen-dependent tumour.

C

Dosage

- For hirsutism in females: 50 mg daily for short courses during each menstrual cycle, usually combined with oestrogenic (e.g. ethinyloestradiol) treatment.
- To treat deviant sexual behaviour in males, 50 mg twice daily.
- In female acne, a low dose of 2 mg in combination with ethinyloestradiol is taken from day 1 to day 21 of the menstrual cycle and repeated after a 7-day interval.
- Prostatic cancer, for long-term therapy, 50 mg once or three times daily depending upon response. To reduce the severity of acute testosterone surges or 'flares' in patients receiving initial LHRH antagonist therapy for this condition, 300 mg daily in 2–3 divided doses.

Nursing implications

- When administered to male patients:
  - reduction in sperm count and therefore infertility usually occurs
  - gynaecomastia (breast enlargement) and tenderness of the breast may occur.
- When administered to females, galactorrhoea and breast enlargement may occur.
- The Dianette combination with ethinyloestradiol is contraceptive and may be used as such in patients with acne who also require an oral contraceptive.
- Common symptoms during the first few weeks of treatment include tiredness, fatigue and lassitude. Such symptoms usually disappear within the first few months of treatment.
- Weight gain is a common problem with prolonged administration of cyproterone acetate.
- It should be administered with caution or avoided in patients with adrenal dysfunction or diabetes mellitus.
- Relative contraindications to treatment include a history of thrombosis or embolism and a history of depression.
- With long-term treatment, hypochromic anaemia may occur.

Storage

Preparations containing cyproterone acetate are stored at room temperature.

CYTARABINE (Alexan, Cytosar)

Also described as cytosine arabinoside and Ara-C.

Presentation

Injection – 40 mg in 2 ml, 100 mg in 5 ml, 1 g (1000 mg) in 10 ml and 100 mg, 500 mg dry pellet vials

Actions and uses

Cytarabine is a cytotoxic drug which is thought to act by inhibiting an enzyme required for synthesis of DNA which in turn is an essential step in the growth and division of the cell itself. Since cancer cells grow and divide at a rapidly increased rate when compared to 'normal' host cells, they are naturally most vulnerable to the actions of such a drug.

- Cytarabine is used in the treatment of acute leukaemias, especially acute myeloid leukaemias in adults.
- It also exerts an antiviral action but is now rarely, if ever, used in the treatment of infections due to herpes virus.

Dosage

Cytarabine is given by intravenous infusion and intravenous, subcutaneous and intrathecal injection, perhaps in combination with a variety of other cytotoxic agents. Since treatment schedules vary from time to time as our knowledge of cancer chemotherapy and optimum use of cytotoxic drugs develops, it is advisable to consult up-to-date drug dosage schedules in use at individual institutions. Seek advice from local oncology services or from the hospital pharmacy.

Nursing implications

- Patients often experience nausea, vomiting, diarrhoea and oral ulceration. Nurses must pay particular attention to meeting the nutritional needs of these patients and ensuring adequate oral hygiene.
- Suppression of bone marrow function with resultant increased risk of haemorrhage, anaemia and infection is an important dose-limiting side effect. Patients should be advised to report any unusual bleeding such as bruising, epistaxis, haematuria. In addition, early signs of infection should be reported.
- Less frequently, skin rashes, abdominal pain, chest and joint pain and neurotoxicity or nephrotoxicity are reported.
- Patients with impaired liver function are at increased risk of dose-related side effects.
- In common with most cytotoxic chemotherapy, animal studies have demonstrated adverse effects on fetal development such that treatment is contraindicated in pregnancy and any woman receiving the drug should be encouraged to take adequate contraceptive measures.
- Nurses should be aware of the risks posed by cytotoxic drugs. Some are irritant to the skin and mucous surfaces and care must be exercised when handling them. In particular, spillage or contamination of personnel or the environment must be avoided. If cytotoxic drugs are handled regularly, it is theoretically possible that repeated skin contact or inhalation may produce systemic toxic effects in nurses who have developed hypersensitivity to them. Most hospitals now operate a centralized (pharmacy-organized) additive service. While this reduces the risk of exposure to cytotoxic drugs, it is essential that nurses recognize and understand the local policy on their safe handling and disposal. The Health and Safety Executive has decreed that such a policy should be in place wherever cytotoxic drugs are administered. These should be adapted, wherever possible, to care of patients in the community.

Storage

- Injection solution and dry pellets are preferably stored in a refrigerator.
- Reconstituted solutions may be retained for up to 48 hours.
- Any solution in which a slight haze has developed must be immediately discarded.
- Intravenous infusions are given in 0.9% sodium chloride or 5% glucose injection.

DACARBAZINE (DTIC)

Presentation
Injection – 100 mg, 200 mg

Actions and uses
Dacarbazine is a cytotoxic drug with limited uses which include malignant melanoma and, in combination with other cytotoxic drugs, soft tissue sarcomas and Hodgkin's disease.

Dosage
In common with other cytotoxic drugs, the dosage of dacarbazine is likely to change in line with clinical experience. Consult local chemotherapy drug regimens for up-to-date advice on dose.

Nursing implications
- Bone marrow depression producing anaemia, haemorrhage due to thrombocytopenia and infection due to suppression of white cell production may arise and is a major factor limiting the use of this cytotoxic drug. Patients should be advised to report any signs of bleeding or bruising.
- Frequent, often distressing side effects include anorexia, intense nausea and vomiting. Nurses should regularly assess patients' nutritional needs and give advice regarding oral hygiene.
- Other less common adverse effects include diarrhoea, muscle pain, tiredness, alopecia, facial flushing, paraesthesia and altered liver function.
- It is extremely important to note that dacarbazine is a very irritant drug and contact with the skin or eyes must be avoided.
- Nurses should be aware of the risks posed by cytotoxic drugs. Some are irritant to the skin and mucous surfaces and care must be exercised when handling them. In particular, spillage or contamination of personnel or the environment must be avoided. If cytotoxic drugs are handled regularly, it is theoretically possible that repeated skin contact or inhalation may produce systemic toxic effects in nurses who have developed hypersensitivity to them. Most hospitals now operate a centralized (pharmacy-organized) additive service. While this reduces the risk of exposure to cytotoxic drugs, it is essential that nurses recognize and understand the local policy on their safe handling and disposal. The Health and Safety Executive has decreed that such a policy should be in place wherever cytotoxic drugs are administered. These should be adapted, wherever possible, to care of patients in the community.

Storage
- Dacarbazine injection must be stored in a refrigerator and protected from light.
- Solutions are prepared by adding 9.9 ml to each 100 mg vial or 19.7 ml to each 200 mg vial using water for injection.
- Prepared solutions are stable for 72 hours under refrigeration.

DALTEPARIN (Fragmin)

Presentation
Injection ampoules – 10 000 unit in 1 ml and in 4 ml
Injection syringes – 2500 and 5000 unit in 0.2 ml

Actions and uses
Dalteparin is a product of heparin fractionation and the section on Heparin, Low Molecular Weight (p. 168) should be consulted for an account of this class of injectable anticoagulants.

Dalteparin has the following uses.

- Prevention of deep venous thrombosis (DVT) in 'at-risk' groups.
- Treatment of established DVT.
- Treatment of pulmonary embolism (PE).

Dosage
Prophylaxis of DVT: adult dose is 2500–5000 unit subcutaneously once daily depending upon relative risk (highest after orthopaedic surgery). Highest dose (5000 unit/day) may be split so that half the initial dose is given 1–2 hours preoperatively and the remainder 12 hours later.
Treatment of established DVT: single daily subcutaneous dose based on 200 unit/kg once daily or, to reduce risk of bleeding, 100 unit/kg 12-hourly.
Treatment of PE (unlicensed use): single daily subcutaneous dose based on up to 400 unit/kg or, to reduce risk of bleeding, 200 unit/kg 12-hourly.
Use in conjunction with haemodialysis or haemofiltration (to reduce risk of clotting): 35 unit/kg by IV bolus followed by 13 unit/kg/h by IV infusion. Alternatively, if procedure <4 hours, single IV bolus dose of 5000 unit.

Nursing implications
See section on Heparin, Low Molecular Weight (p. 168).

Storage
- Dalteparin injection solution and syringes are stored at room temperature.
- They are intended for single dose use only.

DANAZOL (Danol)

Presentation
Capsules – 100 mg and 200 mg

Actions and uses
Danazol, which is chemically related to testosterone, inhibits the production of gonadotrophic hormones normally secreted by the pituitary. The major effect is to suppress maximum levels of oestrogen which are normally required to stimulate function of the ovaries and endometrium during the menstrual cycle. Danazol is therefore described as producing a hypo-oestrogenaemic effect which is useful in the following situations.

- The treatment of endometriosis, including preparation prior to hysteroscopic endometrial ablation.
- The treatment of cyclical mastalgia, gynaecomastia and fibrocystic mastitis.
- Dysfunctional uterine bleeding presenting as menorrhagia.

Dosage
It is important to note that the therapeutic effect of danazol is controlled by careful dosage adjustment, according to individual response.
Endometriosis: the usual adult dose is 400 mg daily starting on the first day of menstruation and continued for 6–9 months.
Preoperatively: 400–800 mg daily for up to 6 weeks prior to ablation surgery.
Dysfunctional uterine bleeding: 200 mg daily starting on the first day of menstruation and continuously thereafter.
Breast disease: 200–400 mg daily for 3–6 months.

Nursing implications
- It is important to exclude pregnancy in patients with amenorrhoea.
- The drug's androgenic properties can produce side effects of acne, oily skin, fluid retention, hirsutism, deepening voice and clitoral hypertrophy.

D

D

- Other side effects include flushing, reduction in breast size, skin rash, anxiety, dizziness, vertigo, headache, nausea and hair loss.
- Due to the risk of fluid retention, the drug should be used with great caution in patients with heart disease, kidney disease or epilepsy.
- If patients have impaired liver function, the dosage may have to be reduced.

Storage
Danazol capsules are stored at room temperature.

DANTROLENE (Dantrium)

Presentation
Capsule – 25 mg, 100 mg
Injection – 20 mg per vial (supplied in UK to hospitals only)

Actions and uses
Dantrolene is an antispastic drug which acts directly on muscles to prevent the release of calcium from within the muscle cell itself which is a prerequisite for skeletal muscle contraction.

It is used in the treatment of conditions associated with spasticity of skeletal muscular origin. It is also used specifically to treat muscle spasm related to malignant hyperthermia, which may be a complication of anaesthesia or, more recently highlighted by the media, an adverse reaction to the CNS stimulant popularly known as Ecstasy.

Dosage
Skeletal muscular spasticity: 25 mg daily increased as required to a total dose of 100 mg four times daily.
Malignant hyperthermia, including reactions to Ecstasy: 1 mg/kg by IV infusion repeated to a total dose of 10 mg/kg.

Nursing implications
- Dantrolene, predictably, causes feelings of muscle weakness as well as dizziness, drowsiness and diarrhoea.

- It should not be used in patients who may be disabled if spasticity is abolished (i.e. a degree of which contributes to mobility).
- It is also contraindicated in patients with liver impairment or in the event of lung dysfunction which might be compromised by skeletal muscle inhibition.
- Patients should be advised that dantrolene can affect the performance of skilled tasks, for example driving and operating machinery.

Storage
Dantrolene capsules are stored at room temperature.

DEMECLOCYCLINE

Presentation
Capsules – 150 mg

Actions and uses
Demeclocycline is demethylchlortetracycline, an antibiotic of the tetracycline group. Its major use, however, is in the treatment of the syndrome of inappropriate ADH secretion (SIADH) in which it blocks the action of antidiuretic hormone (ADH, vasopressin) on the renal tubules. The function of this hormone is to maintain plasma volume by stimulating reabsorption of free water by the kidney. Under certain circumstances, an excess of ADH may be produced, leading to a dilutional hyponatraemia (reduced plasma sodium concentration).

Dosage
Treatment of inappropriate ADH secretion (SIADH) in adults: a total daily dose of 600 mg is taken in 2–4 divided doses.

Nursing implications
- In common with all tetracyclines, this drug is associated with gastrointestinal upsets (nausea, vomiting, GI pain, diarrhoea) in a proportion of patients.

- Absorption is impaired in the presence of food and, in particular, milk and antacids so patients should be advised to take this medication before meals.
- Demeclocycline is well recognized as a cause of photosensitivity reactions which may limit its use. Patients should be advised of this side effect.

Storage
- Demeclocycline tablets are stored at room temperature.
- Protect from light.

DESMOPRESSIN (DDAVP, Desmotabs, Desmospray)

Presentation
Intranasal solution –
100 microgram/ml
Nasal spray – 10 microgram/metred
0.1 ml dose
Injection – 4 microgram in 1 ml
Tablets – 100 microgram,
200 microgram

Actions and uses
Desmopressin is a chemical derivative of vasopressin, the antidiuretic hormone (ADH), produced by the posterior pituitary gland. It has a much longer action than ADH and does not possess the marked vasoconstrictor effect of the natural hormone. It is therefore a more convenient and safer alternative in the treatment of diabetes insipidus.

Very high doses of desmopressin have been given by intravenous injection as a means of stimulating clotting factor VIII synthesis in deficiency states (haemophilia and Von Willebrand's disease). This use is highly specialized and only carried out under the haematologist's supervision.

Dosage
Note that dosage is variable in the individual and adjusted in order to produce sufficient diuresis each day so that water overload is prevented. The following is a guide.

Diabetes insipidus
- Injection: 1–4 microgram daily for adults (up to 0.4 microgram for children) by IV, IM or SC injection.
- Oral: 100 microgram three times daily (adults and children) initially to a daily dose range of 200–1200 microgram.
- Intranasal: 10–40 microgram daily in 1–2 doses (5–20 microgram/day for children).
- Diagnosis: 2 microgram by IM or SC injection or 20 microgram intranasally (adults and children).

Nocturnal enuresis
- Oral: 200–400 microgram at bedtime.
- Intranasal: 20–40 microgram at bedtime.

Nursing implications
- The wide variation of dosage between individuals and in the same subject during long-term maintenance therapy must be stressed. It is therefore important to monitor urine output during therapy.
- The risk of hyponatraemic convulsions may be minimized by the strict adherence to prescribed dosage. Those patients who have been prescribed this drug for primary nocturnal enuresis should be advised to avoid a high fluid intake and if vomiting or diarrhoea is experienced they should be instructed to cease dosing until fluid balance returns to normal.
- The poor oral bioavailability of this drug is reflected in the major differences between oral, intranasal and injectable dosages.
- The method of administration of the intranasal forms of desmopressin vary and require careful patient education in order to achieve optimum control. The nurse has therefore an important task in confirming patient compliance.
- Desmopressin lacks the potent vasoconstrictor action of ADH

---

and is much less likely to produce hypertension or constriction of the coronary arteries. Nevertheless, patients with cardiovascular disease should be carefully monitored.
- Following pituitary surgery for diabetes insipidus, desmopressin may only be required for a relatively short period.

Storage

Desmopressin preparations are stored in the refrigerator.

DEXAMETHASONE (Decadron)

Presentation

Tablets – 0.5 mg, 2 mg
Injection – 8 mg in 2 ml, 100 mg in 5 ml
Also in combination in eye drop, ear drop and intranasal preparations.

Actions and uses

Dexamethasone is a potent member of the corticosteroid group used widely by the topical and systemic routes. See the section on Corticosteroids (p. 107) for a full account of the actions and uses of these important drugs.

When used systemically, dexamethasone is approximately seven times more potent than prednisolone and 25–30 times more potent than hydrocortisone on a mg-for-mg basis.

Dosage

Doses vary considerably with the nature and severity of the illness being treated and it is not therefore appropriate to quote specific instances.

Nursing implications
- See the section on Corticosteroids (p. 107).
- Intravenous bolus injections are given slowly over 30 seconds to 1 minute or infusion in glucose 5% or sodium chloride 0.9% (50–500 ml) continuously or intermittently.

- Perineal itching or burning discomfort may develop during or soon after IV bolus injection. A few patients also complain of chills, headaches and flushing. These effects are a form of hypersensitivity which are very short-lived.

Storage
- Preparations containing dexamethasone are stored at room temperature.
- Protect from light.

DEXTROMORAMIDE (Palfium)

Presentation

Tablets – 5 mg and 10 mg
Suppositories – 10 mg

Actions and uses

Dextromoramide is a potent opioid drug used in the treatment of severe pain. Its actions and uses are in fact similar to those of conventional morphine preparations but it is less sedative than morphine and has a somewhat shorter duration of action (i.e. 2–3 hours only). Dextromoramide, especially by the sublingual route, is often used to provide a brief period of analgesia in order to cover a painful procedure or to manage breakthrough pain when it arises.

Dosage

Adults: orally or sublingually, 5 mg increased as required and repeated 2–4 hourly according to the patient's response. Rectally, 10 mg suppository should be administered 2–4 hourly according to patient response.
Children: as above, dosage based on 80 microgram (0.08 mg)/kg body weight.

Nursing implications
- Dextromoramide produces side effects which are typical of the narcotic analgesics generally. These include dose-related sedation (though less so than with morphine), nausea, constipation and respiratory depression.

- In common with other drugs of this type, it has major abuse potential and as such it is classified as a Controlled Drug requiring specific prescribing, ordering, supply, storage and administration procedures.
- Note that sublingual administration ensures a rapid onset of action and bypasses first-pass metabolism by the liver during absorption. This is a particularly useful route if rapid onset, short-term analgesia is required, e.g. to assist with a painful procedure such as a dressing change, bathing or other movement which evokes severe pain.

Storage

- Dextromoramide is stored in a double-locked (Controlled Drug) cupboard.
- It is stored at room temperature but excessive heat must be avoided when storing rectal suppositories which may readily melt.

DIAMORPHINE (Heroin)

Presentation

Injection – various strengths from 5 mg to 500 mg per ampoule for reconstitution with water for injections.

Actions and uses

Diamorphine is the most potent opioid (opiate or narcotic) analgesic which is used in the treatment of severe and overwhelming pain. It is in fact an inactive prodrug of morphine which, following injection, is converted via an intermediate metabolite which very rapidly distributes to brain tissues. The rapid rate with which the metabolite enters the CNS explains the very high potency of diamorphine compared to other opioid analgesics. When taken orally, however, diamorphine is virtually completely metabolized to morphine by the liver during first pass and so has no special advantages over morphine by this route. Diamorphine is the drug of first choice when parenteral analgesia is indicated in severe and often chronic pain, particularly that associated with cancer.

Dosage

Dosage varies widely depending on the condition under treatment and the individual's response to the drug. Initial doses (given as a guideline only) would be 5–10 mg by subcutaneous, intramuscular or intravenous routes, repeated 3–4 hourly as required according to the patient's response and increased appropriately as tolerance develops. In the control of pain associated with advanced cancer, gram quantities may be necessary. In this case it may be administered by continuous subcutaneous infusion often in combination with antiemetic drugs.

Nursing implications

- It is vital that special attention is paid to the range of dosage of this drug used in practice. Although very high doses, even gram quantities, may be administered in patients with advanced cancer-related pain, it is unlikely that bolus doses on an 'as-required' basis will exceed 5–10 mg when used postoperatively or for short-term pain control.
- Vigilance is essential. Packaging of diamorphine ampoules is standard across the range of strengths and on more than one occasion an inappropriately high dosage has been administered with fatal results.
- This drug causes profound respiratory depression when administered in high dose to patients in the initial stages. **It is only in chronic pain and after repeated dosing that tolerance to the respiratory depressant and sedative effect develops.**
- The nature of the analgesia produced by diamorphine is such that euphoria or a feeling of well-being is evoked. This may be of particular value in the treatment of chronic pain which can lead to despair and

depression in the affected patient. It is also, however, the basis for the popularity of heroin as a drug of abuse.

- Parenteral diamorphine, commonly administered by continuous subcutaneous infusion, is often preferred for patients with chronic severe pain when the oral route is no longer available. When transferring from oral morphine a suggested dose of diamorphine by injection of one-third the oral morphine dosage is suggested.
- The solubility of diamorphine is exceedingly high so that even very large doses can be dissolved in a fraction of 1 ml, so facilitating subcutaneous bolus administration.
- Constipation is such a common side effect that it is essential that all patients receiving regular dosing are also prescribed a stimulant laxative (e.g. co-danthramer). Constipation is the most common cause of nausea and vomiting in such patients.

Storage
- Diamorphine ampoules are stored at room temperature in a double-locked (Controlled Drug) cupboard.
- Solutions readily break down by a process known as hydrolysis to form morphine. Injections can be prepared on a daily (even 48-hourly) basis when administered by continuous infusion.

DIAZEPAM (Diazemuls, Stesolid, Valium)

Note: this drug can only be prescribed under the NHS in its generic form.

Presentation
Tablets – 2 mg, 5 mg, 10 mg
Oral solution – 2 mg in 5 ml
Injection – 10 mg in 2 ml in aqueous solution or emulsified form
Rectal solution – 5 mg and 10 mg

Actions and uses
Diazepam is a member of the Benzodiazepine group. See p. 47 for an account of the actions and uses of this group generally.

In clinical practice diazepam has the following uses.

- It may be taken orally during the day for the treatment of anxiety, including delirium tremens associated with acute alcohol withdrawal.
- In large doses it may be taken as a hypnotic.
- It may be administered intravenously or intramuscularly for the control of acute muscle spasm in such conditions as tetanus or status epilepticus.
- It may be given orally for the relief of muscle spasm associated with chronic neurological abnormalities such as cerebral palsy and disseminated sclerosis.
- It may be given intravenously for sedation immediately prior to minor surgical, dental and investigative procedures.
- It may be administered by the rectal route as an alternative to the oral or injectable routes, especially if used during febrile illness in patients with a history of febrile convulsions.
- Rectal solution is an alternative to injections in the control of convulsions.

Dosage
- For the treatment of anxiety and acute alcohol withdrawal: adult dosage ranges from 5 to 40 mg per day given once, twice, three or even four times daily by either the oral or intramuscular routes.
- Rarely for the treatment of insomnia: single adult dose ranging from 5 to 30 mg taken on retiring.
- In acute muscle spasm including tetanus in adults and children: 100–300 microgram (0.1–0.3 mg)/kg body weight by intravenous injection every 1–4 hours or via nasoduodenal tube.
- Status epilepticus in adults: 10–20 mg administered intravenously at a rate of 2.5 mg over 30 seconds and repeated, as required, at half to one-hourly intervals. A continuous IV infusion of up to 3 mg/kg body weight over 24 hours may be given by way of follow-up when deemed necessary.

- Status epilepticus in children: dose is based on 200–300 microgram (0.2–0.3 mg)/kg or 1 mg per year of age by direct IV injection.
- Rectal route in status: adults and children, 10 mg or 5 mg if frail elderly or <3 years of age. Repeat as required after 5 minutes until control is achieved.
- Control of muscle spasm associated with chronic neurological disorders: dosage adjusted on an individual basis to try to obtain the best relief from spasm without inducing excess sedation.
- When used intravenously for sedation prior to dental, surgical or investigative procedures, doses of 5–20 mg are given. It must be emphasized that intravenous diazepam should only be used when facilities for resuscitation are available as **respiratory arrest may occur**.

Nursing implications
- See the section on Benzodiazepines (p. 47).
- During intravenous injection (usual rate 5 mg/min) the patient can be expected to become drowsy and develop slurred speech. This is generally an indication that the optimum dose has been administered.
- Patients who have received intravenous diazepam should remain under observation for at least an hour after the procedure has been completed as they may be quite markedly sedated.
- As emphasized above, there is always the danger of respiratory arrest with intravenous administration of diazepam.
- Injection solution is irritant and may cause redness around the injection site and thrombophlebitis. It should be noted that for this reason the intravenous use of Diazemuls, containing emulsified diazepam, is preferred. The fat emulsion provides a protective coating along the venous tract and hence reduces the degree of irritancy.

Storage
- Preparations containing diazepam are stored at room temperature.
- Injection should not be mixed with other drugs in the same syringe or infusion solution since diazepam is poorly soluble in aqueous solution.
- Therefore, injections are preferably administered undiluted though if intravenous infusion is necessary, it may be added to sodium chloride 0.9% or glucose 5% injection.
- Such infusion solutions should be used within 6 hours of preparation.

D

DIAZOXIDE (Eudemine)

Presentation
Tablets – 50 mg
Injection – 300 mg in 20 ml

Actions and uses
Diazoxide has two main actions. It is a potent arteriolar vasodilator which, given intravenously, produces a rapid fall in blood pressure. It has therefore been used in the treatment of hypertensive crises but has now largely been replaced by other drugs which allow more effective control of markedly elevated BP.

It raises blood glucose level and has been used as an oral hyperglycaemic agent to reverse severe hypoglycaemia.

Dosage
In accelerated or so-called malignant hypertension, diazoxide is only effective by the intravenous route, when in adults 300 mg (5 mg/kg in children) is administered rapidly over no less than 30 seconds. Patients should be lying flat during administration. The duration of action is usually 4–6 hours. It may be given as required up to four times in 24 hours.

In the treatment of hypoglycaemia in adults and children, the dose is 5 mg/kg daily taken in 2–3 divided doses but ultimately titrated against the blood glucose response.

Nursing implications
- As mentioned above, the effect of this drug is so rapid and profound that patients should

be supine during administration. Despite this, profound hypotension is not uncommon.
- Pain may arise at the injection site.
- Repeated dosage may produce the following effects.
  - Hyperglycaemia, so that blood/urine should be tested for glucose excess. Treatment with oral hypoglycaemic drugs may be necessary.
  - Salt and water retention, so that symptoms of heart failure must be excluded.
  - Hyperuricaemia, although joint pain is rarely noted.
- There have been reports that when the drug is used in hypertensive crises during childbirth, delivery may be delayed unless oxytocin is concurrently administered.
- Long-term dosage is usually not recommended because of the possible occurrence of hyperglycaemia, salt and water retention, hypertrichosis, skin rash, leucopenia, thrombo-cytopenia, extrapyramidal effects, hyperuricaemia.

Storage
- Diazoxide injection is stored at room temperature.
- It must be given undiluted and never mixed with other drugs.
- Tablets are stored at room temperature.

DICLOFENAC (Arthrotec, Diclomax, Voltarol)

Also available in combination with misoprostol which provides protection of the gastric mucosa, so limiting the risk of erosion and ulceration.

Presentation
Tablets – 25 mg, 50 mg
Tablets, dispersible – 50 mg
Tablets, slow release – 75 mg, 100 mg
Capsules, slow release – 75 mg, 100 mg
Suppositories – 12.5 mg, 25 mg, 50 mg, 100 mg
Injection – 75 mg in 3 ml

Actions and uses
Diclofenac is a non-steroidal antiinflammatory drug and the section on NSAIDs (p. 250) should be consulted for a full account of its actions.

In practice, diclofenac is used in the treatment of:

- rheumatoid and osteoarthritis
- ankylosing spondylitis
- acute gout
- other inflammatory pain associated with acute or chronic injury
- postoperative pain
- renal colic associated with ureteric spasm.

Dosage
The adult oral dose range is 25–50 mg three times a day or 75 mg (once or twice) or 100 mg once daily as slow-release tablets. Up to 100 mg may be administered at night by the rectal route and 75 mg by intramuscular injection once or twice daily.

Nursing implications
- See the section on NSAIDs (p. 250).
- Note that co-administration with misoprostol, a prostaglandin, affords a degree of protection of the gastric mucosa in patients prone to severe gastrointestinal upsets in association with NSAID therapy.

Storage
Diclofenac preparations are stored at room temperature.

DICYCLOMINE (Merbentyl)

Presentation
Tablets – 10 mg, 20 mg
Syrup – 10 mg in 5 ml

Actions and uses
Dicyclomine is an anticholinergic drug which has a specific antispasmodic action on the smooth muscle of the gastrointestinal tract. It is therefore used for the following conditions:

- irritable colon
- spastic constipation
- infant colic

- spasm associated with colitis
- diverticulitis and other gastrointestinal disorders.

Dosage

Adults: 10–20 mg three times daily taken before or after meals.
Children >6 months: 5–10 mg three or four times daily taken 15 minutes before feeds.

Nursing implications

- As an anticholinergic drug typical side effects include dry mouth, thirst, blurred vision, constipation, anorexia, nausea and urinary hesitancy.
- Dizziness, tiredness and fatigue may also occur.
- Caution is necessary in patients with narrow angle glaucoma and symptoms of prostatism, hiatus hernia or reflux oesophagitis.

Storage

- Dicyclomine preparations are stored at room temperature. Liquid should, however, be protected from light by storing in amber glass bottles.
- For ease of administration, if required, the liquid may be diluted immediately before use with an equal quantity of water.

DIDANOSINE (Videx)

Presentation

Tablets – 25 mg, 100 mg

Actions and uses

This drug is an antiviral nucleoside derivative which specifically inhibits replication of retroviruses such as HIV. It is used in the treatment of AIDS and AIDS-related complex or symptomatic HIV infection in patients intolerant of first-line zidovudine or when zidovudine alone has proved clinically ineffective, in which case combination therapy may be tried. The result is delay in emergence of HIV resistance to zidovudine and hence progression of HIV status.

Dosage

Adults only: 125 mg twice daily if <60 kg body weight or 200 mg twice daily if heavier.

Nursing implications

- Each dose is taken as two tablets (hence standard tablet strengths) irrespective of body weight, chewed thoroughly or first crushed or dispersed in water, in order to aid absorption.
- Pancreatitis is a potentially severe side effect of this drug and serum amylase levels must be monitored during treatment, which should be discontinued if levels are elevated, even in the absence of symptoms, until this condition is clinically excluded.
- Avoid treatment in patients with previous liver or pancreatic dysfunction while receiving didanosine.
- Gastrointestinal upsets with nausea, vomiting, diarrhoea (occasionally severe), skin rash, confusion, weakness, pruritus, chills and fever are relatively common.
- Peripheral neuropathy, especially in the advanced stages of HIV, may be of sufficient severity to warrant discontinuation of treatment or dosage reduction, at the very least.
- Serious side effects include convulsions and pneumonia.

Storage

Didanosine preparations are stored at room temperature.

DIFLUCORTOLONE (Nerisone)

Presentation

Ointment – 0.1%, 0.3%
Cream – 0.1%
Oily cream – 0.1%, 0.3%

Actions and uses

This potent topical corticosteroid (see p. 107) is used in the treatment of inflammatory skin conditions such as psoriasis, eczema and dermatitis.

D

Dosage
Cream, oily cream and ointment are applied one to three times daily to affected areas.

Nursing implications

- Although applied topically, significant amounts may be absorbed through the skin to produce at least some of the typical side effects described in the section on Corticosteroids (p. 107). Therefore, patients should be advised to apply sparingly. When using concentrated ointment or oily cream, it is recommended that the weekly dose be restricted to 60 g.
- Children (>4 years only) should not receive more than 3 weeks continuous application of 0.1% diflucortolone topical preparations of any kind.

Storage
- Store all preparations at room temperature but under cool, dry conditions.
- These products have a shelf life of 5 years from the date of manufacture.

DIFLUNISAL (Dolobid)

Presentation
Tablets – 250 mg, 500 mg

Actions and uses
Diflunisal is a NSAID based on aspirin but causing fewer gastrointestinal upsets than aspirin and having a much longer duration of action such that twice daily dosing is permissible. The section on NSAIDs (p. 250) should be consulted for a full account of its actions.

In practice diflunisal is used in the treatment of:

- rheumatoid arthritis and osteoarthritis
- other inflammatory pain associated with acute or chronic injury
- postoperative pain.

Dosage
Adults only: dosage range is 250–500 mg twice daily and, on occasions, up to 500 mg three times daily.

Nursing implications

- As a result of a possible link, however remote, with Reye's syndrome (a serious neurological condition), all aspirin-like drugs or salicylates should be avoided in children under 12 years.
- For an account of the nursing implications generally, see the section on NSAIDs (p. 250).
- **Note** the relatively high incidence of skin rashes (occasionally severe) associated with diflunisal.

Storage
Diflunisal tablets are stored at room temperature.

DIGOXIN (Lanoxin)

Presentation
Tablets – 62.5 microgram (0.0625 mg), 125 microgram (0.125 mg) and 250 microgram (0.25 mg)
Injection – 100 microgram (0.1 mg) in 1 ml, 500 microgram (0.5 mg) in 2 ml
Oral elixir – 50 microgram (0.05 mg) in 1 ml delivered using the oral pipette provided

Actions and uses
Digoxin is a cardiac glycoside based on a natural substance (digitalis) which was first isolated from the common foxglove plant over two centuries ago. It is renowned for its stimulant action on myocardial contractility (its positive inotropic effect) for which it is now, however, little used with the exception of the few patients with heart failure who remain severely symptomatic on standard first-line therapy (usually consisting of a diuretic plus ACE inhibitor).

Digoxin has an important action also on the rate of conduction of impulses between the atrium and left ventricle of the heart in that it suppresses conduction across the atrioventricular (AV) node. This action (described as a negative chronotropic effect) results in its use mainly in the treatment of atrial fibrillation in which it reduces the ventricular response to a too rapid atrial beat, so maintaining an effective cardiac output.

Digoxin is therefore now rarely used in patients who are in sinus rhythm.

Dosage

In acute atrial fibrillation requiring rapid control, digoxin may be administered in an initial 'loading' dose in order to hasten its onset of action. The loading dose may be administered by the oral or intravenous (but never the intramuscular) routes depending upon the degree of urgency.

Emergency intravenous loading dose (adults): 250–500 microgram administered over 10–20 minutes under ECG monitoring repeated every 4–8 hours according to the response to a maximum total dose of 1000 microgram. Alternatively 750–1000 microgram may be administered by IV infusion over 2–4 hours.

A safer, oral loading dose for adults is 250–500 microgram in three doses 8-hourly for 24 hours.

Adult maintenance doses are in the range 62.5–500 microgram as a single daily dose depending upon age and renal function.

Ultimately the maintenance dose is dependent upon plasma digoxin concentration which should be in the range 1.2–2.6 nanomol or 1–2 microgram per litre depending upon the units normally expressed by the biochemistry laboratory.

Children's dosages (guide only)

- <1 year, loading dose 20 microgram/kg 8-hourly (oral); maintenance 10 microgram/kg daily.
- 1–5 years, loading 200 microgram 8-hourly (oral), maintenance 10 microgram/kg daily.
- 6–12 years, loading 375 microgram 8-hourly (oral), maintenance 250 microgram per day.

Nursing implications

The nurse's role in monitoring patients on digoxin therapy is particularly important for two reasons.

1. Non-cardiac side effects (see below) are most likely to be observed by the nurse and therefore warning may be given and the dose changed before life-threatening complications arise.
2. The nurse has an active role to play in the day-to-day manipulation of drug dosage. It is generally accepted that digoxin should be withheld, at least until medical staff are consulted, if the apical pulse rate is less than 55 per minute.

   - Other symptoms of excessive dosage include sudden loss of appetite, diarrhoea, nausea and vomiting or the appearance of yellow-green halo-like visual disturbances.
   - Gynaecomastia may be a particularly disturbing side effect which arises as a result of the sex steroid-like structure of digoxin.
   - Cardiac side effects include bradycardia (already mentioned) but progressing if unnoticed to heart block, paroxysmal atrial tachycardia and ventricular arrhythmias of any kind.
   - Note that the frail and elderly are most likely to have reduced renal function (digoxin is excreted unchanged by the kidney) and are therefore most at risk from toxicity. Lower standard doses are generally required in such patients.
   - As hypokalaemia predisposes to toxicity, diuretics used with digoxin should be potassium sparing or potassium supplements should also be given.

Storage

- Digoxin preparations are stored in a dry place at room temperature.
- The drug should be protected from light.
- Oral elixir must never be diluted for ease of administration. Digoxin is poorly soluble and such dilutions are likely to contain precipitate.

D

- Intravenous infusions (emergency loading dosage regimen only) are prepared in glucose 5% or sodium chloride 0.9% minibags, 50–100 ml.

DIHYDROCODEINE (DF 118, DHC Continus)

Presentation
Tablets – 30 mg, 40 mg
Tablets, sustained release (Continus) – 60 mg, 90 mg, 120 mg
Elixir – 10 mg in 5 ml
Injection – 50 mg in 1 ml

Actions and uses
Dihydrocodeine is an opioid analgesic used in the treatment of moderate to severe pain. It is not as potent as morphine and certain of the other potent opioids and has a clear maximum or ceiling dose above which further pain relief is unlikely to be achieved. It is often a useful short-term measure when analgesia greater than that provided by paracetamol or low-dose codeine plus aspirin or paracetamol combinations is required. However, more potent analgesics may often be necessary, when persevering with a drug such as this is wholly unjustified.

Dihydrocodeine (alone or in combination with paracetamol and/or a NSAID) is often a useful short-term measure in controlling postoperative pain, especially associated with relatively minor procedures.

Dosage
Adults.

- Orally: 30 mg 4–6 hourly or 40–80 mg 8-hourly as required using conventional tablets or 60–120 mg 12-hourly in sustained-release form.
- By intramuscular or deep subcutaneous injection: up to 50 mg repeated 4–6 hourly as required.

Children >4 years: by any route, up to 1 mg/kg body weight repeated 4–6 hourly as required.

Nursing implications
- As an opioid drug of moderate potency, dihydrocodeine commonly causes sedation, confusion, constipation and nausea.
- Note that as a result of its abuse potential, injection is classified as a Controlled Drug and must comply with special ordering, storage and administration regulations.

Storage
- Oral preparations of dihydrocodeine are stored at room temperature and protected from light.
- Injection ampoules are stored at room temperature in a double-locked Controlled Drug cupboard.

DIHYDROTACHYSTEROL (AT 10)

Presentation
Oral solution – 250 microgram/ml in 15 ml oral ampoules

Actions and uses
This drug is a highly potent metabolite of vitamin D or calciferol (discussed on p. 388) which is used principally in the treatment of hypocalcaemic tetany associated with hypoparathyroidism.

Dosage
Adults only: 750–1250 microgram per day initially depending on the age of the patient and the severity of the disorder. The dosage should subsequently be adjusted (after a few days) according to individual needs.

Nursing implications
See the section on Calciferol (p. 388) but bear in mind the marked potency of this drug compared to calciferol.

Storage
- Dihydrotachysterol liquid is stored at room temperature.
- Protect from light.

DILTIAZEM (Adizem, Britiazim, Dilzem, Slozem, Tildiem)

Presentation
Tablets – 60 mg
Capsules (sustained release) – 60 mg,
90 mg, 120 mg, 180 mg, 200 mg,
240 mg, 300 mg
Tablets (sustained release) – 90 mg,
120 mg

Actions and uses
Diltiazem blocks the movement of calcium into cardiac muscle and vascular smooth muscle cells, an action which explains its description as a 'calcium channel blocker' or calcium antagonist and which results in reduced muscle activity or tone. Thus cardiac muscle cells become less excitable, with consequent reduction in heart work and atrioventricular (AV) nodal conduction. At higher doses, peripheral vasodilatation occurs with reduction in vascular resistance and a fall, therefore, in blood pressure.

As a result of the above, diltiazem is used in the treatment of angina pectoris and hypertension.

Dosage
The total adult daily dose is widely variable from 180 to 480 mg daily. Dose and frequency depend upon the nature of the preparation prescribed and may be taken once, twice or three times in the day.

Nursing implications
- The introduction over the years of a bewildering range of diltiazem preparations has created major confusion among patients and doctors alike. This is exemplified by the description of standard, slow and even slower release products; see above. In fact, it should not be assumed that all preparations which are labelled slow or sustained release are biologically equivalent.
- To avoid confusion, therefore, it is strongly recommended that diltiazem be prescribed as a recognized branded product so that patients will receive consistency in terms of bioavailability and activity. Nurses may find themselves in the position whereby they must promote rationalization of therapy and reassure patients accordingly.
- Diltiazem depresses cardiac function and care should be exercised when it is prescribed with other cardiac depressant drugs (e.g. beta-blockers). Note that digoxin also depresses AV nodal conduction.
- Patients with mild bradycardia or a prolonged P-R interval on ECG should be carefully monitored.
- The heart rate should be carefully monitored in elderly patients and those with kidney and/or liver impairment.
- Diltiazem should not be used in patients with advanced heart block, sick sinus syndrome or severe bradycardia.
- The peripheral vasodilator effect of diltiazem may manifest as flushing, dizziness, headache and ankle oedema, but patients should be reassured that such effects will rapidly diminish during continued treatment.

Storage
- Diltiazem tablets and capsules may be stored at room temperature.
- Note that slow-release tablets, if scored, can be halved only. Otherwise slow- or modified-release products must not be crushed or dissolved for ease of administration. If in doubt, seek advice from the pharmacy.

DIPYRIDAMOLE (Persantin)

Presentation
Tablets – 25 mg, 100 mg, 200 mg slow-release

Actions and uses
Dipyridamole is both an inhibitor of platelet aggregation and a direct vasodilator. It has in the past been used as a coronary vasodilator but is now more likely to be administered in conjunction with aspirin as an antithrombotic agent since both drugs

D

block platelet plugging by mechanisms which are complementary. Traditionally, dipyridamole has had a role in preventing thrombotic episodes in patients who have received prosthetic heart valves. More recently, a large-scale European stroke prevention study (designated ESPSII) has shown substantial benefit in terms of cerebral reinfarction or mortality from stroke when dipyridamole was given together with low-dose aspirin. As a result, it is possible that increasing emphasis will be placed on the role of dipyridamole in stroke prevention.

Dosage

To decrease platelet aggregation, 100 mg taken 3–4 times daily.
Stroke: 200 g twice daily SR capsules

Nursing implications

- Since it is a peripheral vasodilator, treatment may (at least in the early stages) be associated with postural dizziness, flushing and headache.
- Other side effects, which include skin rash, gastric upset and diarrhoea, are relatively uncommon.

Storage

Dipyridamole tablets are stored at room temperature.

DISOPYRAMIDE (Dirythmin SA, Rythmodan)

Presentation

Capsules – 100 mg, 150 mg
Tablets, slow release – 150 mg, 250 mg
Injection – 50 mg in 5 ml

Actions and uses

Disopyramide has a number of effects on the heart muscle and the conducting tissues of the heart, which make it useful in the treatment of the supraventricular and ventricular tachyarrhythmias. These effects are:

- prolongation of the refractory period of cardiac muscle
- decrease in excitability of cardiac muscle
- decrease in conduction velocity.

Dosage

- Intravenously: 2 mg/kg body weight given over 5 minutes (to a maximum of 150 mg irrespective of body weight) followed by maintenance IV infusion at a dosing rate 400 microgram (0.4 mg/kg)/h, to a maximum of 800 mg in 24 hours.
- Oral dose range for adults is 300–800 mg/day divided into 3–4 equal doses.
- Alternatively, an oral dose of 250–450 mg twice daily may be given using slow-release tablets.
- Seek specialist advice if use in children is contemplated.

Nursing implications

- Disopyramide has pronounced anticholinergic side effects and its use may result in typical symptoms such as dry mouth, blurred vision and urinary retention, the latter being especially important in elderly men, particularly those with prostatism.
- Nausea, diarrhoea and dizziness may also occur.
- Heart failure may be precipitated in patients with poor left ventricular function.
- Serious rhythm disturbances may occur in patients who develop hypokalaemia or heart block.
- Too rapid intravenous injection may cause profuse sweating.

Storage

- Disopyramide capsules, tablets and injections are stored at room temperature.
- When administered by intravenous infusion, the injection solution is added to sodium chloride, glucose or compound sodium lactate/ Ringer's solution.

DOBUTAMINE (Dobutrex)

Presentation

Injection – 250 mg vials

Actions and uses

Dobutamine is an inotropic drug which stimulates heart muscle indirectly, i.e. it causes release of noradrenaline leading to an increase in the force of myocardial contractility and hence improved cardiac output. It is administered by continuous intravenous infusion in the treatment of low-output heart failure (cardiogenic shock), the commonest cause of which is a major heart attack complicated by extensive loss of myocardial function. Inotropes of this type are used as a means of providing circulatory support during recovery in the intensive care period.

Dosage

Dosage varies from 2.5 to 10 microgram/kg/min and up to 40 microgram/kg/min in severe cases.

Nursing implications

Note that tachycardia and acute elevation of blood pressure may indicate excessive dosage. Staff should be informed accordingly.

Storage

- Dobutamine injection is stored at room temperature.
- Injection solution is reconstituted by adding water for injections or glucose 5% to the vial.
- Reconstituted solution may be stored in a refrigerator for up to 48 hours or at room temperature for 6 hours.
- This solution is further diluted by addition to solutions of sodium chloride, dextrose, dextrose/saline, or compound sodium lactate injection.
- Infusion solutions must be used within 24 hours of preparation; they may develop a slight pink discolouration which does not necessarily indicate an alteration in potency.

DOCUSATE SODIUM (Dioctyl)

Presentation

Tablets – 100 mg
Syrup – 12.5 mg in 5 ml, 50 mg in 5 ml

Actions and uses

Docusate is a stool softener which exerts a mild laxative effect. Its action

on dry impacted stools results in increased fluid uptake, stool mobility and defecation. Docusate is therefore used mainly in the treatment of constipation, often in combination with a stimulant laxative (e.g. co-danthrusate is such an example). Very occasionally, ear drops containing docusate have been used to aid the removal of ear wax.

Dosage

Adults: up to 600 mg per day in three divided doses.
Children:

- infants: up to 37.5 mg per day in three divided doses
- older children: up to 75 mg per day in three divided doses.

The syrup may be given by the rectal route as an enema:

- adults: 15–40 ml
- children: 7.5–15 ml
- infants: 5–10 ml (above doses as syrup 12.5 mg in 5 ml).

Nursing implications

- The action of docusate is purely physical and localized in the gut. There are few if any problems associated with its use.
- Oral preparations act within 1–2 days.
- For an optimum effect, doses should be taken with plenty of fluid.
- Note that the oral liquid is sugar free which may have important implications for treating diabetic patients.

Storage

Preparations containing docusate sodium are stored at room temperature.

DOMPERIDONE (Motilium)

Presentation

Tablets   10 mg
Suspension – 5 mg in 5 ml
Suppositories – 30 mg

Actions and uses

Domperidone has similar actions and uses to metoclopramide, though it does not produce the same degree of side effects in CNS and is often preferred, especially for younger patients, as a result. It has two main uses.

- As an antiemetic. This action results from increased upper gut motility coupled with inhibition of the chemoreceptor trigger zone (CTZ). The CTZ is located in the floor of the fourth ventricle in the brain and acts as an important stimulant to the vomiting reflex.
- Treatment of dyspepsia associated with gastrooesophageal reflux disease. This action is a direct result of increased oesophageal and gastric motility and hence clearance of the gastric contents.

Dosage

Adults: 10–20 mg every 6–8 hours by the oral route or 60 mg rectally every 6–8 hours.

Children: use is confined to treatment of emesis associated with cancer chemotherapy or radiotherapy. The rectal route is used with dosage based on body weight: 10–15 kg (15 mg twice daily); up to 25 kg (30 mg twice daily); up to 35 kg (30 mg three times daily); over 35 kg (30 mg four times daily).

Nursing implications

- In the treatment of dyspeptic symptoms (e.g. heartburn), it is advisable to take the medication half an hour before meals and on retiring at night.
- For treatment of emesis in children, suppositories can be cut (lengthwise) to provide 15 mg dose.
- While it is generally considered that this drug produces few, if any, side effects, patients should nevertheless be carefully assessed for occurrence of the typical dystonic reactions associated most often with metoclopramide (see p. 220).
- Children are very sensitive to metoclopramide-induced dystonic reactions, hence the restriction of domperidone to control nausea and vomiting (see Dosage section above).

Storage

- Preparations containing domperidone are stored at room temperature.
- Do not store suppositories close to a heat source – they will readily melt.

E

EFORMOTEROL (Foradil, Oxis)

Presentation
Inhalation therapy – 6 and 12 microgram as Turbohaler or 12 microgram capsules for use in a breath-actuated inhaler device.

Actions and uses
Eformoterol is a direct-acting bronchodilator of the sympathetic beta-2 agonist type which combines the rapid onset (10–15 minutes) of salbutamol or terbutaline with a long duration (12 hours) of action. In the latter context it resembles other long-acting bronchodilators such as salmeterol.

Eformoterol is indicated when a bronchodilator with this action profile is warranted (i.e. prolonged action, regular use) in the management of asthma or reversible chronic obstructive pulmonary disease.

Dosage
Eformoterol is currently only licensed for use in adults but this may change in time. Dosage may be taken once daily (e.g. to cover overnight wheeze) or twice daily to provide permanent cover against wheeze in brittle patients.

Unit dose is 6–12 microgram (using the Turbohaler) or 12–24 microgram using the breath-actuated device.

Nursing implications
- Eformoterol is likely to be associated with the side effects reported with rapid-onset short-acting beta-2 agonists and the section on Salbutamol should be consulted (p. 325).
- Due to its long duration of action, any side effects may persist even if treatment is withdrawn.
- Patients should be advised not to take eformoterol for the relief of acute attacks and always comply with the dose prescribed and the manufacturer's instructions.
- If the prescribed dose of inhaled eformoterol does not relieve symptoms, the advice of a doctor should be sought immediately.

Storage
Eformoterol inhaler devices are stored at room temperature. They should not be stored in a moist environment such as a bathroom cabinet.

ENALAPRIL (Innovace)

Presentation
Tablets – 2.5 mg, 5 mg, 10 mg, 20 mg

Actions and uses
See section on ACE Inhibitors (p. 4). In practice, enalapril is licensed for use in the following situations:

- chronic heart failure
- essential or renovascular hypertension
- secondary prevention after myocardial infarction or in at-risk patients with poor left ventricular function.

Dosage
Adult dose range is 2.5–20 mg as a single daily dose. Lower dosage is used initially and even up to 40 mg may be required in the treatment of cardiac failure.

Nursing implications
See section on ACE Inhibitors
(p. 4).

Storage
Enalapril tablets are stored at room temperature.

E | EPIRUBICIN (Pharmorubicin)

Presentation
Injection – 10 mg, 20 mg, 50 mg

Actions and uses
Epirubicin is a cytotoxic drug and a member of the anthracycline group of antibiotics. Although possessing antibacterial activity, it is used in practice for its antitumour action. In this respect it resembles other anthracyclines, daunorubicin and doxorubicin, but is generally better tolerated and somewhat safer than these agents. Its uses to date have included the management of breast, ovarian, lung, gastric and colorectal cancers and lymphomas, leukaemias and multiple myeloma.

Dosage
This is largely determined by specific indication and current dosage regimens which may change from time to time. The existing schedule should be consulted for up-to-date details of dosage and route of administration.

It is administered by the intravesicular route under specialist supervision in the treatment of transitional cell carcinoma of the bladder.

Injection vials are reconstituted using water for injections or sodium chloride 5 ml to each 10 mg of epirubicin and administered as a slow intravenous bolus injection over 3–5 minutes directly into the drip tubing of a running IV saline infusion. Alternatively, a rapid IV infusion in saline solution may be given over 30 minutes.

Nursing implications
- The two prominent adverse effects of the anthracycline antibiotics, particularly during prolonged use, are:
  1. bone marrow suppression
  2. serious cardiotoxicity.
  These require close monitoring of bone marrow and cardiac function.
- Reversible hair loss is very common, as are gastrointestinal upsets, hyperpyrexia and mucositis presenting a week or more after dosing.
- **Note**: this drug is irritant – avoid extravasation and report leakage from vein to surrounding tissues immediately.
- Nurses should be aware of the risks posed by cytotoxic drugs. Some are irritant to the skin and mucous surfaces and care must be exercised when handling them. In particular, spillage or contamination of personnel or the environment must be avoided. If cytotoxic drugs are handled regularly, it is theoretically possible that repeated skin contact or inhalation may produce systemic toxic effects in nurses who have developed hypersensitivity to them. Most hospitals now operate a centralized (pharmacy-organized) additive service. While this reduces the risk of exposure to cytotoxic drugs, it is essential that nurses recognize and understand the local policy on their safe handling and disposal. The Health and Safety Executive has decreed that such a policy should be in place wherever cytotoxic drugs are administered. These should be adapted, wherever possible, to care of patients in the community.

Storage
- Epirubicin vials are stored at room temperature but exposure to direct sunlight should be avoided.
- Reconstituted solutions retain their chemical stability for up to 48 hours if stored in a refrigerator or 24 hours at room temperature.

EPOETIN (Eprex, Recormon)

Presentation
Injection – 1000, 2000, 4000, 5000 and 10 000 IU vials or prefilled syringes

Actions and uses
Epoetin is recombinant alpha or beta human erythropoietin, i.e. forms of a natural hormone which is produced by genetic biotechnology. Erythropoietin is a protein normally present in low concentrations in plasma which is largely produced as a result of the action of a renal enzyme (erythrogenin) on a plasma protein or preformed and released directly by the kidney. It acts on the bone marrow to stimulate production of erythrocytes and so maintains circulating haemoglobin levels which adequately oxygenate the tissues of the body.

Anaemia as a result of erythropoietin deficiency occurs in chronic renal failure and is associated with significant morbidity, despite the fact that a small proportion (10–15%) of the protein is normally produced by the liver. Replacement therapy is therefore indicated for patients with anaemia of chronic renal failure sufficiently severe to require renal dialysis and other patients with severe symptoms of anaemia though not yet receiving dialysis. Alpha and beta forms are equally active and indeed are interchangeable.

Dosage
- Erythropoietin is usually administered by subcutaneous injection but may also be given by the intravenous route over 2 minutes.
- Dialysis patients: initially 20–50 units/kg body weight three times weekly, increased according to response in increments of 20–25 units/kg at intervals of 4 weeks up to a maximum of 600 units/kg weekly. Once Hb 10–12 g/dl (10–12 g/100 ml) is reached maintenance doses as low as 20–50 units twice weekly can be used.
- Severe symptomatic anaemia in patients not yet requiring dialysis: as above by subcutaneous injection.

Nursing implications
- An influenza-like syndrome is reported in some patients as a result of hypersensitivity, especially when intravenous injections are administered too quickly.
- A dose-dependent rise in blood pressure can occur and may be hazardous for patients with existing hypertension, if poorly controlled. Hypertensive encephalopathy and tonic-clonic convulsions have been reported. Blood pressure must be carefully monitored in all patients.
- There may also be a dose-related rise in blood platelets during the early treatment stage and shunt thrombosis may arise in patients who are prone to complications with arteriovenous shunts.
- Other side effects include hyperkalaemia, raised creatinine, urea and phosphate, skin reactions and palpebral oedema denoting possible allergy to epoetin. Myocardial infarction and anaphylaxis are rare but severe untoward events.
- Note that no more than 1 ml should be administered at any one subcutaneous site.

Storage
- Both alpha and beta epoetin preparations must be stored in a refrigerator and protected from light.
- Alpha epoetin is ready mixed and unpreserved. No more than one dose should therefore be administered from each vial.
- Beta epoetin is diluted and used immediately. Do not mix with any other drug.

ERGOTAMINE (Migril, Cafergot)

NB: These preparations contain ergotamine in combination with caffeine.

Presentation

Tablets – 1 mg and 2 mg
Inhaler – 0.36 mg in each metered dose
Suppositories – 2 mg

Actions and uses

Migraine classically causes severe, throbbing, unilateral headache associated with a change in cerebral perfusion. Ergotamine in clinical practice is found to be effective in the treatment of this condition as it reverses the changes in cerebral vasculature which result in dilatation and the migraine headache.

Dosage

Orally: 1 or 2 mg repeated every 30 minutes until relief is obtained to a maximum of 6 mg in a day and 12 mg in any one week.
Rectally: 2 mg at the onset of an attack, repeated half-hourly to a total of 6 mg per day or 12 mg per week.
Inhalation: one dose repeated after 5 minutes if required to a total of six doses per day or 15 doses per week.

Nursing implications

- If ergotamine is to be effective in the acute attack it should be administered as soon as possible after the onset of either the premonitory symptoms, if they occur, or the headache itself.
- This drug causes generalized vasoconstriction which may produce, in minor cases, coldness of the skin and limbs and in extreme cases gangrene.
- Other side effects include nausea, vomiting, diarrhoea, dizziness, ocular disturbance, muscular weakness, confusion, anxiety, drowsiness and convulsion.
- The drug should be used with great care in patients who suffer from heart diseases as it may produce angina, alter the blood pressure and alter the rhythm of the heart.
- It is important to stress to patients that they must never exceed the maximum advised doses.
- This drug should never be used during pregnancy as it will induce labour.

Storage

All forms of the drug are stored at room temperature.

ERYTHROMYCIN (Erythrocin, Erymax, Ilosone)

Presentation

Tablets – 250 mg, 500 mg
Capsules – 250 mg
Syrup – 125 mg in 5 ml, 250 mg in 5 ml, 500 mg in 5 ml
Injection – 1 g vials

Actions and uses

Erythromycin is an antibiotic with a mainly bacteriostatic action which inhibits growth by inhibiting bacterial protein synthesis. It is effective principally against Gram-negative organisms including staphylococci, streptococci and *Haemophilus influenzae* although resistance is regularly reported and may be a problem in practice. Erythromycin is often used as an alternative to penicillin in patients with known penicillin allergy. It is also used in the treatment of rare but serious infections due to mycoplasma, rickettsia, chlamydia and in the treatment of legionnaire's disease.

Dosage

Oral adult doses: from 250–500 mg and up to 2 g four times a day in severe infection.
Adult intravenous dose: 1 g 8-hourly in 250–500 ml sodium chloride 0.9% injection.
Children <2 years: usual oral dose 125 mg four times a day or 250 mg twice daily based on 30–50 mg/kg per day; 2–7 years, 125–250 mg orally four times a day; >7 years, as for lower adult range.
Intravenous doses in children: 25–50 mg/kg daily in 3–4 divided doses.

Nursing implications

- Mild and occasionally severe gastrointestinal upsets with nausea and vomiting, and diarrhoea may occur. This may be reduced by ensuring that doses are taken with meals.

- The estolate form of erythromycin (Ilosone) has been associated with liver injury which usually manifests as fever, pain and obstructive jaundice. This occurs only very rarely but it is recommended that the dosage of erythromycin estolate be reduced in patients with previously diagnosed liver disease.
- Erythromycin for intravenous administration should be in a final concentration of 1% (i.e. 10 mg per ml) or, for administration via a large vein, up to 5%.
- Erythromycin is a potent inhibitor of the liver's capacity to produce drug-metabolizing enzymes (i.e. the hepatic microsomal enzyme system). This has resulted in the marked potentiation of certain common drugs which are normally extensively metabolized by the liver during absorption and passage into the systemic circulation. This includes theophylline, warfarin and phenytoin. Extreme caution is therefore warranted when erythromycin is prescribed for any patient regularly taking drugs of this type since their sudden and severe toxicity might develop.

Storage

- Erythromycin preparations are stored at room temperature.
- Oral solutions should be used within 14 days of preparation.
- Intravenous erythromycin lactobionate is prepared by first adding water for injections to the vial before addition to the final infusion fluid.

ESMOLOL (Breviblock)

Presentation

Injection – 100 mg in 10 ml, 2.5 g in 10 ml

Actions and uses

Esmolol is a beta-blocker, the section on which should be consulted for a general account of these compounds. However, esmolol is notably different from other beta-blockers in that it has an ultra-short action and is administered only by continuous infusion. Esmolol is used perioperatively for short-term prevention and treatment of supraventricular arrhythmias (atrial fibrillation, atrial flutter and sinus tachycardia) and hypertension in at-risk patients. Because of its very rapid and total inactivation in the circulation, it is administered by continuous intravenous infusion when control is readily titrated against drip rate.

Dosage

Esmolol is administered under specialist supervision when the infusion rate is determined by the individual's response. The usual dose rate is in the range 50–200 microgram/kg/min.

Nursing implications

- See the section on Beta-blockers (p. 51).
- The dosing rate of esmolol is carefully adjusted throughout by patient response so that excessive beta-blockade should not occur.

Storage

- Esmolol injection is stored at room temperature and protected from light.
- Ampoules containing 100 mg in 10 ml are for use undiluted. The 2.5 g vial must be first diluted (5 g to 500 ml) to provide a final concentration of 10 mg in 1 ml. Sodium chloride and glucose injections or mixtures of these are used for dilution. Hartmann's lactated Ringer's solution can also be used but not sodium bicarbonate injection.

ESTRAMUSTINE (Estracyt)

Presentation

Capsules – 140 mg

Actions and uses

This drug is a combination of an oestrogenic substance (oestradiol) and a cytotoxic agent (mustine). It readily concentrates in prostatic tissue and is used for the treatment of cancer of the prostate, particularly when unresponsive to conventional oestrogenic treatment.

Dosage

The daily dose may vary from 140 mg to 1400 mg and it is usually divided to be taken with meals. An average dose is of the order of 560 mg.

E

Nursing implications

- Patients should be advised to take each dose at least 1 hour before or 2 hours after meals. Estramustine should not be taken with dairy products.
- Relatively common side effects include nausea, vomiting and diarrhoea.
- Thrombocytopenia with resultant increased risk of haemorrhage may occur with this drug.
- Other side effects include altered liver function, gynaecomastia and increased risk of myocardial infarction.
- This drug should not be prescribed for patients with active peptic ulcer disease and those with severe liver or cardiac disease.
- It should be used with great caution by patients who already have existing impairment of bone marrow function.
- Nurses should be aware of the risks posed by cytotoxic drugs. Some are irritant to the skin and mucous surfaces and care must be exercised when handling them. In particular, spillage or contamination of personnel or the environment must be avoided. If cytotoxic drugs are handled regularly, it is theoretically possible that repeated skin contact or inhalation may produce systemic toxic effects in nurses who have developed hypersensitivity to them. Most hospitals now operate a centralized (pharmacy-organized) additive service. While this reduces the risk of exposure to cytotoxic drugs, it is essential that nurses recognize and understand the local policy on their safe handling and disposal. The Health and Safety Executive has decreed that such a policy should be in place wherever cytotoxic drugs are administered. These should be adapted, wherever possible, to care of patients in the community.

Storage

Capsules of estramustine should be stored in a refrigerator.

ETHAMBUTOL (Myambutol)

Presentation

Tablets – 100 mg, 400 mg
NB: Ethambutol is often used in combination with isoniazid in the preparation Mynah.

Actions and uses

Ethambutol is an antibacterial drug which is of use only for the treatment of tuberculosis caused by the organism *Mycobacterium tuberculosis*. Its action may be either bacteriostatic (inhibiting growth and replication of the organism) or bacteriocidal (killing the organism), depending upon the concentration achieved in the tissues. If used on its own for the treatment of tuberculosis it will be, in a large number of cases, ineffective as the organism gradually develops resistance; hence its use in combination with other antituberculous drugs.

Dosage

For initial treatment and for prophylaxis against tuberculosis: a single daily oral dose of 25 mg/kg is recommended.
For maintenance treatment a single oral dose of 15 mg/kg body weight is recommended.

E

Nursing implications

- Patients undergoing treatment for tuberculosis receive their drugs for considerable periods of time. The nurse may play an important role in reminding patients that their drug therapy must be taken regularly for as long as recommended, whether or not they themselves feel that they have recovered.
- Ethambutol is generally well tolerated by most patients. Rare side effects include:
  - gastrointestinal upsets
  - an optic neuritis with visual disturbance including colour blindness to green and red. As early changes in visual acuity are largely subjective patients should be advised to report any visual disturbances
  - skin rashes
  - jaundice
  - peripheral neuritis
  - raised serum urate level (which may give rise to joint pain due to gout).
- It is recommended that ethambutol be used with caution by patients with impaired renal function, gout or reduced visual acuity. In this group, regular testing of visual acuity should be performed.

Storage

Ethambutol tablets are stored at room temperature and protected from light.

ETHOSUXIMIDE (Zarontin, Emeside)

Presentation

Capsules – 250 mg
Syrup – 250 mg in 5 ml

Actions and uses

Ethosuximide is a long-established anticonvulsant drug now used only occasionally in the treatment of epilepsy. Epilepsy can be summarized as an altered neurochemical state induced by defect or trauma which leads to an excessive amount of 'electrical' activity in the brain (seizure). It is, in fact, relatively common and, for management purposes, can be divided into a series of brain 'syndromes'. Ethosuximide has long had a role in the management of 'absence' seizures, known previously as 'petit mal' epilepsy, but it does occasionally have wider usage.

Dosage

NB: Individual dosage requirements vary greatly. The following doses are given as a guide only.
Adults: usual maintenance dose range is 1–1.5 g daily.
Children: initial dose is 250 mg in children less than 6 years and 500 mg in older children. The dose should thereafter be gradually increased until an optimum response is achieved.

Nursing implications

- Gastrointestinal upset including nausea, vomiting and anorexia commonly occur with this drug.
- Neurological effects are fairly common and include drowsiness, lethargy, euphoria, dizziness, headache and behavioural disorders such as restlessness, agitation, anxiety and aggression.
- Skin rashes and disorders of the blood may rarely occur.

Storage

Preparations containing ethosuximide are stored at room temperature and protected from light.

ETIDRONATE (Didronel)

Presentation

Tablets – 200 mg, 400 mg (combined with calcium in Didronel PMO)

Actions and uses

Etidronate is classed as a bisphosphonate or diphosphonate, a group of drugs which alter the metabolic activity of bone. Bone is metabolically very active, being constantly destroyed and rebuilt in a process known as remodelling which maintains fresh bone throughout life.

E

In some circumstances, however, the breakdown of bone (which is influenced by the activity of cells called osteoclasts) is relatively greater than new bone synthesis (which is influenced by cells called osteoblasts). Etidronate inhibits osteoclast activity and so redresses this balance.

Etidronate, by this action, inhibits the release of calcium from bone and is used therefore when this occurs excessively. Indications include the treatment of hypercalcaemia of malignancy, Paget's disease and to arrest osteoporosis after the menopause. The latter is the indication for Didronel PMO: it should be noted that in women, oestrogen produced by the ovary is important in stimulating bone synthesis. This is gradually lost once the menopause arrives as ovarian failure develops.

Dosage
Adults:

- Paget's disease: usually 5 mg/kg daily for up to 6 months.
- Osteoporosis: 400 mg is taken orally for 14 days then stopped. Calcium tablets are then taken daily throughout a cycle of 90 days (3 months approximately). The cycle may then be repeated.

Nursing implications
- The absorption of etidronate and indeed other bisphosphonates is very poor and reduced even further by the presence of food in the gut. It should therefore be taken at a time when the least amount of food is present, i.e. midway between meals. Antacids impair absorption and should not be taken at or around the same time.
- Gastrointestinal disturbances are often reported and etidronate should be used with caution in enterocolitis.

- Etidronate should not be used in the presence of severe renal impairment and kidney function should be monitored during treatment.
- A few patients with Paget's disease may complain of a transient increase or 'flare' in bone pain at pagetoid sites.

Storage
Etidronate tablets are stored at room temperature.

ETODOLAC (Lodine)

Presentation
Tablets – 200 mg, 600 mg sustained release
Capsules – 200 mg, 300 mg

Actions and uses
Etodolac is a member of the NSAID group. Consult the section on Non-Steroidal Antiinflammatory Drugs for an account (p. 250).

Dosage
Adults only: 200 mg twice daily or 400–600 mg may be taken as a single daily dose.

Nursing implications
- See the section on NSAIDs (p. 250).
- Etodolac is a relatively new drug and early impressions are that it produces a low incidence of gastrointestinal and renal disturbances.
- Nevertheless it is important that patients treated with this drug should be carefully monitored for any adverse effects.

Storage
Etodolac tablets and capsules are stored at room temperature.

F

FAMCICLOVIR (Famvir)

Presentation
Tablets – 125 mg, 250 mg, 750 mg

Actions and uses
After absorption this drug is converted in the body to its active metabolite, penciclovir. Its actions and uses are identical to those of aciclovir but its absorption and hence bioavailability are far greater so that adequate blood levels are achieved with less frequent oral dosing. Currently, famciclovir is licensed for the treatment of *Herpes zoster* (shingles) infection and acute and recurrent genital herpes infection.

Dosage
Adults only.
Shingles: 250 mg 8-hourly, reduced to 12-hourly in patients with moderate renal impairment (creatinine clearance 30–60 ml/min) or once daily in severe renal impairment. Alternatively, a single daily dose of 750 mg can be administered for 7 days.
Treatment of genital herpes infection: if first attack, 250 mg 8-hourly for 5 days or if recurrent attack, 125 mg 12-hourly for 5 days.
Suppression of genital herpes infection: 250 mg 12-hourly for 6–12 months then reassess need for continued treatment.

Nursing implications
- The nursing implications for aciclovir apply to this drug also.
- Famciclovir is generally well tolerated though a proportion of patients have complained of nausea and headache.

Storage
Store at room temperature.

FAMOTIDINE (Pepcid PM)

Presentation
Tablets – 20 mg, 40 mg

Actions and uses
Famotidine is one of the histamine H2-Receptor Antagonists, the actions and uses of which are described on p. 169.

Dosage
- Treatment of peptic ulcer: 40 mg at bedtime for up to 8 weeks. Prevention of relapse: usually a single bedtime dose of 20 mg which is taken continuously.
- Gastrooesophageal reflux disease (GORD): 20 mg twice daily for up to 3 months or double this dose if there is evidence of erosion or ulceration.
- Prevention of GORD recurrence: 20 mg twice daily.
- All the above are adult dosages.
- Famotidine is unlicensed in children.

Nursing implications
See Histamine H2-Receptor Antagonists (p. 169) for a full account.

Storage
Famotidine tablets are stored at room temperature.

FELBINAC (Traxam)

Topical gel – 3%
Topical foam – 3.17%

Actions and uses

Felbinac is a NSAID intended for topical application in the treatment of sprains and strains and soft tissue injury generally.

Dosage

A generous quantity (ideally 1 g) is applied to the affected site and rubbed in gently 2–4 times a day depending upon degree of severity. At the maximum dosage, a single 100 g tube should last for 4–5 days or more.

F

Nursing implications

- Although many side effects, most notably gastrointestinal upsets, are reported with systemic NSAID therapy, there is little likelihood of problems arising from topical use, unless overused.
- Mild local redness and eczema may occasionally occur and allergic contact dermatitis is a rare possibility.
- Caution is required in patients who react severely to aspirin and systemic NSAIDs (e.g. gastrointestinal bleeding, active ulceration and bronchospasm).

Storage

Felbinac gel and foam are stored at room temperature.

FELODIPINE (Plendil)

Tablets, modified release – 2.5 mg, 5 mg and 10 mg

Actions and uses

Felodipine is a Calcium Antagonist and has the actions and uses described for this group on p. 67.

Dosage

Adults only.
Hypertension: initial dose is as low as 2.5 mg once daily increased gradually according to response up to a maximum of 20 mg once daily above which further response is unlikely. Angina pectoris: initially 5 mg once daily in the morning increased, if necessary, to 10 mg once daily.

Nursing implications

- Patients should be advised to avoid grapefruit juice as drug absorption is greatly enhanced.
- See Calcium Antagonists (p. 67).

Storage

- Felodipine tablets are stored at room temperature.
- Do not crush for ease of administration.

FENBUFEN (Lederfren)

Presentation

Capsules – 300 mg
Tablets – 300 mg, 450 mg

Actions and uses

Fenbufen is a non-steroidal antiinflammatory drug and the section on NSAIDs (p. 250) should be consulted for a full account of its actions. In practice, fenbufen is used in the treatment of:

- rheumatoid arthritis
- osteoarthritis
- ankylosing spondylitis
- acute musculoskeletal and soft tissue injury.

Dosage

The usual adult dose is 600 mg at night and 300 mg in the morning or alternatively 450 mg taken twice daily. Fenbufen is not licensed for use in children.

Nursing implications

The section on NSAIDs (p. 250) should be consulted for a full account of the nursing implications which apply to this drug.

Storage

Fenbufen capsules and tablets are stored at room temperature.

FENOFIBRATE (Lipantil)

Presentation

Capsules – 100 mg, 200 mg (micronized)

Actions and uses

This is a lipid-lowering agent of the fibrate group (see Ciprofibrate, p. 93).

Dosage

Adults: initially 100 mg three times daily taken with food adjusted to the lowest maintenance dose once the blood lipid pattern is within the target range. Usual maintenance dose is in the range 200–400 mg daily in divided doses with food. Alternatively, a single 200 mg dose of a micronized capsule may be taken with the main meal of the day.

Children: as above using conventional capsules and based on 5 mg/kg body weight daily.

Nursing implications

- See under Ciprofibrate (p. 93).
- Fenofibrate is contraindicated in pregnancy and breastfeeding.

Storage

Store at room temperature and protect from excessive moisture.

FENOPROFEN (Fenopron)

Presentation

Tablets – 300 mg, 600 mg

Actions and uses

Fenoprofen is a non-steroidal antiinflammatory drug and the section on NSAIDs (p. 250) should be consulted for a full account of its actions. In practice, it is used in the treatment of:

- mild to moderate inflammatory pain
- rheumatoid arthritis
- osteoarthritis
- ankylosing spondylitis.

Dosage

The usual adult dose is 300–600 mg three or four times per day.

Nursing implications

- The section on NSAIDs (p. 250) should be consulted for a full account of the nursing implications which apply to this drug.

Storage

Fenoprofen tablets are stored at room temperature.

FENOTEROL (Berotec)

Presentation

Inhaler – 100 and 200 microgram/dose of metered aerosol

Actions and uses

This drug has a highly selective action on receptors in bronchial muscle, causing relaxation of muscle tone. It is used, therefore, for the treatment of reversible airways obstruction (bronchospasm) in asthma and other conditions such as bronchitis and emphysema.

Dosage

One or two inhalations (metered doses) three or four times a day or on an as-required basis to relieve wheeze.

Nursing implications

- Rarely this drug may cause palpitation, tachycardia, headache and fine muscle tremor.
- It should be used with care in patients suffering from heart disease, hypertension or hyperthyroidism.

Storage

The pressurized aerosol should be stored at room temperature. The container should never be punctured or incinerated at the end of use.

FENTANYL (Durogesic, Sublimaze)

Presentation

Transdermal patch – 25, 50, 75 and 100 microgram of drug released across the skin barrier per hour from a reservoir built into the patch

Injection – 100 microgram in 2 ml, 500 microgram in 10 ml

Actions and uses

Fentanyl is a rapid-onset, short-acting opioid (narcotic) analgesic (i.e. similar to morphine) which has two main uses in practice.

- Traditionally it has been administered by continuous IV infusion to reduce the dose of anaesthesia required at induction in patients who might otherwise poorly tolerate general anaesthesia at full dosage.
- More recently, it has found favour in the treatment of chronic pain when administered as a skin patch for transdermal systemic analgesia over a prolonged period. In this role, it may be used postoperatively or as an alternative to continuous administration of diamorphine by subcutaneous infusion in cancer patients intolerant of oral analgesic medication.

Nursing implications
- As an opioid drug, fentanyl may produce significant respiratory depression requiring oxygen therapy and, on occasion, the administration of the specific opioid antagonist drug naloxone. Caution is thus warranted in frail elderly patients.
- Other typical opioid side effects are possible but fentanyl is claimed to cause less constipation than is morphine. Nevertheless, concurrent treatment with laxatives is required during chronic treatment.
- The skin (transdermal) patch, once applied, may take up to 12–24 hours to achieve a significant skin depot from which systemic levels are achieved. Similarly, it may take at least as long for the intradermal depot to become depleted when the patch is removed.
- The above should be taken into account when commencing and stopping or changing analgesic therapy; transdermal fentanyl is not suitable for treatment of acute pain or breakthrough pain.
- Fentanyl for IV infusion is compatible with most commonly used intravenous infusion fluids (e.g. glucose and saline solutions).

Storage
- Store injection solution and transdermal patches in the Controlled Drugs cupboard at room temperature.
- Protect from light.
- Do not mix injection solution with intravenous barbiturates for basal anaesthesia.

FILGRASTIM (Neupogen)

Presentation
Injection – 30 million unit per ml in 1 ml and 1.6 ml liquid in vial or prefilled syringe

Actions and uses
Filgrastim is one of a series of human sequence granulocyte-colony stimulating factors (G-CSF) prepared by recombinant DNA technology and not derived from a human source as such. G-CSF stimulates the production by bone marrow of white blood cells called neutrophils which may become deficient (resulting in a state known as neutropenia) as a result of bone marrow suppression. Neutropenia is a frequent dose-limiting, potentially fatal, side effect of many cancer chemotherapy regimens since it predisposes to unprotected infection by even the most innocuous of organisms. Neutropenia may also be congenital in origin.

G-CSF therefore permits much more aggressive use of cancer chemotherapy without fear of the consequences which might arise as a result of marrow depression. Indeed, it permits complete ablation of bone marrow prior to bone marrow transplantation such is the degree to which it stimulates production of new white cells by the reseeded recipient marrow tissue.

Dosage
In cytotoxic-induced neutropenia, filgrastim is administered by subcutaneous injection or intravenous

infusion in a dose 500 000 (½ million) unit per kg daily.

Check local treatment regimens for use in other indications.

Nursing implications

- Hypersensitivity reactions to injections of filgrastim are not uncommon and vary in their severity. They include muscle aches and pains, hypotension, vasculitis, skin rash, proteinuria and changes in liver function.
- A fall in blood platelets (thrombocytopenia) may occur and may be associated with bleeding from the nose and urinary tract, for example.
- Headaches, gastrointestinal upsets and alopecia are also reported.
- There is a risk of tumour growth if administered to patients with tumours of a 'myeloid' (white blood cell) characteristic. Treatment must be immediately discontinued in the event of a leucocytosis (increased production of white cells in excess of normal).
- Administer intravenously over 30 minutes or continuously in glucose 5% injection.
- If concentration of IV infusion is <1.5 mega unit (15 microgram/ml), add albumin solution (to prevent adsorption onto the infusion system) to a final concentration of 2 mg/ml.
- Do not dilute to a final concentration <200 000 unit (2 microgram)/ml.
- DO NOT dilute in sodium chloride solution.

Storage

- Store in a refrigerater.
- Do not freeze. The pack is fitted with a 'freezer indicator' which, if showing red, indicates that it SHOULD NOT be used.

FINASTERIDE (Proscar)

Presentation

Tablets – 5 mg

Actions and uses

Growth of the prostate gland and hence prostatic hypertrophy is dependent upon the conversion of testosterone to its more active metabolite, dihydrotestosterone, within the gland itself by the action of an enzyme, 5-alpha reductase. Finasteride is a potent inhibitor of 5-alpha reductase; it consequently prevents the formation of the active metabolite without interfering with testosterone directly and as a result reduces the gland size in benign prostatic hypertrophy.

Dosage

A single daily dose of 5 mg is taken for a prolonged period of up to 6 months before being reassessed. If a positive response is obtained continuous treatment thereafter is indicated.

Nursing implications

- Patients who do not respond to the above dosage are unlikely to respond to increasingly higher doses and treatment should be abandoned if initially unsuccessful.
- This drug may affect male sexual function. Impotence, decreased libido and reduced volume of ejaculate are reported in up to 5% of patients.
- Finasteride is otherwise well tolerated and does not appear to interact with other drugs.
- The drug is of no benefit in the treatment of prostatic cancer, which should be excluded at the outset and reassessed during treatment.
- Nurses should avoid handling broken or crushed tablets as, theoretically, transcutaneous absorption can occur. This poses particular problems for nurses who are either pregnant or of child-bearing age.

Storage

Finasteride tablets are stored at room temperature and protected from light.

F

Presentation
Tablets – 200 mg

Actions and uses
This drug has an anticholinergic action associated with reduction in tone of the urinary bladder. In practice, it is used for the treatment of disorders associated with spasm of the smooth muscle of the lower urinary tract including treatment of dysuria, urgency, nocturia and painful spasm of the bladder due to catheterization or cystoscopy.

Dosage
200 mg three times a day in adults.

Nursing implications
- Due to its anticholinergic action, flavoxate produces dry mouth and blurred vision and should not be used in patients who suffer from glaucoma.
- It is contraindicated in patients who have gastrointestinal obstruction.
- Other relatively common side effects include nausea, headache and fatigue.

Storage
Flavoxate tablets are stored at room temperature.

FLUCLOXACILLIN (Floxapen)

Presentation
Capsules – 250 mg, 500 mg
Syrup – 125 mg in 5 ml, 250 mg in 5 ml
Injection – vials containing 250 mg, 500 mg and 1 g

Actions and uses
Flucloxacillin is a member of the penicillin group of antibiotics. Its spectrum of action is relatively narrow, however, so that it is used mainly in the treatment of infections due to Gram-positive Streptococcus, especially *Strep. aureus* and *Strep. epidermidis*. Examples include infections of the skin and soft tissue, bone, the respiratory tract and staphylococcal endocarditis.

Penicillin antibiotics are rapidly bactericidal as a result of their ability to inhibit bacterial wall synthesis so that affected organisms are rapidly lysed (ruptured) during their growth phase.

Dosage
Adults.

- Orally: 250–1000 mg four times a day. In serious infection (e.g. endocarditis) 2 g 4-hourly is used.
- Intramuscular or intravenous: as for oral route.
- Intrapleural and intraarticular: 250–500 mg per day.

Children.

- Less than 2 years: one-quarter of the adult dose.
- Over 2 years: one-half of the adult dose.

Nursing implications
- See the section on Penicillin V (p. 275).
- Injections are prepared as follows.
  - Intramuscular injection: vials should be diluted with 1.5–2 ml of water for injection.
  - Intravenous injection: 1 g should be dissolved in 20 ml of water for injection and either given directly over 3–4 minutes or added to 0.9% sodium chloride, 5% dextrose or dextrose/saline mixtures and infused over 4–6 hours.
  - Intraarticular or intrapleural injection: vials should be diluted with 5–10 ml of water for injection.

Storage
- Preparations containing flucloxacillin are stored at room temperature.
- Once reconstituted, injection solution is used immediately or stored in a fridge for up to 24 hours.
- Once reconstituted, the syrup should be used within 7 days.

FLUCONAZOLE (Diflucan)

Presentation

Capsules – 50 mg, 200 mg
Oral suspension – 50 mg in 5 ml,
200 mg in 5 ml
Injection – 50 mg in 25 ml, 200 mg in
100 ml

Actions and uses

Fluconazole (like itraconazole) is a
member of the triazole group of
antifungals which selectively inhibit
fungal synthesis of ergosterol, an
essential component of the cell wall.
Thus leakage of cell contents and
eventual death of the fungus follow.
In practice, fluconazole is used in the
treatment of:

- acute and recurring vaginal candida
  infection
- oral candidiasis and oropharyngeal
  and oesophageal candidiasis
- bronchopulmonary candida
  infections
- systemic candidiasis
- tinea pedis, tinea corporis, tinea
  cruris, tinea versicolor and dermal
  candida infections
- cryptococcal infection including
  meningitis and pulmonary and
  cutaneous infections
- urinary candidiasis
- prevention of opportunistic fungal
  infections in immunocompromised
  patients.

Dosage

Adults.

- Vaginal candidiasis: oral 150 mg
  single dose.
- Mucosal candidiasis: oral 50 mg
  once daily for 1–2 weeks.
- Denture-related candida infection:
  oral 50 mg once daily for 2 weeks in
  combination with oral antiseptic use.
- Systemic (disseminated) candida
  infection: 400 mg initially then
  200–400 mg once daily until clinical
  recovery. May require treatment for
  2 months or longer in cryptococcal
  meningitis infection. Intravenous
  therapy in acutely ill patients.
- Prevention of relapse of
  cryptococcal meningitis in AIDS
  patients: 100–200 mg orally once
  daily may be administered
  indefinitely.

- Prevention of fungal infections in
  'at-risk' or immunocompromised
  groups: 50–100 mg once daily
  orally.
- Tinea and dermal candida
  infections: 50 mg once daily orally
  for up to 6 weeks.

Children: daily doses of up to 12 mg/kg
have been administered with a
maximum 400 mg/day but experience
in children is generally limited.

Nursing implications

- The only common side effect of
  this drug is mild gastrointestinal
  upset (discomfort, nausea,
  diarrhoea).
- Since fluconazole is excreted
  mainly unchanged in the urine
  the dosage interval should be
  prolonged to 48 and 72 hourly
  in patients with moderate and
  severe renal impairment.
  Patients on haemodialysis
  should receive their daily dose
  immediately after dialysis is
  completed.
- Fluconazole potentiates
  warfarin and the oral
  hypoglycaemic (antidiabetic)
  drugs, e.g. chlorpropamide,
  glibenclamide. Close monitoring
  is therefore required to detect
  any increased bleeding or the
  development of hypoglycaemia
  in patients on warfarin and oral
  antidiabetic drugs.
- Concurrent use with phenytoin
  may lead to accumulation and
  phenytoin intoxication.
- Fluconazole significantly
  increases serum levels of
  cyclosporin in patients who
  have undergone renal
  transplantation.

Storage

- Fluconazole capsules, oral
  suspension and injection solution
  are all stored at room temperature.
- Once reconstituted, the oral
  suspension should be refrigerated if
  possible and used within 2 weeks.
- Injection solution is administered
  intravenously undiluted but, if
  required, it can be mixed with

F

common solutions containing sodium chloride and glucose.

FLUDARABINE (Fludara)

Presentation
Injection – 50 mg vial

Actions and uses
This drug is a cytotoxic which inhibits the synthesis of DNA by a complex action on cellular enzyme processes leading ultimately to failure of cell division and inhibition of cellular protein in the growth phase. Fludarabine is used in the treatment of B-cell chronic lymphocytic leukaemia (CLL) unresponsive to first-line treatment with cytotoxic regimens which include an alkylating agent.

Dosage
Check existing cytotoxic dosage schedules in use in the unit concerned. Fludarabine has been administered by intravenous injection in a dose of $25 mg/m^2$ on 5 consecutive days per monthly cycle, usually for six cycles.

Nursing implications
- Common side effects include fever, chills, weakness, malaise, oedema, skin rashes, anorexia, nausea and vomiting.
- Suppression of bone marrow function may result in neutropenia, anaemia and thrombocytopenia with consequent risk of infection, bleeding and fatigue.
- Metabolic upsets may be associated with breakdown of tumour tissue resulting in hyperuricaemia, hyperphosphataemia, hypocalcaemia, hyperkalaemia and metabolic acidosis.
- Urate crystal formation in the renal tract may lead to kidney failure and adequate hydration with good urine output should be maintained during treatment.
- Severe CNS toxicity with blindness, coma and even fatal outcome is a risk with very high-dose therapy.

- Dosage modification is recommended in patients with renal impairment.
- Administration is normally by slow IV bolus injection. After initial reconstitution with water for injections (2 ml per vial), fludarabine is further diluted in 10 ml sodium chloride 0.9% injection. Alternatively, add to 100 ml sodium chloride 0.9% and infuse over 30 minutes.
- Nurses should be aware of the risks posed by cytotoxic drugs. Some are irritant to the skin and mucous surfaces and care must be exercised when handling them. In particular, spillage or contamination of personnel or the environment must be avoided. If cytotoxic drugs are handled regularly, it is theoretically possible that repeated skin contact or inhalation may produce systemic toxic effects in nurses who have developed hypersensitivity to them. Most hospitals now operate a centralized (pharmacy-organized) additive service. While this reduces the risk of exposure to cytotoxic drugs, it is essential that nurses recognize and understand the local policy on their safe handling and disposal. The Health and Safety Executive has decreed that such a policy should be in place wherever cytotoxic drugs are administered. These should be adapted, wherever possible, to care of patients in the community.

Storage
- Fludarabine dry powder vials are stored at room temperature when shelf life is up to 1 year.
- Injections are freshly prepared.

FLUDROCORTISONE (Florinef)

Presentation
Tablets – 0.1 mg (100 microgram)

Actions and uses

Fludrocortisone is a corticosteroid drug which has primarily mineralocorticoid actions. In this respect it promotes sodium retention by the kidney and is used in the treatment of disorders associated with deficiency of adrenal gland function and salt loss, such as Addison's disease. It also has limited use in the management of postural hypotension, presumably maintaining blood pressure on postural change as a result of its sodium-retaining properties.

Dosage

- For replacement of mineralocorticoid function in Addison's disease, 0.1 mg daily or on alternative days is given. Adequacy of dosage is monitored by checking the urea and electrolytes and blood pressure of the patient.
- Higher doses (e.g. 0.3 mg/day) may be used in the management of postural hypotension.

Nursing implications

- Fludrocortisone has mainly mineralocorticoid actions. Insufficient dosing or non-compliance will be manifested by weakness, nausea, vomiting, hypotension and, in extreme cases, shock.
- Excessive dosage will be manifested by hypertension and hypokalaemia.

Storage

Fludrocortisone tablets are stored at room temperature.

FLUMAZENIL (Anexate)

Presentation

Injection – 500 micrograms in 5 ml

Actions and uses

Flumazenil is a specific antagonist of drugs of the benzodiazepine group (i.e. it blocks the sedative effects of such drugs on the central nervous system). In practice, flumazenil is used to reverse anaesthesia or marked oversedation produced by benzodiazepines, permitting a rapid return of consciousness, spontaneous respiration and mobility. Its major roles are in anaesthesia, intensive care units and following acute major benzodiazepine overdosage.

Dosage

Adults: initially, a 200 microgram dose is administered by slow intravenous injection, with further doses at 1–2 minute intervals until recovery is achieved or a maximum total dose of 1–2 mg has been given. In practice, total doses exceeding 300–600 micrograms are rarely required.

Nursing implications

- It is important to note that withdrawal symptoms may be precipitated in patients who have habitually taken drugs of the benzodiazepine group and who are, as a result, dependent on them. This may not always be known and careful monitoring of the patient is essential.
- Note that flumazenil has been investigated under carefully controlled conditions as an aid to weaning benzodiazepine-addicted subjects off their drug. It is stressed that such use should not be attempted except under specialist supervision.
- When used in an anaesthetized patient, prior reversal of any administered neuromuscular blocking drug is necessary since recovery may not otherwise be apparent.
- The action of flumazenil is very short-lived (2–3 hours only) and sedation may rapidly and unexpectedly become reestablished unless repeated dosage is given.
- Patients treated with flumazenil may therefore require prolonged monitoring, particularly if long-acting benzodiazepines have been taken. This may be especially important if a benzodiazepine has been

F

administered for short-term sedation in an outpatient department (e.g. prior to endoscopy) with a view to the patient returning home immediately afterwards.
- Flumazenil may interfere with the action of other central nervous system depressants (although it is relatively specific for the benzodiazepines), including antidepressants, anticonvulsants and neuroleptics.
- Administration has been associated with nausea, vomiting, anxiety, agitation, raised blood pressure, tachycardia and seizures. Such effects may, in fact, be related to benzodiazepine withdrawal symptoms.

Storage

Flumazenil injection is stored at room temperature and protected from light.

FLUOROURACIL (5-Fluorouracil, 5-FU)

Presentation

Injection – 250 mg in 10 ml

Actions and uses

Fluorouracil is a cytostatic drug which inhibits cell division by interfering with cellular DNA and, to some extent, RNA synthesis too. Its action is that of an antimetabolite since it prevents incorporation of pyrimidine bases into the nucleic acid structure. Fluorouracil is used systemically in the palliative treatment of a variety of inoperative solid tumours including those of the breast, gastrointestinal tract, liver, pancreas, endometrium and bladder.

Dosage

Local cytotoxic chemotherapy regimens which include fluorouracil should be checked for up-to-date information on fluorouracil dosage.

Nursing implications
- Diarrhoea, nausea and vomiting commonly occur during treatment and leucopenia usually follows completion of a course of therapy.
- Treatment must be discontinued if white cell counts fall below 3500/mm^3, platelets below 100 000/mm^3 or if stomatitis or oral ulceration develops. Nurses should advise patients of the importance of regular oral hygiene during therapy.
- Severe diarrhoea and gastrointestinal bleeding may also limit its use.
- Fluorouracil for intravenous infusion is prepared by dilution in glucose or sodium chloride solutions or mixtures thereof up to a final concentration not exceeding 1 g in 500 ml.

Storage
- Fluorouracil injection is stored at room temperature and protected from light.
- Solutions for infusion should be freshly prepared.

FLUOXETINE (Prozac)

Presentation

Capsules – 20 mg, 60 mg
Oral liquid – 20 mg in 5 ml

Actions and uses

Fluoxetine is one of a relatively new group of antidepressants known collectively as the SSRIs or selective serotonin reuptake inhibitors, so-called because their action in the CNS is to block the removal of serotonin from nerve endings, so 'boosting' levels in the brain. Serotonin or hydroxytryptamine (as it is also known) has an important 'activating' role in the brain so that a relative lack of its availability appears to be associated with depressive illness. Drugs of this type are especially appropriate in patients with obsessive-compulsive disorder.

Dosage

For adults, the dose ranges from 20 mg to 60 mg taken once in the day. Highest dose is required for patients with resistant depression or obsessive-compulsive symptoms.

Nursing implications

- Gastrointestinal upsets with diarrhoea and nausea and vomiting may be a problem for some patients in the early stages of treatment. These symptoms normally become less troublesome as treatment continues.
- Side effects in the CNS include anxiety, insomnia (also drowsiness), agitation and headache.
- Caution is necessary if prescribed for patients with epilepsy, especially where control is poor.
- Mania and hypomania are uncommon yet serious possible adverse effects of fluoxetine and other antidepressants of this type.
- Muscle/joint pain and weakness are occasionally reported and possibly reflect allergy to the drug.
- Obvious allergic reactions such as skin rashes and major abnormality of liver function (transient rises in some liver enzymes are reported) are a further contraindication to treatment.
- Note that fluoxetine has a very long half-life (up to 1 week). If problems manifest they may persist. Alternate daily dosing has been advocated by some specialists.
- Disturbances of sexual function (ejaculatory delay or failure, anorgasmia and impotence) are side effects which patients may be reluctant to disclose but which nonetheless can pose significant problems.
- Evidence suggests that abrupt withdrawal of SSRI antidepressants may be associated with withdrawal symptoms. Therefore long-term treatment should be discontinued gradually, e.g. halving daily dose for 1–2 weeks, then reverting to alternate daily dosing, then twice weekly.

Storage

- Fluoxetine capsules and oral liquid are stored at room temperature.
- Protect from light.

FLUPENTHIXOL (Depixol, Fluanxol)

Presentation

Tablets – 0.5 mg, 1 mg and 3 mg (as dihydrochloride)
Injection – 20 mg in 1 ml, 40 mg in 2 ml, 200 mg in 10 ml (all as decanoate)

Actions and uses

Flupenthixol is a neuroleptic and antidepressant drug used for its tranquillizing or calming effect in the management of patients with severe behavioural disorders, including depression. It shares many of the actions and uses described for the Phenothiazine major tranquillizers (see p. 281).

Dosage

Adults.

- 1–2 mg by the oral route once daily or up to 6 mg daily in two divided doses.
- As a long-acting intramuscular depot injection it is usually administered every 2–4 weeks in doses of 20–40 mg but up to 50–300 mg.

Nursing implications

See the account under Phenothiazines (p. 281).

Storage

- Flupenthixol tablets and injection should be stored at room temperature.
- Protect from light.

FLUPHENAZINE (Modecate, Moditen)

Presentation
Tablets – 1 mg, 2.5 mg, 5 mg (as hydrochloride)
Injection (oily) – 25 mg in 1 ml in 0.5 ml, 1 ml and 2 ml as the decanoate
– 100 mg in 1 ml concentrate in 0.5 ml and 1 ml as decanoate

Actions and uses
Fluphenazine is a member of the phenothiazine group of drugs and its actions and uses are described in the section on these drugs (p. 281). It may be taken orally or, more frequently, it is administered by deep intramuscular injection. The latter method of administration ensures a prolonged effect lasting several days to some weeks. The use of long-acting intramuscular preparations of fluphenazine allows many schizophrenic patients to be treated at home with their drug being administered at regular clinic visits.

Dosage
Adults.

- Orally: in anxiety 1–2 mg twice daily or in schizophrenia, mania or hypomania and other psychoses up to 10 mg daily in 2–3 divided doses.
- By deep intramuscular injection: 12.5–100 mg is administered in a single dose at intervals varying between 10 days and 4 weeks according to clinical effect.

Nursing implications
- See the section on Phenothiazines (p. 281).
- The muscle twitching and tremors which occur as side effects of the Phenothiazines (see p. 281) are particularly likely to occur with this drug and usually require prophylactic treatment with anti-parkinsonian tablets.

Storage
- Preparations containing fluphenazine are stored at room temperature.

- Solution for injection must be protected from direct sunlight.

FLURBIPROFEN (Froben, Ocufen)

Presentation
Tablets – 50 mg, 100 mg
Capsules (sustained release) – 200 mg
Suppositories – 100 mg
Eye drops – 0.03% in polyvinyl alcohol film

Actions and uses
Flurbiprofen is a non-steroidal antiinflammatory drug and the section on NSAIDs (p. 250) should be consulted for an account of its actions.
In practice, it is used in the treatment of:

- pain in which there is a significant inflammatory component (e.g. acute tissue injury)
- musculoskeletal injury
- rheumatoid and osteoarthritis
- ankylosing spondylitis

Eye drops are administered to inhibit intraoperative miosis as a result of the antiinflammatory action: the drug itself does not possess mydriatic properties.

Dosage
- The usual adult oral dose is 150–300 mg daily in three or four divided doses or 200 mg as sustained-release capsule at night.
- Similar doses are administered rectally when the oral route is compromised.
- Check local procedure for use of eye drops (usually 1 drop ½-hourly starting 2 hours before surgery) with the last drop not less than 30 minutes preoperatively. Following surgery, after 24 hours 1 drop is administered four times daily for at least 1 week after laser trabeculoplasty and for 2–3 weeks in the case of other ophthalmic surgery.

Nursing implications
- See the section on NSAIDs (p. 250).
- Instil eye drops directly into the conjunctival sac as a single dose then discard after use.

- Avoid eye drops in patients with dendritic (herpes virus) keratitis.

Storage

Flurbiprofen tablets and eye drops (single dose units) are stored at room temperature.

FLUTICASONE (Flixonase, Flixotide)

Presentation

Pressurized inhaler – 25, 50, 125 and 250 microgram/metered dose
Diskhaler – dry powder for inhalation containing 50, 100, 250 and 500 microgram for use in a 'Disk'
Accuhaler – containing 50, 100, 250 and 500 microgram per dose
Intranasal spray – 50 microgram per metered dose
Cream – 0.05%
Ointment – 0.005%

Actions and uses

- This drug is a new and potent corticosteroid.
- It is used by inhalation in the prophylaxis of asthma. Since chronic inflammation with hyperresponsiveness of the airways underlies asthma it follows that any drug having potent antiinflammatory activity can modify disease progression. Fluticasone is claimed to be more effective than beclomethasone dipropionate and may prove successful in patients who fail to respond adequately to that drug.
- It is also used by intranasal instillation in the prevention and treatment of seasonal or perennial (allergic) rhinitis.
- Fluticasone propionate ointment and cream are applied topically in the treatment of severe eczema (dermatitis).

Dosage

Adults (inhalation): dosage varies between 100 and 1000 microgram twice daily depending upon the amount required to achieve control of symptoms.

Children (inhalation): doses of between 50 and 100 microgram twice daily are generally required.
Rhinitis in adults: 2–4 sprays into each nostril once daily.
Rhinitis in children: 1/2 adult dose for over 4 years only.
Cream/ointment is applied sparingly twice daily.

Nursing implications

- Corticosteroids are important disease-modifying drugs in asthma. Therefore nurses have an important role in advising patients on the appropriate use of steroids as a preventive measure rather than to relieve bronchospasm.
- Patients should be instructed to keep their inhalers by their bedside and use them on awakening each morning and retiring at night.
- High doses should be given via a large spacer device (Volumatic). This improves airway penetration and reduces local side effects in the mouth and larynx (i.e. oral candidiasis and dysphonia).
- Patients always require careful instruction in the use of their inhaler device in order to optimize therapy. Seek advice from the pharmacy, if necessary.
- Patients should be advised to double their usual dose or use their inhaler four times daily in the event of worsening symptoms or development of a chest cold. Medical advice must be sought coincidentally.
- Note that penetration of the airways by dry powder forms is generally poorer than with pressurized spray inhalers. Consequently, the dose using dry powder drug is generally double that of conventional inhalers.
- Intranasal administration may be associated with irritation, sneezing, bleeding and disturbances of smell.

F

Storage
- Fluticasone preparations are stored at room temperature.
- Powder for inhalation must be stored in a dry place.
- Pressurized inhaler devices must not be incinerated after use.

FLUVASTATIN (Lescol)

Presentation
Capsules – 20 mg and 40 mg

Actions and uses
This drug is a member of the statin group of lipid-lowering drugs used in the treatment of conditions associated with familial hypercholesterolaemia or in the secondary prevention of coronary heart disease (CHD). The role of the statins is increasing as it becomes apparent that lowering total cholesterol levels may benefit patients with carotid disease (ischaemic stroke), peripheral vascular disease and global risk of premature vascular or cardiovascular death (including diabetics).

Dosage
Adults only: dosage ranges from 20 to 80 mg once daily according to cholesterol level and response to treatment.

Nursing implications
- The optimum effect of fluvastatin occurs overnight and nighttime dosing is recommended.
- Gastrointestinal upsets are relatively common but may diminish on continued therapy. Patients should be advised to take their medication with meals which may help to alleviate this problem.
- A diet which is low in fat and cholesterol should be encouraged.
- Headaches and myalgia also occur and blood creatine kinase (CK) levels should be checked to ensure no untoward muscle damage.

- Continuous drug compliance is essential in order to maintain cholesterol at lower levels. Patients should be informed that the effects of the drug may not, however, become apparent for several weeks.
- The potential for liver toxicity requires regular liver function testing.
- 3–6 monthly blood tests are required to monitor cholesterol levels.
- This drug should be avoided in pregnancy.
- Statins may interact with other drugs administered concomitantly, in particular warfarin (increased risk of bleeding) and the oral contraceptives (levels of oestrogen increased in line with high oestrogen-containing oral contraceptives).

Storage
Fluvastatin capsules are stored at room temperature.

FLUVOXAMINE (Faverin)

Presentation
Tablets – 50 mg and 100 mg

Actions and uses
Fluvoxamine is an antidepressant having some similarities to the tricyclic antidepressants. It appears to have a specific action on 5-hydroxytryptamine (serotonin) uptake by nerve fibres in the CNS and thus potentiates the action of this neurotransmitter at nerve endings. Such an effect is thought to be associated with mood elevation and increased activity and fluvoxamine is used in the treatment of depression characterized by persistent lowering of mood and, specifically, in depression associated with obsessive-compulsive disorder.

Dosage
Adults: 100–300 mg daily in a single or two divided doses.

Nursing implications

- Patients with disease of the liver and/or kidney should receive appropriately lower doses.
- Nausea is a common occurrence during the early treatment period and anorexia, constipation, agitation and tremors have also been noted.
- Other side effects include sweating, insomnia, anxiety, weakness and irritability.
- Use with caution in poorly controlled epileptic patients.

Storage

Fluvoxamine tablets are stored at room temperature.

FOLIC ACID

Presentation

Folic acid is available in a number of preparations either alone or in combination with iron and other vitamins.

Actions and uses

Folic acid is indicated for the treatment of megaloblastic anaemia (anaemia associated with large immature red cells in the blood). This type of anaemia may be produced by:

- nutritional deficiency
- pregnancy
- malabsorption.

Folic acid is also used in pregnancy for the prevention of neural tube defects.

Dosage

- In the treatment of megaloblastic anaemia: initially 10–20 mg daily for 14 days. Subsequently 5–10 mg daily.
- For the prophylaxis of megaloblastic anaemia in pregnancy: 200–500 microgram (0.2–0.5 mg) once daily.
- To prevent first occurrence of neural tube defects in women planning a pregnancy, 400 microgram should be taken daily prior to conception and for the first 12 weeks of pregnancy. Women who have not taken folic acid and find that they are pregnant should start to take the recommended daily dose and continue for the first 12 weeks of their pregnancy.
- To prevent recurrence of neural tube defect (where there is a history of spina bifida in the family) 5 mg daily of folic acid should be taken prior to conception and for the first 12 weeks of the pregnancy.

Nursing implications

- No problems are encountered with the administration of this drug.
- Patients should also be given advice on the dietary sources of folic acid.
- It is important to note that when a megaloblastic anaemia is identified, folic acid should never be instituted prior to the elucidation of its cause. Administration of folic acid to patients with megaloblastic anaemia due to vitamin B12 deficiency may result in severe and irreversible neurological symptoms.
- Women who take antiepileptic therapy and are planning a pregnancy should consult their doctor for individual advice regarding folic acid administration and dosage.

Storage

Folic acid is stored at room temperature.

FORMESTANE (Lentaron)

Presentation

Injection – 250 mg vial plus 2 ml diluent depot injection

Actions and uses

Formestane is a selective inhibitor of aromatase in peripheral tissues and so is effective in the treatment of postmenopausal women with advanced breast cancer.

Peripheral tissues are capable of metabolizing natural androgenic sex hormones to oestrogen by the action of an enzyme, aromatase. This provides a stimulus for continued growth of oestrogen-dependent tumours in advanced breast cancer in women after the menopause or in whom an early menopause has been induced.

F

F

Dosage
A single dose of 250 mg by deep intramuscular injection provides a depot effect for up to 2 weeks.

Nursing implications
- Deep intramuscular injection into the gluteal region is advised, using alternate buttocks for successive dosages.
- Local injection site reactions are common and include itching, pain and irritation, burning sensation and appearance of lumps or granulomas. Haematomas are also reported and caution is advised if this drug is administered to an anticoagulated patient.
- Skin rashes, pruritus and increased facial hair growth, as well as alopecia, may occur.
- Other side effects include lethargy, drowsiness, emotional upsets, headaches, dizziness, oedema of the lower leg and thrombophlebitis.
- Some patients complain of nausea, vomiting, constipation, hot flushes, vaginal bleeding, pelvic cramps, muscle cramps and arthralgia.
- Note that this drug is intended for use in postmenopausal women only.

Storage
- The unprepared injection is stored in a refrigerator.
- Reconstitution with sodium chloride diluent provides a fine suspension from which the drug is gradually released into the circulation. Gentle shaking facilitates dispersal of the drug.
- Prepare immediately before use or if necessary, store in a refrigerator for up to 24 hours.

FOSINOPRIL (Staril)

Presentation
Tablets – 10 mg, 20 mg

Actions and uses
See section on ACE Inhibitors (p. 4).

Dosage
Range: 10–40 mg as a single daily dose.

Nursing implications
See section on ACE Inhibitors (p. 4).

Storage
Fosinopril tablets are stored at room temperature.

FRUSEMIDE (Lasix)

Presentation
Tablets – 20 mg, 40 mg, 500 mg
Injections – 20 mg in 2 ml, 50 mg in 5 ml, 250 mg in 25 ml
Mixture – 1 mg, 4 mg, 8 mg and 10 mg all in 1 ml, most available only on 'special' order (see BNF)

Actions and uses
All diuretics act on the kidney to increase excretion of water and electrolytes from the body. The functional unit of the kidney is called a nephron and is composed of a glomerulus and a tubule. The tubule has four sections, each of which has different functions. They are known as the proximal tubule, the loop of Henle, the distal tubule and the collecting tubule. Frusemide is the best known and most commonly used of the diuretics known as 'loop' diuretics. This particular group acts on the loop of Henle and inhibits electrolyte and therefore water reabsorption. Diuretics which act on the loop of Henle tend to have a rapid onset of action and produce a much more marked diuresis than diuretics acting at other parts of the tubule. The indications for use of frusemide therefore are in situations where a rapid loss of body salt and water is necessary, such as acute left heart failure with pulmonary oedema, or where milder diuretics have proved ineffective. It is worth noting that frusemide is not as effective in the management of hypertension as other (thiazide-type) diuretics.

Dosage

Adults.

- Intravenous injection in emergency situations: usual initial dose is between 40 and 120 mg but up to 500 mg may be required in renal failure.
- Intramuscular: may be given in emergency situations or where oral treatment is contraindicated.
- Oral dosage: usually given once per day in the morning – initially 40 mg increased until an appropriate clinical response has been achieved. It is worth noting that doses of up to 2 g orally or 1 g intravenously may be given in patients with chronic renal failure.

Children's oral doses are as follows: 1 year or less, 1–2 mg/kg; 1–5 years, 10–20 mg; 6–12 years, 20–40 mg. Intramuscular or intravenous doses should be half of the recommended oral dose.

Nursing implications

- The nursing implications for Thiazide Diuretics (p. 357) are also applicable to frusemide.
- When high doses are given transient deafness may occur.
- Acute renal failure may be precipitated if frusemide and other 'loop' diuretics are used in combination with gentamicin or other potentially nephrotoxic antibiotics.

Storage

- Frusemide tablets, liquid and injection are stored at room temperature.
- Solutions are sensitive to light and therefore packed in amber-coloured containers.
- Other drugs must not be mixed with frusemide injection in the same syringe and the drug should not be added to glucose solutions before infusion.
- Recommended solutions for intravenous infusion are sodium chloride 0.9% injection or compound sodium lactate (Ringer's)

injection: rate of infusion must not exceed 4 mg/min.

FUSIDIC ACID/SODIUM FUSIDATE (Fucidin)

Presentation

Tablets – 250 mg
Suspension – 250 mg in 5 ml
Injection – 500 mg vials with 50 ml diluent
Ointment and cream – 2%
Gel – 2%
Medicated gauze dressing (tulle) – 2%

Actions and uses

Fusidic acid/sodium fusidate is an antibiotic with specific activity against staphylococci. It has the advantage that it may be given to patients who are sensitive to penicillin and, in addition, it is particularly good at penetrating most tissues including, importantly, bone. It has the disadvantage that when used alone, bacteria rapidly develop resistance so that it is often used in combination with other anti-staphylococcal antibiotics (e.g. erythromycin, flucloxacillin).

Fusidic acid/sodium fusidate is used in all types of staphylococcal infection including skin and soft tissue, wound infection, pneumonia, septicaemia and osteomyelitis.

Dosage

Oral.

- Adults: 500 mg–1 g three times a day.
- Children: <1 year, 50 mg/kg body weight in total daily in three divided doses; 1–5 years, 250 mg three times per day; 5–12 years, 500 mg three times per day.

Intravenous injection.

- Adults: 2 g in total per day in three or four divided doses.
- Children: 20 mg/kg per day in total usually given in three divided doses.

The ointment, gel or medicated gauze dressing should be applied to topical infections three or four times daily if uncovered and less frequently if covered.

F

Nursing implications
- The drug itself is associated with very few side effects other than some reports of jaundice.
- It is usually recommended that patients with liver dysfunction or those receiving high doses of the drug should have periodic liver function tests performed.
- Fucidin for injection should never be given intramuscularly or subcutaneously as severe local tissue reaction and injury may occur.
- Fucidin may be infused in sodium chloride solutions for injection and has also been given safely in plasma and 5% glucose injection. Higher concentrations of glucose may result in formation of an opalescence in which case the infusion should be stopped and advice sought.
- Fucidin should not be infused together with amino acid solutions or with whole blood.

Storage
- Store all preparations at room temperature.
- Suspension should be protected from direct light.
- After reconstitution the injection should be discarded if unused after 24 hours.
- Powder for injections should be reconstituted with the diluent provided and it is customary to then dilute it in 500 ml of either normal saline or 5% dextrose and infuse over 2–4 hours or longer. Other problems with fucidin for infusion are discussed above.

G

GABAPENTIN (Neurontin)

Presentation
Capsules – 100 mg, 300 mg, 400 mg

Actions and uses
Gabapentin is an anticonvulsant which chemically resembles the neurotransmitter gamma-amino butyric acid (GABA) which occurs in the brain. As the importance of GABA as an inhibitory transmitter has become apparent, several newer anticonvulsants have been introduced which mimic or potentiate its action. The result is a 'dampening' of electrical discharge in the brain of which epilepsy is an extreme manifestation. Gabapentin is intended for add-on therapy (i.e. used with established anticonvulsants) in the management of partial seizures, possibly accompanied by generalized seizures.

Dosage
Adults: titrate dosage to individual need using 300 mg daily increments to the usual range of 900–2400 mg, administered on a three times daily basis.

Nursing implications
- The dose of gabapentin must be adjusted for patients with renal impairment. Guidelines should be available from the pharmacy. Note also that elderly people often have reduced kidney function and may therefore require correspondingly lower doses.
- This drug is not generally effective in absence seizures and, indeed, may activate absence seizures in some patients.

- Likely side effects include drowsiness, dizziness, ataxia, fatigue, nystagmus, headache, tremor, diplopia, rhinitis, nausea and vomiting.
- The administration of antacids with gabapentin may reduce the amount absorbed by up to 25% and co-administration should be avoided.
- Gabapentin is a member of a new range of anticonvulsants and it is unlikely that its true toxicity will emerge for some time. As with all new drugs, therefore, extra vigilance is required and all suspected adverse events should be reported to the prescriber.

Storage
Gabapentin capsules are stored at room temperature.

GANCICLOVIR (Cymevene)

Presentation
Capsules – 250 mg
Injection – vial containing 500 mg powder

Actions and uses
Ganciclovir is an antiviral drug which, like aciclovir, inhibits DNA synthesis. It is, however, much more active than aciclovir and, in particular, is effective in the treatment of cytomegalovirus (CMV) infections including retinitis. This is reflected in its common adverse effects on rapidly dividing normal cells to the extent that ganciclovir is reserved for the treatment of severe or life-threatening (or sight-threatening) viral infections, especially in the immunocompromised host.

Dosage

Treatment of CMV infections (intravenous route): initially, 5 mg/kg every 12 hours for a period of 2–3 weeks. Long-term maintenance treatment for patients at risk of relapse may be administered at a dose of 6 mg/kg/day on 5 days/week or 5 mg/kg/day on 7 days/week. Reintroduction of the high initial dose may be necessary if there is progressive CMV retinitis.

Oral maintenance therapy: 1 g three times daily or 500 mg taken six times daily, both regimens taken with food, but only recommended after at least 3 weeks of intravenous therapy.

Nursing implications

- Ganciclovir is notably toxic to the bone marrow and is commonly associated with neutropenia and thrombocytopenia which, if severe, require appropriate dosage reduction.
- Anaemia, fever, skin rashes and liver dysfunction are reported in about 2% of patients.
- Other reported adverse effects include alopecia, pruritus, fluctuations in blood pressure, cardiac arrhythmias, ataxia, sleep disturbances, confusion, tremor and psychosis.
- Nausea and vomiting, gut pain and bloody diarrhoea may prove troublesome. Haematuria is also reported.
- Retinal detachment is reported in AIDS patients treated for CMV retinitis.
- Pregnancy should be avoided and contraceptive advice given.

Storage

- Capsules and vials of ganciclovir must be handled with caution; seek advice from pharmacy. Skin contact, inhalation or ingestion must be avoided.
- Each vial is reconstituted with 10 ml water for injection (without preservative).
- The drug is administered by intravenous infusion over 1 hour

in 100 ml sodium chloride 0.9% or glucose 5%.

GEMFIBROZIL (Lopid)

Presentation

Capsules – 300 mg
Tablets – 600 mg

Actions and uses

Gemfibrozil is a derivative of isobutyric acid and a lipid-lowering substance which has a particular role in the treatment of mixed hyperlipidaemias associated with raised triglyceride levels. Diabetics often fall into this category.

Dosage

Adults: 1200–1500 mg daily in three divided doses adjusted according to response.

Nursing implications

- Gastrointestinal upsets, skin rashes, dizziness, headaches and joint and muscle pains are relatively common side effects.
- Drugs of this type are associated with sexual impotence in males. However, it may be inappropriate to blame drug therapy alone.
- Caution is required when gemfibrozil is prescribed for patients also receiving warfarin since anticoagulant control might be altered.
- It should be avoided in patients with liver disease or gallstones.

Storage

Gemfibrozil tablets and capsules are stored at room temperature.

GENTAMICIN (Genticin, Cidomycin)

Presentation

Injection – 20 mg in 2 ml, 80 mg in 2 ml
Injection, intrathecal – 5 mg in 1 ml
Cream – 3 mg in 1 g (0.3%)
Eye drops/eye ointment/ear drops – 0.3%

Actions and uses

Gentamicin is a member of the aminoglycoside group of antibiotics.

Drugs of this type are notably active against Gram-negative bacilli including the often troublesome pathogen *Pseudomonas aeruginosa*. They are widely used in the treatment of Gram-negative sepsis, which is a particular problem in elderly hospitalized patients and in the immunocompromised. Aminoglycoside antibiotics also have an important role in the management of severe, recurring respiratory infections (often due to Pseudomonas) in cystic fibrosis and in bronchiolitis. They are also used together with broad-spectrum penicillins and cephalosporins in the prevention and treatment of infections in at-risk groups when broad-spectrum cover is required.

The aminoglycosides are specifically bactericidal. They act by inhibiting the synthesis of essential proteins after binding to the bacterial ribosome. Some resistance does occur, as a result of either reduced penetration and transport across the bacterial cell membrane or the production by resistant organisms of enzymes which destroy the drugs by a chemical action. Resistance is, however, relatively uncommon.

Dosage

- Systemic infection: past administration has used a dose of 2–5 mg/kg/day at 8-hourly or 12-hourly intervals but recent evidence suggests that a single daily dose of 7 mg/kg or more administered once daily may be more effective in the treatment of Gram-negative sepsis.
- The usual route of administration is intravenous bolus injection or rapid intravenous infusion.
- Children receive doses as above. Once-daily dosing (3–4 mg/kg) is especially suitable for neonates who excrete the drug very slowly.
- Blood levels of gentamicin are now measured in most centres and it is customary to adjust the dose according to the results of these investigations.
- Dosage of topical applications is as follows.
  - Gentamicin cream should be applied to the skin 3–4 times

daily, though there are good reasons why such application should only be done under specialist supervision.
- Gentamicin eye and ear drops: 1–3 drops should be instilled into the affected eye/ear 2–4 times daily.

Nursing implications

- Experience with the aminoglycoside antibiotics suggests that once-daily (rather than two or three times daily) dosing may be most effective since the bactericidal effect seems to be related to the initial (peak) blood level which is reached after IV administration.
- Aminoglycoside antibiotic therapy is associated with two major side effects. Such drugs are potentially toxic to the tissues of the kidney (nephrotoxicity) and the inner ear (ototoxicity). For this reason it is necessary to monitor blood levels, especially predose (trough levels), in order to limit the possibility of such toxicity. The pharmacy can advise on target blood levels.
- As a result of the above, it is essential that patients who develop hearing loss or difficulty or unexpected loss of balance and coordination be evaluated for possible aminoglycoside toxicity.
- Gentamicin injection is administered by direct IV bolus injection or added to 50–100 ml 0.9% sodium chloride and infused over 30 minutes to 1 hour.
- Although aminoglycosides are synergistic with (potentiate) the action of the penicillin and cephalosporin antibiotics, such combination therapy should never be mixed in the same IV infusion system since they are chemically incompatible.

G

Storage

- Preparations containing gentamicin are stored at room temperature.
- Do not mix injection solutions with any beta-lactam (penicillin or cephalosporin) antibiotic since they are chemically incompatible.

GLIBENCLAMIDE (Euglucon, Daonil)

Presentation

Tablets – 2.5 mg, 5 mg

Actions and uses

Glibenclamide is one of a group of oral hypoglycaemic drugs of the sulphonylurea class. These drugs stimulate pancreatic insulin production by the failing pancreatic beta islet cells which is a feature of type II, non-insulin dependent diabetes mellitus (NIDDM, previously known as 'maturity-onset diabetes' because of its prevalence in adult subjects). Also, in the longer term, they increase the sensitivity to insulin in the periphery by increasing the availability of insulin receptors. This form of diabetes mellitus has a strong hereditary association and is notable in obese individuals who may have other metabolic disorders or risk factors for coronary heart disease and/or stroke. Not surprisingly, therefore, lifestyle and dietary advice, with emphasis on weight loss, is a first-line measure in newly diagnosed subjects before drug therapy is commenced. Glibenclamide has a notably long duration of action to the extent that it is now used less often than other shorter-acting sulphonylureas due to the risk of prolonged hypoglycaemia which is reported, especially in older patients.

Dosage

Adults only: initial dose of 2.5–5 mg is advised with gradual increments to a total of 20 mg as a single morning dose.

Nursing implications

- Patient education regarding diet, lifestyle and drug

compliance is an essential component of diabetic management.
- Patients should be advised to administer the daily dose approximately 30 minutes before a meal in order to obtain the maximum hypoglycaemic effect.
- Attention is again drawn to the prolonged action of glibenclamide and its association with hypoglycaemia, occurring especially late in the day. Elderly subjects, in particular, must be monitored for signs of hypoglycaemia.
- Common side effects include gastrointestinal upsets (nausea, dyspeptic symptoms, diarrhoea or constipation) and allergic skin rashes.
- Liver function may be impaired by drugs of this type though serious liver damage is relatively rare.
- Note that oral hypoglycaemics must not be used in pregnancy in which close control of blood glucose is essential using insulin injections. Poorly controlled diabetes is associated with loss of the fetus, increased risk of stillbirth and congenital abnormalities.

Storage

Tablets are stored at room temperature and protected from light.

GLICLAZIDE (Diamicron)

Presentation

Tablets – 80 mg

Actions and uses

Gliclazide is one of a group of oral hypoglycaemic drugs of the sulphonylurea class. These drugs stimulate pancreatic insulin production by the failing pancreatic beta islet cells which is a feature of type II, non-insulin dependent diabetes mellitus (NIDDM, previously known as 'maturity-onset diabetes' because of its prevalence in adult subjects). Also, in the longer term, they increase the sensitivity to insulin in the periphery by increasing the availability of insulin receptors. This form of diabetes mellitus has a strong hereditary association and is notable in obese individuals who may have other metabolic disorders or risk factors for coronary heart disease and/or stroke. Not surprisingly, therefore, lifestyle and dietary advice, with emphasis on weight loss, is a first-line measure in newly diagnosed subjects before drug therapy is commenced. Gliclazide, being largely excreted by a non-renal (hepatic) mechanism, is often favoured for patients with existing kidney impairment.

Dosage
Adults only: 40–80 mg initially, increasing up to 320 mg daily.

Nursing implications
- Patients should be advised to administer the daily dose approximately 30 minutes before a meal in order to obtain the maximum hypoglycaemic effect.
- Common side effects include gastrointestinal upsets (nausea, dyspeptic symptoms, diarrhoea or constipation) and allergic skin rashes.
- Liver function may be impaired by drugs of this type though serious liver damage is relatively rare.
- With doses in excess of 160 mg daily, it is advised that the dosage be split and given twice daily to coincide with the main meals of the day.
- Note that oral hypoglycaemics must not be used in pregnancy in which close control of blood glucose is essential using insulin injections. Poorly controlled diabetes is associated with loss of the fetus, increased risk of stillbirth and congenital abnormalities.

Storage
Tablets are stored at room temperature and protected from light.

GLIPIZIDE (Glibenese, Minodiab)

Presentation
Tablets – 2.5 mg, 5 mg

Actions and uses
Glipizide is one of a group of oral hypoglycaemic drugs of the sulphonylurea class. These drugs stimulate pancreatic insulin production by the failing pancreatic beta islet cells which is a feature of type II, non-insulin dependent diabetes mellitus (NIDDM, previously known as 'maturity-onset diabetes' because of its prevalence in adult subjects). Also, in the longer term, they increase the sensitivity to insulin in the periphery by increasing the availability of insulin receptors. This form of diabetes mellitus has a strong hereditary association and is notable in obese individuals who may have other metabolic disorders or risk factors for coronary heart disease and/or stroke. Not surprisingly, therefore, lifestyle and dietary advice, with emphasis on weight loss, is a first-line measure in newly diagnosed subjects before drug therapy is commenced.

Dosage
Adults only: 2.5–5 mg initially, increasing gradually up to 40 mg daily.

Nursing implications
- Doses >30 mg should be divided to coincide with two or three main meals per day.
- Patients should be advised to administer the daily dose approximately 30 minutes before a meal in order to obtain the maximum hypoglycaemic effect.
- Common side effects include gastrointestinal upsets (nausea, dyspeptic symptoms, diarrhoea

G

or constipation) and allergic skin rashes.

- Liver function may be impaired by drugs of this type though serious liver damage is relatively rare.
- Note that oral hypoglycaemics must not be used in pregnancy in which close control of blood glucose is essential using insulin injections. Poorly controlled diabetes is associated with loss of the fetus, increased risk of stillbirth and congenital abnormalities.

Storage

Tablets are stored at room temperature and protected from light.

GLYCERYL TRINITRATE (Coro-Nitro, Nitrocine, Nitrolingual, Percutol, Suscard, Sustac, Transiderm-Nitro)

Presentation

Sublingual tablets – usually 500 microgram
Slow-release tablets – 2.6 mg and 6.4 mg (now rarely used)
Sublingual aerosol spray – 400 microgram per metered dose
Buccal tablets – 1 mg, 2 mg, 3 mg and 5 mg
Ointment – 2%
Transdermal patches – 5 mg and 10 mg
Injection – 5 mg in 10 ml, 10 mg in 10 ml, 50 mg in 10 ml, 50 mg in 50 ml

Actions and uses

Glyceryl trinitrate reduces the work of the heart by a complex process. It would appear that its major action is the result of venous dilatation and reduction in the return of blood to the right side of the heart. This leads to a subsequent reduction in venous congestion, the amount of blood the heart must deal with and the work that it must therefore perform (i.e. reduced cardiac preload). Glyceryl trinitrate also dilates the coronary artery bed, if not already maximally dilated, by donating nitro groups (nitric oxide is thought to constitute what is now recognized

as endothelial-derived relaxing factor or EDRF – the 'natural vasodilator' substance). Glyceryl trinitrate is used in the following situations.

- Treatment of acute attacks of angina pectoris.
- Angina prophylaxis, particularly before exercise or other activity which might provoke such an attack.
- The reduction in the venous return to the heart which glyceryl trinitrate produces gives the drug a further use in treatment of severe congestive cardiac failure (often secondary to acute myocardial infarction). For this purpose intravenous infusions or buccal tablets are administered.
- To increase regional blood flow leading to a reduction in thrombophlebitis associated with administration of hypertonic or otherwise irritant intravenous infusions.
- Similarly, as a 0.2% ointment administered rectally, to increase healing rates of anal fissures, so obviating the need for surgical intervention.
- A range of different preparations are available. For acute attacks of angina a sublingual tablet is placed under the tongue and sucked vigorously in this position. Alternatively a metered dose is sprayed into the mouth. For prophylaxis, the drug may be sucked or chewed, stuck to the gum, swallowed whole, sprayed into the mouth, smeared on the skin or stuck to the skin.

Dosage

Acute attacks of angina: one sublingual tablet is administered as described above or one metered dose (400 microgram) sprayed into the mouth. Prophylaxis of angina.

- Sublingual route: one tablet held under the tongue immediately before exercise or one buccal spray, as above.
- Buccal route: one tablet (1, 2, 3 or 5 mg) stuck to the gum.
- Topical route: one dose of ointment (measured on a special ruler)

smeared onto the skin or one skin patch applied to skin.
- Intravenous route (for the treatment of heart failure): the dose range varies according to the individual response and is in the range 10–200 microgram/min infused in 5% dextrose or 0.9% sodium chloride.

Nursing implications
The nurse may contribute greatly towards the management of patients on this drug as follows.
- Ensuring that the patient knows exactly how a particular form of the drug is administered, particularly when confusion exists due to the variety of alternatives available.
- Patients may dislike using preparations containing glyceryl trinitrate because of the side effects of flushing, headaches, syncope and hypotension which are all due to an extension of the pharmacological activity of the drug. Often, however, these effects diminish with continued use of the drug. If they occur after sublingual tablets are sucked during an acute attack of angina, patients should be instructed to terminate the action of the drug by spitting out or swallowing the tablet once the angina is relieved.
- **Should an attack of angina be unresponsive to one or two doses of glyceryl trinitrate and should its duration exceed 15 minutes, a myocardial infarction is a possibility and medical assessment and appropriate treatment must be organized**.
- Tablets deteriorate with age and may become ineffective. Loss of a bitter taste or 'fizzing' in the mouth may give an indication that this has occurred. This is especially important to note in patients who only rarely need to use the drug.

- Experience has shown that nitrate tolerance (a condition in which continuous exposure to glyceryl trinitrate is associated with a reduction in efficacy) will develop if transdermal patches are applied continuously without allowing a (frequently overnight) 'low nitrate' period to intervene.

Storage
- Glyceryl trinitrate tablets need to be prescribed on a 6-weekly basis and tablets discarded 2 months after the container is first opened.
- Diluted ointment (used in the treatment of anal fissure) must be discarded 1 month after preparation.
- Pressurized sprays are otherwise stable during usage.

GOSERELIN (Zoladex)

Presentation
Depot injection – implant containing 3.6 mg and 10.8 mg in a solid, biodegradable base

Actions and uses
Goserelin is a chemical analogue of the hypothalamic hormone LHRH (gonadorelin, GnRH) but it is biochemically substantially more active. Initially, it causes an exaggerated increase in pituitary-derived gonadotrophins (LH, FSH) and oestrogen which, however, rapidly leads to a desensitization of the pituitary gland and ultimate suppression of gonadotrophin release over the following 2 weeks to 1 month period. It is used in the treatment of endometriosis related to the presence of hormonally sensitive endometrial tissue growing outwith the uterine cavity. Similarly, it is used to produce endometrial thinning prior to ablation or resection and in the management of fibroids, together with iron therapy, as a means of reducing anaemia preoperatively.

It also has a role in the management of advanced breast cancer in pre- and perimenopausal women because of its suppressive effects on oestrogen production.

In men with advanced prostatic cancer, goserelin administration is associated with a downregulation of pituitary receptor release of LH which leads to a reduction in serum testosterone levels without the unwanted side effects due to oestrogen therapy in males.

Dosage

The 3.6 mg implant is injected subcutaneously into the anterior abdominal wall every 4 weeks. The base or matrix is biodegradable and designed to release the drug in a gradual, controlled manner. The 10.8 mg implant is administered every 12 weeks in the treatment of prostatic cancer.

Nursing implications

- Common side effects are related to reduction in normal hormonal output.
- Hot flushes, sweating and loss of libido are common and expected side effects of this therapy in both men and women.
- Women may occasionally complain of headaches, mood changes (even depression), vaginal dryness and change in breast size.
- Breast swelling and breast tenderness (gynaecomastia) may occur in men. The nursing implications described for buserelin also apply to this agent.
- The initial oversecretion of pituitary hormones related to the marked activity of goserelin may manifest as a temporary flare-up of symptoms in women and men treated.
- Skin rashes and local (implant site) reactions may be noted but should diminish in severity as treatment continues.

Storage

The goserelin implant is supplied in a single unit sealed package which should be stored in a cool place (below 25°C).

GRANISETRON (Kytril)

Presentation

Tablets – 1 mg, 2 mg
Oral liquid – 1 mg in 5 ml
Injection – 1 mg in 1 ml, 3 mg in 3 ml

Actions and uses

Granisetron is a member of the group of drugs including ondansetron and tropisetron which selectively inhibit the effects of 5-hydroxytryptamine (5-HT, serotonin) at specific binding sites called 5-HT1 receptors. Stimulation of these receptors in the gastrointestinal tract and chemoreceptor trigger zone induces nausea and triggers the vomiting reflex. Drugs of this type are therefore used to prevent and treat nausea and vomiting in patients who are exposed to various emetogenic stimuli, including anticancer drugs and radiotherapy. They are also effective in the control of postoperative nausea and vomiting.

Dosage

Adults.

- Oral: 1 mg twice daily or 2 mg once daily for the duration of cytotoxic chemotherapy with the first dose administered 1 hour before the start of the chemotherapy course.
- Intravenous:
  - Postoperative nausea and vomiting: 1 mg diluted to 5 ml and injected intravenously over 30 seconds.
  - Cancer chemotherapy: 3 mg administered in 20–50 ml sodium chloride or glucose injection over 5 minutes prevents nausea and vomiting for 24 hours in the majority of cases. Up to two further doses can, however, be given if necessary but administered at least 10 minutes apart.

Children.

- Oral: 20 microgram/kg twice daily for up to 5 days with initial dose administered 1 hour prior to chemotherapy.

- Intravenous: 40 microgram/kg
  diluted in 10–30 ml sodium chloride
  or glucose injection over 5 minutes.
  May be repeated once within 24
  hours, at least 10 minutes later.

Nursing implications
- Headaches and constipation
  are the most frequently
  reported side effects.
- Allergic reactions to treatment
  include skin rashes, modest
  rise in liver enzymes and, rarely,
  anaphylaxis.

Storage
- Granisetron tablets and injection
  are stored at room temperature but
  must be protected from light during
  storage.
- Once reconstituted, solutions
  for injection should be used
  immediately and any remaining
  discarded after 24 hours.

G

H

HALCINONIDE (Halciderm)

Presentation
Cream – 0.1%

Actions and uses
This is a very potent corticosteroid (i.e. a local antiinflammatory agent) which is used for local application in the treatment of inflammatory skin conditions including eczema, allergic dermatitis and psoriasis.

Dosage
Apply sparingly to the affected area two, or occasionally three, times per day.

Nursing implications
- Although applied to the skin, it is important to remember that prolonged excessive use can result in significant absorption and occasionally the appearance of typical systemic side effects as described for systemic corticosteroid therapy; see Prednisolone (p. 292).
- Accordingly, very potent topical steroids must be applied *sparingly* and for the minimum possible period, especially to 'sensitive' areas of the skin surface (e.g. the face).

Storage
- Store at room temperature.
- **Do not** dilute as chemical stability may be affected.
- Note the expiry date displayed on the tube.

HALOPERIDOL (Haldol, Serenace)

Presentation
Tablets – 1.5 mg, 5 mg, 10 mg, 20 mg
Capsules – 0.5 mg
Oral liquid – 10 mg in 5 ml
Injection – 5 mg in 1 ml, 10 mg in 2 ml, 20 mg in 2 ml for intramuscular or intravenous use
Depot injection – 50 mg in 1 ml and 100 mg in 1 ml (as decanoate)

Actions and uses
Haloperidol is a neuroleptic drug of the butyrophenone chemical class which nevertheless is closely related to the phenothiazines typified by the reference drug, chlorpromazine. It is used for its tranquillizing or calming effect in severely agitated patients with a range of behavioural disorders including schizophrenia, mania and other forms of psychosis. Haloperidol also possesses a pronounced antiemetic effect for which purpose it is used in the control of nausea and vomiting, especially in cancer patients receiving diamorphine analgesia by continuous subcutaneous infusion. This action is the result of increased upper GI motility and suppression of stimuli arriving at the chemoreceptor trigger (of CNS vomiting) zone. In such cases, its anxiolytic and sedative action is often of additional benefit.

Dosage
Adults.

- The dosage varies widely according to the nature and severity of the disorder under treatment. Initially 1–15 mg daily in single or divided doses with gradual increments up to 200 mg until control is achieved. Thereafter maintenance doses are tailored to individual patient requirements.

- Emergency control of severely disturbed patients is treated by an intramuscular or intravenous injection of 5–30 mg (**not** decanoate) repeated at 6-hourly intervals, depending upon degree of severity and subsequent response.
- Haloperidol decanoate is a depot injection for long-term control administered monthly in a dose of 100–300 mg by deep intramuscular injection.

Nursing implications

- Adverse effects which are associated with the phenothiazine tranquillizers are also commonly encountered with haloperidol. In particular, a degree of unwanted sedation, extrapyramidal (parkinsonian) symptoms and tardive dyskinesia occur. See the section on Phenothiazines (p. 281).
- Photosensitivity reactions (an abnormal positive response to sunlight) occasionally occur and patients should be warned to avoid excessive exposure to strong sunlight.
- The endocrine side effects of the phenothiazines are also associated with haloperidol, as is the depressant action on the bone marrow affecting the production of white blood cells. Since this latter effect makes the patients more susceptible to infection, patients developing apparently minor symptoms suggestive of neutropenia, such as sore throat, should have their white blood cell count checked.

Storage

- All preparations containing haloperidol should be stored at room temperature.
- The drug is very sensitive to light and accordingly oral solution or solutions for injections should be suitably protected during storage.
- Note that haloperidol decanoate injection, if stored for long periods in the cold, may precipitate (turn cloudy), though the injection should

clear on re-storage at room temperature.

HEPARIN (Calciparine, Hep-Flush, Heplok, Hepsal, Minihep, Monoparin, Multiparin, Uniparin, Unihep)

Heparin is available as both the sodium and calcium salt.

Presentation

Injection (intravenous) – 5 ml vials contain 1000, 5000 and 25 000 unit in 1 ml
Injection (subcutaneous) – 5000 unit in 0.2 ml, 12 500 unit in 0.5 ml, 20 000 unit in 0.8 ml
Solution (for addition to intravenous catheters) – 50 unit in 5 ml, 200 unit in 2 ml

Actions and uses

Heparin is a naturally occurring antithrombin – a specialized protein which prolongs the bleeding time in the presence of a plasma co-factor (antithrombin III). Various clotting factors and hence clot formation are inhibited, as follows.

- Thrombin (factor IIa) is bound in an inactive complex, so preventing the conversion of fibrinogen to fibrin.
- Activated factor X (or Xa) is similarly neutralized with the result that the conversion of prothrombin to thrombin is prevented.
- Other effects of heparin include inhibition of platelet aggregation and the binding of fibrinogen to platelet aggregates.

Heparin is given by intravenous injection in the treatment of arterial and venous thrombosis and by subcutaneous injection for the prophylaxis of thromboembolic complications following surgery and myocardial infarction.

Dosage

For the treatment of arterial and venous thrombosis: heparin may be administered by continuous or intermittent intravenous infusion.

- Continuous intravenous infusion: it is normal to administer

1000–1400 unit/h and regularly check the activated thromboplastin time (aPTT) which is the test of choice for anticoagulant effect in patients on heparin. Depending on the results of this test, the dose may be adjusted up or down until appropriate anticoagulation is obtained.

- Intermittent intravenous infusion: 5000–10 000 unit is administered intravenously by bolus injection every 4–6 hours and individual requirements are then adjusted according to the results of the thrombin time.

For the prevention of thromboembolic complications following surgery or myocardial infarction: the drug is administered subcutaneously in a dose of 5000 units 8–12 hourly. Clotting studies are not usually estimated when heparin is given by this route as it does not achieve a full anticoagulant effect but still proves useful in the prevention of thromboembolism. For prevention of clotting in intravenous catheters and cannulae: flush through with low-strength (10–100 unit/ml) solution regularly, e.g. 2–4 times daily and after use of the line.

Nursing implications

- As with all anticoagulant therapy, the two major risks to the patients are:
  - overcoagulation with resultant bleeding
  - undercoagulation with failure to treat or prevent problems of thrombosis or embolism. The nurse may play a very important role in the successful administration of heparin by ensuring that intravenous infusions proceed at the appropriate rate and intermittent intravenous or subcutaneous treatment is administered at appropriate times and in the appropriate dosage.
- It is important to note that subcutaneous injections may be very painful.

- Occasional urticaria, fever and thrombocytopenia may be produced by heparin.
- The drug should never be administered by bolus injection by the intramuscular route.
- Heparin is contraindicated for administration to patients with blood clotting disorders such as haemophilia and patients who have a history of active peptic ulceration or severe, uncontrolled hypertension.
- When symptoms of overcoagulation occur the effect of heparin may be rapidly reversed by the administration of protamine sulphate.
- Intravenous infusions, which are delivered continuously via a volumetric pump or other infusion device, are prepared in sodium chloride or glucose injections.

Storage

Heparin injection vials are stored at room temperature.

HEPARIN, low molecular weight

Presentation

This group includes certoparin (Alphaparin), dalteparin (Fragmin), enoxaparin (Clexane) and tinzaparin (Innohep). Each is available as unit dose ampoules or ready-to-use syringes of varying strengths related to their licensed clinical uses.

Actions and use

Standard (unfractionated) heparin is a complex substance of large molecular structure derived from the intestinal mucosa of cattle, sheep or pigs to yield so-called 'mucous' heparin. As a result of chemical breakdown (depolymerization) of the large unfractionated heparin molecule, a series of smaller fragments are produced which can be separated out according to their individual molecular structures. These are the low molecular weight heparins (LMWHs). They differ from standard heparin in terms of activity, adverse reaction profile and the need for monitoring anticoagulant control.

The specificity of LMWH-ATIII complex for activated factor Xa, in contrast to other circulating proteins, explains its more predictable effect and the occurrence of fewer bleeding complications when compared to standard heparin. The increased risk of bleeding with which standard heparin is associated arises as a result of its antithrombin and antiplatelet actions. Since LMWHs have little direct effect on thrombin, the activated thromboplastin time (aPTT) is unaffected. Measurement of aPTT, routinely used to monitor and adjust standard heparin dosage, is unnecessary when LMWH is used. If required, anticoagulant control is assessed by measuring factor Xa activity (only possible in a limited number of haematology units).

LMWH is indicated for:

- prevention of DVT
- treatment of established DVT
- treatment of unstable angina
- treatment of pulmonary embolism
- prevention of clotting during haemodialysis.

The actual licensed indication varies from product to product and the summary of product characteristics or package insert for each should be carefully checked for the application of each LMWH in different indications.

Dosage

Varies from product to product, but generally as follows.

- Prevention of DVT: 2500–5000 unit once daily by subcutaneous injection, depending upon degree of risk (highest after orthopaedic surgery).
- Treatment of DVT: based on 200 unit/kg once daily as above. Doses above 15 000 unit may be split and administered 12-hourly to reduce risk of bleeding
- Treatment of unstable angina: 100–120 unit/kg 12-hourly for at least 48 hours or until the patient is clinically stable.
- Treatment of PE: based on 175 unit/kg administered once daily (but

doses based on 400 unit per day in two divided doses have been used). Seek advice in severe cases.
- During haemodialysis: 30–40 unit/kg by intravenous bolus injection followed by 10–15 unit/kg/h by intravenous infusion.

Nursing implications

As for all low molecular weight heparins.

Storage

Low molecular weight heparins are stored at room temperature.

HISTAMINE H2-RECEPTOR ANTAGONISTS

Actions and uses

Drugs of this class are so called because they competitively inhibit (block) the histamine-stimulated production and hence secretion of gastric acid by the acid-producing cells of the stomach. This results in a reduction of gastric acid and corresponding rise in intragastric pH associated with increased healing rates for gastric and duodenal ulcers, maintenance of remission (non-recurrence) in peptic ulcer disease, symptomatic improvement in reflux oesophagitis, enhanced activity of pancreatin preparations and prevention of gastric aspiration during anaesthesia (Mendelson's syndrome).

The following drugs of this type are available:

- cimetidine
- ranitidine
- nizatidine
- famotidine.

Dosage

See individual drugs.

Nursing implications

- The dosage regimens for individual drugs may vary and patients require careful instruction in order to derive maximum benefit from therapy.

Many patients, for example, are required to take H2 blockers continuously to prevent ulcer relapse but, in the absence of symptoms they may discontinue treatment without medical consultation. Also these drugs are so effective they are liable to misuse and there are many instances where patients have decided, without medical advice, to start treatment for vague symptoms of indigestion.

- Cimetidine but probably not other drugs may interfere with anticoagulant control and bleeding episodes have followed the administration of cimetidine to patients treated with warfarin. Close monitoring of blood clotting, with possibly an adjustment in warfarin dosage, is therefore essential.
- All drugs are primarily excreted by the kidney and will accumulate in patients with renal impairment in whom reduced dosages are therefore necessary.
- Common side effects of the H2 blockers include gastrointestinal upsets (nausea, constipation, diarrhoea), headaches, dizziness, mental confusion and skin rashes.
- Cimetidine is widely reported to produce breast enlargement and tenderness (gynaecomastia) in males and also male impotence, as a result of its antiandrogenic action.

Storage

See specific drugs.

HORMONE REPLACEMENT THERAPY (HRT)

HRT includes the use of an increasingly wide choice of medications which are either taken orally or applied to the skin surface in the form of a sustained-release (transdermal) patch or topical gel or rub. See the package insert for specific information on available HRT preparations.

Actions and uses

The basis of HRT is the replacement of failing ovarian function in women who reach the menopause and beyond or in younger women with an induced early menopause. At this time, progressive reduction in oestrogen output by the ovaries is associated with 'menopausal symptoms' (often disabling flushing, sweating, abnormal bleeding pattern, mood disturbances, loss of libido, dyspareunia) and in the longer term with osteoporosis (the bone-building cells of the body – osteoblasts – are, in women, driven largely by the action of oestrogen). Also, it has been shown that HRT protects against the occurrence of heart and possibly cerebrovascular and peripheral vascular disease. The latter effect has been attributed to the action of oestrogen in reducing levels of LDL cholesterol.

Dosage

See package inserts for details of the various HRT preparations which are available.

Nursing implications

- It is important to note that oestrogen-only therapy is appropriate for patients who have had a hysterectomy. Patients with an intact uterus should receive combination treatment which includes a progestational agent. Otherwise there is a high risk of endometrial hyperplasia and cancer.
- HRT extended beyond 5–10 years is associated with a significant cancer risk.
- A number of women may discontinue or refuse to take HRT because of cancer risk and side effects such as irregular bleeding, weight gain and oedema, hypertension and sore breasts.

Storage

HRT preparations are stored at room temperature.

HYALURONIDASE (Hyalase)

Presentation
Ampoules containing 1500 IU of hyaluronidase.

Actions and uses
This enzyme breaks down hyaluronic acid which is a natural substance concerned with maintaining the cohesion of cells within soft tissue. Hyaluronic acid may be considered a type of 'cell cement' and hyaluronidase therefore a drug which increases the drainage of fluid from the subcutaneous and intramuscular sites. Hyaluronidase is used in clinical practice as an aid to the dispersal of infusions administered subcutaneously or intramuscularly. In particular, it increases the dispersal of injection solutions following extravasation and has a special role in combination with diamorphine administered via the subcutaneous syringe driver. The latter is often associated with inflammation and swelling at the infusion site if high local concentrations of diamorphine are allowed to accumulate.

Dosage
Adults: in general 1500 IU are sufficient for the administration of 500–1000 ml of most fluids.

Nursing implications
- Hyaluronidase is mixed with the solution to be administered by the subcutaneous or intra-muscular route or, alternatively, it can be prepared in 10 ml water for injections and infiltrated around the injection site.
- It should not be administered to insect bites or stings or at sites where infection or malignancy is present.
- It should not be given intravenously.
- Anaphylaxis is very rare.

Storage
The drug should be stored in a cool, dry place and prepared immediately before use.

HYDRALAZINE (Apresoline)

Presentation
Tablets – 25 mg
Injection – 20 mg powder in 2 ml ampoule

Actions and uses
Hydralazine has a direct action on the small peripheral arteries (arterioles), causing them to dilate. The effect of this is to reduce peripheral vascular resistance and hence blood pressure in hypertension and to relieve the work of the failing heart by reducing cardiac afterload. Administration of the drug may lead to some fluid retention and tachycardia so that it is often given together with a diuretic and/or beta-blocker. Hydralazine is now mainly used in the treatment of hypertension which is unresponsive to first- and second-line drugs and especially in severe hypertension when immediate control of blood pressure is important. It is still sometimes advocated in pregnancy because of its long track record of safety in this situation and also in renal impairment because of its ability to increase kidney blood flow. However, hydralazine has now largely been overtaken by the ACE inhibitors as a treatment for heart failure.

Dosage
- Hydralazine is given by slow intravenous or intramuscular injection or by intravenous infusion in hypertensive emergencies in a dose of 20–40 mg.
- The adult oral dose is 25–50 mg two to four times daily up to a maximum of 200 mg daily.

Nursing implications
- The nurse should be aware that the presence of tachycardia in a patient on hydralazine may be due to the drug therapy.
- Headache and flushing may be caused by the vasodilator action of the drug. As patients often find these side effects difficult to tolerate, there may be a reduction in compliance with treatment.

H

- A rare but serious side effect, most often associated with high dosage and therefore limiting the maximum daily dose to 200 mg, is the development of a syndrome similar to systemic lupus erythematosus. The syndrome is associated with widespread damage to the arterial system reflected in skin rashes, renal and hepatic dysfunction. The development of such features (and in particular a characteristic 'butterfly rash' across the nose and cheeks) is an indication for immediate withdrawal of drug therapy.
- Solutions for injection are prepared by adding 1 ml of water to each ampoule which is then further diluted with sodium chloride 0.9% (normal saline) injection.

Storage
Hydralazine tablets and powder for injection are stored at room temperature and protected from light.

HYDROCHLOROTHIAZIDE (Hydrosaluric)

Presentation
Tablets – 25 mg, 50 mg
Most often used in combination with other diuretics and with beta-blocking drugs.

Actions and uses
See the section on Thiazide and Related Diuretics (p. 357).

Dosage
The daily adult dose range is 25–50 mg twice daily.

Nursing implications
- See the section on Thiazide and Related Diuretics (p. 357).

Storage
Hydrochlorothiazide tablets are stored at room temperature.

HYDROCORTISONE (Hydrocortone, Efcortesol, Efcortelan, Solu-cortef)

Numerous other preparations containing hydrocortisone (often combined with other substances) are available.

Presentation
Tablets – 10 mg, 20 mg
Injection, intravenous or intra-muscular – 100 mg in 1 ml and 500 mg in 5 ml
Injection, intraarticular – 25 mg in 1 ml
Ointment and cream – 0.5%, 1% and 2.5%
Eye drops – 1%
Eye ointment – 2.5%

Actions and uses
See the section on Corticosteroids (p. 107).

Dosage
Dosages vary considerably with the nature and severity of the illness being treated and it is not therefore appropriate to quote specific instances.

Nursing implications
- See the section on corticosteroids (p. 107).
- Intravenous use: sodium succinate or sodium phosphate salts only should be used. Hydrocortisone acetate is for intraarticular injection only.
- Intravenous injections are given slowly over a period of 1 minute to several minutes. Generalized hypersensitivity reactions (chills, rigors, etc.) may occur and an uncomfortable, even painful, perineal burning or itching has been described.
- Intravenous infusions are prepared by adding the required dose to the required volume of 5% dextrose or 0.9% sodium chloride injection. The volume of diluent varies from 100 ml to 1 litre.

Storage
Preparations containing hydrocortisone are stored at room temperature.

HYDROMORPHONE (Palladone)

Presentation
Capsules – 1.3 mg, 2.6 mg
Capsules, sustained release – 2 mg,
4 mg, 8 mg, 16 mg, 24 mg

Actions and uses
Hydromorphone is a (hydrogenated ketone) derivative of morphine which has been available in the USA for many years but only recently marketed in the UK. It is available in immediate-release and slow-release formulations for the treatment of acute and chronic severe pain respectively. For practical purposes, 1.3 mg immediate-release hydromorphone is approximately equivalent to morphine 10 mg and controlled-release 2 mg hydromorphone to 15 mg morphine MST (12-hourly formulation). In all other respects, hydromorphone resembles oral morphine and, so far, its role would appear to be as an alternative to oral morphine for patients who experience morphine-related confusion, agitation or oversedation.

Dosage
Ranges from 1.3 mg 4-hourly as a conventional capsule to 4 mg every 12 hours as sustained-release capsules. There is no upper dose limit in the treatment of chronic severe pain and the required dose must be carefully titrated against the level of pain. It is not recommended for children under 12 years.

Nursing implications
- Hydromorphone is a useful alternative to oral morphine for patients who are oversedated or develop confusion and agitation on morphine. Such problems may, however, persist.
- In other respects, the nursing implications for oral morphine resemble this drug.

Storage
Hydromorphone capsules are stored at room temperature.

HYDROXOCOBALAMIN-VITAMIN B12 (Neo-Cytamen)

Presentation
Injection – 1000 microgram in 1 ml

Actions and uses
Hydroxocobalamin is a derivative of cyanocobalamin (vitamin B12) and, indeed, the preferred form of the vitamin. It is used for the treatment of megaloblastic anaemia where this has been shown by the appropriate laboratory test to be due to a deficiency of vitamin B12. Deficiency of vitamin B12 occurs where there is a lack of intrinsic factor (a substance produced in the stomach wall) which is essential for the oral absorption of vitamin B12. This condition is known as pernicious anaemia. There may be other types of vitamin B12 deficiency due to other forms of malabsorption and, more rarely, seen in people who follow a strict vegetarian or vegan diet.

Hydroxocobalamin is preferable as the form of vitamin B12 for replacement therapy as it has the advantage over cyanocobalamin in that it does not contain cyanide. This is especially important when vitamin B12 is being given to patients with either tobacco amblyopia or optic atrophy and optic neuritis due to Leber's optic atrophy when cyanide-containing compounds are specifically contraindicated.

Dosage
In pernicious anaemia: initially 250–1000 microgram intramuscularly on alternate days for 1–2 weeks, then 250 microgram weekly until the blood count is normal. Thereafter 1000 microgram every 2–3 months.
For the prophylaxis of megaloblastic anaemia due to gastrectomy or malabsorption syndromes or strict vegetarian/veganism: 250–1000 microgram monthly.

Nursing implications
- Hypersensitivity reactions to hydroxocobalamin do exist, usually presenting as an itching

---

H

skin rash and very exceptionally as anaphylactic shock.

- Particular caution is advised if the intravenous route (used rarely in those with platelet deficiency) is utilized. Add to 100 ml minibag sodium chloride 0.9% and administer over 1 hour but discontinue immediately if the patient complains of feeling uncomfortable and especially if a skin rash develops.
- Hydroxocobalamin has an additional advantage over cyanocobalamin in that it is longer acting and therefore the interval between injections can be at least monthly.

Storage

Store ampoules at room temperature but protect from light.

HYDROXYCHLOROQUINE (Plaquenil)

Presentation

Tablets – 200 mg

Actions and uses

This drug, originally developed as an antimalarial, was later found to be a useful disease-modifying antiarthritic drug (DMARD) for use alongside other drugs with autoimmune disease-modifying activity including gold salts, penicillamine, etc. It is used in the treatment of the arthritides, notably in active rheumatoid arthritis (including juvenile arthritis or Still's disease) and in discoid lupus erythematosus. The mechanism of action is not clearly understood; hydroxychloroquine is not an antiinflammatory analgesic drug.

Dosage

Adults: initially 400 mg twice daily, usually at mealtimes, and if a response is obtained the dose is reduced after several weeks to a maintenance dosage of 200–400 mg per day. Children: dose as above based on 6.5 mg/kg daily.

Nursing implications

- Side effects include reversible corneal opacities and retinopathy with higher doses.
- All patients should have a comprehensive ophthalmic examination prior to commencement of treatment and at regular intervals during treatment.
- Other side effects include gastrointestinal disturbances, depigmentation and loss of hair and skin reactions.

Storage

Hydroxychloroquine tablets are stored at room temperature.

HYDROXYPROGESTERONE HEXANOATE (Proluton Depot)

Presentation

Injection – 250 mg/ml

Actions and uses

This drug is a specific progestational agent (others possess some androgenic activity) used in the treatment of habitual abortion without running the risk of masculinization of a female fetus.

Dosage

For the treatment of habitual abortion: 250–500 mg at weekly intervals during the first half of pregnancy.

Nursing implications

- Administration should be by slow intramuscular injection.
- Local irritation at the injection site is rare.
- Altered liver function may occur and regular liver function tests should be carried out.
- Pregnancy should be monitored throughout the course of treatment.

Storage

Hydroxyprogesterone hexanoate injection is stored at room temperature and protected from light.

HYDROXYUREA (Hydrea)

Capsules – 500 mg

Actions and uses

Hydroxyurea is an orally active cytotoxic drug which interferes with the synthesis of DNA by a mechanism which is not, however, clearly understood. Its role is mainly in the treatment of chronic myeloid leukaemia but also, on occasion, in the treatment of cancer of the cervix (in conjunction with radiotherapy). Rarely, it may be used to treat polycythaemia.

Dosage

Treatment may be either continuous (20–30 mg/kg per day as a single dose) or intermittent (80 mg/kg every third day as a single dose) in an attempt to reduce the incidence of neutropenia.

Nursing implications

- Bone marrow suppression is the major toxicity, usually associated with leucopenia, thrombocytopenia and anaemia. Careful monitoring of full blood count is therefore essential in long-term treatment.
- Hydroxyurea should be used with caution in renal impairment as it predisposes to toxicity; therefore serum creatinine levels should be monitored.
- There is a possible association with gout and serum urate levels should be monitored.
- Side effects include gastrointestinal upsets (anorexia, nausea, vomiting), diarrhoea or constipation, headache, dizziness, drowsiness, skin rashes, abdominal pain, alopecia, hallucinations and convulsions.
- Skin irritation and erythema associated with radiotherapy may be potentiated by hydroxyurea.
- This drug is contraindicated in pregnancy.

Storage

Hydroxyurea capsules are stored at room temperature and protected from light.

HYDROXYZINE (Atarax)

Presentation

Tablets – 10 mg and 25 mg

Actions and uses

Hydroxyzine is a member of the phenothiazine group of major tranquillizers which are of use in the treatment of anxiety. However, in clinical practice it is now used almost exclusively for its coincidental antihistaminic and hence antipruritic action in dermatological conditions. The ability of older phenothiazines to suppress itch, particularly in patients who have associated anxiety, is well known. It is likely that the sedative action of these drugs is important also in this respect.

Dosage

Adults: 25–100 mg taken three or four times daily.
Children.

- Under 6 years: 30–50 mg daily in divided doses.
- Over 6 years: 50–100 mg daily in divided doses.

Nursing implications

- Hydroxyzine is a CNS depressant drug and marked sedation may follow its use, particularly if other sedative drugs are taken.
- In the above context patients should be warned of the dangers of taking alcohol, even in moderate amounts, concurrently with hydroxyzine.
- Some patients may complain of dryness of the mouth.
- Rarely, tremor or abnormal muscle activity is produced. This symptom is indicative of excessive dosage and if it occurs, should be brought to the attention of the doctor.

H

Storage
> Hydroxyzine tablets are stored at room temperature and protected from light.

HYOSCINE BUTYLBROMIDE (Buscopan)

Presentation
> Tablets – 10 mg
> Injection – 20 mg in 1 ml

Actions and uses
> Hyoscine butylbromide is an anticholinergic drug. It has a specific antispasmodic action on the smooth muscle of the gut, renal and biliary tracts and female genital tract. It is therefore used to relieve pain associated with acute spasm, i.e. renal colic, biliary colic, dysmenorrhoea and spasm produced by diagnostic procedures such as gastric or duodenal endoscopy.

Dosage
> - Adults, oral: 20 mg four times a day.
> - Courses lasting 5 days and commencing 2 days before the onset of menstruation are used in the treatment of dysmenorrhoea.
> - By injection: 20 mg intramuscularly or intravenously repeated at half-hourly intervals as required.
> - Children, oral: 10 mg three times daily is the dose range for the 6–12 age group.

Nursing implications
- Patients may frequently suffer the common anticholinergic side effects of dryness of the mouth, visual disturbance and tachycardia.
- Intraocular pressure may be raised; thus the drug is contraindicated in patients with glaucoma and on occasions may precipitate the onset of glaucoma.
- Patients may have difficulty in initiating micturition and occasionally urinary retention may result.
- The drug should not be used in patients with heart disease or intestinal obstruction.

Storage
> Hyoscine-N-butylbromide tablets and injection are stored at room temperature and protected from light.

HYOSCINE HYDROBROMIDE (Scopaderm, Scopolamine)

> The same considerations apply to hyoscine hydrochloride.

Presentation
> Injection – 400 and 600 microgram/ml ampoules
> Transdermal patch – 1.5 mg each

Actions and uses
> Hyoscine (as hydrobromide or hydrochloride) acts as an antimuscarinic, anticholinergic drug. In this respect, it inhibits or blocks the effect of acetylcholine (the neurotransmitter substance) released at nerve endings in the parasympathomimetic nervous system. Thus hyoscine hydrobromide (or hydrochloride) is used in the following situations.
>
> - By subcutaneous or intramuscular injection as part of the preanaes-thetic medication regimen to 'dry up' respiratory secretions prior to surgery.
> - By continuous (or bolus) subcutaneous administration in palliative care to reduce secretions.
> - By application to the skin, and thus transcutaneous absorption, in the form of a transdermal patch in the treatment of nausea and vomiting, particularly of the 'motion sickness' type.
> - Transdermal hyoscine may also be used in the treatment of prolonged hypersalivation.

Dosage
> Injection: dosage varies from between 200 microgram and 600 microgram administered up to 8-hourly if required.
> Transdermal application: a single patch is applied every 3 days for a continuous effect.

Nursing implications

- Hyoscine hydrobromide causes common anticholinergic side effects including dry mouth, blurred vision and tachycardia. Also constipation and urinary hesitancy.
- It should be avoided or used with caution in closed angle glaucoma, prostatism and arrhythmias.
- Local allergic reactions may follow application of the transdermal patch and be related to the drug itself or the adhesive within the patch surface.
- Overdose of hyoscine is associated with CNS overexcitement, resulting in restlessness and hallucinations.

Storage

Hyoscine preparations are stored at room temperature and protected from light.

H

I

IBUPROFEN (Brufen)

Note: Ibuprofen is also available in other proprietary preparations including those available over the counter in chemists' shops.

Presentation
Tablets – 200 mg, 400 mg and 600 mg
Tablets, sustained release – 800 mg
Granules – 600 mg orange flavoured for ease of administration
Suspension – 100 mg in 5 ml

Actions and uses
Ibuprofen is a non-steroidal antiinflammatory drug and the section on NSAIDs (p. 250) should be consulted for a full account of its actions.

In practice, ibuprofen is used for the treatment of:

- mild to moderate pain, especially if an inflammatory component is present
- osteoarthritis
- rheumatoid arthritis.

Dosage
Adults.

- Initial dosage is 200–400 mg three or four times daily.
- Daily doses of up to 1800 mg may be required.
- Alternatively, 1600 mg may be taken at night in sustained-release form or up to 2400 mg daily in two divided doses.

Children: a dosage of 20 mg/kg has been used but the total daily dose should not exceed 500 mg in those weighing less than 30 kg.

Nursing implications
- Side effects include indigestion, nausea and diarrhoea and occasionally gastric bleeding, therefore patients with a history of gastrointestinal problems should avoid this drug.
- Patients should be advised to take this drug with or after meals.
- Prescribing for elderly people should be carried out with caution as they are more susceptible to side effects.
- Patients with congestive cardiac failure on renal impairment should avoid ibuprofen as sodium and water retention may occur.
- Ibuprofen can increase bleeding time but does not appear to affect prothrombin time.
- Ibuprofen is contraindicated in patients who are asthmatic or sensitive to aspirin.

Storage
Ibuprofen preparations are stored at room temperature.

IFOSFAMIDE (Mitoxana)

Presentation
Injection – 1 g and 2 g powder in vials

Actions and uses
Ifosfamide is a cytotoxic drug of the alkylating type in that it damages cellular DNA and inhibits cell replication. It is in fact chemically related to cyclophosphamide and has a broad application in the treatment of malignant disease.

Dosage
This depends upon the type of malignant disease under treatment and the given dosage schedule which applies at the time. Check up-to-date dosage regimens accordingly.

Nursing implications

- The side effect profile of ifosfamide is the same as for cyclophosphamide.
- In particular, it is important that it is administered in conjunction with a generous fluid regimen which includes MESNA. This prevents haemorrhagic cystitis due to direct irritation of the bladder wall.
- Nurses should pay particular attention to mouth care and food and fluid intake.
- Nurses should be aware of the risks posed by cytotoxic drugs. Some are irritant to the skin and mucous surfaces and care must be exercised when handling them. In particular, spillage or contamination of personnel or the environment must be avoided. If cytotoxic drugs are handled regularly, it is theoretically possible that repeated skin contact or inhalation may produce systemic toxic effects in nurses who have developed hypersensitivity to them. Most hospitals now operate a centralized (pharmacy-organized) additive service. While this reduces the risk of exposure to cytotoxic drugs, it is essential that nurses recognize and understand the local policy on their safe handling and disposal. The Health and Safety Executive has decreed that such a policy should be in place wherever cytotoxic drugs are administered. These should be adapted, wherever possible, to care of patients in the community.

Storage

- Ifosfamide vials for injection are stored at room temperature (below 25°).
- Protect from light.
- Intravenous infusions are prepared in glucose or saline solution and used within 12 hours.

Presentation

Injection (intramuscular) – 500 mg + cilastatin 500 mg
Injection (intravenous) – 250 mg + cilastatin 250 mg
Injection (intravenous) – 500 mg + cilastatin 500 mg

Actions and uses

Imipenem is a chemical derivative of the beta-lactam series of antibiotics which includes the penicillins and cephalosporins. It is described as a thienamycin, beta-lactam antibiotic. This drug is administered in combination with cilastatin, a substance which inhibits its enzymic destruction by the kidney. This has two important consequences. First, it enhances the antibacterial effect of imipenem and provides a notably broad spectrum of activity and, second, it prevents the formation of a degradation product which is itself toxic to the renal tissues.

Imipenem is active against a wide range of aerobic and anaerobic Gram-positive and Gram-negative bacteria which is reflected in its many indications. These include septicaemia, pneumonia, intraabdominal and pelvic sepsis and infections of bone, skin and soft tissue and the genitourinary tract. Because of its broad spectrum, imipenem may be used on an empirical basis when the infecting organism cannot be readily predicted and the results of bacteriological screening are awaited.

Dosage

Adults: doses range from 250 mg to 1 g, 6–8 hourly by IV infusion depending upon the severity of infection and sensitivity of the specific pathogen. Alternatively, 500–750 mg 12-hourly may be given by deep intramuscular injection for less serious infections and as a single dose in the treatment of gonococcal urethritis. Children (over 3 months): 15 mg/kg body weight, 6-hourly up to a maximum daily dose of 2 g.

Nursing implications

- Although some chemical differences exist between imipenem

and the penicillins and cephalosporins, crossreactivity in patients with hypersensitivity to these agents may exist.

- Nurses should be aware that anaphylactic and allergic reactions may occur.
- Gastrointestinal upsets (nausea, vomiting, diarrhoea), blood dyscrasias and altered liver and kidney function are relatively common side effects.
- Very high doses have been associated with CNS disturbances including seizures.
- Patients with inflammatory bowel disease may develop acute flares during treatment with this and other broad-spectrum antibiotics.
- Blood levels of imipenem are increased in patients treated concurrently with probenecid. This is in fact useful in prolonging its action when single doses are used in the treatment of gonococcal urethritis.
- The dosage may need to be adjusted downwards in patients with existing renal impairment.

Storage

- Imipenem injection vials are stored at room temperature.
- Solutions for IV infusion are prepared in sodium chloride 0.9% or glucose 5% injection: 500 mg in 100 ml and administered over 30 minutes (up to 1 hour for 1 g dose).

IMIPRAMINE (Tofranil)

Presentation
Tablets – 25 mg
Syrup – 25 mg in 5 ml

Actions and uses
For an account of the actions and uses, see Antidepressant Drugs (p. 31). Imipramine is one of the tricyclic and related antidepressants.

Dosage
For the treatment of depression: doses range from 75 to 200 mg daily usually given in three or four divided doses.

Lower doses, i.e. up to 30 mg daily, may be sufficient in older patients who often have difficulty in tolerating the standard doses described.

For the treatment of enuresis in children: dosage ranges are as follows: 5–12 years, 25 mg taken as a single dose at bedtime; over 12 years, 50 mg taken as a single dose at bedtime.

Nursing implications
See section on Tricyclic Antidepressant Drugs (p. 31).

Storage
- Preparations containing imipramine are stored at room temperature.
- Oral liquid must be protected from light.

INDAPAMIDE (Natrilix)

Presentation
Tablets – 2.5 mg
Tablets, sustained release – 1.5 mg

Actions and uses
Indapamide is a diuretic drug with an action which is closely related to that of the thiazide diuretics (e.g. bendrofluazide). However, its diuretic action is very weak at the doses normally used but its antihypertensive effect, which is the result of its action on the peripheral vasculature, is nonetheless pronounced. As a result, indapamide is used exclusively as an antihypertensive agent (in mild/moderate hypertension) when the metabolic consequences of a clinically significant diuresis must be avoided. It may be particularly useful for elderly people in whom even low doses of diuretics such as bendrofluazide are likely to produce sodium and potassium imbalance or to precipitate gout of hyperglycaemia.

Dosage
Adults only: a single tablet (conventional or sustained release) is taken once daily in the morning.

Nursing implications
- When given for hypertension in the above dosage, side effects

may include nausea, vomiting and headache. Hypotension and its clinical features may also be produced.

- If higher doses are used the diuretic effect becomes more pronounced and all the adverse effects associated with thiazide diuretics may occur, such as hypokalaemia, hyperuricaemia, glucose intolerance and insulin resistance and elevation of serum cholesterol and calcium.

Storage

Indapamide tablets are stored at room temperature.

INDOMETHACIN (Indocid)

Presentation

Capsules – 25 mg, 50 mg, 75 mg (sustained release)
Suspension – 25 mg in 5 ml
Suppositories – 100 mg
Injection – 1 mg powder in vial specifically indicated as a treatment for maintaining the patent ductus arteriosus in the newborn

Actions and uses

Indomethacin is a potent non-steroidal antiinflammatory drug and the section on NSAIDs (p. 250) should be consulted for a full account of its actions.

In practice, indomethacin is used for the treatment of:

- osteoarthritis
- rheumatoid arthritis
- ankylosing spondylitis
- acute gout
- severe chronic inflammatory pain (e.g. associated with malignancy)
- specifically in the newborn with respiratory disorder associated with congenital heart disease in order to prevent closure of the patent ductus arteriosus and allow shunting of blood from left to right across the heart.

Dosage

Adults.

- The usual adult dose range is 25 mg twice or three times daily up to 200 mg per day in divided doses.

- A sustained-release capsule on a once- or occasionally twice-daily dosage regime can be used.
- One suppository (100 mg) inserted at night is often useful in relieving the troublesome morning stiffness in joints affected by rheumatoid arthritis.

Neonates: maintenance of the patent ductus arteriosus: three doses are given at 12-hourly to 24-hourly intervals based on age and urinary output.

Nursing implications

- The section on NSAIDs (p. 250) should be consulted for a full account of the nursing implications which apply to this drug.
- A specific problem with indomethacin is the production of headache, dizziness and gastrointestinal disturbances in a proportion of patients. This may be sufficiently severe to warrant a change to an alternative NSAID.

Storage

- Indomethacin preparations are stored at room temperature.
- Liquid preparations must be protected from light.

INDORAMIN (Doralese)

Presentation

Tablets – 20 mg

Actions and uses

This drug was originally developed as an antihypertensive. It reduces peripheral vascular resistance by blocking alpha sympathetic tone in the peripheral vasculature but it has now been largely superseded in this role. The action of indoramin on bladder outflow obstruction (it also reduces alpha sympathetic tone in the bladder neck and urethral sphincter) has led to its use almost exclusively in the symptomatic treatment of benign prostatic hypertrophy when reduced resistance to flow improves hesitancy and urine stream and hence bladder emptying.

Dosage
Usually, 20 mg twice daily or once daily in the evening for frail and/or elderly people.

Nursing implications
As a result of the vasodilatory effects of this drug, flushing, headache, tachycardia and an adverse reduction in blood pressure can occur.

Storage
Indoramin tablets are stored at room temperature.

INOSITOL NICOTINATE (Hexopal)

Presentation
Tablets – 500 mg, 750 mg
Suspension – 1 g in 5 ml

Actions and uses
This drug is a nitrate derivative which therefore increases blood flow within the peripheral vasculature (i.e. similarities with glyceryl trinitrate). Its use, however, is confined to improving peripheral blood flow in vascular insufficiency associated with peripheral vascular disease. Indications include Raynaud's phenomenon and intermittent claudication.

Dosage
Adults: 500 mg – 1 g two or three times per day.

Nursing implications
- As a vasodilator it causes flushing, headache and palpitations.
- As a nitrate it can cause significant gastrointestinal upset.

Storage
Tablets and liquid preparations are stored at room temperature.

INSULIN PREPARATIONS

Presentation
Insulin is available today mainly as the human insulin type. It can be injected as immediate-acting soluble (neutral) insulin or delayed-action insulin designed for twice-daily administration or even long-acting once-daily insulin. See standard references to insulin type, derivation and use in practice.

Insulins are available in their various forms in injection multidose vials, cartridges to fit non-disposable insulin pen injectors or in ready-to-use disposable insulin pens.

All forms of insulin are standardized on 100 unit/ml.

Actions and uses
Insulin is the hormone produced by the islet cells of the pancreas which regulates blood glucose levels. Exogenous (injected) insulin is essential in the management of diabetes mellitus, in which there exists a failure of these endocrine cells to produce natural (endogenous) hormone. Many patients with diabetes controlled by diet alone or a combination of diet and oral hypoglycaemic drug therapy (non-insulin dependent diabetes) may also require insulin injections during an acute illness or at the time of surgery or if they develop ketosis.

Dosage
The dose of insulin varies considerably from patient to patient. It is, however, likely that most patients will be controlled on a total daily dose of less than 50–100 units. The dosage may be administered by intramuscular or subcutaneous routes. Usually, a twice-daily regime is used but single daily doses of very long-acting types, more frequent doses with meals and snacks and even continuous infusions have also been employed.

Nursing implications
- The nurse's role is vital in instructing new patients or supervising existing patients in the management and assessment of insulin therapy and control of insulin-dependent diabetes mellitus.
- In situations where patients present with an altered level

of consciousness due to either hypoglycaemia or hyperglycaemia, insulin should not be administered until medical assessment confirms diagnosis.

Storage
- Insulins should be stored in a cool place, preferably in a refrigerator.
- It is good practice in hospital wards to add the date of first use to the label of a multidose vial of insulin and to discard any drug remaining after 3 months.

INTERFERONS

Presentation
Three types of interferon exist, designated:

- interferon alfa (Intron, Roferon-A, Viraferon, Wellferon)
- interferon beta (Axonex, Betaferon, Rebif)
- interferon gamma (Immukin).

All are in injection form with a wide range of strengths available, reflecting the varied uses for these agents. They are available as dry powder ampoules for single use, multidose vials and pre-packed ready-to-use syringes.

Actions and uses
Interferons possess both antiviral and tumour-inhibiting properties. They represent a group of natural substances (cytokines) released by all cells of the body which do not act directly on viral or cancer cells but trigger normal functions which counter viral and tumour cell invasion and proliferation. Their action is complex and still not clearly understood. It involves activation of phagocytosis and of cell-mediated immunity. An expanding range of indications for the interferons is developing. Theoretically, at least, they could be used to treat a host of viral infections or malignancies (and, indeed, have a developing role in the treatment of neurodegenerative diseases) but the cost is prohibitive and they are used only where benefit has been clearly established. This applies to the following indications at present.

- Multiple sclerosis to reduce severity and frequency of relapses in relapsing-remitting disease and in secondary progressive MS (interferon beta).
- Chronic hepatitis C infection (interferon alpha).
- Hairy cell leukaemia, chronic myelogenous leukaemia, multiple myeloma, non-Hodgkin's lymphoma (interferon alpha).
- Condylomata acuminata – venereal wart infection due to papilloma viral invasion of the external genitalia/perianal region (interferon alpha by intralesional injection).
- Kaposi's sarcoma in patients with AIDS (interferon alpha).
- As an adjunct to antibiotic therapy to reduce risk of infection in chronic granulomatous disease (interferon gamma).

Dosage
Since there is a series of complex treatments which might vary from time to time, the up-to-date literature should be checked in every case.

Nursing implications
- Interferons are usually administered by subcutaneous injection.
- It should be noted that injection of any foreign protein, including interferon, may be associated with flu-like symptoms, occasionally severe enough to warrant co-administration of an antipyretic such as aspirin or paracetamol.
- Also, as a foreign protein, interferon might produce an acute allergic reaction in susceptible individuals. Hypotension and cardiac arrhythmias have been reported and patients with ischaemic heart disease or recent myocardial infarction must be carefully monitored during treatment.
- Some patients may experience central nervous system effects, usually confusion, which can take several weeks to resolve on stopping treatment.
- A modified dose is required for patients with kidney impairment.

Storage

- Vials containing interferon must be stored in a refrigerator.
- Injections are normally prepared by reconstitution with water for injection immediately before use but may also be stored in a refrigerator if used within 24 hours.

IPRATROPIUM BROMIDE (Atrovent, Rinatec)

Presentation

Metered aerosol – 20 microgram and 40 microgram per dose
Nebulizer solution – 250 microgram in 1 ml
Nasal spray – 0.03% delivering 21 microgram per dose

Actions and uses

Ipratropium bromide is a drug with anticholinergic actions. When inhaled via an aerosol, it exerts a direct effect on the airways, causing bronchodilation and relief from the symptoms of wheeze and breathlessness due to airways obstruction in diseases such as asthma, emphysema and chronic bronchitis. The drug also has antisecretory activity and, in particular, reduces secretory excess in patients with rhinorrhoea associated with perennial rhinitis.

Dosage

Obstructive airways disease.

- Adults: one or two inhalations (20–40 microgram) three or four times daily. If necessary up to four inhalations may be given four times daily to obtain maximum benefit.
- Children: under 6 years, one inhalation three times daily; 6–12 years, one or two inhalations three times daily.
- In severe breathlessness solution may be administered via a nebulizer in which case it supplements the action of salbutamol or other beta-agonists when nebulized together. The usual dose is 0.4–2 ml administered up to three times a day in children or four times a day in adults.

Rhinorrhoea: adults only, 1–2 sprays into the nostrils up to four times daily.

Nursing implications

- This drug has minor anticholinergic side effects and may produce a dry mouth, urinary retention and constipation.
- Systemic toxic effects rarely occur.

Storage

- Ipratropium bromide inhaler is stored at room temperature.
- As with all pressurized aerosols, the container should never be punctured or incinerated after use.

IRBESARTAN (Aprovel)

Presentation

Tablets – 75 mg, 150 mg, 300 mg

Actions and uses

Irbesartan is one of a relatively new series of antihypertensives which act by blocking the action of angiotensin II (a circulating vasoconstrictor substance) at its target receptors in the vascular endothelium. Thus, angiotensin II-induced increase in vascular tone and hence peripheral vascular resistance is blocked, leading to vasodilatation and reduction in BP. Drugs of this type are collectively termed angiotensin II (AT1 receptor) antagonists. They act on the same system as the ACE inhibitors but at a different site. It remains to be seen if the AT1 receptor antagonists will eventually be used for the range of indications of the ACE inhibitors, notably in the treatment of heart failure or, indeed, in addition to the ACE inhibitors in difficult cases. Trials are currently under way.

Dosage

Adults only: initially 150 mg once daily (75 mg in the frail elderly) increased as required to a maximum 300 mg once daily.

Nursing implications

- The AT1 receptor antagonists are a useful alternative for patients who experience disabling side effects due to the action of ACE inhibitors in the body tissues. Thus they may be used for patients who develop a persistent dry cough on ACE inhibitor therapy or if potentially severe allergic reactions (e.g angiooedema affecting the airway) occur.

- Like ACE inhibitors, they may produce headaches and dizziness and are also associated with musculoskeletal pain.
- Caution should be used in patients receiving potassium supplements or potassium-conserving diuretics since these drugs can themselves reduce potassium excretion by the kidney.

Storage

Irbesartan tablets are stored at room temperature.

IRINOTECAN (Campto)

Presentation

Injection – 40 mg in 2 ml vial

Actions and uses

Irinotecan is a cytotoxic drug used at present as a second-line agent in the treatment of metastatic colorectal cancer. However, it may well replace first-line treatment with fluorouracil in the future. Its action on the cell is complex but can be summarized as the result of inhibition of topoisomerase 1, an enzyme responsible for maintenance of the DNA strand, resulting in single-strand DNA damage during S-phase of the cell cycle.

Dosage

Dose is based on 350 mg/m^2 by IV infusion over 30–90 minutes every 3 weeks until disease progression or unacceptable toxicity results. A lower dose of 300 mg/m^2 or even 250 mg/m^2 is used if significant dose-related neutropenia occurs.

Nursing implications

- Like most cytotoxic drugs, irinotecan has a range of toxic

effects which are dose related and generally predictable. These should be discussed with the patient before commencing therapy.

- Neutropenia is very common and requires that weekly blood counts be carried out during treatment. Febrile neutropenia (temperature >38°C) is potentially serious and requires urgent intervention. Patients must be made aware of the need to report fever immediately.
- Diarrhoea may be particularly severe (especially if previous abdominal/pelvic radiotherapy has been used) and often occurs more than a day or so after administration of irinotecan so that patients must again be warned in advance. It is important that patients take fluid and electrolyte supplements (e.g. Rehidrat) and antidiarrhoeal drugs (e.g. loperamide) as soon as diarrhoea develops.
- Nausea and vomiting is very predictable and treatments must be covered by concurrent antiemetic therapy, usually ondansetron (or a related drug) administered before irinotecan infusion. Uncontrolled emesis in the presence of diarrhoea is potentially life threatening and requires hospitalization with intensive management.
- An acute cholinergic syndrome is described in which diarrhoea is associated with severe abdominal cramping, salivation, sweating, lachrymation and myosis. Treatment with the anticholinergic atropine is required, as is cover with atropine on future dosing.
- Liver dysfunction may occur and it is important to monitor the serum transaminases and bilirubin during treatment.
- Nurses should be aware of the risks posed by cytotoxic drugs. Some are irritant to the skin and mucous surfaces and care must be exercised when handling

them. In particular, spillage or contamination of personnel or the environment must be avoided. If cytotoxic drugs are handled regularly, it is theoretically possible that repeated skin contact or inhalation may produce systemic toxic effects in nurses who have developed hypersensitivity to them. Most hospitals now operate a centralized (pharmacy-organized) additive service. While this reduces the risk of exposure to cytotoxic drugs, it is essential that nurses recognize and understand the local policy on their safe handling and disposal. The Health and Safety Executive has decreed that such a policy should be in place wherever cytotoxic drugs are administered. These should be adapted, wherever possible, to care of patients in the community.

Storage
- Irinotecan vials have a shelf life of 2 years when stored at room temperature.
- Once reconstituted and the infusion prepared, it should be administered within 12 hours if kept at room temperature or 24 hours if kept in a refrigerator.

IRON (Oral)

Presentation
A range of preparations contain iron, either on its own or in combination with folic acid and/or vitamins. Oral iron in the ferrous state (Fe) is available for administration either as the fumarate, succinate, gluconate, sulphate or as a sodium ironedetate complex. The forms most often prescribed are:

- ferrous fumarate capsules 305 mg (100 mg Fe)
- ferrous fumarate syrup 140 mg in 5 ml (45 mg Fe in 5 ml)
- ferrous fumarate tablets 210 mg (68 mg Fe)
- ferrous gluconate tablets 300 mg (35 mg Fe)
- ferrous sulphate, dried tablets 200 mg (65 mg Fe).

Controlled-release preparations of iron are available but not recommended for prescribing in the British National Formulary. It is argued that they are not necessarily better tolerated but rather are more likely to carry iron beyond the optimum absorbing surface of the bowel, so reducing their efficacy.

Actions and uses
Iron is used in two situations:

- where patients, due to inadequate diet or disease of the gut, have been shown by laboratory testing to be deficient in iron
- where patients are known to be at risk of developing iron deficiency anaemia, such as in pregnancy.

Dosage
The dosage of any iron preparation may be expressed in terms of the elemental iron (Fe) which it provides.

- For the treatment of iron deficiency anaemias: 100–200 mg of elemental iron (Fe) daily for 3–6 months is required in adults.
- For the prevention of iron deficiency anaemias during pregnancy: up to 100 mg of elemental iron (Fe) per day is recommended.
- Children: <6 years (45–90 mg Fe daily); higher doses for older children.

Nursing implications
- Iron is irritant to the gastro-intestinal tract. It may produce nausea, vomiting, constipation or diarrhoea. These symptoms may be so troublesome that patients do not take their treatment.
- The nurse can play an important role in encouraging good compliance by emphasizing the importance of continuing with therapy.
- Alternative preparations of iron are worth trying if a particular iron salt is associated with severe side effects.

- Patients may find the GI side effects are less severe if they take iron with food.
- Iron always produces a black stool which can alarm patients who should be forewarned and reassured accordingly.
- In excessive dosage, iron is an extremely dangerous compound, especially to children. This must be emphasized so that the importance of keeping iron preparations out of the reach of children is understood. Parents should be advised to take their children immediately to hospital for treatment should they accidentally swallow any number of iron tablets.

Storage

Iron preparations are stored at room temperature. The importance of storage out of the reach of children is again stressed.

IRON (Parenteral)

Presentation

Iron-hydroxide sucrose complex (Venofer) – 100 mg elemental iron (Fe) in 5 ml ampoule
Iron sorbitol (Jectofer) – 100 mg elemental iron (Fe) in 2 ml ampoule

Actions and uses

Iron salts are usually administered by the oral route but injections are required on occasion. The indications for parenteral iron are identical to those for oral iron but it is a potentially toxic form of therapy and must only be given when the oral route has failed, e.g. due to malabsorption, persistent non-compliance, disabling gastrointestinal upsets or when there is continuing severe blood loss. Jectofer brand is for **intramuscular** use only. Venofer brand is for **intravenous** use only.

Dosage

- Intramuscular dosing: use Jectofer brand. The total replacement dose required is determined by reference to tables produced by the manufacturer and related to body weight and observed haemoglobin. The total dose may then be administered as a series of daily or alternate day intramuscular injections of 1.5 mg/kg body weight (maximum 100 mg per dose) administered in alternate muscle sites.
- Intravenous dosing: use Venofer brand. The total dose is again calculated as for Jectofer, above. A series of short IV infusions (1 hour) are then administered, each containing 100 mg (occasionally 200 mg if urgent replacement required) in sodium chloride 0.9% minibag.

Nursing implications

- Gloves should be worn when administering this drug.
- To prevent irritation to the tissues and staining of the skin at injection site, several precautions should be taken.
  - The needle should be changed after the drug is drawn into the syringe.
  - The injection should be given deep into the muscle of the outer upper quadrant of the buttock to reduce pain and prevent staining. (The arm and thigh should not be used as there is insufficient muscle depth.)
  - Needle gauge and length are important; a 21 gauge needle which is no less than 40 mm should be used and this may need to be longer for obese patients.
  - The 'Z' track technique should be used; this entails gently pulling the skin and subcutaneous tissue to one side prior to the injection.
  - The injection should be given slowly and steadily and the needle should not be withdrawn immediately; this enables this rather viscous substance to be accommodated in the muscle mass.
  - The injection site should not be massaged.

- Parenteral iron is potentially toxic and should only be used when the oral route has been tried and found to be totally unsuccessful.
- The administration of parenteral iron (especially by the IV route) may lead to hypersensitivity reactions including fever, urticaria, skin rash, muscle pain, lymphadenopathy and occasionally anaphylactic shock which is potentially fatal.
- Test doses (e.g. very slow initial infusion rate over 15 minutes) should be given and facilities for emergency resuscitation and the administration of intravenous adrenaline, antihistamines and corticosteroids should be available.
- Intravenous iron (Venofer) is administered over approximately 1 hour in sodium chloride 0.9% 100 ml. Slow IV boluses can be given but should be avoided if at all possible. The solution is strongly alkaline and therefore potentially very irritant.

Storage

Jectofer and Venofer ampoules are stored at room temperature.

ISONIAZID

Presentation

Tablets – 50 mg, 100 mg
Injection – 50 mg in 2 ml
NB: Isoniazid is generally used in combinations containing other drugs. These are as follows:

- isoniazid and rifampicin (Rifadin, Rifinah, Rimactazid)
- isoniazid, pyrazinamide and rifampicin (Rifater).

Actions and uses

Isoniazid is an antibacterial drug used for the treatment of tuberculosis caused by the organism *Mycobacterium tuberculosis*. Its action may be either bacteriostatic (inhibiting growth and replication of the organism) or bactericidal (killing the organism), depending on the concentration achieved in the tissues. If used on its own for the treatment of tuberculosis, it is generally ineffective as the organism gradually develops resistance to it and therefore it is usually used in combination with other antituberculous drugs.

Dosage

For oral, intramuscular or intravenous administration.

- Adults: 300 mg daily or 15 mg/kg thrice weekly if an intermittent regimen.
- Children: 5–10 mg/kg daily or 15 mg/kg thrice weekly in an intermittent regimen.

Nursing implications

- As patients will be required to take therapy regularly for 6 months or more, even when symptoms are alleviated, the nurse plays an important role in encouraging compliance.
- Gastrointestinal upset, including nausea and vomiting, commonly occurs in patients receiving this drug.
- Isoniazid is associated with a high incidence of neurological side effects, the most common of which is peripheral neuropathy (altered sensation and motor function of the limbs). Peripheral neuropathy may be prevented by giving concurrent pyridoxine 25 mg orally daily or on alternate days.
- Other neurological side effects include mental disturbance, convulsion, incoordination, encephalopathy and alcohol intolerance. Unless the patient is receiving an unusually high dose of the drug, the occurrence of these side effects is an indication for change of treatment.
- Isoniazid interferes with the metabolism of naturally occurring pyridoxine. This may cause peripheral neuropathy and, more rarely, anaemia or a deficiency syndrome known as pellagra which is characterized by diarrhoea, dementia and

- dermatitis of the light exposed areas of the skin.
- Other side effects include disorders of the blood such as haemolytic anaemia, aplastic anaemia or agranulocytosis, skin rashes and metabolic disturbances such as hyperglycaemia and acidosis.
- The drug should be used with caution in patients with liver disease, epilepsy or reduced renal function.
- Isoniazid should be given with caution to patients receiving phenytoin as it increases the effects of phenytoin and may precipitate phenytoin toxicity.

Storage

The drug may be stored at room temperature.

ISOSORBIDE DINITRATE
(Cedocard, Isocard, Isoket, Isordil, Sorbichew, Sorbid SA, Sorbitrate)

Presentation

Tablets – 10 mg, 20 mg
Tablets – 5 mg (sublingual and chewable)
Tablets – 20 mg, 40 mg (sustained release)
Capsules – 20 mg, 40 mg (sustained release)
Injection – 0.05% and 0.1% in 10 ml, 50 ml and 100 ml, usually to be diluted before use
Transdermal spray – 30 mg per metered dose

Actions and uses

This drug reduces heart work in a similar manner to glyceryl trinitrate. It is a vasodilator which acts predominantly on the venous return, so relieving congestion at the right side of the heart and reducing cardiac preload. Circulation in the coronary arteries is also maximized. Isosorbide dinitrate itself is metabolized by the liver to isosorbide mononitrates and in practice the mononitrate is probably used more often when administered orally. However, isosorbide dinitrate

can also be taken by the buccal route (chewed or allowed to dissolve under the tongue) in the treatment of angina pectoris, applied to the skin surface and administered by intravenous infusion in acute coronary care (unstable angina, heart failure). Its advantage over glyceryl trinitrate is that it has a longer duration of action (up to 12 hours with slow-release preparations).

Dosage

- The usual oral adult dose for prevention of angina is 10 mg three or four times a day or 20 mg twice daily of a sustained-release preparation. Alternatively, up to two sprays (60 mg) can be applied to the chest wall and gently rubbed in twice daily.
- In an acute attack, 5 mg is taken sublingually or chewed.
- Continuous intravenous infusions are administrated in acute unstable angina and after myocardial infarction to reduce the possibility of cardiac failure (a frequent cause of late mortality). The dose must be carefully titrated against the individual's cardiac output.

Nursing implications

- The side effects of this drug result from generalized vasodilation and are similar to those of glycerol trinitrate. They include flushing, dizziness and throbbing headache. These effects will diminish over the first week or so of treatment and eventually become much less troublesome.
- See comments under isosorbide mononitrate regarding the need to avoid nitrate tolerance.

Storage

- Isosorbide dinitrate tablets and injection may be stored at room temperature.
- The topical spray should be kept in a cool place and **definitely not** incinerated after use.

ISOSORBIDE MONONITRATE (Elantan, Imdur, Ismo, Monit, Mono-Cedocard)

Presentation
Tablets – 10 mg, 20 mg, 40 mg
Tablets – 40 mg, 60 mg (sustained release)
Capsules – 25 mg, 50 mg (sustained release)

Actions and uses
This drug is one of the active metabolites of isosorbide dinitrate, the difference being that it passes through the liver after absorption without being substantially metabolized. It is often preferred, therefore, to isosorbide dinitrate for oral use in the prophylaxis of angina pectoris because its effects are more predictable.

Dosage
Usually 20 mg is taken two or three times a day. Alternatively a single daily dose of 25 mg, 40 mg, 50 mg or 60 mg, carefully titrated against individual need, may be taken using a sustained-release preparation.

Nursing implications
- As for isosorbide dinitrate.
- So-called nitrate tolerance may develop with loss of effectiveness if standard tablets or capsules are taken through the day and late in the evening. This can be overcome using a once-daily sustained-release preparation which is designed to provide a low nitrate period overnight.
- Alternatively, ensure that the last dose of a standard preparation is taken by 6 pm. This also provides the required low nitrate period overnight.

Storage
Isosorbide mononitrate tablets and capsules are stored at room temperature.

ISOTRETINOIN (Isotrex, Roaccutane)

Presentation
Capsules – 5 mg, 20 mg
Topical gel – 0.05%

Actions and uses
Isotretinoin is a chemical derivative of vitamin A and, like etretinate and acitretin, belongs to the family known as the retinoids. However, its major use is in the treatment of severe acne which is unresponsive to antibiotic therapy.

Dosage
Oral.

- Adults only: an initial dose of 0.5 mg/kg/day is taken once or twice daily for a few weeks then adjusted according to the response.
- If poor response, increase to 1 mg/kg daily.
- If poorly tolerated, reduce to 0.1–0.2 mg/kg daily.
- Single courses of up to 4 months are given.

Topical gel: apply thinly once or twice daily.

Nursing implications
- Vitamin A derivatives are strongly teratogenic and fetal malformations are highly likely in the event of pregnancy. Pregnancy must be excluded in women of child-bearing age at the outset and patients actively counselled thereafter to ensure that adequate contraceptive measures are always taken. Therapeutic abortion is offered if pregnancy occurs. Furthermore, pregnancy must be avoided for at least 4 weeks after treatment is discontinued since isotretinoin is stored for prolonged periods in the body tissues.
- It is important to note that treatment with isotretinoin must be arranged through a specialist clinic and supplies of the drug in the UK are restricted to

hospitals or designated community pharmacies.

- Vitamin A compounds are poorly tolerated by some patients (hence the need for careful dosage adjustment). Dryness of the skin, erythema, pruritus and alopecia are common and erosion of mucous surfaces is possible.
- Other side effects include headache, nausea, drowsiness, joint pain and myalgia.
- Hepatotoxicity occurs and liver function tests should be carried out regularly to detect early liver damage. Concurrent use of hepatotoxic drugs and alcohol should be discouraged and treatment avoided in the event of existing liver impairment.
- A further metabolic effect results in an unfavourable shift in the blood lipid profile and hyperlipidaemia. This may have important consequences for patients who have a history of angina or myocardial infarction and other risk factors for coronary heart disease.
- Care is also required in patients with diabetes in whom altered glucose tolerance may develop.
- Isotretinoin must not be used in patients with renal failure.

Storage
Isotretinoin capsules are stored at room temperature and protected from light.

ISPAGHULA (Fybogel, Regulan)

Presentation
Sachets – 3.5 g
Granules – 165 g canister

Actions and uses
See also the nursing implications section. Ispaghula falls into the bulk-forming group of laxatives. The ispaghula husk, like bran, is a natural dietary fibre supplement and it is used in those disorders of the bowel thought to be associated with reduced dietary fibre, i.e.:

- diverticular disease
- spastic or irritable colon
- chronic constipation associated with low-residue diet.

Dosage
One sachet (3.5 g) or two 5 ml spoonfuls of granules taken twice daily after meals, stirred into a glass of cold water.

Nursing implications
- There are no specific problems associated with this drug other than mild bloating and flatulence.
- A generous fluid intake should be encouraged to ensure maximum response.
- This drug is contraindicated in cases of intestinal obstruction, atonic colon and faecal impaction.

Storage
Sachets and granules containing ispaghula husk are stored at room temperature.

ITRACONAZOLE (Sporanox)

Presentation
Capsules – 100 mg
Oral liquid – 50 mg in 5 ml

Actions and uses
Itraconazole (like fluconazole) is a member of the triazole group of antifungals which selectively inhibit fungal synthesis of ergosterol, an essential component of the cell wall. Thus leakage of cell contents and eventual death of the fungus follow. In practice itraconazole is used for:

- vulvovaginal candidiasis
- pityriasis versicolor
- dermatophytic infection, e.g. due to Trichophyton spp., Microsporum spp., including tinea pedis, tinea cruris and tinea corporis
- oropharyngeal candidiasis
- aspergillus infection of the lung.

Dosage

- Vulvovaginal candidiasis: 200 mg 12-hourly for a single day.
- Pityriasis versicolor: 200 mg once daily for 7 days.
- Tinea corporis and tinea cruris: 100 mg once daily for 2 weeks.
- Tinea pedis, tinea manuum: 100 mg once daily for 1 month.
- Oropharyngeal candidiasis: 100 mg once daily (200 mg if immunocompromised) for 2 weeks.

Much higher doses are used under specialist supervision for serious aspergillus infection of the lung.

Nursing implications

- Itraconazole should not be taken with food or fluid.
- Common side effects of this drug include mild gastrointestinal upset, such as nausea and diarrhoea, headache and dizziness.
- Rare cases of hepatitis and cholestatic jaundice have been reported.
- Itraconazole potentiates warfarin and close monitoring of clotting time is important in anticoagulated subjects.
- Concurrent use with phenytoin may lead to accumulation of itraconazole.
- Concurrent use with cimetidine, ranitidine, omeprazole and related drugs may impair the absorption of itraconazole.

Storage

Itraconazole capsules are stored at room temperature and protected from light.

K

KETAMINE (Ketalar)

Presentation
Injection – 200 mg/20 ml,
500 mg/10 ml, 1 g/10 ml vials

Actions and uses
Ketamine (Ketalar) is a non-opioid
general anaesthetic agent used in
subanaesthetic doses in the treatment
of neuropathic 'opioid-resistant'
pain. It is a specific inhibitor of the
N-methyl-D-aspartate (NMDA)
receptor through which glutamate,
an excitatory neurotransmitter in the
CNS, is activated in these difficult
pain syndromes. There remains
general disagreement as to whether
or not the strong opioids are of any
value in neuropathic pain, with the
possible exception of methadone
which also inhibits the NMDA
receptor. Ketamine is therefore used
in addition to a strong opioid to
establish pain control and to
reduce the opioid dosage
requirement.

Dosage
Injection solution can be taken orally
diluted in fruit juice, instilled rectally
if the oral route is unavailable or
administered by continuous
subcutaneous infusion (CSI) via the
syringe driver. The response to
ketamine is first established using
a test dose, 5 mg orally/rectally or
2.5 mg by subcutaneous bolus.
Suggested starting doses are 15 mg
6-hourly (oral/rectal) or 25 mg/24 hours
by CSI titrated according to response.
Breakthrough pain is managed by
additional doses based on 10% of
the total daily dose. The average
oral dose is in the range 75–250 mg
daily.

Nursing implications
- It is important to note that the
  addition of ketamine is likely to
  affect the requirement for oral
  morphine or subcutaneous
  diamorphine (or other
  opioid analgesia) such that a
  reduction in opioid dosage by
  one-third is recommended
  when ketamine is introduced.
- A relatively high incidence
  of hallucinations and other
  psychotic-like reactions have
  been noted with this drug when
  used as a general anaesthetic.
  Careful titration of dosage is
  therefore essential to reduce the
  likelihood of sudden-onset
  adverse behavioural effects of
  this type.
- In practice, however, it is
  generally possible to arrive at an
  effective analgesic dose without
  incurring these side effects but
  careful monitoring is necessary.

Storage
Ketamine injection vials are stored at
room temperature.

KETOCONAZOLE (Nizoral)

Presentation
Capsules – 200 mg
Oral suspension – 100 mg in 5 ml
Cream – 2% (only prescribable for
treatment of seborrhoeic dermatitis or
pityriasis versicolor)
Shampoo – 240 mg in 120 ml bottle
for use twice weekly

Actions and uses
Ketoconazole is an antifungal drug
which is available for application to

skin and scalp but which is also effective when administered by the oral route for systemic treatment of fungal infections. It is used in the treatment of the following disorders.

- Treatment of fungal infections of skin and hair by dermatophytes and/or yeasts, i.e. dermatomycosis, pityriasis versicolor, chronic mucocutaneous candidosis.
- Treatment of yeast infections of the mouth (*Candida albicans*).
- For treatment of systemic mycoses, i.e. systemic candidosis, paracoccidioidomycosis, histoplasmosis, coccidioidomycosis, etc.
- Recurrent vaginal candidosis.
- It may be used prophylactically in 'at-risk' groups, i.e. those with reduced immunity due to cytotoxic therapy for malignant disease.

In practice, newer and safer alternatives exist (see liver impairment, below) so that the use of ketoconazole by the oral route is now largely restricted.

Dosage
Adults.

- Initially 200 mg once daily is given. The dose may be doubled if a satisfactory response is not achieved. The treatment is continued for at least 1 week after symptoms have cleared and the usual duration of treatment varies widely according to the condition under treatment, i.e. 10 days for oral thrush, 6 months for systemic infections with paracoccidioidomycosis, coccidioidomycosis and histoplasmosis.
- Shampoo is used twice weekly for 2–4 weeks to treat seborrhoeic dermatitis or once daily for up to 5 days for scalp infection with pityriasis versicolor. It is also used every 1–2 weeks as prophylaxis.
- For the treatment of recurrent vaginal candidosis: 200 mg twice daily for 5 days.

Children: the single daily dose is calculated on the basis of 3 mg/kg. See adult use of topical preparations.

Nursing implications

- The commonest problem associated with this drug is gastrointestinal upset, predominantly nausea.
- Reports of severe liver impairment and the need to monitor liver function when treatment exceeds 14 days have now largely limited its use in practice.
- Skin rash and pruritus are also fairly common.
- Any drug which reduces the acid content of the stomach, such as antacids, cimetidine, ranitidine and anticholinergic drugs, will impair the absorption of ketoconazole. Therefore at least 2 hours should be allowed between administration of ketoconazole and any of these agents.
- Ketoconazole tablets should be taken with meals when gastric acidity is high.
- The drug should be avoided in pregnancy.

Storage
Ketoconazole preparations are stored at room temperature.

KETOPROFEN (Orudis, Oruvail)

Presentation
Capsules – 50 mg, 100 mg
Capsules – 100 mg, 150 mg, 200 mg sustained release
Injection – 100 mg in 2 ml
Suppositories – 100 mg

Actions and uses
Ketoprofen is a non-steroidal antiinflammatory drug and the section on NSAIDs (p. 250) should be consulted for a full account of its actions. In practice, ketoprofen is used for the treatment of:

- mild to moderate pain, especially if an inflammatory component is present
- osteoarthritis
- rheumatoid arthritis.

Dosage

Oral: the usual adult dose is 50–100 mg twice daily although 50 mg three or four times daily is used occasionally. In a few cases some patients achieve adequate control with a single (usually bedtime) dose of 100–200 mg sustained-release capsule. Intramuscular: acute inflammatory pain, 100 mg deep IM injection 4-hourly up to a maximum dose of 200 mg in one day and for no longer than 3 days.
Rectal: a single suppository inserted at night to supplement daytime oral dosing.

Nursing implications

The section on NSAIDs (p. 250) should be consulted for a full account of the nursing implications which apply to this drug.

Storage

Ketoprofen preparations are stored at room temperature.

KETOROLAC (Toradol)

Presentation

Tablets – 10 mg
Injection – 10 mg and 30 mg in 1 ml ampoules

Actions and uses

The actions and uses of this potent NSAID are described under the group heading (see NSAIDs, p. 250). Ketorolac is, however, licensed only for short-term use (up to 2 days by injection or 7 days orally) and restricted to the treatment of moderate-to-severe postoperative pain. This should be noted in the light of severe adverse reactions to the drug during long-term use (see below).

Dosage

Adults only.

- By intravenous or intramuscular injection, a dose of 10 mg initially with further doses of 10–30 mg 4–6 hourly as required up to a total of 90 mg daily. Maximum treatment duration of 2 days.

- Orally, 10 mg 4–6 hourly as required for pain up to 40 mg daily in total. Treatment duration should not exceed 7 days.
- The (unlicensed) role of this drug in palliative care, often administered via the syringe driver, is acknowledged.

Nursing implications

- Patients should be advised that immediate pain relief is unlikely and 30 minutes may elapse before the effects of an injection of this drug are experienced.
- The following dosage restrictions apply in the case of elderly patients: do not exceed 60 mg by injection and do not give oral therapy more frequently than 6–8 hourly.
- Serious and even fatal reactions have been associated with this drug and long-term use is not recommended. Patients especially at risk include those with a history of asthma, haemorrhagic stroke, actively bleeding peptic ulcer, where there is a high risk of haemorrhage associated with surgery, those on current anticoagulant therapy and patients with renal impairment, hypovolaemia or dehydration.
- See also the section under NSAIDs (p. 250).

Storage

- Ketorolac preparations are stored at room temperature and protected from light.
- Though normally administered by bolus IV injection, the drug may be diluted in sodium chloride 0.9% or glucose 5% for more prolonged IV administration.

KETOTIFEN (Zaditen)

Presentation

Tablets – 1 mg
Capsules – 1 mg
Elixir – 1 mg in 5 ml

K

Actions and uses

Ketotifen is an antiallergic drug which stabilizes the mast cell, the breakdown of which is the cause of the allergic reaction. It is used in the prevention of allergic asthma (in which mast cell degradation is associated with inflammatory bronchospasm) and in allergic rhinitis and conjunctivitis (hay fever).

Dosage

Adults: 1–2 mg twice daily with food. Children (over 2 years): 1 mg twice daily with food.

Nursing implications

- It is important to note that this drug is for prophylactic use only and will not be of any benefit in the treatment of an established attack of bronchospasm.
- The nurse may play an important role in encouraging patients to persevere with the therapy in the early stages when symptomatic benefit may not be obtained. It has been found in practice that symptomatic benefit is only established after several weeks of treatment.
- In addition, patients should be encouraged to persist with this therapy despite disturbing symptoms in the early treatment period of drowsiness, dizziness and dry mouth. These symptoms will become less troublesome as treatment continues.
- Patients should be advised that driving and the performance of skilled tasks may be adversely affected during treatment with this drug.

Storage

Ketotifen preparations are stored at room temperature.

KLEAN-PREP

Klean-Prep is the trade name for a complex mixture of laxative and electrolytes. It is recognized by this title and described as such in the following text.

Presentation

Powder for reconstitution containing polyethylene glycol, sodium sulphate, sodium chloride, sodium bicarbonate and potassium chloride.

Actions and uses

Once reconstituted, the Klean-Prep mixture is swallowed. It acts as an osmotic laxative designed to completely empty the bowel contents within 4 hours or more, thus facilitating colonoscopy or X-ray or surgery of the lower bowel. The complex formulation should neither remove electrolytes from within the body nor increase the possibility of potentially harmful absorption of electrolytes.

Dosage

Adults: amounts of 250 ml are swallowed at 10-minute intervals until the bowel effluent is clear or else the maximum dose of 4 litres has been drunk.

Nursing implications

- Not surprisingly, patients may experience difficulty in swallowing such large volumes of liquid. The following actions may help the patient:
  - the solution should be reconstituted with warm water
  - fruit juice swallowed at the same time or mixed with Klean-Prep may assist some patients
  - if swallowing is not possible, administration via a nasogastric tube at a rate of 20–30 ml per minute can be tried.
- Patients should be instructed to fast for at least 4 hours before administration.
- Nausea, abdominal bloating, cramps and anal irritation are often associated with ingestion of such large volumes of fluid and patients should be reassured accordingly.

Storage

Klean-Prep powder for reconstitution is stored at room temperature.

L

LABETALOL (Trandate)

Presentation
Tablets – 50 mg, 100 mg, 200 mg, 400 mg
Injection – 100 mg in 20 ml

Actions and uses
Labetalol is a beta-adrenoreceptor blocking drug and the section on Beta-blockers (p. 51) should be consulted for a full account of this aspect of its actions. However, labetalol also possesses alpha-sympathetic blocking activity, so causing vasodilatation in the peripheral circulation. This adds to its capacity to reduce blood pressure so that labetalol's main use is in the treatment of hypertension and co-existing angina pectoris.

Dosage
- In hypertensive emergencies it may be given by slow intravenous injection (50 mg given over a period of at least 1 minute) or by intravenous infusion of a solution containing 200 mg in 200 ml given at a rate of 2 mg per minute. The maximum intravenous dosage is 300 mg.
- The usual adult oral maintenance dose is 300–600 mg per day in three divided doses. Up to 2.4 g daily may be given in divided doses to establish control of hypertension.

Nursing implications
- See the section on Beta-blockers (p. 51).
- Its additional alpha-blocking actions make it likely to produce postural hypotension. Patients must be warned of this and instructed on how to avoid its effects by changing posture slowly.
- When patients receive intravenous doses of this drug they should be in a supine position to avoid hypotension.
- Labetalol has a number of side effects not seen with other beta-blocking drugs including difficulty with micturition, epigastric pain, blurred vision, a lichenoid skin rash and tingling sensations affecting the scalp.

Storage
Labetalol tablets and injection may be stored at room temperature. The injection solution is, however, sensitive to light.

LAMIVUDINE (Epivir)

Presentation
Tablets – 150 mg
Oral solution – 10 mg in 1 ml

Actions and uses
Lamivudine is one of a new generation of antiretroviral drugs which have been developed since the first drug of this type, zidovudine, was introduced for the treatment of HIV infection. These drugs block an essential phosphorylation reaction by which the element phosphorus is incorporated into the viral DNA. Lamivudine is used in a drug cocktail to delay the progession of HIV in infected patients. It is now accepted that the optimum treatment to ensure disappearance of measurable virus from the blood of an infected patient is to combine two different antiretroviral agents (synergy is reported) with one drug of the viral protease inhibitor type.

Dosage

Adults: 150 mg twice daily.
Children: not yet licensed but has been tried on a weight-for-age basis.

Nursing implications

- Common side effects include headache, malaise, fatigue, insomnia, cough and nasal irritation, muscle pain and gastrointestinal upsets.
- More serious is the occurrence of pancreatitis and peripheral neuropathy.
- Full blood counts and liver function tests should be carried out because of the risk of anaemia, neutropenia, thrombocytopenia and liver disease.
- The excretion of lamivudine is reduced in patients with renal impairment and an appropriate dosage reduction is necessary in the event of moderate-to-severe kidney failure.
- Lamivudine is readily removed by haemodialysis.
- Avoid use during the first trimester of pregnancy.
- This drug is contraindicated in breastfeeding.

Storage

Store in a cool place, preferably a refrigerator if prolonged storage is likely.

LAMOTRIGINE (Lamictal)

Presentation

Tablets – 25 mg, 50 mg, 100 mg, 200 mg
Dispersible tablets – 5 mg, 25 mg, 100 mg

Actions and uses

Lamotrigine is an anticonvulsant which stabilizes the conducting tissue in the CNS by inhibiting release of certain excitatory neurotransmitter substances, notably glutamate whose presence is thought to be associated with the generation of seizure activity. It is used as sole anticonvulsant or add-on therapy of simple partial or complex partial seizures and as a second-line agent in refractory generalized tonic-clonic seizures and in Lennox–Gastaut syndrome.

Dosage

- Monotherapy for adults: initially 25 mg daily for 2 weeks, increased to 50 mg daily for a further 2 weeks, then increased by 50–100 mg every 1–2 weeks until control is achieved. The usual maintenance dose is 100–200 mg daily in a single or two divided doses.
- Combination therapy with sodium valproate for adults: initially 25 mg on alternate days for 2 weeks, thereafter increased by 25–50 mg every 1–2 weeks. Usual maintenance dose is 100–200 mg daily, as for monotherapy.
- Combination therapy with enzyme-inducing drugs (e.g. carbamazepine) for adults: initially 50 mg daily for 2 weeks, then 50 mg twice daily for a further 2 weeks, thereafter increased by 100 mg every 1–2 weeks. Usual maintenance dose is 200–400 mg daily in 2 divided doses.

Nursing implications

- It is important to warn patients to seek medical advice immediately if a rash or flu-like symptoms develop as withdrawal of the drug may be necessary.
- This is a relatively new drug and active monitoring and reporting of all suspected adverse reactions should be encouraged.
- Side effects so far reported include maculopapular skin rash (up to 10% of patients affected) and rarely angiooedema and Stevens–Johnson syndrome.
- Central side effects include diplopia, blurred vision, dizziness, drowsiness incoordination and headache.
- Gastrointestinal upsets are also reported.
- The metabolism of lamotrigine is increased by other anticonvulsants which stimulate liver microsomal enzyme

production, e.g. carbamazepine, phenobarbitone, phenytoin.
- Lamotrigine has weak antifolate activity and should be avoided in pregnancy.
- Lamotrigine should be used with caution in patients with renal or hepatic impairment. It is both metabolized by the liver and excreted via the kidney.

Storage

Lamotrigine tablets are stored at room temperature in a dry place.

LANSOPRAZOLE (Zoton)

Presentation

Capsules – 15 mg, 30 mg
Sachets – 30 mg

Actions and uses

Lansoprazole belongs to the group of drugs which inhibit the proton pump. Their action and uses can be described as follows.

The production of gastric acid, which takes place in the parietal cells of the stomach lining or mucosa, depends upon the generation of hydrogen ion (H^+) by an intracellular mechanism called the proton pump. The pump is activated in response to secretion of the hormone gastrin and by the action of histamine on a specific histamine H2 receptor on the cell's surface. Hence the histamine H2 receptor antagonists such as cimetidine and ranitidine reduce acid output by one of these mechanisms.

The proton pump inhibitors, on the other hand, can bring about almost complete suppression of gastric acid, whether produced in response to histamine or gastrin. For this reason, drugs such as lansoprazole are very much more potent than the histamine H2 receptor antagonists which they have now largely replaced in the following indications.

- Treatment and prevention of peptic ulcer disease.
- Eradication of *Helicobacter pylori*, a Gram-negative bacterium which is implicated in most cases of gastric

and duodenal ulceration. Lansoprazole is administered in combination with at least two antibiotics from metronidazole, amoxycillin and clarithromycin.
- Treatment and prevention of gastrooesophageal reflux disease.
- Prevention of NSAID-induced gastritis, bleeding and peptic ulceration.
- Other conditions in which acid suppression is indicated.

Dosage

- Usual dose in the treatment of active disease is 30 mg once daily.
- Half this dose may be used in children and in maintenance treatment aimed at preventing disease recurrence.
- Twice-daily dosage with 30 mg lansoprazole is used in *Helicobacter pylori* eradication regimen. The drug is administered for 2 weeks and continued at this dose for a further period of up to 1 month where active bleeding was present.

L

Nursing implications

- Allergic reactions to lansoprazole include skin rash, pruritus and urticaria.
- Diarrhoea and headaches, sometimes severe enough to warrant discontinuation of treatment, have also been reported.
- Other GI side effects include constipation, nausea and vomiting, and abdominal pain.
- Muscle aches and pains and neuropathic symptoms are rarely reported.
- The absorption of drugs which are dependent on gastric acidity (e.g. ketoconazole) may be impaired by concurrent treatment with lansoprazole.
- Interactions with drugs metabolized by the liver (e.g. phenytoin, warfarin) may also be reduced.

Storage

Lansoprazole capsules and sachets are stored at room temperature.

LATANOPROST (Xalatan)

Presentation
Eye drops – 125 microgram in 2.5 ml (0.005%)

Actions and uses
Latanoprost is a prostaglandin derivative which increases the outflow of aqueous humour from the eye, so reducing its accumulation and associated rise in intraocular pressure. It is a long-acting drug so that once-daily administration in ocular hypertension and open angle glaucoma is possible.

Dosage
Instil one drop in the affected eye once daily, preferably in the evening.

Nursing implications
- DO NOT exceed the standard dose. This is likely to lead to a **reduction** in the efficacy of latanoprost.
- Eye drops tend to increase the brown pigment of the iris and patients should be advised accordingly.
- Side effects may include ocular irritation and change in the texture of the eyelashes.
- Avoid in breastfeeding and pregnancy.

Storage
Use within 4 weeks of opening.

LENOGRASTIM (Granocyte)

Presentation
Injection – 33.6 mega unit (263 microgram) and 13.4 mega unit (105 microgram) dry powder vials

Actions and uses
Lenograstim is a leucocyte growth factor. It is specifically one of the granulocyte-colony stimulating factors (G-CSFs) which regulate the formation and development of neutrophils (phagocytic, granulocytic WBCs) essential for normal host defence. Lenograstim is used to prevent or reverse neutropenia and hence the risk of bacterial infections in at-risk groups. This includes patients undergoing cytotoxic chemotherapy in which life-threatening neutropenia may occur and in conjunction with cytotoxic bone marrow ablation therapy associated with bone marrow transplantation.

Dosage
- Treatment is administered by subcutaneous injection or continuous subcutaneous infusion or by intravenous infusion over 30 minutes.
- Route of administration and dosage are determined by specific indication. Check package insert or accompanying literature.

Nursing implications
- The initial dose of G-CSF should not be administered until 24 hours after cytotoxic chemotherapy has been given.
- Daily doses are then administered until the expected neutrophil nadir has passed and the count has recovered to within the normal range of 2.0–7.5 × 10^9 cells/litre. This may take up to 14 days to achieve with a maximum treatment course for lenograstim of 28 days. Dosage may be titrated downwards during this period as a sustained response is apparent.
- Pain affecting the bones and joints is the most frequently encountered side effect which may respond to treatment with simple analgesics. Others include headache, fever, skin rashes, fatigue and injection site reactions, though treatment is in general well tolerated.

Storage
Store in a refrigerator.

LERCANIDIPINE (Zanidip)

Presentation
Tablets – 10 mg

Actions and uses
Lercanidipine is a member of the Calcium Antagonist group (see p. 67).

It is similar to nifedipine and amlodipine in this respect. Lercanidipine is licensed specifically for the treatment of isolated systolic hypertension (ISH), a common finding in elderly hypertensives in particular.

Dosage
Adults: 10–20 mg once daily, taken about 15 minutes before one of the main meals of the day.

> **Nursing implications**
> See the section on Calcium Antagonists (p. 67).

Storage
Tablets are stored at room temperature.

LEVODOPA-CONTAINING PREPARATIONS (Madopar, Sinemet)

Presentation
Levodopa is now rarely given alone. It is usually given with an inhibitor of dopa-decarboxylase, the enzyme which is responsible for the conversion of levodopa to the active neurotransmitter dopamine. It is therefore very unlikely that any nurse will encounter levodopa other than in the form of co-beneldopa (dopa-decarboxylase inhibitor is beneldopa) or co-careldopa (dopa-decarboxylase inhibitor is careldopa). The combination ensures that the maximum amount of levodopa (dopamine precursor) crosses the blood–brain barrier, so reducing substantially the quantities which would otherwise be required (and which were associated with considerable side effects as a result of peripheral conversion).

Madopar capsule preparations contain:

- levodopa 50 mg + benserazide 12.5 mg = co-beneldopa 12.5/50 or Madopar 62.5
- levodopa 100 mg + benserazide 25 mg = co-beneldopa 25/100 or Madopar 125
- levodopa 200 mg + benserazide 50 mg = co-beneldopa 50/200 or Madopar 250

Madopar dispersible tablet preparations contain:

- levodopa 50 mg + benserazide 12.5 mg = co-beneldopa 12.5/50 or Madopar 62.5 dispersible
- levodopa 100 mg + benserazide 25 mg = co-beneldopa 25/100 or Madopar 125 dispersible

Madopar CR capsule preparation contains:

- levodopa 100 mg + benserazide 25 mg = co-beneldopa 25/100 or Madopar 125 controlled/modified release

Sinemet tablet preparations contain:

- levodopa 50 mg + carbidopa 12.5 mg = co-careldopa 12.5/50 or Sinemet 62.5
- levodopa 100 mg + carbidopa 10 mg = co-careldopa 10/100 or Sinemet 110
- levodopa 100 mg + carbidopa 25 mg = co-careldopa 25/100 or Sinemet Plus
- levodopa 250 mg + carbidopa 25 mg = co-careldopa 25/250 or Sinemet 275

Sinemet CR tablet preparations contain:

- levodopa 100 mg + carbidopa 25 mg = co-careldopa 25/100 or Half Sinemet CR
- levodopa 200 mg + carbidopa 50 mg = co-careldopa 50/200 or Sinemet CR

Actions and uses
In Parkinson's disease it has been shown that certain (nigrostriatial) areas of the brain are depleted of a substance known as dopamine. It has further been shown that treatment with substances which increase concentrations of dopamine in these areas leads to an improvement in symptoms, including tremor, rigidity and dyskinesias. Levodopa is a precursor of dopamine which is converted in the body to dopamine. It is used, therefore, for the treatment of Parkinson's disease.

Dosage
Dosage must be carefully titrated to the individual's requirement. It is therefore highly variable as Parkinson's

disease develops inexorably. Eventually, very frequent (1–2 hourly) dosage may become necessary to maintain control of the disease in its advanced stages.

Nursing implications

- Side effects are usually dose related and do occur at some time in most patients. During the initiation of therapy nausea, vomiting, anorexia, weakness and hypotension (commonly postural) may occur.
- To reduce the likelihood of nausea and vomiting the nurse can advise patients to take the drug immediately after food. Occasionally, however, an antiemetic drug may be necessary.
- At any stage in the treatment the following other side effects may occur: psychiatric disturbance including elation, depression, anxiety, agitation, aggression, hallucination and delusion.
- Involuntary movements, commonly in the form of oral dyskinesia or similar writhing movements of the limbs. These effects are usually dose related and may disappear after a reduction in the dose. They are particularly likely to occur in elderly people.
- Abnormalities in liver function tests and other biochemical blood values may occur.
- Patients on levodopa may notice a darkening in colour with a reddish tinge of the urine. They should be reassured that this does not imply any renal damage.

Storage

Madopar and Sinemet preparations are stored at room temperature.

LIGNOCAINE INTRAVENOUS INJECTION

Presentation

Intravenous – 2%
For infusion – 20%

Actions and uses

Lignocaine suppresses the conduction of electrical impulses through heart muscle and may be given intravenously to treat serious ventricular dysrhythmias.

Dosage

Bolus dosage at onset of treatment: 1 mg/kg given over 5 minutes. This may be repeated once or twice if necessary at 5–10 minute intervals. Maintenance regime: initially 2 mg per minute, increasing to 3 mg per minute and a maximum of 4 mg per minute if necessary. This regime is usually continued for 48 hours and prior to discontinuation, loading doses of oral antidysrhythmic are given.

Nursing implications

- Lignocaine is often given in emergency situations such as cardiac arrest. It is important to note that the 20% solution is never appropriate for bolus injection.
- Calcium chloride or gluconate cannot be injected into a solution containing lignocaine or the calcium salt will precipitate in a solid form.
- Too rapid or excessive intravenous dosage may be associated with the following side effects: nervousness, dizziness, blurred vision, tremor and convulsions, nausea, hypotension and bradycardia and, respiratory depression (with very high doses).
- Patients with impaired liver function are more likely to develop adverse side effects.

Storage

- Lignocaine preparation may be stored at room temperature.
- Lignocaine 20% solution for cardiac use must be added to glucose 5% (1 g added to 500 ml of infusion fluid) to give a final concentration of 0.2%.

LISINOPRIL (Carace, Zestril)

Presentation
Tablets – 2.5 mg, 5 mg, 10 mg, 20 mg

Actions and uses
See section on ACE Inhibitors (p. 4).

Dosage
Range: 10–40 mg as a single daily dose.

Nursing implications
See section on ACE Inhibitors (p. 4).

Storage
Lisinopril tablets are stored at room temperature.

LITHIUM PREPARATIONS (Camcolit, Li-Liquid, Liskonium, Litarex, Priadel)

Presentation
Tablets – 250 mg, 400 mg
Controlled-release tablet – 450 mg, 564 mg, 200 mg, 400 mg
Liquid – 5.4 (520 mg) and 10.8 mmol (1040 mg) in 5 ml

Actions and uses
Lithium, by an unknown mechanism, has been found to be useful for the treatment of depression, mania, hypomania and self-mutilating disorder. In particular, it controls both the manic and depressive phases of manic-depressive psychosis and continuing treatment reduces the recurrence of depressive and manic phases in patients who have already been found to have endogenous depression.

Dosage
For the treatment of depression in adults the precise dosage is that which maintains the plasma lithium level in the range 0.4–1.0 mmol/l.

Nursing implications
- On commencement of therapy clients may experience lack of coordination and concentration, which may affect driving, and they should be advised accordingly.
- Clients should be advised on the importance of compliance; withdrawal of therapy will cause manic symptoms to recur.
- Treatment is usually taken once per day and it is important that all patients receiving the drug have their dosage carefully monitored to keep them within the above range.
- Side effects, which are mainly seen if an excess dose is being taken, include anorexia, nausea, vomiting, diarrhoea, thirst, polyuria, fatigue, malaise, dizziness, confusion, hypotension and cardiac dysrhythmias.
- Patients should be advised on the importance of an adequate fluid and sodium intake.
- The drug should be used with caution in patients with renal failure or cardiac disease.
- Lithium may alter thyroid function, rendering the patient clinically hypothyroid. This may be detected as the formation of a goitre (thyroid swelling). However, regular monitoring with clinical and biochemical testing should avoid the development of this effect.
- Elderly patients require lower doses of this drug.

Storage
Preparations containing lithium are stored at room temperature.

LOFEPRAMINE (Gamanil)

Presentation
Tablets – 70 mg

Actions and uses
Lofepramine is a member of the tricyclic antidepressant group and the section on Antidepressant Drugs (p. 31) should be consulted.

Dosage
Adults: usually 70 mg twice or three times daily but higher doses are used in severe resistant depression.

L

Nursing implications
See the section on Antidepressant Drugs (p. 31).

Storage
Lofepramine tablets are stored at room temperature. Protect from light.

LOMUSTINE (CCNU)

Presentation
Capsules – 10 mg, 40 mg

Actions and uses
Lomustine is a cytotoxic drug of the alkylating agent group. It inhibits cell growth and cell division by combining with and preventing important changes required for cell growth and development. It may be used alone, with radiotherapy or in combination with other cytotoxic drugs in the treatment of the following conditions:

- brain tumours
- bronchogenic carcinoma
- malignant melanoma
- Hodgkin's disease.

It has been occasionally given for non-Hodgkin's lymphoma, myeloma, tumours of the gut, kidney, testis, ovary, cervix, uterus and breast.

Dosage
The drug is taken orally. The dose for adults and children is up to 120–130 mg/m^2 as a single dose repeated every 6–8 weeks.

Nursing implications
- Bone marrow suppression is an important side effect and the resultant leucopenia and thrombocytopenia leave the patient at risk of severe infection and haemorrhage.
- Other side effects include anorexia, nausea, vomiting, alopecia, stomatitis and altered liver function.
- White blood cell counts, platelet counts and liver function tests are normally monitored during treatment.

- Nurses should be aware of the risks posed by cytotoxic drugs. Some are irritant to the skin and mucous surfaces and care must be exercised when handling them. In particular, spillage or contamination of personnel or the environment must be avoided. If cytotoxic drugs are handled regularly, it is theoretically possible that repeated skin contact or inhalation may produce systemic toxic effects in nurses who have developed hypersensitivity to them. Most hospitals now operate a centralized (pharmacy-organized) additive service. While this reduces the risk of exposure to cytotoxic drugs, it is essential that nurses recognize and understand the local policy on their safe handling and disposal. The Health and Safety Executive has decreed that such a policy should be in place wherever cytotoxic drugs are administered. These should be adapted, wherever possible, to care of patients in the community.

Storage
Lomustine capsules are stored at room temperature. It is important to note that they should be stored in the original container and protected from light and moisture.

LOPERAMIDE (Imodium)

Presentation
Capsules – 2 mg
Syrup – 1 mg in 5 ml

Actions and uses
Loperamide has a direct action on the nerves which control muscular movement of the intestinal wall. Its overall effect is to slow the passage of substances through the intestine and its use is therefore in the treatment of diarrhoea.

Dosage
Adults: 4 mg initially followed by 2 mg after each loose stool. The

maximum daily dosage should not
exceed 16 mg.
Children: 4–8 years require 1 mg four
times per day; 9–12 years require 2 mg
four times per day.
It is recommended that all the above
doses be given until the diarrhoea is
controlled.

Nursing implications
- The drug is very poorly
  absorbed from the gut and
  therefore produces little in the
  way of side effects.
- Continued use after diarrhoea
  has been controlled may
  produce constipation.
- Persistent diarrhoea may be
  indicative of a serious
  underlying condition and
  therefore patients should be
  made aware of the importance
  of seeking medical advice
  should their symptoms persist.

Storage
- Loperamide preparations are stored
  at room temperature.
- For ease of administration the syrup
  may be diluted with water just
  before use.
- The commercial syrup is sugar free
  and is therefore suitable for patients
  who are disaccharide intolerant.

LORAZEPAM

Presentation
Tablets – 1 mg, 2.5 mg
Injection – 4 mg in 1 ml

Actions and uses
Lorazepam is a member of the
Benzodiazepine group (p. 47). In
practice it is used for the control of
status epilepticus and for the control
of anxiety. Because of its short
duration of action it is sometimes used
as an alternative to diazepam for
sedation prior to minor operative or
dental procedures.

Dosage
Status epilepticus: adults require 4 mg
by slow IV bolus injection.
For the treatment of anxiety: adults
receive 1–4 mg daily in divided doses.

For sedation prior to minor surgical or
dental procedures: 2–4 mg is given as
a single dose, 1 or 2 hours before the
procedure begins.

Nursing implications
See the section on Benzodiazepines
(p. 47).

Storage
Store at room temperature.

LOW MOLECULAR WEIGHT HEPARIN/HEPARINOID (LMWH)

Presentation
This new group of injectable
anticoagulants include the following
compounds, listed by approved (and
trade) name and presentation.
- Dalteparin (Fragmin) – prefilled
  syringes of 2500 unit/0.2 ml,
  5000 unit/2 ml, 10 000 unit/0.4 ml,
  15 000 unit/0.6 ml, 18 000
  unit/ 0.72 ml. Ampoules of
  2500 unit/ml – 1 ml and 4 ml.
  10 000 unit/ml – 1 ml,
  25 000 unit/ml – 4 ml.
- Enoxaparin (Clexane) – 100 mg/
  10 000 unit/ml. Prefilled syringes of
  0.2, 0.4, 0.6, 0.8 and 1 ml.
- Tinzaparin (Innohep) – prefilled
  syringes of 10 000 unit/ml
  including 0.35 ml, 0.45 ml, 2 ml,
  and 20 000 unit/ml including
  0.5 ml, 0.7 ml, and 0.9 ml. Vials
  containing 20,000 units in 2 ml and
  40,000 units in 2 ml.
- Danaparoid (Orgaron), a
  heparinoid – 750 IU ampoules.

Actions and uses
Standard (unfractionated) heparin is a
complex substance of large molecular
structure derived from the intestinal
mucosa of cattle, sheep or pigs to
yield so-called 'mucous' heparin. As a
result of chemical breakdown
(depolymerization) of the large heparin
molecule, a series of smaller fragments
are produced which can be separated
out according to their individual
molecular structures. These are the
low molecular weight heparins
(LMWHs). They differ from standard
heparin in terms of activity, adverse

reaction profile and the need for monitoring anticoagulant control.

LMWHs, after binding to antithrombin III (ATIII), activate this natural anticoagulant. The LMWH-ATIII complex has a specific inhibitory effect on activated factor Xa and little, if any, effect on thrombin. It therefore produces a more consistent anticoagulant effect without the same degree of bleeding risk which is associated with standard heparin. As a result, it is rarely necessary to monitor anticoagulant control, which can only be carried out by measuring the activated factor Xa activity.

LMWHs have been gradually replacing standard heparin since the late 1990s. They are currently used for the following indications.

- For prevention of deep vein thrombosis during and after surgery (various types but particularly if the risk of haemorrhage is high).
- Treatment of DVT and pulmonary embolism.
- In association with haemodialysis.
- Treatment of unstable angina and non-Q wave infarction.

Dosage

- Varies according to indication and commercial LMWH in use. Check accompanying manufacturer's literature.
- LMWHs are administered by subcutaneous injection once, or occasionally twice, a day.

Nursing implications

- LMWHs are usually administered by subcutaneous injection, alternating the site between right and left anterolateral and posterolateral abdominal wall.
- The risk of bleeding is not eliminated by use of LMWHs. All heparins should be avoided in patients at major risk including recent haemorrhagic stroke, thrombocytopenia, active peptic ulceration and uncontrolled or uncontrollable hypertension.
- Caution is necessary in severe liver disease.
- Platelet count should be monitored. A temporary fall in platelet count is not uncommon but if thrombocytopenia develops, treatment must be discontinued.
- Thrombocytopenia occurs in around 4% of patients treated with heparin for 1 week or more. It is due to hypersensitivity to which cross-reactivity to different heparins exists. Danaparoid, which is not chemically a heparin but rather a unique substance (a heparinoid) possessing anti-factor Xa activity, has been substituted in such cases.
- Caution is required in surgical procedures involving epidural or spinal anaesthesia. Preoperative doses may be omitted to limit risk of intraspinal haemorrhage.

Storage

All LMWHs are stored at room temperature. Protect from light.

M

MEBEVERINE (Colofac)

Presentation
Tablets – 135 mg

Actions and uses
Mebeverine is an anticholinergic drug which relieves colonic spasm by a direct action on the smooth muscle of the colon. It is used to relieve abdominal pain, cramps, flatulence and diarrhoea which are frequent symptoms of irritable bowel syndrome and also the gastrointestinal spasm associated with diverticular disease, gastritis, duodenitis, etc.

Dosage
The usual dose is 135 mg taken three times daily around 20 minutes before a meal.

Nursing implications
- Although mebeverine is anticholinergic, it causes few typical anticholinergic side effects unless taken in excessive dosage. These may include dry mouth, blurred vision or urinary retention.
- This drug should be avoided in pregnancy and breastfeeding.

Storage
Mebeverine tablets are stored at room temperature.

MEDROXYPROGESTERONE (Farlutal, Provera, Depo-Provera, Premique, Premique Cycle)

Presentation
Tablets – 2.5 mg, 5 mg, 10 mg, 100 mg, 200 mg, 250 mg, 400 mg, 500 mg
Injection – 500 mg suspension in 2.5 ml vial
Depot injection – 150 mg suspension in 1 ml prefilled syringe
Also combined with conjugated oestrogen in HRT products.

Actions and uses
Medroxyprogesterone, as the name suggests, is a progestational hormone which is used as follows.

- As a depot contraceptive administered by deep intramuscular injection every 3 months.
- In the control of dysfunctional (anovulatory) uterine bleeding.
- Treatment of endometriosis of mild-to-moderate degree.
- Treatment of secondary amenorrhoea.
- Treatment of breast cancer in postmenopausal women.
- Treatment of endometrial, prostatic and renal cell carcinoma.
- Medroxyprogesterone is also included as progestational hormone together with conjugated oestrogens in the combined HRT preparations Premique and Premique Cycle.

Medroxyprogesterone has the advantage of possessing fewer of the androgenic side effects which are associated with other progestational agents.

Dosage
As a depot contraceptive injection: administer 150 mg (1 ml) by IM injection during the first 5 days of a cycle or within 5 days post partum if not breastfeeding or after 6 weeks post partum if breastfeeding. Repeat every 12 weeks thereafter.
Treatment of endometriosis: 10 mg orally three times daily starting on the first day of the cycle and taken continuously for 3 months.

Secondary amenorrhoea: 2.5–10 mg daily for 5 days starting on the assumed 16th to 21st day of the cycle and repeated for three consecutive cycles.
Breast cancer: 1 g to 1.5 g Farlutal orally daily or Provera 400–800 mg orally daily.
Endometrial, prostatic and renal cell carcinoma: 100–500 mg Farlutal orally daily or 200–400 mg Provera orally daily.
Dysfunctional uterine bleeding: 2.5–10 mg taken daily for 5–10 days then repeated on two consecutive cycles.

Nursing implications
- Note that the oral bioavailability of the Farlutal and Provera brands is different. Therefore it must be ensured that the prescribed dose is compatible with the particular brand being used.
- Typical side effects of the progestational hormones include gastrointestinal upsets, acne-like skin eruptions, breast tenderness, galactorrhoea and weight gain. Such effects are, however, less likely to occur with this drug than with other progestational agents.

Storage
All products are stored at room temperature.

MEFENAMIC ACID (Ponstan)

Presentation
Tablets – 500 mg
Capsules – 250 mg
Paediatric suspension – 50 mg in 5 ml

Actions and uses
Mefenamic acid is a member of the NSAID group (p. 250). It is now used primarily as an analgesic for short-term or intermittent treatment of pain and, in particular, in the management of painful/heavy periods (dysmenorrhoea/menorrhagia) when in practice almost any NSAID will effectively reduce pain and blood loss.

Dosage
Adults: for all indications, 250–500 mg three times daily.
Children: over 6 months, 50 mg; 2–4 years, 100 mg; 5–8 years, 150 mg; 9–12 years, 200 mg. All children's doses are also taken 8-hourly.

Nursing implications
- Mefenamic acid produces all the side effects which are normally associated with NSAIDS including dyspepsia, gastritis, duodenitis, gastrointestinal bleeding and ulceration.
- It has also been associated with side effects including diarrhoea and colitis.
- In the elderly, in particular, mefenamic acid may precipitate acute renal failure and it is important to ensure adequate hydration in this group beforehand.
- Haemolytic anaemia has also been reported.
- Mefenamic acid is specifically neurotoxic in overdosage.

Storage
Store at room temperature.

MEFLOQUINE (Lariam)

Presentation
Tablets – 250 mg

Actions and uses
Mefloquine is an antimalarial drug that is chemically derived from quinine. It is currently favoured for prevention of malaria for travellers abroad staying for up to 1 year in highly endemic areas in which there is documented resistance to chloroquine by falciparum malaria. It is also used in the treatment of acute falciparum malaria where resistance to first-line drugs is likely to exist. The side effects of mefloquine, which have received widespread publicity, may limit its use in practice.

Dosage
Treatment: dosage varies according to body weight and immune status.

The data sheet or summary of product characteristics should be consulted. Prophylaxis for adult travellers visiting risk areas: a single dose of 250 mg is taken on the same day each week, commencing 1 week before departure and continuing for at least 4 weeks after returning. Children take a proportion of the adult dose according to age; seek advice on individual cases.

Nursing implications

- Patient education regarding compliance is essential.
- Mefloquine has received widespread publicity as a result of the often bizarre side effects with which it has been associated. The most unusual of these include depression, anxiety, confusion, hallucinations, panic attacks, restlessness, agitation, aggression, mood swings, paranoia and psychosis.
- Nausea, vomiting, diarrhoea, abdominal pain, dizziness, vertigo, headache and sleep disturbances are relatively much more common.
- Flushing and fluctuations in BP and heart rate are a likely problem for patients with hypertension and/or heart disease.
- Skin rashes, muscle weakness, loss of appetite, blood disorders and changes in liver function have also been reported.
- Caution is necessary in patients with a history of seizures and mental illness.
- Mefloquine should be avoided in pregnancy.
- Driving and other skilled tasks should also be avoided.

Storage
Store at room temperature. Protect from moisture.

MEGESTROL ACETATE (Megace)

Presentation
Tablets – 40 mg, 160 mg

Actions and uses
Megestrol acetate is a progestational hormone. In clinical practice it is used to block the growth of oestrogen-dependent neoplasms, such as endometrial and breast cancers. It also possesses some androgenic/anabolic activity and as such is used to stimulate appetite in malnourished, frail or cachectic cancer sufferers.

Dosage
Breast cancer: 160 mg daily in single or divided doses.
Endometrial cancer: 40–320 mg daily with divided doses in the higher range.
Malnourished/cachectic patients: 160–320 mg daily as a single or two divided doses.

Nursing implications

- In breast and endometrial cancer, treatment must be administered for at least 2 months in order to be effective, therefore patient education regarding compliance is crucial.
- Nausea and other gastrointestinal upsets are relatively common.
- Weight gain can be anticipated due to the anabolic actions of the drug. Hence its use in malnourished or cachectic patients.
- Allergic skin reactions, including urticaria, are reported.
- Megestrol acetate should be avoided in those with a history of thromboembolic disease and in severe liver impairment.

Storage
Store at room temperature.

MELOXICAM (Mobic)

Presentation
Tablets – 7.5 mg, 15 mg
Suppositories – 7.5 mg, 15 mg

Actions and uses
Meloxicam is a non-steroidal antiinflammatory drug and the section on NSAIDs (p. 250) should be consulted for a full account of its actions. It differs from other NSAIDs, however, in that it has a relatively selective action

M

on the inflammatory response and less so on the mechanism by which gastric mucosal protection is maintained. The implication of this is that it is less likely than other NSAIDs to produce the severe gastrointestinal side effects with which the group as a whole is associated.

In practice meloxicam is used for the treatment of:

- mild to moderate pain, especially if an inflammatory component is present
- osteoarthritis
- rheumatoid arthritis.

Dosage

Licensed for use in adults only. Initial dosage is 7.5 mg increased as necessary to 15 mg taken once daily.

Nursing implications
- The section on NSAIDs (p. 250) should be consulted for a full account of the nursing implications which apply to this drug.
- A lesser degree of gastrointestinal side effects might be expected but such problems are not eliminated by use of this drug.

Storage

Meloxicam tablets and suppositories are stored at room temperature. Do not store suppositories close to a heat source (e.g. radiator).

MELPHALAN (Alkeran)

Presentation

Tablets – 2 mg, 5 mg
Injection – 50 mg dry powder ampoules plus diluent

Actions and uses

Melphalan is a member of the nitrogen mustard group of cytotoxic drugs and belongs to the class known as the alkylating agents. After conversion to a highly reactive compound, irreversible binding to guanine components on the DNA strand takes place. The result is that the double strands of DNA become crosslinked so that cell division cannot take place. Melphalan is used as follows.

- In multiple myeloma, which is probably its major use.
- In advanced ovarian adenocarcinoma.
- It has also been used for the treatment of advanced breast cancer.
- Administered by regional arterial perfusion in localized malignant melanoma and soft tissue sarcoma of the extremities.
- Neuroblastoma of childhood in association with autologous bone marrow transplantation.
- In polycythaemia rubra vera.

Dosage

- In multiple myelomatosis the oral dose schedule is 0.15 mg/kg daily for 4 days given in combination with prednisolone. It is repeated at intervals of 6 weeks.
- For treatment of other tumours, regimes are variable; the up-to-date literature should be consulted.

Nursing implications
- Severe bone marrow suppression may occur even at low dose ranges, resulting in a risk of infection or haemorrhage.
- Nausea, vomiting and alopecia also occur but are more frequent with higher dosage.
- Melphalan is highly irritant and precautions should be taken to avoid contact with skin and eyes.
- Nurses should be aware of the risks posed by cytotoxic drugs. Some are irritant to the skin and mucous surfaces and care must be exercised when handling them. In particular, spillage or contamination of personnel or the environment must be avoided. If cytotoxic drugs are handled regularly, it is theoretically possible that repeated skin contact or inhalation may produce systemic toxic effects in nurses who have developed hypersensitivity to them. Most hospitals now

operate a centralized (pharmacy-organized) additive service. While this reduces the risk of exposure to cytotoxic drugs, it is essential that nurses recognize and understand the local policy on their safe handling and disposal. The Health and Safety Executive has decreed that such a policy should be in place wherever cytotoxic drugs are administered. These should be adapted, wherever possible, to care of patients in the community.

Storage
- Melphalan tablets are stored at room temperature.
- The injection should be stored in a cool place and for this purpose refrigeration may be preferred.
- The injection must be protected from light.

MEPTAZINOL (Meptid)

Presentation
Tablets – 200 mg
Injection – 100 mg in 1 ml

Actions and uses
Meptazinol is a potent, non-narcotic analgesic used in the treatment of moderate-to-severe pain, e.g. postoperatively, after myocardial infarction, in obstetrics, etc. It is a step 2 drug on the analgesic step-ladder which places it alongside other analgesics such as dihydrocodeine and pethidine. Meptazinol does not appear to produce significant dependence, respiratory depression or cardiovascular disturbances which may be disadvantageous with opioids such as morphine. It is not, however, comparable with morphine in anything but low-range morphine dosage.

Dosage
Adults.

- Orally: 200 mg 4-hourly.
- Intravenous/intramuscular injection: 50–100 mg repeated every 2–4 hours.

- A dose of 100 mg meptazinol produces analgesia comparable to 15 mg morphine or 100 mg pethidine.

Nursing implications
- Although meptazinol is reported to be associated with little, if any, dependence, it is intended for short-term pain relief and the possibility of meptazinol abuse should not be overlooked.
- In common with opioid analgesics meptazinol may produce nausea and constipation requiring remedial antiemetic and laxative therapy.
- There is no evidence that the newborn are adversely affected by meptazinol administered during labour and the respiratory depression associated with pethidine does not appear to occur.

Storage
Meptazinol tablets and injection are stored at room temperature.

MERCAPTOPURINE (Puri-Nethol)

Presentation
Tablets – 50 mg

Actions and uses
Mercaptopurine is essentially a cytotoxic. It is also the drug which is generated by the liver metabolism of a related drug, azathioprine, which, as the trade name (Imuran) suggests, is used exclusively as an immunosuppressant in clinical practice.

Mercaptopurine is one of the antimetabolites which inhibits a number of different enzymes involved in the early stages of purine synthesis which is an essential prerequisite to the synthesis of cellular DNA. Subsequently cell division, which relies upon successful functioning of intact DNA, is blocked.

Mercaptopurine is used in the maintenance treatment of acute lymphoblastic leukaemia (ALL). Its other uses include in acute myelogenous leukaemia (AML) and chronic granulocytic leukaemia (CGL).

Dosage

The oral daily dose for adults is usually in the range 2.5–5 mg/kg body weight. Children's doses are as for adults.

Nursing implications

- Bone marrow suppression is an important side effect. It may produce anaemia, bleeding due to thrombocytopenia and infection due to suppression of white cell production. Regular blood tests are frequently carried out during treatment to detect its onset.
- This drug commonly causes gastrointestinal problems including anorexia, nausea, vomiting, diarrhoea and oral ulceration.
- Mercaptopurine may rarely cause severe, potentially life-threatening liver damage so that blood tests of liver function should be carried out regularly.
- The drug allopurinol, which is used in the treatment of hyperuricaemia and gout prophylaxis, alters the metabolism of mercaptopurine in such a way that the effect of a particular dose of mercaptopurine may be markedly increased in patients who are given both drugs. The dose of mercaptopurine should be reduced to approximately one-quarter of that intended if patients are already on or are commenced on allopurinol.
- Nurses should be aware of the risks posed by cytotoxic drugs. Some are irritant to the skin and mucous surfaces and care must be exercised when handling them. In particular, spillage or contamination of personnel or the environment must be avoided. If cytotoxic drugs are handled regularly, it is theoretically possible that repeated skin contact or inhalation may produce systemic toxic effects in nurses who have developed hypersensitivity to them. Most hospitals now operate a centralized (pharmacy-organized) additive service. While this reduces the risk of exposure to cytotoxic drugs, it is essential that nurses recognize and understand the local policy on their safe handling and disposal. The Health and Safety Executive has decreed that such a policy should be in place wherever cytotoxic drugs are administered. These should be adapted, wherever possible, to care of patients in the community.

Storage

Store at room temperature. Protect from light.

MEROPENEM (Meronem)

Presentation

Injection – 250 mg, 500 mg, 1 g dry powder vials
Intravenous infusion kits – 500 mg, 1 g dry powder vials with 100 ml bag of 0.9% sodium chloride

Actions and uses

Meropenem is a carbapenem antibiotic, a member of the group of beta-lactam antibiotics. It is only used parenterally. Meropenem has a bactericidal action, interfering with bacterial cell wall synthesis. It readily penetrates bacterial cell walls, is stable to beta-lactamases and has a marked affinity for the penicillin-binding proteins. Meropenem is similar to imipenem but differs in that it is stable to the renal enzyme which inactivates imipenem.

Meropenem is active against a wide range of aerobic and anaerobic Gram-positive and Gram-negative bacteria which is reflected in its many indications including:

- pneumonias
- urinary tract infections
- intraabdominal infections
- gynaecological infections
- skin infections
- meningitis

- septicaemia
- empiric treatment, when the infecting organism cannot be readily predicted and the results of bacteriological screening are awaited.

Dosage

Meropenem can be given as an IV bolus over 5 minutes or by IV infusion over 15–30 minutes.
Adults.

- 500 mg IV every 8 hours for pneumonia, UTI, gynaecological infections and skin infections.
- 1 g IV every 8 hours for nosocomial pneumonias, peritonitis, presumed infections in neutropenic patients, septicaemia.
- Up to 2 g IV every 8 hours in cystic fibrosis.
- 2 g IV every 8 hours for meningitis.

Children: 3 months–12 years, 10–20 mg/kg every 8 hours depending on the severity and type of infection. If the child is over 50 kg, use the adult dose. Doses of up to 40 mg/kg every 8 hours have been used in children with cystic fibrosis. In meningitis 40 mg/kg every 8 hours is recommended.

Nursing implications

- In common with other antibiotics, meropenem can cause skin reactions, including thrombo-phlebitis at the injection site.
- Other side effects include oral candidiasis, nausea, vomiting and diarrhoea (pseudo-membranous colitis has been reported).
- Blood dyscrasias and disturbed liver function can also occur.
- Unlike imipenem, meropenem has not been associated with CNS toxicity.
- Probenecid competes with meropenem for excretion, therefore blood levels of meropenem will increase if probenecid is given concurrently.

Storage

Store at room temperature.

MESALAZINE
(Asacol, Pentasa, Salofalk)

Presentation

Tablets – enteric coated 250 mg, 400 mg, slow release 500 mg
Modified-release granules – 1 g/sachet
Suppositories – 250 mg, 500 mg, 1 g
Enema – 1 g, 2 g

Actions and uses

Mesalazine is chemically aminosalicylic acid, a component of sulphasalazine which is formed after administration of sulphasalazine. Mesalazine possesses an antiinflammatory action and is used in the maintenance of remission of ulcerative colitis for patients who are intolerant of sulphasalazine.

Dosage

Adults only.

- Orally: 1.5–4 g in divided doses in acute disease. 750 mg – 2.4 g daily in divided doses as maintenance therapy.
- Rectal: 750–1500 mg daily in divided doses with the last dose at night on retiring.

Note that 400 mg mesalazine is theoretically the dose available from a 1 g dose of sulphasalazine.

M

Nursing implications

- Tablets are specially formulated to release the active ingredient in the terminal ileum and colon and it is most important that patients swallow these whole and that they are not crushed for ease of administration.
- Since mesalazine is chemically related to aspirin, it should be avoided in patients with a history of aspirin sensitivity.
- Side effects are mainly gastro-intestinal and include nausea, diarrhoea and abdominal pain.
- Mesalazine appears to be a safe alternative to sulphasalazine in pregnancy. It is also of value in males who develop low sperm counts and infertility during sulphasalazine therapy.
- Delivery characteristics: enteric-coated mesalazine

preparations may vary therefore preparations should not be interchanged.
- Blood disorders occur rarely but patients should be advised to report to their doctors any unexplained bleeding, bruising, purpura, sore throat, fever or malaise occurring while they are taking this medication.
- Mesalazine is contraindicated in moderate-to-severe renal impairment.

Storage
Mesalazine preparations may be stored at room temperature. They should be protected from direct sunlight.

MESNA (Uromitexan)

Presentation
Tablets – 400 mg, 600 mg
Injection – 400 mg in 4 ml, 1 g in 10 ml

Actions and uses
The cytotoxic agents ifosfamide and cyclophosphamide are well known to cause urothelial toxicity, manifesting as haemorrhagic cystitis. This is caused by acrolein, a metabolite of ifosfamide and cyclophosphamide. Mesna is excreted in the urine, reacts with acrolein and reduces the urotoxic effects of these drugs. Mesna is routinely used for the prophylaxis of urothelial toxicity in patients receiving ifosfamide and in patients receiving cyclophosphamide by the IV route at high dose. It is also used where patients have previously had urothelial toxicity with cyclophosphamide.

Dosage
- Adults: the dose of mesna given is dependent on the dose of ifosfamide or cylophosphamide and the route of mesna administration. Product literature should be referred to for accurate dosage guidelines. As an example, for intermittent ifosfamide therapy, oral mesna 40% of the ifosfamide dose should be given 2 hours prior to and repeated 2 and 6 hours after the ifosfamide dose. Alternatively, IV mesna, 20% of the ifosfamide dose can be given with the IV ifosfamide dose and followed by oral mesna 40% of the IV ifosfamide dose 2 and 6 hours after the ifosfamide has been administered. See example below.
- Mesna IV injection should be given over 15–30 minutes. Mesna can also be given as a concurrent continuous infusion with ifosfamide infusion. Mesna and ifosfamide are chemically compatible with 0.9% sodium chloride.
- Children and high-risk patients (high-risk patients include those who have had previous irradiation of the small pelvis, occurrence of cystitis during previous cyclophosphamide or ifosfamide therapy or a history of urinary tract lesions) may require shorter intervals between doses and/or an increased number of doses.

Nursing implications
- Side effects are uncommon at recommended doses but include gastrointestinal upset, fatigue, headache, joint pains and depression, irritability, rarely hypersensitivity reactions.

Example of mesna dosing with ifosfamide

	−2 hours	0 hours	2 hours	4 hours	6 hours	8 hours
Ifosfamide		1 g IV				
Mesna	400 mg orally		400 mg orally		400 mg orally	
		200 mg IV	400 mg orally		400 mg orally	
		200 mg IV		200 mg IV		200 mg IV

- The injection can be given orally in a flavoured drink such as orange juice or cola which may be stored in a sealed container in a refrigerator for up to 24 hours.

Storage
- Mesna is stored at room temperature.
- Protect injection from light.

METFORMIN (Glucophage)

Presentation
Tablets – 500 mg, 850 mg

Actions and uses
Metformin is a biguanide drug used in the treatment of Type II diabetes.

Dosage
Adults: 500 mg three times a day or 850 mg twice a day with meals. Doses as high as 3 g per day can be used but a maximum of 2 g per day is preferred.

Nursing implications
Metformin causes GI upset with nausea, vomiting and diarrhoea.

Storage
The drug is stored at room temperature.

METHADONE (Physeptone)

Presentation
Tablets – 5 mg
Mixture – 1 mg in 1 ml (for methadone maintenance)
Oral concentrate – 10 mg in 1 ml, 20 mg in 1 ml for dilution
Linctus – 2 mg in 5 ml
Injection – 10 mg in 1 ml

Actions and uses
Methadone is a narcotic analgesic with a long duration of action and its general actions and uses are described in the section dealing with these drugs (p. 238).

Methadone has an additional specific use in that it is less addictive than other narcotic analgesics such as morphine and diamorphine and if used when patients are being weaned off these drugs, it may lead to a reduction in the severity of withdrawal symptoms.

Dosage
- For analgesia: adults should receive 5–10 mg 6–8 hourly initially, increasing if necessary to 30 mg 6-hourly.
- For methadone maintenance in addicts: the dose is widely variable.
- Avoid in children.
- Methadone linctus is indicated for cough in terminal illness at a dose of 2.5 ml every 4–6 hours. This is not routinely recommended.

Nursing implications
See the section on Narcotic Analgesics (p. 238).

Storage
- The drug should be stored in a locked (Controlled Drug) cupboard.
- The drug should be stored at room temperature.

METHOTREXATE

Presentation
Tablets – 2.5 mg, 10 mg
Injection – 5 mg in 2 ml, 50 mg in 2 ml, 200 mg in 8 ml, 500 mg in 20 ml, 1 g in 40 ml, 5 g in 200 ml, 1 g in 10 ml, 5 g in 50 ml

Actions and uses
Methotrexate is a folate antagonist widely used in cancer chemotherapy and for a number of other conditions. It acts by inhibiting the enzyme dihydrofolate reductase. This enzyme is required to convert folic acid into tetrahydrofolic acid which in turn is required for the synthesis of DNA and cell division. Methotrexate therefore reduces cell growth and multiplication by depriving cells of tetrahydrofolic acid.
It is used in the treatment of acute lymphoblastic leukaemia. Initial

M

treatment is usually with other drugs but once the leukaemia is under control, methotrexate is used as maintenance therapy. It is also used for the prevention and treatment of meningeal leukaemia.

Other malignancies which have been reported to respond to treatment with methotrexate include:

- choriocarcinoma and related trophoblastic diseases
- lymphosarcoma
- Burkitt's lymphoma
- tumours of the head and neck.

Methotrexate is occasionally used in the treatment of severe cases of psoriasis and rheumatoid arthritis which do not respond to conventional therapy.

Dosage

The drug may be given by oral, intramuscular, intravenous, intraarterial, intraarticular and intrathecal routes. The doses vary widely according to the route of administration, type of malignant disease under treatment and with the variety of other cytotoxic or immunosuppressant drugs which are used in combination. Because of the wide variety of dosage regimes, none are specifically stated here. However, it should be noted that intrathecal doses are very much smaller than doses given by other routes. Courses of treatment with methotrexate are very often followed by the administration of calcium folinate which is a methotrexate antagonist. This has been found to reduce the incidence of associated toxic effects.

M

Nursing implications

- The principal toxic effects are suppression of the bone marrow and gastrointestinal disturbance. The former effect leads to leuco-penia and thrombocytopenia and a resultant increased risk of severe infection or haemorrhage.
- One of the earliest manifestations of toxicity is oral discomfort and ulceration. Other gastrointestinal effects include nausea, vomiting and diarrhoea.
- Megaloblastic anaemia, skin rashes, alopecia, altered ovarian and testicular function, enteritis with bleeding episodes and intestinal perforation may occur.
- Damage to specific tissues such as the kidneys, liver, lungs and nervous system have been reported. Liver damage is thought to occur more commonly with long-term oral therapy and renal damage is thought to be more common in intermittent high-dose regimes. Intrathecal therapy is the commonest cause of neurotoxicity.
- The drug has produced abortion and a wide range of fetal abnormalities and must not be taken during pregnancy.
- Routine monitoring should include full blood counts, liver function tests and renal function.
- **1 g in 10 ml, 5 g in 50 ml and 500 mg in 20 ml are NOT for intrathecal use**.
- Interactions: NSAIDs, including aspirin, and probenecid can reduce the excretion of methotrexate, therefore use with caution. Some antibiotics, e.g. co-trimoxazole, trimethoprim and sulphonamides increase the risk of toxicity.
- Nurses should be aware of the risks posed by cytotoxic drugs. Some are irritant to the skin and mucous surfaces and care must be exercised when handling them. In particular, spillage or contamination of personnel or the environment must be avoided. If cytotoxic drugs are handled regularly, it is theoretically possible that repeated skin contact or inhalation may produce systemic toxic effects in nurses who have developed hypersensitivity to them. Most hospitals now operate a centralized (pharmacy-organized) additive service. While this reduces the risk of exposure to cytotoxic drugs, it is essential that nurses recognize and understand the local policy on their safe handling and disposal. The Health and Safety Executive has decreed that such a policy

should be in place wherever cytotoxic drugs are administered. These should be adapted, wherever possible, to care of patients in the community.

Storage
Preparations of methotrexate are stored at room temperature.

METHOTRIMEPRAZINE (rINN Levomepromazine) (Nozinan)

Presentation
Tablets – 25 mg
Injection – 25 mg in 1 ml

Actions and uses
Methotrimeprazine is a member of the phenothiazine group. It is therefore a neuroleptic or major tranquillizer and has a limited role in the treatment of severe anxiety, schizophrenia and manic depressive psychosis. In practice, however, the main role for this drug is as an anxiolytic and antiemetic when used in combination with diamorphine (or a related opioid analgesic) in pain control. In particular, it is widely used in the control of pain in terminal cancer when it is often mixed with diamorphine in the same syringe and delivered by continuous subcutaneous infusion via a syringe driver.

Dosage
Oral: doses vary from as low as 25 mg to as high as 1 g daily with a maximum of 37.5 mg daily for children. In pain control, the injectable route is most often used.
Injection: usually 12.5–50 mg by IM or IV injection administered every 6–8 hours. Doses of 25–200 mg may be administered by continuous SC infusion over 24 hours in combination with diamorphine.

Nursing implications
- The nursing implications for Phenothiazines (p. 281) apply to this drug.
- In particular, methotrimeprazine may produce severe postural

hypotension and close monitoring of ambulant patients is necessary.
- When given by the IV route, methotrimeprazine injection must first be diluted with an equal volume of sodium chloride 0.9% injection.

Storage
Methotrimeprazine tablets and ampoules may be stored at room temperature. They must, however, be protected from light. Note that on exposure to light the injection solution will develop a pink or yellow discolouration in which case it should be discarded.

METHYLDOPA (Aldomet)

Presentation
Tablets – 125 mg, 250 mg, 500 mg
Injection – 250 mg in 5 ml

Actions and uses
Methyldopa reduces the blood pressure through a direct action on the centres controlling blood pressure in the brain. It is metabolized to alpha-methylnoradrenaline which stimulates central inhibitory alpha-adrenoceptors, resulting in a drop in arterial blood pressure. Methyldopa is available for use orally on a regular basis but may be given intravenously in hypertensive emergencies. It has been used for many years safely in obstetrics and is therefore often used for control of hypertension in pregnancy. It can also be used safely in asthmatics and for those with heart failure.

Dosage
Adult dose: 250 mg two to three times daily, rising to a maximum of 3 g per day in three divided doses.
Adult emergency intravenous dose: 250–500 mg 6-hourly as required given in 100 ml 5% dextrose and infused over 30–60 minutes.
Children: orally, initially 10 mg/kg body weight daily in 2–4 divided doses adjusted according to response to a

M

maximum of 65 mg/kg or 3 g per day. Intravenously, 20–40 mg/kg daily in four divided doses, maximum of 65 mg/kg or 3 g per day.

Nursing implications
- Although methyldopa is a very effective drug in the treatment of hypertension, the major problem with its use is the large number of potentially serious side effects which may occur and it is in the early detection of these side effects that the nurse can make a major contribution.
- Neurological side effects: depression is by far the most important, but paraesthesia, parkinsonism, involuntary muscle twitching, nightmares, confusion, light-headedness and dizziness may also occur.
- Cardiovascular: postural hypotension, fluid retention, worsening of existing angina and bradycardia.
- Gastrointestinal: nausea, vomiting, distension, excess flatus, constipation, dry mouth, black tongue and very rarely pancreatitis.
- Blood: haemolytic anaemia, leucopenia, granulocytopenia, thrombocytopenia.
- Other side effects include nasal stuffiness, a raised blood urea, gynaecomastia/galactorrhoea, impotence in males, loss of libido, skin rashes, drug fever and abnormal liver function tests.

Storage
Methyldopa tablets and injection are stored at room temperature. Protect from light.

METHYLPHENIDATE (Ritalin)

Presentation
Tablets – 5 mg, 10 mg, 20 mg

Actions and uses
Methylphenidate is used for attention deficit hyperactivity disorder in children who have failed to respond to psychotherapy. It should only be prescribed under specialist advice. Methylphenidate is a mild CNS stimulant although its exact mode of action has yet to de determined.

Dosage
Children over 6 years: initially 5 mg once or twice daily increasing as necessary by weekly increments of 5–10 mg in the daily dose to a maximum of 60 mg daily in divided doses.

Nursing implications
- It is important not to give the drug for at least 4 hours before bedtime because of the potential risk of insomnia.
- Side effects include nervousness, decreased appetite, gastro-intestinal upset and headache.
- Treatment should be discontinued if there is no response after 1 month.
- Treatment should be discontinued periodically to assess the child's condition as drug therapy is only one component of treatment.

Storage
Methylphenidate is stored at room temperature. Protect from moisture.

METHYLPREDNISOLONE (Medrone, Depo-Medrone, Solu-Medrone)

Presentation
Tablets – 2 mg, 4 mg, 16 mg, 100 mg
Intravenous or intramuscular injection – 40 mg, 125 mg, 500 mg, 1 g, 2 g
Long-acting intramuscular and intraarticular injection – 40 mg in 1 ml, 80 mg in 2 ml, 120 mg in 3 ml

Actions and uses
Methylprednisolone is a Corticosteroid Drug (p. 107). Its rapid onset of action following intravenous injection makes it particularly useful in the management of emergencies such as severe shock and anaphylaxis. Methylprednisolone can be given by various routes including the periarticular, intrabursal and intralesional routes.

M

Dosage

Oral: this varies widely with the nature and severity of the condition being treated.

Intravenous or intramuscular injection: varies depending on the condition being treated, initial dose being from 10 to 500 mg. Doses of up to 250 mg IV should be given over at least 5 minutes, higher doses should be given over at least 30 minutes.

Intraarticular injection: dosages vary between 4 and 80 mg according to the size of the joint under treatment.

Nursing implications

See the section on Corticosteroid Drugs (p. 107).

Storage

Preparations containing methylprednisolone are stored at room temperature.

METHYSERGIDE (Deseril)

Presentation

Tablets – 1 mg

Actions and uses

Methysergide is a 5-hydroxytryptamine (serotonin) antagonist and a vasoconstrictor. It is licensed for the prophylaxis of migraine and other types of headache. It is also used for the control of profuse diarrhoea associated with carcinoid disease where excess 5-hydroxytryptamine is produced, leading to increased gastrointestinal motility.

Dosage

Adults.

- For the treatment of carcinoid syndrome: up to 20 mg per day may be required according to individual patient response.
- For the prophylaxis of migraine: 1 or 2 mg three times a day with meals.

Nursing implications

- This drug is now rarely used for migraine prophylaxis and should

only be administered under hospital supervision.

- This drug on rare occasions may cause extensive fibrosis involving the heart, pleura, lung and retroperitoneal tissues. It should therefore be given in short courses only and should not be administered for long periods.
- Common side effects include nausea, epigastric pain, dizziness, drowsiness, restlessness, muscle cramps and psychological effects. Vomiting, muscle weakness, ataxia, weight increase, oedema, tachycardia and postural hypotension may also occur.
- The vasoconstrictor effect may lead to cold extremities.
- The drug should be used with great caution in patients with peripheral vascular disease, coronary heart disease, peptic ulceration and reduced kidney or liver function.

Storage

The drug should be stored at room temperature.

METIPRANOLOL (Minims Metipranolol)

Presentation

Eye drops – 0.1%, 0.3%

Actions and uses

Metipranolol is a beta-blocking drug and it has the actions and uses of other drugs described in the section on beta-adrenoreceptor blocking drugs (p. 51). In practice, however, metipranolol is only used in the form of eye drops for the treatment of raised intraocular pressure and chronic open angle glaucoma. Topical beta-blockers lower raised intraocular pressure by an unknown mechanism which is associated with a reduction in aqueous humour production.

Dosage

Glaucoma: one drop is instilled into the affected eye twice daily, therapy being initiated with 0.1% strength drops and increased in time as necessary.

Nursing implications
- Despite the fact that this drug is administered externally, sufficient may be absorbed from the cornea to produce systemic side effects in susceptible patients (see Beta-Adrenoreceptor Blocking Drugs, p. 51). Thus patients with obstructive airways disease (particularly asthmatics) and those with uncontrolled heart failure should not be treated with beta-blocker eye drops.
- Other patients in whom metipranolol must be used with caution include those with sinus bradycardia and second- or third-degree heart block.
- Use in glaucoma is restricted to those allergic to preservatives or to those wearing soft contact lenses.

Storage
Metipranolol eye drops may be stored at room temperature. They have a relatively short life during use and a risk of bacterial contamination after opening exists. Normally eye drops of any kind should not be used after 1 week for a hospitalized patient or after 4 weeks for others.

METOCLOPRAMIDE
(Gastrobid Continus, Gastromax, Maxolon)

Presentation
Tablets – 10 mg
Modified-release tablets – 15 mg
Modified-release capsules – 15 mg, 30 mg
Oral solution – 5 mg in 5 ml
Paediatric liquid – 1 mg in 1 ml
Injection – 10 mg in 2 ml, 100 mg in 20 ml

Actions and uses
Metoclopramide has two major modes of action.

- It has a direct action on the gut, increasing normal gut motility

(peristalsis) and increasing gastric emptying time.
- It is a dopamine receptor antagonist acting centrally at the chemoreceptor trigger zone.

It has the following uses.

- It can be used to control vomiting associated with gastrointestinal disease, drug therapy (particularly cytotoxic drugs), radiotherapy, migraine and in the postoperative period.
- In diagnostic radiology metoclopramide is used to speed the passage of barium through the stomach and also as an aid to duodenal intubation.

Dosage
Adults: orally or parenterally, 10 mg three times a day.
Children: orally or parenterally:

- up to 1 year: 1 mg twice daily
- 1–3 years: 1 mg 2–3 times daily
- 3–5 years: 2 mg 2–3 times daily
- 5–9 years: 2.5 mg three times daily
- 9–14 years: 5 mg three times daily
- **do not exceed 500 microgram/kg/day**.

For diagnostic procedures a single dose of metoclopramide is given 5–10 minutes before the examination. Dosage is as follows.

- Adults: 10–20 mg
- Child under 3 years: 1 mg
- Child 3–5 years: 2 mg
- Child 5–9 years: 2.5 mg
- Child 9–14 years: 5 mg

Nursing implications
- It is important to note that metoclopramide is of little benefit in the prevention or treatment of motion sickness or in the treatment of nausea and vertigo due to Ménière's disease or other labyrinthine disturbances.
- Metoclopramide blocks the action of dopamine in the central nervous system and produces a range of symptoms and signs similar to those seen in Parkinson's disease. This effect is

particularly likely to occur in children and young adults and where higher dosages are used. The effects include facial muscle spasm, trismus, a rhythmic protrusion of the tongue, bulbar speech, muscle spasm around the eyes, rolling of the eyeballs and an unnatural positioning of the head and shoulders.

- In patients under 20 years old, use is restricted to severe intractable vomiting of known cause, vomiting of radiotherapy and cytotoxics, aid to gastrointestinal intubation and premedication.
- Because drugs of the Phenothiazine group (p. 281) also produce similar effects, meto-clopramide and phenothiazines should only be given together with great caution.
- Metoclopramide stimulates the production of prolactin by the pituitary. This may lead to an increase in breast size in males and galactorrhoea in females.
- Metoclopramide and antimuscarinic drugs should be avoided as the latter drugs antagonize the effects of metoclopramide on the gut.
- Metoclopramide should be used with caution in pregnancy and breastfeeding.

Storage
Preparations containing metoclopramide are stored at room temperature. Liquid preparations are sensitive to light and ampoules containing injection solution which show a yellow discolouration should be discarded.

METOLAZONE (Metenix)

Presentation
Tablets – 5 mg

Actions and uses
See the section on Thiazide and Related Diuretics (p. 357). Metolazone has additional diuretic properties because of its further action on the proximal renal tubule where some reabsorption of sodium takes place. This makes it an extremely potent diuretic so that it is generally reserved for the treatment of heart failure which is refractory to first-line thiazide diuretics.

Dosage
Oedema: the usual adult dose is 5–20 mg once daily; the duration of action is approximately 12–24 hours. Hypertension: initially 5 mg daily reducing to 5 mg on alternate days.

Nursing implications
See the section on Thiazide and Related Diuretics (p. 357).

Storage
Metolazone tablets are stored at room temperature. Protect from light.

METOPROLOL (Betaloc, Lopresor)

Presentation
Tablets – 50 mg, 100 mg
Modified-release tablets – 200 mg
Injection – 5 mg in 5 ml

Actions and uses
Metoprolol is a cardioselective Beta-blocker and its actions are described in the section dealing with these drugs (p. 51).

Dosage
The adult dose range is 100–400 mg per day which is usually given in two equal doses. Sustained-release tablets of metoprolol may be given as a single daily dose.

Orally.

- Hypertension: 100–200 mg daily in 1–2 doses.
- Angina: 50–100 mg 2–3 times daily.
- Arrhythmias: 50 mg 2–3 times daily up to 300 mg per day in divided doses.
- Migraine prophylaxis: 100–200 mg daily in divided doses.
- Thyrotoxicosis: 50 mg four times daily.

IV injection.

- Arrhythmias: 5 mg (rate of 1–2 mg per minute) repeating if required after 5 minutes to a total dose of 10–15 mg.

M

- In surgery to control arrhythmias: 2–4 mg by slow IV injection to a maximum of 10 mg.

Nursing implications
See the section on Beta-Adrenoreceptor Blocking Drugs (p. 51).

Storage
Metoprolol tablets and injection are stored at room temperature. Protect injection from light.

METRONIDAZOLE (Flagyl)

Presentation
Tablets – 200 mg, 400 mg, 500 mg
Oral suspension – 200 mg in 5 ml
Suppositories – 500 mg and 1 g (for vaginal and rectal administration)
Injection – 0.5% for intravenous infusion
Gel – 0.75%, 0.8%
Cream – 0.75%, 1%

Actions and uses
Metronidazole has been found to be effective in the treatment of both protozoal and bacterial and parasitic infections in man. It is active against a wide range of organisms including Bacteroides, Clostridia, anaerobic cocci and *Gardnerella vaginalis*. Its main uses are as follows.

- Prevention of postoperative infections
- Treatment of anaerobic infections
- Treatment of urogenital trichomoniasis
- Treatment of bacterial vaginosis
- Treatment of amoebiasis
- Treatment of giardiasis
- Treatment of acute ulcerative gingivitis
- Treatment of anaerobically infected leg ulcers and pressure sores
- Treatment of acute dental infections
- Treatment of antibiotic-associated colitis
- Topically to reduce the odour produced by anaerobic bacteria in fungating tumours and for rosacea

Dosage
Surgical prophylaxis.

- Adults: 400 mg orally (or 500 mg IV) 8-hourly during 24 hours preceding surgery, then IV or rectal administration until patient can take oral form again.
- Child: 7.5 mg/kg 8-hourly.

Anaerobic infections.

- Adults: orally, 800 mg initially then 400 mg 8-hourly or 500 mg 8-hourly. Rectally, 1 g 8-hourly for 3 days. Intravenously, if oral route compromised, 500 mg 8-hourly.
- Child: orally or IV 7.5 mg/kg 8-hourly. Rectally: 5–10 years, 500 mg 8-hourly for 3 days; 1–5 years, 250 mg 8-hourly for 3 days; under 1 year old, 125 mg 8-hourly for 3 days.

Urogenital trichomoniasis.

- Adults, orally: 400 mg twice daily for 7 days.
- Child 1–3 years, orally: 50 mg 8-hourly.
- Child 3–7 years, orally: 100 mg 12-hourly.
- Child 7–10 years, orally: 100 mg 8-hourly.

Bacterial vaginosis.

- Orally: 400–500 mg twice daily for 5–7 days or 2 g as a single dose.

Amoebiasis. Dose varies depending on susceptibility of patients and site of infection. For invasive intestinal disease in susceptible patients:

- Adults, orally: 800 mg 8-hourly for 5 days.
- Child, 1–3 years, orally: 200 mg 8-hourly for 5 days.
- Child, 3–7 years, orally: 200 mg 6-hourly for 5 days.
- Child, 7–10 years, orally: 400 mg 8-hourly for 5 days.

Gardiasis.

- Adults, orally: 2 g once a day for 3 days.
- Child, 1–3 years, orally: 500 mg once a day for 3 days.
- Child, 3–7 years, orally: 600–800 mg once a day for 3 days.
- Child, 7–10 years, orally: 1 g once a day for 3 days.

Leg ulcers and pressure sores.

- Orally: 400 mg 8-hourly for 7 days.

Acute ulcerative gingivitis.

- Adult, orally: 200–250 mg 8-hourly for 3 days.
- Child, 1–3 years, orally: 50 mg 8-hourly for 3 days.
- Child, 3–7 years, orally: 100 mg 12-hourly for 3 days.
- Child, 7–10 years, orally: 100 mg 8-hourly for 3 days.

Acute dental infections.

- Orally: 200 mg 8-hourly for 3–7 days.

Topically.

- Rosacea: apply once or twice daily.
- Malodorous tumours and skin ulcers: once or twice daily.

Nursing implications
- Patients should be warned that a common effect of taking this drug with alcohol is severe nausea and vomiting. Patients should therefore be advised not to drink alcohol during therapy and for 48 hours after completing their course.
- It is important to note that this drug may cause darkening of the urine. The patient should be warned of this possibility to prevent anxiety.
- Gastrointestinal effects are common. These include anorexia, nausea, an abnormal taste in the mouth and dryness of the tongue.
- Peripheral neuropathy and seizures have been reported with intensive or prolonged therapy.
- Blood disorders can occur, e.g. leucopenia.
- Reduce dose in severe hepatic impairment.
- It is very important to note that the drug has no effect on diseases caused by *Candida albicans* (thrush).
- Flagyl infusion is compatible with cefotaxime, ceftazidime and cefuroxime.

- Metronidazole should be used with caution in pregnancy and breastfeeding.

Storage
- The drug is stored at room temperature. Protect from light.
- Do not store suppositories close to a heat source (e.g. radiator).

METYRAPONE (Metopirone)

Presentation
Capsules – 250 mg

Actions and uses
Metyrapone acts on the adrenal cortex to inhibit production of hydrocortisone (cortisol) by a specific effect on the chemical process called 11-beta-hydroxylation. Use of metyrapone leads to increased ACTH (adreno-corticotrophic hormone) production and its use is associated with an increase in the urinary excretion of precursors of cortisol which, if not detected, indicates either failure of the adrenal cortex or hypopituitarism, or both.

Metyrapone, since it inhibits cortisol production, has also been used in the treatment of Cushing's syndrome, a disorder in which there is excess cortisol production.

Dosage
Differential diagnosis of ACTH-dependent Cushing's syndrome: 750 mg every 4 hours for 6 doses. Child: 15 mg/kg (minimum 250 mg) every 4 hours for six doses.
Management of Cushing's syndrome: dosage adjusted according to individual needs, usually 0.25–6 g daily.
Treatment of resistant oedema due to increased aldosterone secretion: 3 g daily in divided doses.

Nursing implications
- Metyrapone may produce nausea and vomiting. Doses should be taken with food.
- Special care is necessary if major impairment of pituitary function exists.

M

- The measurement of urinary steroid output, which is the basis for the metyrapone test, may be affected by certain drugs which the patient might be taking concurrently, e.g. anticonvulsants, antidepressants, neuroleptics, hormones and antithyroid agents.
- Metyrapone is contraindicated in pregnancy and breastfeeding.

Storage

Metyrapone capsules are stored at room temperature.

MEXILETINE (Mexitil)

Presentation

Capsules – 50 mg, 200 mg
Modified-release capsules – 360 mg
Injection – 250 mg in 10 ml

Actions and uses

Mexiletine is an antiarrhythmic drug which is used to abolish or prevent serious ventricular arrhythmias in patients who have had a myocardial infarction. It is usually given by intravenous injection initially and subsequently orally for the long-term prophylaxis of these rhythm disturbances.

Dosage

The adult intravenous loading dose is 100–250 mg by bolus injection at a rate of 25 mg/min. This is followed by intravenous infusion containing 500 mg in 500 ml. The first 250 ml is given over 1 hour, the second 250 ml is given more slowly over 2 hours. Further maintenance infusions may be given using 250 mg in 500 ml at a rate of 0.5 mg/min. For oral maintenance therapy an initial loading dose of 400 mg is followed by 200–250 mg three or four times a day. Alternatively 360 mg twice daily as slow-release capsules may be administered.

Nursing implications

- This drug requires careful monitoring for adverse effects which tend to be dose related.

- ECG monitoring is required with IV administration. When the drug is being administered intravenously the patient should also be observed for light-headedness, confusion, drowsiness, dizziness, diplopia, blurred vision, nystagmus, dysarthria, ataxia, paraesthesias, convulsions, hypotension, bradycardia, atrial fibrillation, nausea, vomiting, dyspepsia, an unpleasant taste and hiccoughs. Such effects are both less frequent and milder with oral therapy.
- The injection may be added to several infusion solutions including sodium chloride 0.9%, sodium chloride 0.9% with potassium chloride 0.3% or 0.6%, dextrose 5%, sodium bicarbonate 1.4% and sodium lactate.

Storage

Mexiletine capsules and injection are stored at room temperature. Protect the injection from light.

MICONAZOLE (Daktarin)

Presentation

Oral gel – 24 mg/ml
Cream – 2%
Dusting powder – 2%
Spray powder – 0.16%
Denture lacquer – 50 mg/g
Intravaginal cream – 2%
Pessaries – 100 mg
Vaginal capsule – 1.2 g

Actions and uses

Miconazole is an imidazole antifungal agent (see Clotrimazole, p. 101) used to prevent and treat oral and intestinal infections. It is also used for fungal skin infections and to treat vaginal and vulval candidiasis.

Dosage

Prevention and treatment of oral fungal infections, oral gel:

- adult: 5–10 ml in the mouth four times daily

- child under 2 years: 2.5 ml twice daily
- child 2–6 years: 5 ml twice daily
- child over 6 years: 5 ml four times daily.

Fungal skin infections: apply cream, dusting powder or spray powder twice daily.
Vaginal and vulval candidiasis: intravaginal cream, 5 g inserted daily for 10–14 days or twice daily for 7 days; pessaries, 100 mg inserted daily for 14 days or twice daily for 7 days; vaginal capsule, 1.2 g inserted at night as a single dose.

Nursing implications
See Clotrimazole (p. 101).

Storage
Miconazole preparations are stored at room temperature.

MIDAZOLAM (Hypnovel)

Presentation
Injection – 10 mg in 5 ml, 10 mg in 2 ml, 50 mg in 50 ml

Actions and uses
Midazolam is a benzodiazepine used as an IV sedative for minor procedures and in intensive care and for induction of anaesthesia in high-risk and elderly patients. Unlike diazepam, midazolam is water soluble and is used where a faster recovery time is desirable.

Dosage
Sedation: IV injection over 30 seconds 2 mg followed after 2 minutes by increments of 0.5–1 mg as required to achieve adequate sedation.
Premedication: IM injection 70–100 microgram/kg 30–60 minutes before surgery.

Sedation of patients in intensive care: IV infusion 30–300 microgram/kg over 5 minutes then 30–200 microgram/kg/h.

Nursing implications
- Excessive sedation can occur with high intravenous doses.
- Doses should be reduced in elderly people.
- The dose should be reduced in the intensive care setting if hypovolaemia, vasoconstriction or hypothermia occurs.
- Patients receiving concurrent opioids often require lower doses of midazolam.
- Abrupt withdrawal after prolonged administration (>14 days) may lead to withdrawal symptoms.

Storage
Midazolam injection is stored at room temperature.

MINOCYCLINE (Aknemin, Minocin)

Presentation
Tablets – 50 mg, 100 mg
Capsules – 50 mg, 100 mg
Modified-release capsules – 100 mg

Actions and uses
General notes on the actions and uses of Tetracyclines (p. 355) apply to minocycline. In addition, the drug has been found to be of particular use for the prevention of meningitis due to *Neisseria meningitidis* in the families of carriers of the disease; however, it is no longer recommended for this indication because of side effects.
   Perhaps the most common use for this drug is in the treatment of acne vulgaris.

Dosage
The adult dose is 100 mg every 12 hours. It is worth noting that food appears to have less effect on the absorption of minocycline than tetracyclines in general and therefore the drug may be taken with food.

- For acne: 100 mg daily in one or two divided doses for 6 weeks or longer.
- For gonorrhoea: 200 mg initially then 100 mg every 12 hours for at least 4 days in men, sometimes longer in women.

Nursing implications
- For nursing implications see the section on Tetracyclines (p. 355).
- It is worth noting that neurological side effects are particularly prominent with this drug as compared to other tetracyclines. These effects cause light-headedness, dizziness and vertigo.
- Tetracyclines should be avoided in children under 12 years.

Storage
The drug is stored at room temperature. Protect from light.

MINOXIDIL (Loniten)

Presentation
Tablets – 2.5 mg, 5 mg and 10 mg
Topical solution – 2% and 5%

Actions and uses
Minoxidil is a vasodilating antihypertensive agent used for severe hypertension in patients who are resistant to other antihypertensive drugs. It causes direct peripheral vasodilatation of the arterioles which is accompanied by increased cardiac output, tachycardia and fluid retention. A beta-blocker and a diuretic therefore must be prescribed alongside minoxidil. Minoxidil can also be used, applied topically, to stimulate hair growth. It is only successful in a small proportion of adults and continued application is required.

Dosage
Hypertension: 5 mg (or 2.5 mg in the elderly) daily in one or two doses, increased gradually by 5–10 mg every 3 or more days to a maximum of 50 mg daily.
Male-pattern baldness in men and women: 1 ml of the topical solution should be applied twice a day to dry hair and scalp. The 5% solution is for use by men only.

Nursing implications
- Side effects as mentioned above include tachycardia and fluid retention.

- Hypertrichosis is a side effect of oral therapy, therefore it should not be used in women.
- In the treatment of baldness, if no improvement is seen after 1 year discontinue use.
- Do not use in phaeochromocytoma.

Storage
Minoxidil preparations are stored at room temperature.

MIRTAZAPINE (Zispin)

Presentation
Tablets – 30 mg (scored)

Actions and uses
Mirtazapine is an antidepressant. For an account of the actions and uses see Antidepressant Drugs (p. 31). It acts centrally, blocking presynaptic alpha-2-adrenoceptors, increasing central transmission of noradrenaline and 5-hydroxytryptamine (serotonin).

Dosage
Adults only, initially 15 mg daily increasing as necessary up to 45 mg daily according to clinical response. Ideally mirtazapine should be taken as a single dose at night but the dose can be divided throughout the day.

Nursing implications
- See Antidepressant Drugs (p. 31).
- Sedation is common during initiation of therapy.
- Mirtazapine can cause increased appetite and weight gain.
- Blood dyscrasias can occur and patients should be advised to consult a doctor with symptoms such as fever and sore throat.

Storage
Mirtazapine tablets are stored at room temperature. Protect from light.

MISOPROSTOL (Cytotec)

Presentation
Tablets – 200 microgram

Actions and uses

Misoprostol is a prostaglandin analogue indicated for the treatment of duodenal and gastric ulcers and the prophylaxis of NSAID-induced ulcers. It acts by inhibiting acid secretion and by increasing bicarbonate and mucus secretion, thereby protecting the gastroduodenal mucosa.

Dosage

Adults only.

- In benign gastric and duodenal ulceration and NSAID-induced ulceration, 800 microgram daily in 2–4 divided doses for 4–8 weeks should be given.
- In the prophylaxis of NSAID-induced gastric and duodenal ulcer, 200 microgram 2–4 times daily should be taken at the same time as the NSAID.

Nursing implications

- Use of this drug should be avoided in women of child-bearing age (can be used to induce medical abortion although this is an unlicensed use).
- Severe diarrhoea can be a side effect, as are other gastrointestinal symptoms.
- Abnormal vaginal bleeding has been reported.

Storage

Misoprostol tablets are stored at room temperature.

MITOXANTRONE
(Novantrone, Onkotrone)

Presentation

Injection – 20 mg in 10 ml, 25 mg in 12.5 ml, 30 mg in 15 ml

Actions and uses

Mitoxantrone is a cytotoxic agent structurally related to doxorubicin. Its mechanism of action has not been clearly defined but it results in cell death and is active against a variety of neoplastic conditions including advanced breast cancer, non-Hodgkin's lymphoma, adult acute non-lymphocytic leukaemia and inoperable primary hepatocellular carcinoma.

Dosage

Advanced breast cancer, non-Hodgkin's lymphoma and hepatoma.

- Single agent dosage: 14 mg/m^2 of body surface area single IV infusion repeated at 21-day intervals. Use 12 mg/m^2 if the patient has inadequate bone marrow reserves.
- Combination therapy: reduce the above dose by 2–4 mg/m^2 according to expert advice.

Acute non-lymphocytic leukaemia.

- Single agent dosage in relapse: 12 mg/m^2 single IV dose daily for 5 consecutive days.
- Combination therapy: e.g. mitoxantrone with cytosine arabinoside, previously untreated patients, mitoxantrone 10–12 mg/m^2 IV for 3 days combined with cytosine arabinoside 100 mg/m^2 IV for 7 days according to expert advice.
- Paediatric leukaemia: dose according to expert advice.

M

Nursing implications

- The main side effects are myelosuppression and mucositis, nausea and vomiting. Alopecia and tissue necrosis can also occur.
- Mitoxantrone can cause cardiotoxicity. Cardiac function should be monitored if the total dose exceeds 160 mg/m^2.
- Nurses should be aware of the risks posed by cytotoxic drugs. Some are irritant to the skin and mucous surfaces and care must be exercised when handling them. In particular, spillage or contamination of personnel or the environment must be avoided. If cytotoxic drugs are handled regularly, it is theoretically possible that repeated skin contact or inhalation may produce systemic toxic effects in nurses who have developed hypersensitivity to them. Most hospitals now operate a centralized (pharmacy-organized)

additive service. While this reduces the risk of exposure to cytotoxic drugs, it is essential that nurses recognize and understand the local policy on their safe handling and disposal. The Health and Safety Executive has decreed that such a policy should be in place wherever cytotoxic drugs are administered. These should be adapted, wherever possible, to care of patients in the community.

Storage

Mitoxantrone is stored at room temperature.

MOCLOBEMIDE (Manerix)

Presentation

Tablets – 150 mg, 300 mg

Actions and uses

For an account of the actions and uses see Antidepressant Drugs (p. 31) and Monoamine Oxidase Inhibitors (p. 228). This drug is a reversible inhibitor of the enzyme monoamine oxidase type A (hence RIMA). Its action in the brain results in accumulation of high levels of the monoamine neurotransmitters noradrenaline and 5-hydroxytryptamine (serotonin) which is associated with mood elevation and the reversal of depression. Moclobemide is therefore used in the treatment of major depressive illness unresponsive to tricyclic and related antidepressants as an alternative to the traditional monoamine oxidase inhibitors (MAOIs). Because of its specific and reversible action on type A receptors it is much less likely to produce the serious hypertensive episodes which occur with other MAOIs when certain well-known foodstuffs containing tyramine (e.g. cheeses, yeast extracts, soya-based products, etc.) are eaten. Similarly the drug is much less likely to interact with monoamine decongestants present in various cough and cold remedies.

Dosage

Initially 150 mg twice daily increased according to response up to a maximum dose of 600 mg daily.

Nursing implications

- This drug is preferably taken with or immediately after food to limit possible gastrointestinal upsets.
- As noted above, the various well-known interactions involving traditional MAOIs appear to be much less likely to occur with this drug. Caution is nevertheless advised and excessive ingestion of foods rich in tyramine should be avoided. Similarly, patients should avoid cough and cold remedies containing monoamines such as ephedrine, pseudoephedrine and phenylpropanolamine, which can generally be purchased over the counter.
- In common with traditional MAOIs, this drug should be used with caution in agitated or excited patients (unless additional sedation is used) and in patients with severe liver disease and thyrotoxicosis.
- Moclobemide is likely to exacerbate an existing acute confusional state and increase the risk of dangerously elevated BP in patients with phaeochromocytoma. It is therefore contraindicated in such cases.
- Common side effects include sleep disturbances, agitation, restlessness, dizziness, nausea, headaches, confusion and a rise in liver enzymes.

Storage

Moclobemide tablets are stored at room temperature.

MONOAMINE OXIDASE INHIBITORS (Isocarboxazid, Phenelzine, Tranylcypromine)

Actions and uses

(See individual drugs and Antidepressant Drugs (p. 31)).

When the enzyme monoamine oxidase, which is present in many tissues in the body, is inhibited by the group of drugs known as monoamine oxidase inhibitors there is a resultant increase in the concentration of 5-hydroxytryptamine and catecholamines in the central nervous system. This leads to marked effects on mental function ranging from feelings of well-being and increased energy to, in some patients, psychosis. This group of drugs is therefore used for the treatment of depression. However, they have many serious side effects and for this reason are usually only used when other drugs, such as tricyclic antidepressants, have been found to be ineffective.

Dosage

See specific drugs.

Nursing implications

- Severe headache and dangerous hypertensive crisis may be precipitated in patients taking monoamine oxidase-inhibiting drugs by the ingestion of certain foodstuffs. These include cheese, yoghurt, pickled herrings, broad beans, yeast extracts, meat extracts (Bovril, Marmite, etc.), wines and beers. The nurse may play an important role in both educating patients about food intake and monitoring their diets.
- The nurse may also play an important role in warning patients that they must never indulge in self-medication of any kind, particularly those sold for coughs and colds, as these contain chemicals which may lead to serious hypertension and headache if they are taken at the same time as MAOIs.
- A number of other drugs are extremely dangerous if they are given at the same time as monoamine oxidase inhibitors. The nurse may play an important role in identifying such potential combinations. The major groups of drugs contraindicated for concurrent administration with monoamine oxidase inhibitors are as follows.
  - Other antidepressants: if tricyclic and monoamine oxidase-inhibiting drugs are given together mental excitement and hyperpyrexia may occur. Allow a 2-week washout period between stopping an MAOI and starting another anti-depressant and vice versa (with some antidepressants the washout period is shorter; check product literature in each case).
  - Antihypertensives: hypotensive effect enhanced.
  - Narcotic analgesics: the coincident administration of pethidine and MAOIs may lead to respiratory depression, restlessness, coma and hypotension. Avoid con-comitant use and for 2 weeks after the MAOI has been discontinued.
  - Antiepileptics: MAOIs lower the seizure threshold.
  - Drugs which stimulate the sympathetic nervous system, e.g. ephedrine, phenylephrine and the amphetamines, may produce serious (and even fatal) rises in blood pressure which result in brain haemorrhage.
- A common side effect produced by monoamine oxidase-inhibiting drugs is hypotension. Symptoms of dizziness on standing, indicating postural hypotension, may occur. It is important to remember that hypertensive crises can still occur in patients who have been rendered hypotensive by the drug.
- Other side effects include cardiac dysrhythmias, dizziness, headache, anxiety, tremor, convulsions and liver toxicity.
- **It is advisable that all patients receiving monoamine oxidase-inhibiting drugs be issued with a warning card which provides a complete list of substances which they may accidentally take and which may lead to the effects described above.**

M

Storage
See individual drugs.

MONTELUKAST (Singulair)

Presentation
Tablets – 10 mg
Chewable tablets – 5 mg

Actions and uses
Montelukast is a leukotriene receptor antagonist, binding to leukotriene receptors in the lung and inhibiting their actions. Leukotrienes are released from inflammatory cells and cause bronchoconstriction, increased mucus secretion, oedema, inflammatory cell infiltration and airways smooth muscle proliferation. Montelukast acts to prevent these effects, thereby improving lung function. This drug is used to treat asthma and to prevent asthma which is predominantly exercise induced. It is licensed for add-on therapy where the patient's asthma is not controlled with inhaled corticosteroids and beta-2 agonists.

Dosage
Adults: 10 mg daily at night.
Child, 6–14 years old: 5 mg daily at night.

Nursing implications
- Montelukast is **not** a treatment for an acute asthmatic attack and patients should be advised of this.
- Side effects include headache, gastrointestinal disturbances and hypersensitivity.
- Montelukast should be used with caution in pregnancy and breastfeeding.

Storage
Montelukast tablets are stored at room temperature and protected from light.

MORPHINE (as Hydrochloride, Sulphate or Tartrate)

Presentation
Morphine sulphate is available in numerous preparations, often in combination with other drugs and in varying strengths. The following are only examples of the many preparations in common use.
Tablets – 10 mg, 20 mg, 50 mg
Tablets, MST Continus – 10 mg, 30 mg, 60 mg and 100 mg as slow release
Injection – 15 mg and 30 mg in 1 ml
Suppositories – 10 mg,15 mg, 20 mg and 30 mg
Oral solutions – 10 mg in 5 ml
Unit dose vials (for oral use) – 10 mg in 5 ml, 30 mg in 5 ml

Actions and uses
See the section on Narcotic Analgesics (p. 238). Morphine is one of the most commonly used narcotic analgesics and like all the other drugs in this class, it acts upon specific receptors in the central nervous system, causing an analgesic effect. It also causes euphoria and mental detachment. Morphine is frequently used postoperatively by injection and orally in the treatment of severe pain in palliative care where it is not unusual to see the use of very high doses.

Dosage
NB: The following doses are given as a guideline only and both initial dosage and maintenance dosage may vary considerably depending on the condition under treatment and the development of tolerance to the drug in the patient.
Adults.

- Orally: standard preparations, 10–20 mg 4–6 hourly as required. Slow-release tablets (MST Continus) 30–100 mg twice daily.
- By subcutaneous or intramuscular injection: 15–30 mg 4–6 hourly as required for pain.
- Intravenous injections may cause a rapid fall in blood pressure. They should be administered slowly and the dosage recommended is 10–20 mg 4–6 hourly as required.

Children:

- Up to 1 month: 150 microgram/kg 4–6 hourly.
- Up to 1 year: 200 microgram/kg 4–6 hourly.
- 1–5 years: 2.5–5 mg 4–6 hourly.
- 6–12 years: 5–10 mg 4–6 hourly.

Nursing implications
See the section on Narcotic
Analgesics (p. 238).

Storage
- Preparations may be stored at room
  temperature.
- By law this drug must be kept
  in a locked (Controlled Drug)
  cupboard.

MOXONIDINE (Physiotens)

Presentation
Tablets – 200 microgram,
400 microgram

Actions and uses
Moxonidine is a centrally acting
antihypertensive agent indicated for
the treatment of mild to moderate
essential hypertension. Unlike other
centrally acting antihypertensives,
moxonidine interacts with imidazoline
receptors leading to reduced
activity of sympathetic nerves and a
fall in blood pressure. It is generally
used where other commonly used
antihypertensives have failed to reduce
blood pressure.

Dosage
Adults: initially, 200 microgram each
morning, increased after 3 weeks to
400 microgram daily in one or two
divided doses if necessary. The dose
can be further increased after
another 3 weeks to a maximum of
600 microgram daily.

Nursing implications
- 400 microgram single dose
  should not be exceeded.
- In moderate renal impairment a
  maximum of 200 microgram in a
  single dose and 400 microgram
  daily should be used.
- Side effects include dry mouth,
  headache, fatigue, sleep
  disturbance and dizziness.

Storage
Moxonidine tablets are stored at room
temperature.

MULTIVITAMINS (Pabrinex)

Presentation
Capsules
Intravenous high potency (IVHP)
injection
Intramuscular high potency (IMHP)
injection

Actions and uses
There are numerous oral vitamin and
multivitamin preparations available for
sale over the counter but relatively few
are prescribable at NHS expense.

Parenteral multivitamins (Pabrinex)
can be administered by either the
intramuscular route or by short
intravenous infusion. Only the IV
preparation is used to any extent now.

- Oral vitamins and multivitamin
  supplements are frequently
  prescribed and even more
  frequently purchased directly for
  use as tonics. There is no real
  evidence that they are of any
  benefit for this purpose.
- In patients who have a documented
  history and clinical signs of
  inadequate diet, oral or parenteral
  preparations may be usefully
  prescribed to aid physical recovery.
- In patients with impaired
  absorption of foodstuffs due either
  to disease of the gallbladder,
  pancreas or gut, parenteral vitamin
  preparations are an essential
  component of therapy.
- Parenteral multivitamins have been
  shown to be useful in the
  management of delirium tremens, a
  state of agitated confusion caused
  by acute cessation of prolonged
  heavy drinking. It should be noted
  that Pabrinex contains primarily a
  number of the vitamin B complex
  compounds and vitamin C.

Dosage
The dosage of oral preparations varies
according to the proprietary brand and
nurses are advised to consult
manufacturers' literature. Parenteral
therapy is as follows.

- Intravenous: the contents of a pair
  of ampoules are given on each
  occasion, preferably diluted with
  50–100 ml of sodium chloride 0.9%
  injection or 5% dextrose, infused
  over 15–30 minutes.

M

- For use in patients with delirium from alcohol, narcotics or barbiturates, the contents of 2–3 pairs of IV high-potency ampoules 8-hourly.
- For psychosis following narcosis or ECT or in toxicity from acute infections, the contents of one pair of IV high-potency or IM high-potency ampoules twice daily for up to 7 days.
- In patients on chronic intermittent haemodialysis to maintain levels of vitamin C the contents of one pair of IV high-potency ampoules should be given every 2 weeks.
- Children:
  - Under 6 years: 25% adult dose
  - 6–10 years: 33% adult dose
  - 10–14 years: 50–66% adult dose
  - 14 years: adult dose.

Nursing implications

- The ill effects caused by administration of an excess of vitamins are discussed more fully under the individual headings (see the sections covering Vitamin A (p. 386), Vitamin B Complex (p. 387), Vitamin C (p. 387), Vitamin D (p. 388) and Vitamin E (p. 388).
- Parenteral administration of Pabrinex has a number of problems.
  - With repeated injections anaphylactic shock may occur and appropriate measures such as the injection of adrenaline and soluble glucocorticoids or antihistamines should be readily available during administration of this therapy.
  - Pabrinex contains pyridoxine and this may antagonize levodopa therapy for Parkinson's disease.
  - Perhaps the most important point for the nurse to note is that the intramuscular preparation should never be given intravenously.
- For parenteral administration, two ampoules are always used as each

ampoule contains different vitamins. Thiamine, riboflavin and pyridoxine are in one ampoule and nicotinamide and ascorbic acid in the other.

Storage

Ampoules of Pabrinex are stored at room temperature. Protect from light. Some oral vitamin preparations require storage below 15°C but most preparations are stored at room temperature.

MUPIROCIN (Bactroban)

Presentation

Ointment – 2%
Nasal ointment – 2%

Actions and uses

Mupirocin is an antibacterial agent active against Gram-positive organisms including *Staphylococcus aureus* and methicillin-resistant *Staphylococcus aureus* (MRSA). *Pseudomonas aeruginosa* is resistant but some Gram-negative organisms are susceptible to its actions, e.g. *Haemophilus influenzae*. Mupirocin is only used topically. Applied intranasally, it is used to eliminate the nasal carriage of staphylococci, particularly in MRSA in hospitals. Mupirocin ointment is also used for skin infections such as impetigo and folliculitis.

Dosage

Topically: apply to affected area up to three times a day for up to 10 days. Intranasally: apply a small amount of ointment into each nostril 2–3 times a day. For MRSA eradication in hospital, apply three times a day for 5 days, sampling to confirm eradication 2 days after the course is completed.

Nursing implications

- For MRSA eradication the course may be repeated if the first sample is still positive but no further courses should be given to avoid resistance developing.
- As a general rule in hospitals, mupirocin is reserved for the eradication of intranasal MRSA.

Storage

Mupirocin preparations are stored at room temperature.

MYCOPHENOLATE MOFETIL (Cellcept)

Preparations

Capsules – 250 mg
Tablets – 500 mg
Infusion – 500 mg powder

Actions and uses

Mycophenolate is an antiproliferative immunosuppressant agent licensed to prevent acute renal or cardiac transplant rejection when used in combination with cyclosporin and corticosteroids. Mycophenolate acts by inhibiting the proliferation of T and B lymphocytes, suppressing the body's immune response and thereby facilitating organ acceptance rather than rejection. It should only be used under specialist advice.

Dosage

Renal transplant: orally, 1 g twice daily starting within 72 hours of the transplant. If the oral route cannot initially be used mycophenolate can be given by IV infusion, 1 g twice daily for up to 14 days, converting to oral dosing as soon as possible.

Follow manufacturer's instructions for reconstitution and administration of the infusion.

Cardiac transplant: orally 1.5 g twice daily started within 5 days of the transplant.

Nursing implications

- The infusion is licensed for the prevention of acute renal transplant rejection only.
- Side effects include gastrointestinal upsets, hypertension, blood dyscrasias and infection.
- Patients should have a full blood count every week during the first 4 weeks of therapy, then twice a month for months 2 and 3, then monthly for the first year.
- Patients should be advised of the signs of bone marrow suppression, i.e. infection, unexpected bruising or bleeding.
- Mycophenolate is contraindicated in pregnancy and breastfeeding.

Storage

Mycophenolate preparations are stored at room temperature.

N

NABILONE (Cesamet)

Presentation
Capsules – 1 mg

Actions and uses
Nabilone is an antiemetic drug which is chemically related to substances called cannabinoids which are found in cannabis resin. It is used in the management of vomiting associated with anticancer therapy which has not responded to other conventional antiemetics.

Dosage
Adults over 18 years old: 1–2 mg taken the night before anticancer therapy and repeated 1–3 hours prior to the first dose of anticancer drug administered. Then 1 or 2 mg twice daily throughout each cycle of anticancer therapy. It can be continued for 48 hours after the cycle is completed.

Nursing implications
- The major problem with this drug is that it will be liable to misuse since it resembles cannabis and for this reason it is restricted to prescription in hospitals only. The nurse may therefore play a valuable role in ensuring that dosages are taken and that tablets are not allowed to accumulate in the home.
- Alertness may be impaired. This is a particular problem if other sedative drugs such as alcohol are also taken. Therefore, patients should be advised to avoid driving and the performance of other skilled tasks.
- Patients should be made aware of nabilone's ability to cause mood and behavioural changes.
- Patients with a history of psychotic illness may react adversely and should be carefully monitored.

Storage
Nabilone capsules are stored at room temperature.

NABUMETONE (Relifex)

Presentation
Tablets – 500 mg
Suspension – 500 mg in 5 ml

Actions and uses
This drug is converted after absorption to its active metabolite which is a NSAID (see p. 250). It has antiinflammatory and analgesic properties and is used in the treatment of osteoarthritis and rheumatoid arthritis.

Dosage
Adults: usually 1 g taken as a single dose at bedtime. This may be supplemented by an additional 500 mg to 1 g dose in the morning.
Elderly: 500 mg–1 g daily.

Nursing implications
See NSAIDs (p. 250).

Storage
Nabumetone tablets and suspension are stored at room temperature and should be protected from light.

NADOLOL (Corgard)

Presentation
Tablets – 40 mg, 80 mg

Actions and uses
Nadolol is a non-selective beta-adrenoreceptor blocking drug and its actions and uses are described in the section dealing with these drugs (p. 51). It is used in the management of hypertension, angina, arrhythmias, migraine and thyrotoxicosis.

Dosage
The usual adult dose is in the range 40–240 mg daily as a single dose or in two divided doses, depending upon the indication.

Nursing implications
See the section on Beta-Adrenoreceptor Blocking Drugs (p. 51).

Storage
Nadolol tablets are stored at room temperature.

NAFTIDROFURYL (Praxilene)

Presentation
Capsules – 100 mg
Injection – 200 mg in 10 ml

Actions and uses
This drug acts on the cardiovascular system to produce vasodilation. It is used in clinical practice for the following disorders.

- For the treatment of peripheral vascular insufficiency including Raynaud's syndrome, intermittent claudication, night cramps and frostbite.
- It is also used to improve blood supply to the brain in cerebro-vascular insufficiency.

Dosage
Orally: 100–200 mg three times per day.

Nursing implications
- Assess patients for improvement after 3–6 months.

- Nausea, epigastric pain, rash, hepatitis and hepatic failure are recognized side effects.

Storage
Naftidrofuryl is stored at room temperature. Protect from light.

NALBUPHINE (Nubain)

Presentation
Injection – 10 mg in 1 ml and 20 mg in 2 ml

Actions and uses
For nalbuphine's actions and uses see the section on Narcotic Analgesics (p. 238). It is indicated for the treatment of moderate-to-severe pain, premedication, perioperative analgesia and myocardial infarction. Nalbuphine is similar in efficacy to morphine for pain relief but causes less nausea and vomiting.

Dosage
Moderate–severe pain: subcutaneous, intramuscular or intravenous injection: for a 70 kg patient, 10–20 mg adjusting dose as required; for a child, up to 300 microgram per kg can be given and repeated once or twice if required.
Premedication: subcutaneous, intramuscular or intravenous injection: 100–200 microgram/kg.
Induction: intravenous injection 0.3–1 mg/kg given over 10–15 minutes.
Intra-operative analgesia: intravenous injection 250–500 microgram/kg given at 30-minute intervals.
Myocardial infarction: slow intravenous injection of 10–20 mg repeated after 30 minutes if necessary.

Nursing implications
- See the section on Narcotic Analgesics (p. 238).
- Though nalbuphine is reported to be associated with little if any dependence, it is intended for short-term pain relief and the possibility of abuse should not be overlooked.

N

- In common with opiate analgesics, nalbuphine may produce nausea and constipation requiring remedial antiemetic and laxative therapy.

Storage

Nalbuphine injection is stored at room temperature. Protect from light.

NALIDIXIC ACID (Negram, Uriben)

Presentation

Tablets – 500 mg
Suspension – 300 mg in 5 ml

Actions and uses

Nalidixic acid is a quinolone antibiotic. This drug has a bactericidal action inhibiting DNA synthesis. It has been found to be particularly effective against the Gram-negative organisms which commonly cause urinary tract infections. It is important to remember that infections due to *Pseudomonas aeruginosa* are rarely, if ever, effectively treated by nalidixic acid. Nalidixic acid can also be used for some gastrointestinal Gram-negative infections.

Dosage

Adults.

- For acute urinary tract infections: 1 g four times a day.
- For prolonged treatment of chronic infections: 500 mg four times a day.

Children: children under 3 months of age should rarely, if ever, be given this drug as their livers are incapable of metabolizing it. Older children should receive 50 mg/kg body weight in total daily, given in divided doses.

Nursing implications

- Nalidixic acid should be taken on an empty stomach or an hour before food.
- As noted above, the drug should rarely, if ever, be given to children under the age of 3 months.

- If given to infants, raised intracranial pressure manifest by drowsiness, convulsions and papilloedema may occur.
- Use with caution in children or adolescents as there may be a risk of arthropathy.
- Avoid use in pregnancy.
- Use with caution in patients with a history of epilepsy or any condition predisposing to convulsions. The CSM has warned that quinolones may induce convulsions whether or not the patient has a history of convulsions and that taking NSAIDs concomitantly may induce convulsions.
- The CSM has also advised, in relation to tendon damage, that at the first sign of any inflammation or pain whilst taking a quinolone, the treatment should be discontinued and the affected limb rested until symptoms have subsided.
- Discontinue the drug if psychiatric, neurological or hypersensitivity reactions occur.
- Side effects include skin rash, visual disturbance, headache, dizziness and gastrointestinal symptoms such as nausea, vomiting and abdominal pain. Renal impairment and hepatic dysfunction have also been reported.
- Photosensitivity reactions, urticaria, pruritus, fever and blood disorders may occur in patients who prove to be hypersensitive to the drug. Discontinue if photosensitivity occurs.
- The drug interacts with several drugs including:
  – warfarin – leading to a danger of bleeding unless the dosage is carefully monitored and reduced appropriately
  – analgesics – possible increased risk of convulsions with NSAIDs
  – cyclosporin – increased risk of nephrotoxicity.

- Nalidixic acid may interfere with urinary tests for 17-ketosteroids, vanilmandelic acid and glycosuria.

Storage
The drug is stored at room temperature.

NALOXONE (Narcan, Narcan Neonatal)

Presentation
Injection – 40 microgram in 2 ml, 400 microgram in 1 ml, 800 microgram in 2 ml

Actions and uses
Naloxone is indicated for the reversal of opioid-induced respiratory depression and for treating opioid overdosage. It is an opioid antagonist acting directly at opiate receptors to reverse the effects of opioid drugs. It is particularly useful for reversing respiratory depression but also the sedative effects of opioids and reversing any lowering of blood pressure that may have occurred with the opioid drug. It is used in anaesthesia where it can be used to immediately reverse opioid-induced respiratory depression. Naloxone is very short acting. Repeated doses may be required. It is important to note that the analgesic effect of the opioid will also be reversed.

In the emergency treatment of poisoning, naloxone is used to manage opioid overdose in cases where the patient is comatose or has bradypnoea. Repeated doses may be required depending on the patient's respiratory rate or depth of coma.

Dosage
Adults.

- Opioid overdose: IV injection (SC or IM only if IV access is unavailable) 0.4–2 mg repeated every 2–3 minutes to a maximum of 10 mg. By continuous IV infusion, 2 mg in 500 ml sodium chloride 0.9% or glucose 5%, adjusting rate according to response.
- Reversal of respiratory depression: IV injection of 100–200 microgram

every 2–3 minutes if required until respiratory depression is reversed. Further doses can be given IM.

Child.

- Opioid overdose: IV injection 10 microgram/kg; if no response, give 100 microgram/kg.
- Reversal of respiratory depression: dose as for opioid overdose. Divided doses via SC or IM route may be used if there is no IV access.

Neonate.

- Reversal of respiratory depression: SC, IM or IV injection 10 microgram/kg repeated every 2–3 minutes or at birth, a single dose of 200 microgram (60 microgram/kg) by IM injection.

Nursing implications
- It is important to note that the effects of some opioids, e.g. buprenorphine, will be only partially reversed.
- Naloxone should be used with caution in patients with cardiovascular disease or in those patients who are taking cardiotoxic drugs.
- Side effects include nausea and vomiting, tachycardia and fibrillation.
- Naloxone will precipitate withdrawal in patients dependent on opiates.

N

Storage
Naloxone is stored at room temperature, protected from light.

NALTREXONE (Nalorex)

Presentation
Tablets – 50 mg

Actions and uses
Naltrexone is an opioid antagonist used to help prevent relapse of former opioid addicts. It should be used only under specialist advice.

Dosage
Initially, 25 mg daily increased to 50 mg each day. The weekly dose may be given in divided doses, e.g. 100 mg

on a Monday and Wednesday, 150 mg on a Friday.

> ## Nursing implications
> - Naltrexone therapy should only be initiated in specialist clinics.
> - Side effects include nausea and vomiting, anxiety, nervousness, sleeping difficulties, abdominal pain, headache, joint pains, depression.
> - Avoid this drug during pregnancy and breastfeeding.

Storage
Naltrexone tablets are stored at room temperature, protected from light.

NAPROXEN (Naprosyn, Nycopren, Synflex)

Note: Also combined with misoprostol in Napratec.

Presentation
Tablets – 250 mg, 275 mg, 500 mg
Tablets (enteric coated) – 250 mg, 375 mg, 500 mg
Tablets (sustained release) – 500 mg
Suspension – 250 mg in 10 ml
Suppositories – 500 mg

Actions and uses
See the section on NSAIDs (p. 250).

Dosage
Oral

Pain and inflammation in rheumatic disease.

- Adults: 250 mg or 500 mg twice a day or 1 g once daily.
- Child over 5 years for juvenile arthritis: 5 mg/kg twice a day.

Acute musculoskeletal disorders and dysmenorrhoea.

- Adults: 500 mg initially, then 250 mg three or four times a day as required. Maximum daily dose after the first day is 1.25 g.
- Child: not recommended for children under the age of 16.

Acute gout.

- Adult: 750 mg initially then 250 mg three times a day until gout attack has subsided.

- Child: not recommended for children under the age of 16.

Rectal
500 mg twice a day or once in the evening for adults only.

> ## Nursing implications
> See the section on NSAIDs (p. 250).

Storage
Naproxen preparations are stored at room temperature.

NARATRIPTAN (Naramig)

Presentation
Tablets – 2.5 mg

Actions and uses
Naratriptan is a 5-HT1 (5-hydroxytryptamine) agonist, similar to sumatriptan. It is used in the treatment of acute migraine attacks. Acting at 5-HT1 receptors, it causes vascular contraction in intracranial blood vessels, reversing any dilatation or oedema in these vessels which is thought to cause migraine attacks.

Dosage
Adults only: a single 2.5 mg dose should be taken at the onset of a migraine attack. A second dose can be taken only if symptoms recur after an initial response. There should be a minimum of 4 hours between doses and a maximum of 5 mg taken in 24 hours.

> ## Nursing implications
> See Sumatriptan (p. 344).

Storage
Naratriptan tablets are stored at room temperature.

NARCOTIC ANALGESICS

Narcotic or opioid analgesics comprise a group of drugs derived from opium, and termed opium alkaloids, and synthetic compounds based on the opium alkaloids. They include the following drugs.

Alfentanil
Buprenorphine
Codeine
Dextromoramide
Dextropropoxyphene
Diamorphine
Dihydrocodeine
Dipipanone
Fentanyl
Hydromorphone
Meptazinol
Methadone
Morphine
Nalbuphine
Papaveretum
Pentazocine
Pethidine
Phenazocine
Remifentanil
Tramadol

Actions and uses

Narcotic analgesic drugs have a powerful analgesic action mediated by their direct effect on specific receptor sites in the central nervous system. They are used for the treatment of conditions associated with acute or chronic severe pain such as myocardial infarction, childbirth, postoperative pain and the pain associated with malignant disease. They are also used regularly for preoperative medication. Apart from analgesia, these drugs also cause euphoria, respiratory depression, depression of the cough reflex, nausea and vomiting, constipation, tolerance and dependence.

Within this group of drugs there is a range of efficacy. For example, dextropropoxyphene is a relatively mild analgesic commonly given in combination with paracetamol for mild-to-moderate pain. Diamorphine is one of the most potent narcotic analgesics, frequently used in large doses for the pain of malignant disease; its main advantage over morphine is its solubility so large doses can be given in small volumes.

See individual drug entries for specific actions and uses.

Dosage

See individual drugs.

Nursing implications

- The most important point for the nurse to note is that the use of many of the drugs in this group is strictly controlled by law. The legal aspects of prescribing these drugs must be adhered to.
- Narcotic analgesics produce a dose-related depression of neurological function resulting in sedation, drowsiness and sleepiness. They may eventually produce profound depression of respiratory function and therefore must be used with great caution in patients who already have poor respiratory function or in those in whom the sedative effect may be enhanced, such as patients with liver cirrhosis.
- Many analgesics in this group produce severe nausea and vomiting and for this reason antiemetics should always be co-prescribed.
- Narcotic analgesics influence the motility of the gut and cause constipation. This is a major problem which may give rise to great discomfort, especially in elderly and bedridden patients. Laxatives should always be prescribed with regular potent narcotic analgesics.
- Narcotic analgesics must be used with extreme caution in patients who are also receiving MAOIs (p. 228) as the combination of these two types of drug may produce serious cardiovascular reactions.
- The most serious problem encountered with patients who receive these drugs is the production of physical dependence and addiction. Nurses play an important role in giving patients support when such drugs are being withdrawn after short-term use, in identifying patients who may be becoming dependent on these drugs and in providing support to those who are being

N

weaned off prolonged use of these drugs.

- In addition to physical dependence, the phenomenon of tolerance may arise in patients receiving prolonged treatment with these analgesics. The term 'tolerance' basically means that with prolonged treatment patients receive less benefit from doses which were previously effective. This may mean that the frequency of administration and dosage may have to be increased as duration of therapy progresses. Many patients receiving prolonged narcotic analgesia are suffering from chronic pain due to malignancy and the nurse's role in identifying the relative efficacy of their treatment regimes is important. This will enable the need for change in therapy to be brought to the attention of the medical staff.
- See individual drug entries for specific nursing implications.

Storage
See specific drugs.

NEBIVOLOL (Nebilet)

Presentation
Tablets – 5 mg

Actions and uses
Nebivolol is a cardioselective beta-adrenoceptor blocking drug. The section on Beta-blockers (p. 51) should be consulted for a full account of its actions and uses. Nebivolol is indicated for the treatment of essential hypertension.

Dosage
Adults only: 5 mg daily. Elderly patients should start on 2.5 mg daily, increasing to 5 mg if necessary.

Nursing implications
See the section on Beta-blocker Drugs (p. 51).

Storage
Nebivolol tablets are stored at room temperature.

NEDOCROMIL (Rapitil, Tilade)

Presentation
Pressurized inhaler – 2 mg per metered dose
Eye drops – 2% solution

Actions and uses
Nedocromil is a specific anti-inflammatory drug with an action in the lung. In asthma there is a tendency for a variety of cells present within the bronchial mucosa to break down on exposure to certain environmental trigger factors (animal dander, cigarette smoke, house dust mite, etc.), resulting in the release of chemicals which provoke bronchospasm. Nedocromil inhibits the release of such substances. It is administered by inhalation for the prevention of asthmatic attacks and as eye drops for the prevention and treatment of allergic conjunctivitis and vernal keratoconjunctivitis.

Dosage
Inhaled.

- Adults and children over 6 years old: 4 mg by inhalation 2–4 times daily.

Eye drops.

- Seasonal and perennial conjunctivitis: adults and children over 6 years old, apply twice a day increasing to four times a day if necessary. Treat for a maximum of 12 weeks for seasonal allergic conjunctivitis.
- Vernal keratoconjunctivitis: adults and children over 6 years old, apply four times a day.

Nursing implications
- It is important to recognize that this is a prophylactic drug. It must be taken regularly and never to treat an asthmatic attack.
- The action of nedocromil is somewhat similar to that of sodium cromoglycate which is

the drug of choice for young children.

- Occasionally headaches and nausea have been reported and some patients may complain of an unpleasant bitter taste.
- Transient burning and stinging can occur with the eye drops.
- In common with other pressurized containers, metered aerosols should not be punctured or incinerated after use.

Storage
Nedocromil preparations are stored at room temperature. Eye drops have a relatively short life during use and a risk of bacterial contamination after opening exists. Normally eye drops of any kind should not be used after 1 week for a hospitalized patient or after 4 weeks for others.

NEFAZODONE (Dutonin)

Presentation
Tablets – 50 mg, 100 mg, 200 mg

Actions and uses
Nefazodone is an antidepressant. For an account of its actions and uses see Antidepressant Drugs (p. 31). Nefazodone inhibits serotonin reuptake and selectively blocks serotonin type 2 receptors. It is used to treat all types of depression, including depression which is accompanied by anxiety or sleep disturbances.

Dosage
Adults only: start with a dose of 50–100 mg twice daily increasing to 200 mg twice daily to a maximum of 300 mg twice daily. Titrate the dose carefully and slowly in the elderly.

Nursing implications
- See the section on Antidepressant Drugs (p. 31).
- If the patient is being transferred from another CNS medication use a starting dose

of 50 mg twice daily and titrate up at weekly intervals until an effective dose has been reached.
- Use lower doses in patients with liver disease or severe renal impairment.
- Interaction with MAOIs: nefazodone should not be started until 2 weeks after stopping an MAOI; conversely, an MAOI should not be started until at least 1 week after stopping nefazodone.
- Avoid concomitant use with terfenadine due to increased risk of arrhythmias.

Storage
Nefazodone tablets are stored at room temperature.

NEFOPAM (Acupan)

Presentation
Tablets – 30 mg
Injection – 20 mg in 1 ml

Actions and uses
Nefopam is an analgesic drug which acts by a direct effect on the central nervous system. It is chemically unrelated to the narcotic analgesic drugs and it is indicated for the management of moderate-to-severe pain which is not amenable to treatment with mild analgesics but is not felt to be of sufficient severity to require narcotic analgesia.

Dosage
Adults only.

- Orally: 30–90 mg three times per day.
- By intramuscular injection: 20 mg four times per day (see nursing implications for administration procedure).

Nursing implications
- When this drug is given by intramuscular injection care must be taken to ensure that accidental intravenous injection

is avoided. The injection should always be given while the patient is lying down as there is a risk of syncope. The patient should remain lying down for 15–20 minutes after receiving the injection and then sit or stand up slowly.

- Common side effects include nausea, vomiting, blurred vision, nervousness, light-headedness, dry mouth, drowsiness, sweating, insomnia, headache and tachycardia.
- Patients with a history of fits should not receive this drug.
- The metabolism and excretion of nefopam may be impaired in patients with liver or kidney disease.
- Avoid concomitant use with MAOIs.

Storage

The drug is stored at room temperature.

NELFINAVIR (Viracept)

Presentation

Tablets – 250 mg
Oral powder – 50 mg/g

Actions and uses

Nelfinavir is indicated for use in combination with other antiretroviral agents to treat patients with the HIV infection. It is a protease inhibitor, acting on the HIV protease enzyme to prevent the production of essential proteins.

Dosage

Adults: 750 mg three times a day or 1.25 g twice a day.
Child age 3–13 years: 25–30 mg/kg three times a day.

Nursing implications

- Treatment of HIV is expensive and the drugs can cause serious side effects, so they should be prescribed only under expert advice.
- The timing of commencement of therapy should be decided by those expert in the management of HIV and depends on symptoms, viral load and the CD4 count and should be weighed against drug toxicities and the likely development of drug resistance.
- Resistance to antiretroviral drugs is reduced by using combination therapy.
- Most antiretroviral agents are used in pregnancy although teratogenic effects are not yet fully understood. Mothers are advised not to breastfeed their infants as HIV can pass from mother to infant via the breast milk.
- Side effects include diarrhoea and other gastrointestinal symptoms.
- Lipidodystrophy can be a problematic side effect; body fat redistribution can occur as can hyperlipidaemia, insulin resistance and diabetes mellitus.
- The tablets should be taken with or after food.
- The powder may be mixed with water, milk formula feeds or puddings, not with acidic foods or juices due to taste.
- Nelfinavir interacts with a variety of drugs. Concomitant use should be avoided with amiodarone, quinidine, rifampicin, St John's wort, terfenadine, pimozide, midazolam and simvastatin.
- It is also important to advise women on the combined oral contraceptive pill that additional contraceptive measures should be taken as nelfinavir may interfere with the pill's metabolism.

Storage

Nelfinavir preparations are stored at room temperature.

NEOMYCIN (Nivemycin)

Presentation

Tablets – 500 mg

NB: Neomycin is included in a vast range of preparations for topical use including ointments, creams, eye drops and ear drops. It is usually combined with other medicaments, particularly other antibiotics and corticosteroids.

Actions and uses

Neomycin is an antibiotic of the aminoglycoside group which resembles gentamicin (p. 158). It is not absorbed orally and is too toxic for systemic use. It is therefore only useful in the following situations.

- It may be given in an attempt to sterilize the gut. This is useful before bowel surgery and also may lead to a decrease in protein absorption from the bowel which is useful in patients with cirrhosis of the liver when they develop encephalopathy.
- It is an effective antibiotic for the treatment of superficial infections of the skin, eye and ear.

Dosage

To attempt bowel sterilization.

- Adults: 1 g every 4 hours for 2–3 days preoperatively.
- Children: under 6 years, not recommended; 6–12 years, ½–1 tablet every 4 hours for 2–3 days preoperatively; over 12 years, 2 tablets every 4 hours for 2–3 days preoperatively.

Hepatic coma: up to 4 g daily in divided doses for a maximum of 14 days.

Nursing implications
- Systemic adverse effects are unlikely as very little of the drug is absorbed.
- Despite the fact that the drug is very poorly absorbed, a large number of patients develop skin rashes due to hypersensitivity.
- Side effects also include gastrointestinal upsets, ototoxicity and nephrotoxicity. It is contraindicated in intestinal obstruction and renal impairment.

- Nurses who are sensitive to the drug develop severe skin rashes if they handle it. Therefore the wearing of protective gloves is advised.

Storage

Neomycin tablets are stored at room temperature.

NEOSTIGMINE (Prostigmin)

Presentation
Tablets – 15 mg neostigmine bromide
Injection – 2.5 mg in 1 ml

Actions and uses
Neostigmine is an anticholinesterase, preventing the action of the enzyme that destroys acetylcholine in the body. This in effect leads to a prolongation of acetylcholine action which is to stimulate the parasympathetic component of the autonomic nervous system. It has the following uses in clinical practice.

- For the treatment of myasthenia gravis.
- As an antidote to non-depolarizing or competitive (curariform) muscle relaxants used in surgery.

Dosage
For the treatment of myasthenia gravis.

- Adults: a daily dose of 5–20 tablets by mouth or 1–2.5 mg by SC or IM injection is commonly given but doses higher than these may be needed in some patients.
- Children: the doses should be decided by the attending physician. A guideline is as follows.
  - Neonates: 50–250 microgram by injection or 1–5 mg orally every 4 hours.
  - Older children: 200–500 microgram by injection as required or 15–90 mg daily orally.

As an antidote to curariform drugs: 50–70 microgram/kg intravenously over 1 minute (maximum dose of 5 mg). Atropine 0.4–1.25 mg should normally be given some minutes before this injection.

Nursing implications
- Side effects include excess salivation, anorexia, nausea, vomiting, abdominal cramp and diarrhoea. Bradycardia and hypotension may occur along with an increase in bronchial secretions. Rarely weakness, paralysis, convulsion and coma may occur.
- It is important to note that the major symptom of overdosage with this drug is increased muscular weakness. When used for the treatment of myasthenia gravis, the patient may become weak and it is then difficult to differentiate whether this is due to inadequate or excessive treatment. In this situation the intravenous administration of edrophonium chloride (Tensilon) will produce a rapid and short-lived improvement in muscle power if inadequate dosage is the cause of weakness but will not have this effect if overdosage is the cause of weakness.
- The drug should never be given to patients who are known to suffer from intestinal or urinary obstruction.
- Patients with bradycardia, bronchial asthma, heart disease, epilepsy, hypotension and parkinsonism should not receive this drug.

Storage
- Store at room temperature.
- All preparations should be protected from light.
- Tablets should be stored in well-closed containers.

NETILMICIN (Netillin)

Presentation
Injection – 15 mg in 1.5 ml, 50 mg in 1 ml, 100 mg in 1 ml, 150 mg in 1.5 ml, 200 mg in 2 ml

Actions and uses
Netilmicin is a member of the aminoglycoside group of antibiotics. Its actions and uses are similar to those of Gentamicin (p. 158). It is administered only by injection and may be favoured since it produces a lower incidence of ototoxicity than do other aminoglycosides.

Dosage
As for gentamicin, though slightly higher doses may be used.

Nursing implications
- See the section on Gentamicin (p. 158).
- Administration is by IM injection, slow IV injection or IV infusion in glucose 5% solution, glucose 10% solution or sodium chloride 0.9% solution.

Storage
Netilmicin injections are stored at room temperature.

NICARDIPINE (Cardene)

Presentation
Capsules – 20 mg, 30 mg
Sustained-release capsules – 30 mg, 45 mg

Actions and uses
Nicardipine has the actions and uses described for Nifedipine (p. 247). It is indicated for the treatment of mild-to-moderate hypertension and the prophylaxis of chronic stable angina.

Dosage
20–40 mg three times daily or 30–60 mg sustained-release capsules twice daily.

Nursing implications
The nursing implications for Nifedipine (p. 247) also apply to this drug.

Storage
Nicardipine capsules are stored at room temperature.

NEVIRAPINE (Viramune)

Presentation
Tablets – 200 mg
Suspension – 50 mg in 5 ml

Actions and uses
Nevirapine is indicated for use in combination with at least two other antiretroviral agents to treat patients with the HIV infection. It is a non-nucleoside reverse transcriptase inhibitor which acts on the reverse transcriptase enzyme, preventing viral RNA from being processed.

Dosage
Adult: 200 mg daily for 14 days increased to 200 mg twice a day if there is no rash present.
Child 2 months–8 years: 4 mg/kg daily for 14 days increased to 7 mg/kg twice a day (to a maximum of 400 mg daily) if there is no rash present.
Child 8–16 years and under 50 kg: 4 mg/kg daily for 14 days increased to 4 mg/kg twice a day (to a maximum of 400 mg daily) if there is no rash present.

Nursing implications
- Treatment of HIV is expensive and the drugs can cause serious side effects, so they should be prescribed only under expert advice.
- The timing of commencement of therapy should be decided by those expert in the management of HIV and depends on symptoms, viral load and the CD4 count and should be weighed against drug toxicities and the likely development of drug resistance.
- Resistance to antiretroviral drugs is reduced by using combination therapy.
- Most antiretroviral agents are used in pregnancy although teratogenic effects are not yet fully understood. Mothers are advised not to breastfeed their infants as HIV can pass from mother to infant via the breast milk.
- Nevirapine can cause skin rash, including Stevens–Johnson

syndrome and toxic epidermal necrolysis. It usually occurs shortly after starting therapy, therefore low doses are initially prescribed then gradually increased. The drug should be discontinued permanently if a severe rash occurs.
- Nevirapine can also cause raised liver function tests and hepatitis, which again usually occur shortly after starting therapy. LFTs should be monitored before treatment, every 2 weeks for the first 2 months, then after 1 month, then every 3–6 months. Discontinue nevirapine permanently if abnormal LFTs are accompanied by hypersensitivity reactions or suspend use if no hypersensitivity reaction is present.
- Note that if treatment is suspended for more than 7 days, it should be recommenced at the starting dose (as above) and dosage increased gradually.
- Avoid concomitant use with St John's wort and ketoconazole.
- Nevirapine reduces the plasma concentration of saquinavir, therefore avoid concomitant use. Nevirapine also reduces the plasma concentration of indinavir and possibly amprenavir.
- It is also important to advise women on the combined oral contraceptive pill and other hormonal contraceptives that additional contraceptive measures should be taken as nelfinavir may interfere with the hormone metabolism.

Storage
Nevirapine preparations are stored at room temperature.

NICLOSAMIDE (Yomesan)

Presentation
Tablets – 500 mg

N

Actions and uses

This antihelminthic drug is used for the treatment of the following tapeworm infections.

- Beef tapeworm (*Taenia saginata*)
- Pork tapeworm (*Taenia solium*)
- Fish tapeworm (*Diphyllobothrium latum*)
- Dwarf tapeworm (*Hymenolepis nana*)

Dosage

For the treatment of beef, pork and fish tapeworm.

- Adults and children over 6 years: 2 g
- Children 2–6 years: 1 g
- Children under 2 years: 500 mg

For the treatment of dwarf tapeworm.

- On the first day adults and children over 6, 2 g; children 2–6 years, 1 g; children under 2 years, 500 mg.
- For the subsequent 6 days: adults and children over 6, 1 g daily; children 2–6 years, 500 mg daily; children under 2 years, 250 mg daily.

Nursing implications

- A laxative given 2 hours after treatment with this drug ensures a rapid and complete expulsion of the worm which would otherwise be excreted in pieces during the next few days. It is felt that in the treatment of *Taenia solium* a laxative is essential.
- The drug may be given without danger to patients with liver, biliary or kidney disease.

Storage

The drug is stored at room temperature. Protect from light.

NICORANDIL (Ikorel)

Presentation

Tablets – 10 mg, 20 mg

Actions and uses

Nicorandil is a potassium channel activator indicated for the prevention and treatment of angina. It acts by opening potassium channels leading to arterial vasodilatation and, via its nitrate component, causes venous vasodilatation. Hence both the preload and afterload are reduced and blood flow in the heart is improved.

Dosage

Adults: 10–30 mg twice a day.

Nursing implications

- Nicorandil may cause dizziness and weakness. Patients should be advised not to drive or operate machinery until they have established the severity of their side effects.
- Other side effects include transient headache, flushing, nausea and vomiting.
- Nicorandil interacts with sildenafil, with hypotension occurring. They must not be used together.

Storage

Nicorandil tablets are stored at room temperature.

NICOUMALONE (rINN Acenocoumarol) (Sinthrome)

Presentation

Tablets – 1 mg

Actions and uses

Like warfarin, but rarely used, nicoumalone or acenocoumarol is an anticoagulant agent.

A number of substances present in blood which play an important part in preventing bleeding by forming clots are produced by the liver from vitamin K. Nicoumalone inhibits the synthesis of these substances (known as clotting factors) and therefore reduces the ability of the blood to clot. Its principal uses are for the prevention and treatment of thromboembolic states such as deep venous thrombosis and pulmonary embolus. It is also used to prevent the formation of clot in cardiovascular disease either on artificial heart valves or in the atria of patients who have atrial dysrhythmias.

Dosage

Adults only.

- Loading dose: day 1, 8–12 mg; day 2, 4–8 mg; day 3, dosage should be adjusted according to result of blood clotting test.
- Maintenance dose: varies according to individual response and should be decided after reference to the results of blood clotting test. Usually 1–8 mg daily.

Nursing implications

- See Warfarin (p. 391).
- The daily maintenance dose of nicoumalone is, as noted above, determined by the results of clotting studies. As the effects of bleeding due to overcoagulation or thrombosis due to undercoagulation can be so rapidly catastrophic, strict adherence to the recommended dose is mandatory and the nurse may play an important role in ensuring that patients are aware of this.
- The effects of nicoumalone may be influenced by a number of factors listed below and the nurse may play an important role by identifying their occurrence and alerting both the patient and medical staff. The following circumstances may lead to a requirement for alteration in dosage.
  - Acute illness such as chest infection or viral infection.
  - Sudden weight loss.
  - The concurrent administration of other drugs: a number of drugs may affect the patient's dosage requirements. See the section on Warfarin (p. 391).
- The occurrence of haemorrhage in a patient on nicoumalone is an indication for immediate withdrawal of the drug and if the haemorrhage is at all serious or repetitive, the patient should be referred immediately to hospital for further assessment and, if necessary, they may be given vitamin K which accelerates a return to normal clotting function.

- Nicoumalone is relatively contraindicated in patients with severe liver or kidney disease, haemorrhagic conditions or uncontrolled hypertension. It should also be used with great caution immediately after surgery or labour.
- Nausea, loss of appetite, headache and allergic reactions may occur.

Storage

The tablets are stored at room temperature.

NIFEDIPINE (e.g. Adalat; there are many other brands)

Presentation

Capsules – 5 mg and 10 mg
Modified-release tablets – 10 mg, 20 mg, 30 mg, 40 mg, 60 mg
Modified-release capsules – 10 mg, 20 mg, 30 mg, 60 mg

Actions and uses

Nifedipine is a calcium channel blocker; see the actions and uses described for this group of drugs on p. 67. It has three main actions.

1. It decreases the work done by the heart in two ways:
   - it directly affects heart muscle, depressing its activity
   - it dilates peripheral vessels, reducing the pressure against which the heart has to work.
2. It lowers raised blood pressure by its action on peripheral blood vessels which results in vasodilatation.
3. It improves peripheral perfusion in patients with vascular insufficiency.

These properties make it useful for the treatment of angina pectoris, hypertension and Raynaud's phenomenon.

Dosage

For angina and hypertension: the dose depends on the preparation used, varying from 20 mg to 90 mg daily. Plain capsules are taken three times a day but modified-release preparations are taken only once or twice daily.

Nursing implications
- See the section on Calcium Antagonists (p. 67).
- Note that different modified-release preparations exist and that these are not necessarily interchangeable.
- Headaches and flushing may be expected in patients on this drug. Lethargy or tiredness may also occur.
- There is some evidence that occasionally, after an acute myocardial infarction, the drug may divert blood to healthy rather than damaged muscle and so increase the extent of damage.
- Sometimes angina may be paradoxically exacerbated and require the drug to be stopped.
- Patients should be advised to avoid drinking grapefruit juice as this may affect the metabolism of nifedipine.

Storage
The drug is stored at room temperature. It is light sensitive so always protect from light.

NIMODIPINE (Nimotop)

Presentation
Tablets – 30 mg
Infusion – 10 mg in 50 ml

Actions and uses
Nimodipine is a calcium channel blocker. For the actions and uses of this group of drugs see p. 67. Nimodipine acts preferentially on cerebral vessels, increasing cerebral perfusion and, unlike other drugs of this group, it is used only for the management of ischaemic neurological deficits following subarachnoid haemorrhage (SAH).

Dosage
Prevention of ischaemic neurological deficits following SAH: orally 60 mg

every 4 hours starting within 4 days of a SAH and continued for 21 days. Treatment of ischaemic neurological deficits following SAH: IV infusion via central catheter, 1 mg/h initially increasing after 2 hours to 2 mg/h with monitoring for a fall in blood pressure. If the patient has unstable blood pressure or weighs less than 70 kg, start with an infusion rate of 500 microgram/h or less. Continue treatment for at least 5 days (maximum of 14 days) change to oral therapy and complete the 21-day course.

Nursing implications
- See the section on Calcium Channel Blockers (p. 67).
- Nimodipine solution reacts with polyvinylchloride (PVC) so use polyethylene, polypropylene or glass infusion devices.

Storage
Nimodipine preparations are stored at room temperature. The solution is light sensitive and should always be protected from light, particularly direct sunlight.

NISOLDIPINE (Systor MR)

Presentation
Modified-release tablets – 10 mg, 20 mg, 30 mg

Actions and uses
Nisoldipine is a calcium channel blocker. For the action and uses of this group of drugs see p. 67. It is indicated for angina and hypertension.

Dosage
10–40 mg daily before breakfast.

Nursing implications
See the section on Calcium Channel Blockers (p. 67).

Storage
Nisoldipine preparations are stored at room temperature.

NITRAZEPAM (Mogadon)

Presentation
Tablets – 5 mg
Suspension – 2.5 mg in 5 ml

Actions and uses
Nitrazepam is a member of the Benzodiazepine group (p. 47). It has a pronounced sedative effect and is taken at night as a hypnotic.

Dosage
5–10 mg on retiring, 2.5 mg for elderly patients. Not recommended for children.

Nursing implications

- See the section on Benzodiazepines (p. 47).
- It is essential to emphasize that nitrazepam is particularly likely to cause a hangover effect with drowsiness and headache the following day. This may be particularly severe when high dosage is used in elderly patients and may lead to frank confusion. It is recommended that the elderly should only very rarely receive a dose exceeding 5 mg of this drug if side effects are to be avoided.

Storage
Preparations containing nitrazepam are stored at room temperature.

NITROFURANTOIN (Macrobid, Macrodantin, Furadantin)

Presentation
Tablets – 50 mg and 100 mg
Capsules – 50 mg and 100 mg
Modified-release capsules – 100 mg

Actions and uses
Nitrofurantoin is bactericidal, i.e. it kills organisms in the body if the concentration of the drug obtained is sufficiently high. At lower concentrations it is bacteriostatic, i.e. it inhibits growth and further multiplication of bacterial cells. It is so rapidly excreted from the body that it is only of use in bacterial infections of the bladder. It is debatable whether sufficient concentration is obtained in the kidney for it to be useful in pyelonephritis and it is certainly not useful for infections of other organs of the body. It is usually effective against *E. coli*, Klebsiella and Enterobacter but resistance is a greater problem with Proteus and *Pseudomonas aeruginosa*.
It is used both in the treatment of urinary tract infections and for prophylaxis against urinary tract infections.

Dosage
For the treatment of urinary tract infections.

- Adults: 50–100 mg four times a day with meals for 7 days.
- Children over 3 months: for acute UTI, 3 mg/kg/day in divided doses for 7 days.

For the prophylaxis of urinary tract infection.

- Adult: 50–100 mg at night
- Child over 3 months: 1 mg/kg at night

N

Nursing implications

- Nausea, vomiting and diarrhoea occur commonly. The incidence and severity of these effects may be reduced if the drug is taken with meals or milk.
- An uncommon but important side effect is peripheral neuropathy. Patients should be continually asked to report symptoms of numbness or tingling of the feet and if such symptoms occur the drug should be immediately withdrawn before irreversible and more severe changes occur.
- Haematological adverse effects can occur including agranulocytosis, thrombocytopenia and aplastic anaemia.
- The drug may rarely damage the lungs, especially in elderly patients, producing pneumonitis and pulmonary fibrosis. Symptoms such as chills, fever

---

and cough should be investigated.

- The drug should not be given to patients who have severe renal damage as it may accumulate in the body and produce severe toxic effects.
- Hepatic reactions can occur, including cholestatic jaundice and hepatitis.
- Avoid use in pregnancy and breastfeeding.

Storage

The drug is stored at room temperature. Protect from light and moisture.

NIZATIDINE (Axid, Zinga)

Presentation

Capsules – 150 mg, 300 mg
Injection – 100 mg in 4 ml

Actions and uses

See Histamine H2-Receptor Antagonists (p. 169).

Dosage

Adults only. Treatment of peptic ulcer.

- Orally: 150 mg twice a day or 300 mg at night for up to 8 weeks. Maintenance dose of 150 mg at night.
- Short-term IV: intermittent infusion in hospital inpatients, 100 mg (given over 15 minutes) three times a day or continuous infusion at a rate of 10 mg/h to a maximum of 480 mg in 24 hours.

Gastrooesophageal reflux disease.

- Orally: 150–300 mg twice daily for up to 12 weeks.

Nursing implications

The nursing implications described for Histamine H2-Receptor Antagonists (p. 169) apply.

Storage

Nizatidine preparations are stored at room temperature. Protect injection from light.

NON-STEROIDAL ANTIINFLAMMATORY DRUGS (NSAIDs)

Actions and uses

This group of drugs relieve pain and reduce inflammation in a variety of diseases affecting the joints, tendons, cartilage and muscle. Thus they are useful in such disorders as rheumatoid arthritis, osteoarthritis, ankylosing spondylitis and gouty arthritis. If given in lower doses for minor painful conditions, they are effective analgesics but simple analgesics such as paracetamol are equally effective and do not have the potentially serious side effects of this group of drugs. For convenience the drugs may be classified according to their chemical structure.

- Salicylates, e.g. aspirin, benorylate
- Benzene acetic acid derivatives, e.g. diclofenac, aceclofenac
- Propionic acid derivatives, e.g. flurbiprofen, ibuprofen, ketoprofen, naproxen
- Oxicams, e.g. piroxicam, meloxicam
- Indole/indene derivatives, e.g. indomethacin
- Pyrazolones, e.g. azapropazone, phenylbutazone
- Anthranilic acid derivatives, e.g. mefenamic acid
- Others, e.g. etodolac, nabumetone

NSAIDs act by inhibiting the action of cyclooxygenases, enzymes involved in the synthesis of prostaglandins and thromboxanes. Prostaglandins are involved in processes which lead to inflammation, pain and fever, hence the usefulness of NSAIDs in managing these conditions.

It is now believed that NSAIDs inhibit both cyclooxygenase-1 (COX-1) and cyclooxygenase-2 (COX-2). It is the inhibition of COX-2 which produces the antiinflammatory action of NSAIDs whereas the inhibition of COX-1 produces adverse gastrointestinal effects. Several drugs have been developed which selectively inhibit COX-2 but they are not completely free of gastrointestinal side effects and long-term safety is not yet known.

NSAIDs are usually taken orally. Some can be injected intravenously or intramuscularly or applied topically.

Dosage
See individual drugs.

Nursing implications

- As mentioned above, this group of drugs are very effective analgesics but they have potentially serious side effects and perhaps the major role to be played by the nurse in the management of patients who are in possession of these drugs is to ensure that they are taken in the correct dosage and only for the problems for which they are prescribed.
- These drugs frequently have gastrointestinal side effects which may range from loss of appetite, nausea, vomiting and diarrhoea to gastric bleeding which may be either chronic and go unnoticed or be acute and result in haematemesis or melaena. In patients with chronic painful disorders, adequate nutrition is absolutely essential and it is important that the nurse monitors the nutrition of patients on these drugs and where necessary encourages patients to try to overcome any associated anorexia. As a substantial number of patients on these drugs will gradually develop an anaemia, it is important that the nurse observes all patients for the clinical signs of anaemia such as pallor, tiredness and dyspnoea on exertion. Note that there is an increased risk of gastrointestinal bleeding or ulceration if NSAIDs are taken concurrently with corticosteroids.
- These drugs are relatively contraindicated in patients with peptic ulceration and they may exacerbate the symptoms of this problem.
- Asthma may be precipitated in a few patients who are hypersensitive to drugs of this type. This occurs most commonly in the salicylate group but it may also rarely occur with the other groups. An important point to note is that patients who suffer from salicylate-induced asthma may not have their symptoms relieved by changing to one of the other chemical groups. Other hypersensitivity reactions include fever, angiooedema and rash.
- All drugs in this group may cause salt and water retention. This may exacerbate or produce hypertension or cardiac failure. This effect is rarely seen in salicylates except when high dosage is given for the treatment of rheumatic fever.
- Most antiinflammatory drugs are metabolized to some extent by the liver and/or are excreted as metabolites or unmetabolized drugs by the kidney. They will therefore tend to accumulate in patients who have impaired liver or kidney function and be more likely to produce toxic effects.
- Some NSAIDs can cause nephrotoxicity and can even provoke renal failure in patients with preexisting renal impairment.
- Other side effects include CNS effects such as headache, vertigo and dizziness, hepatotoxicity and haematological effects including thrombocytopenia and neutropenia.
- NSAIDs are carried in the blood attached to sites on proteins circulating in the blood. They have the capacity to displace other drugs from these proteins. The actual active component of any drug is that part which lies free in the plasma rather than that part which is bound to the protein; any displacement of a

drug from the protein will lead to an increased effect. This is especially important with anticoagulants such as warfarin. If NSAIDs are given to patients who are receiving warfarin or other anticoagulants, the anticoagulant may be displaced from the proteins and therefore be proportionately more active. This may lead to bleeding and may be especially dangerous if NSAIDs' other side effects such as peptic ulceration or gastrointestinal bleeding occur coincidentally. Sulphonylureas may also be displaced with resultant increase in effect and this may cause hypoglycaemia.

- Other interactions include an increase in plasma concentration of lithium, methotrexate, cardiac glycosides and phenytoin and an increased risk of nephrotoxicity with ACE inhibitors, cyclosporin, tacrolimus and diuretics. NSAIDs can also reduce the antihypertensive effects of some drugs, including beta-blockers and diuretics. NSAIDs possibly increase the risk of convulsions with quinolone antibiotics.

Storage
See specific drugs.

NORETHISTERONE (Primulot N, Utovlan, Micronor HRT, Noristerat)

Norethisterone is present in combination products with other hormonal preparations used in hormone replacement therapy and contraception.

Presentation
Tablets – 1 mg and 5 mg
Injection – norethisterone enantate 200 mg in 1 ml

Actions and uses
Norethisterone is a progestogen derived from testosterone. It has some androgenic activity and is metabolized into oestrogenic products. It has many indications for use including hormone

replacement therapy and oral and parenteral contraception. See the section on Progestogens and Oestrogens (p. 297/257) and dosage below.

Dosage
Oral
Endometriosis: 10–15 mg daily for 4–6 months. Start on day 5 of menstrual cycle.
Dysfunctional uterine bleeding and menorrhagia: 5 mg three times a day for 10 days to arrest the bleeding, and to prevent bleeding, 5 mg twice a day from days 19–26 of the cycle.
Dysmenorrhoea: 5 mg three times a day from day 5–24 for 3–4 cycles.
Postponement of menstruation: 5 mg three times a day starting 3 days before anticipated onset.
Progestogenic opposition of menopausal oestrogen HRT: 1 mg daily on days 15–26 of each 28-day oestrogen HRT cycle.
Breast cancer: 40–60 mg daily.

Deep IM injection of norethisterone enantate
Give very slowly into gluteal muscle. For short-term contraception, 200 mg within first 5 days of cycle or immediately after parturition. The contraceptive effect lasts for 8 weeks after which time the dose may be repeated.

Nursing implications
See the sections on Progestogens (p. 297) and Oestrogens (p. 257) and Medroxyprogesterone (p. 207).

Storage
Norethisterone preparations are stored at room temperature.

NORFLOXACIN (Utinor)

Presentation
Tablets – 400 mg

Actions and uses
Norfloxacin is a quinolone antibiotic chemically related to nalidixic acid, ciprofloxacin and ofloxacin. Its spectrum of activity is similar to that of other drugs but norfloxacin is used

mainly in the treatment of urinary tract infections.

Dosage

Urinary tract and other systemic infection.

- Adults: a dose of 400 mg twice daily is given for 3 days in uncomplicated lower urinary tract infections, for 7–10 days in more resistant cases and for up to 12 weeks in chronic relapsing cases.

Nursing implications

- In common with other broad-spectrum antibiotics, disturbances of gastrointestinal function are possible.
- A few patients may develop allergy to norfloxacin. This usually presents as skin rashes but in more severe cases breathlessness, tachycardia, angiooedema and even anaphylaxis may occur.
- Central nervous system side effects include restlessness, agitation, hallucinations and confusion. Convulsions have been reported in a few cases and treatment in epileptics should be avoided. The CSM has warned that quinolones may induce convulsions whether or not the patient has a history of convulsions and that taking NSAIDs concomitantly may induce convulsions.
- The CSM has also advised, in relation to tendon damage, that at the first sign of inflammation or pain whilst taking a quinolone, the treatment should be discontinued and the affected limb rested until symptoms have subsided.
- Since norfloxacin has been shown to impair development of joint tissue in immature animals, it should be avoided in infants and young children if possible.
- Avoid exposure to excessive sunlight and discontinue if photosensitivity occurs.

- Discontinue the drug if psychiatric, neurological or hypersensitivity reactions occur.
- Avoid use in pregnancy.
- Norfloxacin interacts with several drugs including:
  - warfarin, leading to a risk of bleeding unless the dosage is carefully monitored and reduced appropriately
  - analgesics – possible increased risk of convulsions with NSAIDs
  - cyclosporin – increased risk of nephrotoxicity
  - theophylline – possible increased risk of convulsions, increased plasma theophylline concentrations.

Storage

Norfloxacin tablets are stored at room temperature. Protect from light.

NORTRIPTYLINE (Allegron)

Presentation

Tablets – 10 mg, 25 mg

Actions and uses

Nortriptyline is a tricyclic antidepressant drug. Its actions and uses are described in the section on these drugs (p. 31).

Dosage

For the treatment of depression.

- Adult dose ranges vary from 10 to 25 mg three to four times daily. Maximum 150 mg daily.
- Elderly: 30–50 mg daily in divided doses.

Children, for nocturnal enuresis (maximum treatment period of 3 months).

- 7 years: 10 mg at night.
- 8–11 years: 10–20 mg at night.
- Over 11 years: 25–35 mg at night.

Nursing implications

See the section on Tricyclic Antidepressant Drugs (p. 31).

Storage

Preparations containing nortriptyline may be stored at room temperature.

NYSTATIN (Nystan, Mycostatin)

Presentation

Tablets – 500 000 units
Suspension – 100 000 units in 1 ml
Pastilles – 100 000 units
Pessaries – 100 000 units
Vaginal cream – 100 000 units in 4 g
Cream and ointment – 100 000 units in 1 g

Actions and uses

This antifungal drug is used most commonly in clinical practice to eradicate infection due to *Candida albicans* either in the gut or the genital tract.

Dosage

- Orally: one tablet or 1 ml of suspension three or four times daily.
- Vaginally: One or two pessaries at night.

- Topical applications should be administered two to four times daily.
- Nystatin solutions have been used in a variety of strengths for, e.g., bladder/wound irrigation, inhalation via nebulizer, soaks for dentures, etc. Advice on special mixtures of this type should be sought from pharmacy departments.

Nursing implications

- It is important to note that the drug is not absorbed after oral administration and is not used for systemic infections.
- The drug rarely produces side effects but can cause nausea and vomiting, oral irritation and sensitization, rash and urticaria.

Storage

The drug is stored at room temperature.

N

O

OCTREOTIDE (Sandostatin)

Presentation
Injection – 50 microgram in 1 ml,
100 microgram in 1 ml,
500 microgram in 1 ml, 1 mg in 5 ml
Depot injection – 10 mg, 20 mg,
30 mg vials

Actions and uses
Octreotide is an analogue of
somatostatin (hypothalamic
release-inhibiting hormone) which
inhibits the release of growth
hormone and peptides from the
gastroenteropancreatic endocrine
system. It is used in patients with
acromegaly and in the control of
symptoms in patients with
gastroenteropancreatic endocrine
tumours. Octreotide can also be used
following pancreatic surgery to
prevent complications and, although
unlicensed, it is used to stop variceal
bleeding.

Dosage
For the treatment of symptoms of
gastroenteropancreatic endocrine
tumours: 50 microgram SC once or
twice daily initially. Increase dose
gradually according to response up to
200 microgram SC three times a day.
If a rapid response is required it can be
administered IV after dilution with
sodium chloride 0.9% solution to a
concentration of 10–50%. ECG
monitoring is required.
Acromegaly: 100–200 microgram SC
three times a day.

Nursing implications
- Gastrointestinal side effects and
  steatorrhoea can occur.
- Hyper- and hypoglycaemia can
  also occur.

- The injection site should be
  rotated as pain and irritation
  can occur.
- It should be used with caution
  in patients with growth
  hormone-secreting pituitary
  tumours as tumour expansion
  can occur.
- Octreotide affects gallbladder
  activity. Ultrasound examination
  of the gallbladder is recommended before the start of treatment and every 6–12 months
  while treatment continues.

Storage
Octreotide preparations are stored in a
refrigerator at a temperature between
2°C and 8°C. May be stored at room
temperature for up to 14 days. Protect
from light.

OESTRADIOL (Estradiol)

Presentation
Transdermal patch – 25, 50 and 100
microgram released from a reservoir
over 24 hours

Actions and uses
Oestradiol is a natural oestrogen used
in hormone replacement therapy
(HRT). It can be taken orally, applied
topically or implanted under the skin.
Patches are commonly used in HRT
and several brands are available,
e.g. Estraderm TTS (Transdermal
Therapeutic System). Patches provide a
means of achieving gradually, and at a
relatively constant rate, blood levels of
the natural oestrogen 17 beta-
oestradiol via the transdermal route
from application of an impregnated
patch to the skin. This obviates the
need for frequent oral administration

and mimics to some extent the natural release of oestrogen from the functioning ovary. Skin patches of oestradiol are used as a method of hormone replacement after ovarian failure, i.e. in menopausal women or younger women after hysterectomy and oophorectomy. This route is associated with more natural control. See also an account of Oestrogens (p. 257) and Oestradiol Valerate (p. 256).

Dosage

A single patch is applied to the skin twice weekly at 3–4 day intervals, starting with an average dose of 50 microgram/24 h and increasing up to 100 microgram/24 h as required according to the response. The patch should produce oestradiol levels similar to those seen during early follicular release.

Nursing implications

- Patients require careful instructions in application of patches. Each patch is applied to an area of dry, smooth skin below the waist. Patches must never be applied to the breast since high local concentrations may predispose to malignancy. Patches are of course contraindicated in oestrogen-dependent cancers.
- Each patch is applied to the skin and pressed firmly to the site using the warm palm of the hand for at least 10 seconds.
- If applied correctly, oestradiol patches will remain in situ despite normal mechanical friction and hot and cold bathing. It should never be necessary to stick patches with adhesive tape.
- See also notes on Oestrogens (p. 257). This form of therapy, however, provides relatively very low systemic levels of oestradiol and is much less likely than oral oestrogen therapy to increase cardiovascular risk. It can therefore be used when other risk factors exist, including

---

cigarette smoking and hypertension.
- Women with an intact uterus must also receive progestogen for 10–13 days per month.
- Occasionally an allergic contact skin rash occurs in sensitive patients for which an inactive component of the patch may be responsible.

Storage

Oestradiol skin patches are stored at room temperature. Each patch is enclosed in a protective pouch which is removed immediately before application.

OESTRADIOL VALERATE (Progynova)

Also combined with norgestrel in Cyclo-Progynova.

Presentation

Present in many hormone replacement preparations and as Progynova tablets 1 mg and 2 mg.

Actions and uses

Oestradiol valerate is an oestrogenic substance. The general actions and uses of oestrogens are described in the section on these drugs (see below). Oestradiol valerate in clinical practice is used for the alleviation of menopausal symptoms and the prophylaxis and treatment of postmenopausal sequelae of oestrogen withdrawal such as osteoporosis and senile vaginitis.

Dosage

For the treatment of menopausal symptoms: 1–2 mg daily continuously. Oesteoporosis prophylaxis: 2 mg daily continuously.

Nursing implications

- See the section on Oestrogens (p. 257).
- When used as hormone replacement therapy in women with an intact uterus (i.e. who have not undergone hysterectomy) it is necessary to counter uterine hyperplasia and

> an increased risk of cancer by combining this drug with a progestogen, hence the use of Cyclo-Progynova.

Storage
The drug is stored at room temperature.

OESTRIOL (Ortho-Gynest, Ovestin)

Presentation
Tablets – 1 mg
Vaginal cream – 0.01%
Vaginal pessary – 0.5 mg

Actions and uses
Oestriol is a natural oestrogen used orally and topically to treat genitourinary symptoms of oestrogen deficiency.

Dosage
For genitourinary symptoms of oestrogen deficiency, orally: 0.5–3 mg daily, reducing to 0.5–1 mg daily. Topical therapy for vaginal atrophy: one pessary or one applicatorful of cream inserted into the vagina each evening until symptoms improve, then reduce to twice-weekly application.

Nursing implications
- See the section on Oestrogens (p. 257).
- Patients should be advised to take the total daily oral dose at one time.
- The minimum effective dose of topical oestrogens should be used.
- In some cases oral progestogen may be required for 10–14 days a month to prevent endometrial hyperplasia.

Storage
The drug is stored at room temperature.

OESTROGENS

This group of drugs includes:

Dinoestrol
Ethinyloestradiol
Mestranol
Oestradiol/oestradiol valerate
Oestriol
Oestrogens conjugated (equine)
Oestrone sulphate
Piperazine
Quinestradiol
Quinestrol
Stilboestrol

Presentation
See individual drugs.

Actions and uses
The contribution of oestrogens to oral contraceptive therapy is discussed in the section on Contraceptives (Oral) (p. 105).
   Oestrogens are used widely for a number of disorders including:

- Obstetric problems:
  - habitual and threatened abortion
  - suppression of lactation
  - puerperal depression
- Gynaecological problems:
  - menstrual irregularities
  - functional uterine bleeding
  - endometriosis
  - menopausal symptoms
  - premenstrual tension
  - endometrial carcinoma
  - atrophic or senile vaginitis
- Treatment of cancer:
  - mammary carcinoma
  - endometrial carcinoma
  - prostatic carcinoma
- Prevention of bone resorption: oestrogens are used for the prevention and treatment of osteoporosis in postmenopausal women.

Dosage
See specific drugs.

Nursing implications
- The nursing implications of the oestrogen component of contraceptive therapy are discussed in the section on Contraceptives (Oral) (p. 105).
- The use of oestrogens in other clinical situations is associated with the following problems.

- In females, increased uterine growth, withdrawal bleeding and amenorrhoea.
- Breast tenderness, gynaecomastia and loss of sexual characteristics in males.
- Nausea, vomiting, depression, headache and dizziness may commonly occur.
- Salt and water retention leading to hypertension and weight gain may occur.
- Treatment with oestrogens occasionally produces jaundice due to liver damage.
- Rare side effects include hypercalcaemia, skin rashes, e.g. urticaria and erythema muitiforme.
- Oestrogens may stimulate the growth of malignant tumours and are contraindicated in patients with a history of neoplastic disease of the breast or genital tract.
- Oestrogens should not be administered to patients with a history of liver disease or previous thromboembolic disorders.
- The administration of oestrogens to diabetic patients may alter insulin or oral hypoglycaemic requirements.
- The administration of oestrogens to epileptics may lead to an increase in fit frequency and the need to alter their anticonvulsant regime.

Storage

See specific drugs.

OESTROGENS, CONJUGATED (Premarin)

Also combined with norgestrel in Prempak C and medroxyprogesterone acetate in Premique.

Presentation

Tablets – 0.625 mg, 1.25 mg, 2.5 mg
Vaginal cream – 0.625 mg/g

Actions and uses

The actions and uses of oestrogenic hormones in general are described in the section on Contraceptives (Oral) (p. 105).

The oral preparation of this drug is used for the treatment of symptoms due to postmenopausal oestrogen deficiency and for the prevention of postmenopausal osteoporosis.
The vaginal cream is used for the treatment of atrophic vaginitis, atrophic urethritis and kraurosis vulvae.

Dosage

For the oral treatment of postmenopausal oestrogen deficiency and osteoporosis prophylaxis: 0.625–1.25 mg (depending on response) daily continuously (Premarin). Topical application: 1–2 g daily inserted into the vagina for 3 weeks starting on day 5 of cycle followed by one rest week.

Nursing implications

- See the section on Oestrogens (p. 257).
- When used as hormone replacement therapy in women with an intact uterus (i.e. who have not undergone hysterectomy) it is necessary to counter uterine hyperplasia and an increased risk of cancer by combining this drug with a progestogen, hence the use of Prempak C.

Storage

Tablets and vaginal cream are stored at room temperature.

OFLOXACIN (Exocin, Tarivid)

Presentation

Tablets – 200 mg, 400 mg
Infusion – 100 mg in 50 ml, 200 mg in 100 ml
Eye drops – 0.3%

Actions and uses

Ofloxacin is an aminoquinolone antibiotic chemically related to nalidixic acid, ciprofloxacin and enoxacin. Its spectrum of activity includes Staphylococcus spp., Neisseria spp., Gram-negative microorganisms (including *Pseudomonas aeruginosa*), *Haemophilus influenzae*, Chlamydia and Legionella. As a result, ofloxacin may be used in the treatment of upper and lower infections of the urinary tract, lower respiratory tract infections, skin and soft tissue infections and in various forms of venereal disease.

Dosage
Oral
Adults: 200–400 mg once daily and up to 400 mg twice daily in severe infections. Lower urinary tract infections, e.g. cystitis, are generally treated with doses in the lower range. A single dose of 400 mg may be sufficient in uncomplicated urethral and cervical gonorrhoea. For other indications, courses of between 5 and 10 days are normally required.

IV infusion (administer 200 mg dose over at least 30 minutes)
Complicated UTI: 200 mg daily.
Lower respiratory tract infection: 200 mg twice daily.
Septicaemia: 200 mg twice daily.
Skin and soft tissue infections: 400 mg twice daily.
Up to 400 mg twice daily may be given in severe or complicated infections.

Eye drops
One or two drops into affected eye every 2–4 hours for first 48 hours of therapy, then one or two drops four times a day for a maximum of 10 days.

Nursing implications
- In common with other broad-spectrum antibiotics, disturbances of gastrointestinal function are possible.
- A few patients may develop allergy to ofloxacin. This usually presents as skin rashes but in more severe cases breathlessness, tachycardia, angiooedema and even anaphylaxis may occur.
- Central nervous system side effects include restlessness, agitation, hallucinations and confusion. Convulsions have been reported in a few cases and treatment in epileptics should be avoided. The CSM has warned that quinolones may induce convulsions whether or not the patient has a history of them and that taking NSAIDs concomitantly may induce convulsions.
- The CSM has also advised, in relation to tendon damage, that at the first sign of inflammation or pain whilst taking a quinolone, the treatment should be discontinued and the affected limb rested until symptoms have subsided.
- Use with caution in children and adolescents as there is a risk of arthropathy.
- Avoid exposure to excessive sunlight and discontinue if photosensitivity occurs.
- Avoid use in pregnancy and use with caution in hepatic and renal impairment.
- The drug should be discontinued if euphoria, anxiety, neurological or hypersensitivity reactions occur.
- Ofloxacin interacts with:
  - anticoagulants, enhancing the anticoagulant effect
  - cyclosporin, increasing the risk of nephrotoxicity
  - theophylline, with a possible increased risk of convulsions.

Storage
Ofloxacin preparations are stored at room temperature. Protect infusion from light.

OLANZAPINE (Zyprexa)

Presentation
Tablets – 2.5 mg, 5 mg, 7.5 mg, 10 mg
Orodispersible tablets (placed in mouth or dispersed in water) – 5 mg, 10 mg

Actions and uses
Olanzapine is an atypical antipsychotic. Like all other antipsychotics, it is considered to act by interfering with dopaminergic transmission in the brain by blocking dopamine receptors. Olanzapine is a thienobenzodiazepine derivative which is licensed for the treatment of schizophrenia and maintenance of clinical improvement

during continuation therapy in patients who have shown an initial treatment response. This drug has affinity for a number of neurotransmitter receptors and is similar to clozapine in its mixed receptor activity.

May cause fewer extrapyramidal side effects than typical antipsychotic agents.

Dosage

Recommended starting dose is 10 mg daily. Adjust maintenance dose according to individual clinical status within the range 5–20 mg daily.

Nursing implications

- Common side effects include weight gain and somnolence (caution patients on driving and operating machinery), dizziness, peripheral oedema, orthostatic hypotension and anticholinergic effects (caution advised in patients with prostatic hypertrophy, paralytic ileus or related conditions).
- Blood dyscrasias occasionally occur.
- Use a lower starting dose in patients with hepatic or renal impairment.
- Patients with hepatic impairment should be monitored for raised liver enzymes; if this occurs dose reduction should be considered.
- Use with caution if co-prescribed with drugs known to increase the QT interval.
- Metabolism of olanzapine may be increased by smoking or carbamazepine, therefore higher doses may be required.
- Olanzapine is contraindicated in angle closure glaucoma and breastfeeding.

Storage

Olanzapine tablets are stored at room temperature.

OLSALAZINE (Dipentum)

Presentation

Capsules – 250 mg
Tablets – 500 mg

Actions and uses

Olsalazine is chemically aminosalicylic acid. Having an antiinflammatory action, it is used in the treatment and in the maintenance of remission of mild ulcerative colitis.

Dosage

Acute attack: 1 g daily in divided doses increased if necessary to a maximum of 3 g daily (maximum single dose 1 g). Maintenance of remission: 500 mg twice a day.

Nursing implications

- Olsalazine preparations should be taken after meals.
- Since olsalazine is chemically related to aspirin, it should be avoided in patients with a history of aspirin sensitivity.
- Side effects are mainly gastrointestinal, including nausea, diarrhoea (particularly watery diarrhoea) and abdominal pain.
- Blood disorders occur rarely but patients should be advised to report to their doctors any unexplained bleeding, bruising, purpura, sore throat, fever or malaise occurring while they take this medication.
- It is contraindicated in moderate-to-severe renal impairment.
- Use with caution during pregnancy and breastfeeding.

Storage

Olsalazine preparations are stored at room temperature.

OMEPRAZOLE (Losec)

Presentation

Dispersible tablets – 10 mg, 20 mg, 40 mg
Capsules – 10 mg, 20 mg and 40 mg, containing enteric-coated granules

Actions and uses

Omeprazole is described as an inhibitor of the proton pump, an intracellular mechanism located in acid-secreting cells of the gastric mucosa which is essential for production of gastric acid. It therefore inhibits acid output and, if given in sufficiently high dosage, can actually 'switch off' gastric acid output completely. Omeprazole is currently used in the treatment of peptic ulcer disease, NSAID-associated peptic ulcer disease and reflux oesophagitis which has proved resistant to more conventional treatment with drugs such as cimetidine or ranitidine. It has also been licensed for long-term mainten-ance therapy. It is of particular value in Zollinger–Ellison syndrome, a serious condition associated with a gastrinoma which gives rise to excessive gastric acid production. Omeprazole is also used in combination with antibiotics to eradicate *Helicobacter pylori*; many different regimes are used.

Dosage
Oral
Adults
- Duodenal ulcer: 20 mg daily for 4 weeks, increasing to 40 mg daily in severe or recurrent cases. Mainte-nance for recurrent duodenal ulcer: 20 mg daily. Prevention of relapse in duodenal ulcer: 10 mg daily increas-ing to 20 mg if symptoms return.
- Gastric ulcer: 20 mg daily for 8 weeks, increasing to 40 mg daily in severe or recurrent cases.
- Zollinger–Ellison syndrome: doses up to 60 mg once, or even twice, daily are required.
- Reflux oesophagitis: 20 mg daily for 4 weeks and up to 8 weeks if not adequately healed. 40 mg may be required in refractory cases. Thereafter 20 mg daily maintenance therapy can be used.
- Long-term management of acid reflux disease: 10 mg daily, increasing to 20 mg daily if symptoms return.
- Acid-related dyspepsia: 10–20 mg daily for 2–4 weeks as necessary.
- NSAID-associated duodenal and gastric ulcer and gastroduodenal erosions: 20 mg daily for 4 weeks or 8 weeks. Prophylaxis in patients with a history of NSAID-associated gastrointestinal symptoms who are to remain on an NSAID: 20 mg daily.
- Gastric acid reduction during general anaesthesia: two doses of

40 mg, the first on the evening before surgery, the second 2–6 hours before surgery.

Child over 2 years
Severe ulcerating reflux oesophagitis: 0.7–1.4 mg/kg daily for 4–12 weeks (maximum of 40 mg daily) must be initiated by a hospital paediatrician.

IV infusion
(Not recommended for children.)
- Gastric acid reduction during anaesthesia: 40 mg, with infusion completed 1 hour before surgery.
- Benign gastric ulcer, duodenal ulcer and gastrooesophageal reflux: 40 mg daily, changing to oral therapy as soon as possible.

Nursing implications
- The tablets may be swallowed whole or dispersed in water, mixed with fruit juice or yoghurt. The capsules can be opened and the contents mixed with fruit juice or water although the granules themselves must not be crushed or chewed.
- Headaches, nausea, diarrhoea and skin rashes have been reported.
- Omeprazole should be used with caution in patients with liver disease, in pregnancy and breastfeeding.
- Nurses should be aware that these types of drugs can mask any signs of gastric cancer.
- Interactions: omeprazole can enhance the effects of warfarin and phenytoin. These drugs decrease gastric acidity and therefore may increase gastrointestinal infection risk.

Storage
Omeprazole preparations are stored at room temperature.

ONDANSETRON (Zofran)

Presentation
Tablets – 4 mg, 8 mg
Melt tablets – 4 mg, 8 mg
Syrup – 4 mg in 5 ml

Suppositories – 16 mg
Injection – 4 mg in 2 ml, 8 mg in 4 ml

Actions and uses

Ondansetron is a member of the group of drugs including granisetron and tropisetron which selectively inhibit the effects of 5-hydroxytryptamine (5-HT, serotonin) at specific binding sites called 5-HT$_3$ receptors. Stimulation of these receptors in the gastrointestinal tract and chemoreceptor trigger zone induces nausea and triggers the vomiting reflex. Drugs of this type are therefore used to prevent and treat nausea and vomiting in patients who are exposed to various emetogenic stimuli, including anticancer drugs and radiotherapy. More recently, they have been shown to be similarly effective in the control of postoperative nausea and vomiting.

Dosage
Adults

The dose used depends on the severity of the nausea and vomiting and emetogenicity of the chemotherapy or radiotherapy regime. Routinely for patients receiving emetogenic chemotherapy, an 8 mg dose is given IV immediately prior to chemotherapy (or 8 mg orally or 16 mg rectally 1–2 hours prior to chemotherapy) followed by 8 mg orally or 16 mg rectally, every 12 hours. As emesis may be delayed or prolonged after chemotherapy, treatment with ondansetron can be continued for up to 5 days after a course of chemotherapy, the oral or rectal route being routinely used.

For highly emetogenic chemotherapy, dosing is slightly different and it is often necessary to administer ondansetron by a route other than orally, i.e. via IV or IM injection or rectally. A single 8 mg dose by injection should be given immediately prior to chemotherapy. If necessary two further injections should be given 2–4 hours apart. Alternatively, ondansetron can be given by continuous infusion at a rate of 1 mg/h for up to 24 hours. A higher dose of 32 mg in 50–100 ml of infusion fluid can also be administered over at least 15 minutes, immediately prior to chemotherapy. All followed by 8 mg

orally or 16 mg rectally every 12 hours for up to 5 days.

Postoperative nausea and vomiting:

- Prevention, orally: 16 mg 1 hour before anaesthesia or 8 mg 1 hour before anaesthesia followed by two doses of 8 mg at intervals of 8 hours. Injection, IM or slow IV: 4 mg at induction of anaesthesia.
- Treatment: single 4 mg dose by IM injection or slow IV injection.

Children

IV injection or infusion: 5 mg/m^2 single dose, immediately prior to chemotherapy, then 4 mg orally 12 hours later and twice daily for up to 5 days.

Postoperative nausea and vomiting, for children over 2 years:

- Prevention: slow IV injection of 100 microgram/kg (to a maximum of 4 mg) at or prior to induction of anaesthesia.
- Treatment: slow IV injection, 100 microgram/kg (to a maximum of 4 mg).

Nursing implications

- Ondansetron may be of benefit where cytotoxic therapy is likely to cause severe nausea and vomiting. Drugs used for such therapy may include the following: cisplatin, cyclophosphamide, carboplatin, doxorubicin and daunorubicin.
- Radiotherapy can also be associated with moderate nausea and vomiting.
- Since 5-HT also increases gut motility, ondansetron, as might be expected, slows gut transit and produces constipation. As many cancer patients are also treated with strong morphine-like analgesics which also cause constipation, laxative therapy is generally required (if not already given).
- Other side effects of ondansetron include headache, facial flushing and a feeling of warmth in the head and epigastrium which can be

explained by the effect on 5-HT at these sites.

- Ondansetron is metabolized in the liver therefore patients with moderate-to-severe hepatic impairment should receive no more than 8 mg per day.
- Dexamethasone sodium phosphate is routinely used to enhance the antiemetogenic effects of ondansetron.
- When given by intravenous infusion, ondansetron may be added to sodium chloride 0.9%, glucose 5% solutions or Ringer's solution.

Storage

Ondansetron preparations are stored at room temperature and solutions must be protected from light during storage. Prepared infusions are, however, stable for 24 hours even in the presence of direct light.

ORCIPRENALINE (Alupent)

Presentation

Tablets – 20 mg
Syrup – 10 mg in 5 ml
Metered aerosol – 750 microgram per dose

Actions and uses

This drug is a partially selective beta-receptor agonist. It causes relaxation of the smooth muscle in the walls of the large airways (bronchi) and therefore may be used to treat reversible airways obstruction (bronchospasm) due to asthma or other diseases such as bronchitis and emphysema. Orciprenaline is not as safe as the selective beta-2 receptor agonists and therefore is not routinely used.

Dosage
Adults

Orally: 20 mg four times a day.
Inhaled: 0.75–1.5 mg repeated if necessary after at least 30 minutes. Maximum of 9 mg (12 puffs) daily.

Child

Orally:

- Up to 1 year old: 5–10 mg three times a day.

- 1–3 years old: 5–10 mg four times a day.
- 3–12 years old: 40–60 mg daily in divided doses.

Inhaled:

- Up to 6 years old: 750 microgram up to four times a day.
- 6–12 years old: 0.75–1.5 mg up to four times a day.

Nursing implications

- Patients, as well as being instructed in the correct use of the metered aerosol, must be warned never to exceed the prescribed dosage of this drug.
- It is worth noting that the beta-blocking drugs antagonize the action of orciprenaline and, therefore, their concurrent administration is undesirable.
- Transient side effects after administration include palpitation, tachycardia, headache, nausea and abdominal discomfort.
- The drug should be used with caution in those also receiving monoamine oxidase inhibitors or tricyclic antidepressants.
- The drug should be used with great care in patients with heart disease, hypertension or thyrotoxicosis.
- See also Salbutamol (p. 325) for cautions and side effects.

Storage

- Preparations containing orciprenaline are stored at room temperature.
- The syrup should be protected from light.
- The pressurized aerosols should never be punctured or incinerated after use.

ORLISTAT (Xenical)

Presentation
Capsules – 120 mg

Actions and uses
Orlistat is a new antiobesity drug. It acts by inhibiting gastrointestinal

lipases, reducing the absorption of fats in the diet and increasing the excretion of these dietary fats. It should only be used for obese patients with a body mass index (BMI) greater than or equal to 30 kg/m^2 or for overweight patients with a BMI greater than 28 kg/m^2 with other risk factors.

Dosage
Adults only: 120 mg before, during or up to 1 hour before each main meal of the day up to a maximum of three times a day.

Nursing implications
- Orlistat must only be taken in conjunction with a calorie-controlled diet.
- Patients must show that they are dedicated to losing weight and should only be started on orlistat if diet alone has previously produced a weight loss of at least 2.5 kg over a period of 4 consecutive weeks.
- Treatment should be discontinued if at least 5% of body weight has not been lost after 12 weeks.
- If a meal is missed or contains no fat, the corresponding dose should be missed.
- Orlistat is contraindicated in chronic malabsorption syndrome, cholestasis, breastfeeding and pregnancy.
- Any diabetic drug treatment should be monitored during therapy and INR should also be monitored if the patient takes anticoagulants.
- Orlistat also interacts with pravastatin, increasing the risk of pravastatin side effects.
- Absorption of fat-soluble vitamins A, D, E and K may be impaired.
- Patients should be advised that they must adhere to dietary recommendations.
- Adverse effects include gastrointestinal symptoms, e.g. flatulence, faecal urgency, fatty or oily stools, abdominal pain and rectal discomfort, also headache, anxiety and fatigue.

Storage
Orlistat is stored at room temperature.

ORPHENADRINE (Biorphen, Disipal)

Presentation
Tablets – 50 mg
Oral solution – 25 mg in 5 ml, 50 mg in 5 ml

Actions and uses
The actions and uses of this drug are identical to those described for Benzhexol (p. 47). It is an antimuscarinic agent indicated for parkinsonism and drug-induced extrapyramidal symptoms.

Dosage
In adults, orally: 150–400 mg in total given in three divided doses.

Nursing implications
The nursing implications of Benzhexol (p. 47) apply to this drug.

Storage
This drug is stored at room temperature.

OXAZEPAM

Presentation
Tablets – 10 mg, 15 mg, 30 mg

Actions and uses
Oxazepam is a member of the benzodiazepine group. Its principal use is in the treatment of anxiety.

Dosage
Not recommended for children.

- 10–30 mg three times daily with occasionally an additional 10 or 30 mg dose at night.
- For insomnia-associated anxiety: 15–25 mg (maximum 50 mg) at bedtime.

Nursing implications
See the section on Benzodiazepines (p. 47).

Storage
Oxazepam tablets are stored at room temperature.

OXCARBAZEPINE (Trileptal)

Presentation
Tablets – 150 mg, 300 mg, 600 mg

Actions and uses
Oxcarbazepine is a new anticonvulsant, indicated for use in patients with partial seizures with or without secondarily generalized tonic-clonic seizures. Oxcarbazepine is metabolized by the liver to its active metabolite. It is thought to act via blockage of voltage-sensitive sodium channels, thereby stabilizing hyperexcited neuronal membranes, inhibiting neuronal firing and diminishing impulses at the synapses. It may also act by increasing potassium conductance and by modulating calcium channels.

Dosage
Adults: start with a dose of 600 mg/day in two divided doses. Increase if necessary by a maximum of 600 mg/day at weekly intervals to 2400 mg/day.
Children (over 6 years only): start with a dose of 8–10 mg/kg/day in two divided doses. Increase if necessary by a maximum of 10 mg/kg/day at weekly intervals to a maximum of 46 mg/kg/day.

Nursing implications
- Adverse effects include fatigue, asthenia, CNS disturbances, gastrointestinal disturbances, hyponatraemia (monitor sodium concentrations in at-risk patients) and skin reactions.
- Oxcarbazepine does interact with several drugs due to its ability to induce and inhibit certain hepatic enzymes. It can cause an increase in plasma concentrations of phenobarbitone and phenytoin and a decrease in plasma concentration of carbamazepine. Conversely, oxcarbazepine's active metabolite plasma concentration can be decreased on concomitant use with carbamazepine, phenobarbitone, phenytoin or valproic acid.
- Other interactions include a possible rendering ineffective of the oral contraceptive. Patients must be warned of this and advised on other non-hormonal contraceptive methods.
- In renal impairment (creatinine clearance less than 30 ml/min) start at half the usual starting dose.
- Contraindicated in breastfeeding, use with caution and under expert advice in pregnancy.
- The tablets are scored and can be broken in half to aid swallowing.

Storage
Oxcarbazepine preparations are stored at room temperature.

OXETHAZAINE/OXETACAINE (Mucaine)

Presentation
Suspension – 10 mg in 5 ml

Actions and uses
Oxethazaine is a local anaesthetic drug which is taken in an antacid mixture to anaesthetize the lower oesophagus. It is used in the management of oesophagitis, heartburn and hiatus hernia and also after radiotherapy to the throat.

Dosage
5–10 ml of suspension 3–4 times daily before meals and at bedtime.
Not recommended for children.

Nursing implications
Adverse effects are rare but include constipation, dry mouth and nausea.

Storage
Oxethazaine suspension is stored at room temperature.

OXITROPIUM (Oxivent)

Presentation
Aerosol inhaler – 100 microgram/metered dose
Autohaler – 100 microgram/metered dose

Actions and uses
Oxitropium, like Ipratropium (p. 184), is an antimuscarinic bronchodilator used in the management of chronic asthma and reversible airways obstruction.

Dosage
Adult: 200 microgram 2–3 times daily.
Child: not recommended.

Nursing implications
See Ipratropium (p. 184).

Storage
Oxitropium preparations are stored at room temperature.

OXPENTIFYLLINE/PENTOXIFYLLINE (Trental)

Presentation
Tablets – 400 mg (slow release)

Actions and uses
Oxpentifylline is a vasodilator which is also said to make red blood cells more able to alter their shape and therefore to penetrate narrowed and damaged vessels, improving oxygen supply. It is recommended for use in peripheral vascular disease including Raynaud's disease, intermittent claudication, chilblains and night cramps.

Dosage
Adults: 400 mg two or three times a day (slow-release tablets).

Nursing implications
- Symptoms which may be experienced during administration of this drug include nausea, gastric upset, dizziness, flushing and malaise.
- Oxpentifylline is contraindicated in cerebral haemorrhage, extensive retinal haemorrhage, acute MI, pregnancy and breastfeeding.

- The drug should be used with great caution in patients who already have hypotension or who are receiving antihypertensive drugs or have heart disease, renal impairment or severe hepatic impairment.

Storage
The drug is stored at room temperature.

OXPRENOLOL (Trasicor)

Presentation
Tablets – 20 mg, 40 mg, 80 mg, 160 mg and 160 mg modified release

Actions and uses
See the section on Beta-Adrenoreceptor Blocking Drugs (p. 51). Oxprenolol is a 'non-selective' drug. It is used for hypertension, angina, arrhythmias and anxiety.

Dosage
Hypertension and angina: 80–320 mg daily in 2–3 divided doses.
Arrhythmias: 40–240 mg daily in 2–3 divided doses.
Anxiety: 40–80 mg in one or two divided doses.
With modified-release tablets, for hypertension and angina: initially 160 mg daily increased to a maximum of 320 mg daily.

Nursing implications
See the section on Beta-Adrenoreceptor Blocking Drugs (p. 51).

Storage
Oxprenolol tablets are stored at room temperature.

OXYBUTYNIN (Cystrin, Ditropan)

Presentation
Tablets – 3 mg, 5 mg; 2.5 mg and 5 mg and 10 mg modified release
Elixir – 2.5 mg in 5 ml

Actions and uses
Oxybutynin is an antimuscarinic drug, antagonizing acetylcholine at

muscarininc receptors particularly in the bladder. It is indicated for the management of urinary frequency, bladder instability and nocturnal enuresis. Oxybutynin increases bladder capacity and reduces contractions of the detrusor muscle.

Dosage
Adult: 5 mg two or three times a day up to a maximum of 5 mg four times a day.
Elderly: 2.5–3 mg twice a day initially, increasing to 5 mg twice a day according to response and tolerance.
Children over 5: for neurogenic bladder instability, 2.5–3 mg twice a day increasing to 5 mg twice a day (maximum of 5 mg three times a day).
Children over 7: for nocturnal enuresis, 2.5–3 mg twice a day increasing to 5 mg two or three times a day with the last dose taken at bedtime.

Nursing implications
- Oxybutynin is contraindicated in intestinal obstruction, severe ulcerative colitis or toxic megacolon, significant bladder outflow obstruction, glaucoma and myasthenia gravis.
- It should be used with caution in hepatic and renal impairment, neuropathy, hyperthyroidism, cardiac disease, prostatic hypertrophy and hiatus hernia with reflux oesophagitis.
- Adverse effects include typical antimuscarinic effects, e.g. dry mouth, constipation, blurred vision.
- Oxybutynin increases the antimuscarinic effects of other drugs such as antidepressants and antipsychotics.

Storage
Oxybutynin preparations are stored at room temperature.

OXYCODONE (Oxynorm, Oxycontin)

Presentation
Capsules – 5 mg, 10 mg and 20 mg
Oral solution – 5 mg in 5 ml
Concentrated oral solution – 10 mg in 1 ml
Modified-release tablets – 10 mg, 20 mg, 40 mg and 80 mg

Actions and uses
The actions and uses of this drug are described in the section on Narcotic Analgesic Drugs (p. 238). Oxycodone is similar to morphine in its efficacy and side effect profile. It is indicated for use in moderate-to-severe pain in palliative care and postoperatively.

Dosage
Capsules and oral solutions: 5 mg every 4–6 hours increased as required to a usual maximum of 400 mg daily.
Modified-release tablets: start with 10 mg every 12 hours increased as required to a usual maximum of 200 mg every 12 hours.
Not recommended for children.

Nursing implications
The nursing implications of narcotic analgesic drugs in general are described in the section on these drugs (p. 238).

Storage
Oxycodone preparations are stored at room temperature.

OXYTETRACYCLINE (Terramycin)

Presentation
Tablets – 250 mg
Oxytetracycline is also included in compound ointments and creams.

Actions and uses
See the section on Tetracycline (p. 355).

Dosage
Orally: 250–500 mg four times a day.
For acne: 500 mg twice a day.

Nursing implications
See the section on Tetracycline (p. 355).

Storage
The drug is stored at room temperature.

OXYTOCIN (Syntocinon)

Presentation
Injection – 5 units in 1 ml, 10 units in 1 ml

Actions and uses
Oxytocin, of which Syntocinon is a synthetic derivative, is a hormone normally found in the posterior lobe of the pituitary gland in the brain. It stimulates the contraction of the pregnant uterus. It may be administered by intravenous infusion to induce labour and (often in combination with ergometrine as 'Syntometrine') for the treatment of missed abortion or postpartum haemorrhage.

Dosage
Intravenously to induce labour: most maternity units have a documented procedure for the administration of this drug to induce labour and therefore no specific doses are given here.

For the treatment of postpartum haemorrhage or missed abortion: again, nurses are recommended to acquaint themselves with the treatment schedule of the centres to which they are attached.

Nursing implications
- High doses may cause excessive uterine contraction and dosage should therefore be carefully monitored to prevent distress to the fetus and other complications, including uterine rupture. Uterine spasm can occur at low doses.
- Other adverse effects include nausea and vomiting, arrhythmias, rash and anaphylaxis.
- When high doses of Syntocinon are given with large volumes of electrolyte-free fluid, water intoxication may occur. Initially headache, anorexia, nausea, vomiting and abdominal pain may be the presenting features and this progresses to lethargy, drowsiness, unconsciousness and grand mal-type seizures. The concentration of blood electrolytes may be markedly disturbed.

Storage
The drug should be stored in a refrigerator.

O

P

PACLITAXEL (Taxol)

Presentation
Injection – 30 mg in 5 ml, 100 mg in 16.7 ml, 300 mg in 50 ml

Actions and uses
This drug is a novel cytotoxic which blocks the mitotic phase of the cell cycle by impairing microtubular assembly and reorganization during interphase. The result is that normal cell division cannot take place. The current licensed indication for paclitaxel is in the treatment of metastatic ovarian carcinoma in which cisplatin and carboplatin regimens have proved ineffective. It is also licensed for use in combination therapy with cisplatin for the primary treatment of advanced or residual ovarian cancer, for metastatic breast cancer where anthracycline therapy has failed or is inappropriate and non-small cell lung cancer in combination with cisplatin where surgery or radiation is inappropriate.

Dosage
Primary treatment of ovarian cancer: paclitaxel 135 mg/m² administered over 24 hours followed by cisplatin 75 mg/m². Three weeks between courses.
Secondary treatment of ovarian and breast cancer: paclitaxel 175 mg/m² administered over 3 hours. Three weeks between courses.
Treatment of advanced non-small cell lung cancer: paclitaxel 175 mg/m² administered over 3 hours then cisplatin 80 mg/m². Three weeks between courses.

In all cases, subsequent doses should be adjusted according to patient tolerance.
The injection can be administered in the following intravenous solutions to a final concentration of 0.3–1.2 mg/ml:

- 0.9% sodium chloride
- 5% dextrose
- 5% dextrose and 0.9% sodium chloride
- 5% dextrose in Ringer's injection.

Nursing implications
- The occurrence of severe hypersensitivity reactions (hypotension, dyspnoea, rash, angiooedema, etc.) to this drug is such that steroid and complete antihistamine (H1 and H2) cover is essential. Thus doses of oral dexamethasone 20 mg and chlorpheniramine 10 mg IV or diphenydramine 50 mg IV plus cimetidine 300 mg IV or ranitidine 50 mg IV are required. The steroid should be given 12 and 6 hours prior to chemotherapy and the antihistamines 30–60 minutes before.
- Bone marrow suppression (mainly neutropenia but also anaemia and thrombocytopenia) is a life-threatening and hence dose-limiting adverse event.
- Peripheral neuropathy (commonly paraesthesia) generally occurs but more severe neurotoxicity is a signal that dosage reduction of as much as 20% is required with future doses.
- Gastrointestinal side effects including mucositis, nausea and vomiting and diarrhoea are very common. Alopecia occurs in almost all patients.
- A rise in liver enzymes (transaminases, alkaline phosphatase and bilirubin) has been noted

P

and this drug should be used with caution in patients with preexisting liver impairment.

- Cardiac arrhythmias (ventricular tachycardia, AV block) are uncommon side effects, but have occurred and warrant appropriate therapy and monitoring during subsequent doses.
- Nurses should be aware of the risks posed by cytotoxic drugs. Some are irritant to the skin and mucous surfaces and care must be exercised when handling them. In particular, spillage or contamination of personnel or the environment must be avoided. If cytotoxic drugs are handled regularly, it is theoretically possible that repeated skin contact or inhalation may produce systemic toxic effects in nurses who have developed hypersensitivity to them. Most hospitals now operate a centralized (pharmacy-organized) additive service. While this reduces the risk of exposure to cytotoxic drugs, it is essential that nurses recognize and understand the local policy on their safe handling and disposal. The Health and Safety Executive has decreed that such a policy should be in place wherever cytotoxic drugs are administered. These should be adapted, wherever possible, to care of patients in the community.

Storage
- Paclitaxel vials are stored at 'cool' room temperature and protected from light.
- If refrigerated, a precipitate may form but the drug should redissolve when gently shaken on returning to room temperature.
- Prepared infusions are stable for up to 27 hours at room temperature. Do not refrigerate.
- A hazy appearance is quite normal and due to the solubilizing agent which is present in the vial. Solutions must be filtered via a 0.22 micron filter during administration.

- A reaction with PVC is possible and this material must be avoided when preparing and mixing the injection.

PAMIDRONATE or Disodium Pamidronate (Aredia)

Presentation
Injection – 15 mg, 30 mg, 90 mg powder vials

Actions and uses
Pamidronate is chemically a bis(di-)phosphonate compound which is used in the management of hypercalcaemia due to malignant disease, notably associated with myeloma, lymphoma and solid tumours which have spread to bone (bone metastases). It appears to act by inhibiting loss of bone density with subsequent release of calcium into the circulation (bone resorption). The serum calcium usually starts to fall within 48 hours of administration of pamidronate and levels may remain within the normal range for several weeks thereafter.

Other uses for pamidronate include Paget's disease.

Dosage
Hypercalcaemia of malignancy: 15–60 mg in a single dose or divided doses over 2–4 days. Adjust dose according to serum calcium concentration to a maximum of 90 mg per treatment course.
Osteolytic lesions and bone pain in bone metastases associated with breast cancer or multiple myeloma: 90 mg every 3 or 4 weeks.
Paget's disease of the bone: 30 mg weekly for 6 weeks or 30 mg on the first week and 60 mg every second week. Maximum of 360 mg per treatment course. May be repeated after 6 months.

Nursing implications
- Intravenous injections of pamidronate are irritant and must be administered slowly. Never give by bolus injection and never exceed a rate of 60 mg/h (20 mg/h in renal

impairment) or a concentration of 60 mg/250 ml. The recommended infusion solution is sodium chloride 0.9%. Always use a calcium-free solution.

- Patients should be advised that somnolence or dizziness may occur after treatment and should avoid driving or operating machinery.
- Patients may develop transient pyrexia during drug administration.
- Pamidronate produces oliguria in some patients and should be used with extreme caution if renal impairment exists.
- Use in pregnancy, breastfeeding and epilepsy should be avoided.

Storage

Pamidronate injection is stored at room temperature.

PANCREATIN

Presentation

See table below.

Actions and uses

This preparation is a mixture of enzymes normally produced by the pancreas. These enzymes digest starch, fat and protein in the diet. In pancreatic disease, where insufficient enzymes are being produced, food cannot be absorbed. Pancreatin, therefore, is used in cases of malabsorption due to pancreatic deficiency. It is used in cystic fibrosis and, for example, in pancreatectomy and chronic pancreatitis.

Dosage

Note: The true dose is widely variable. It is that which is sufficient generally to prevent steatorrhoea.

Generally, preparations are swallowed whole (unless the preparation is a powder or granules) or the capsules can be opened and the contents sprinkled on food. However, the contents must not be chewed.

Nursing implications

- Irritation of the skin may occur around the mouth and the anus, particularly in very young

Preparation	Dose (applies to adult and child unless otherwise specified)
Creon granules	1 sachet with meals
Creon 10 000 capsules	1–2 capsules with meals
Nutrizym GR capsules	1–2 capsules with meals
Nutrizym 10 capsules	1–2 capsules with meals, 1 capsule with snacks
Pancrease capsules	1–3 capsules with meals, 1 capsule with snacks
Pancrex granules	5–10 g before meals
Pancrex V capsules	Adult and child over 1 year: 2–6 capsules with meals
	Child up to 1 year: 1–2 capsules with feeds
Pancrex V '125' capsules	Neonate: 1–2 capsules with feeds
Pancrex V tablets	5–15 tablets before meals
Pancrex V tablets forte	6–10 tablets before meals
Pancrex V powder	0.5–2 g with meals
	Neonate: 250–500 mg with feeds

High-strength preparations

Creon 25 000 capsules	1 capsule with meals
Nutrizym 22 capsules	1–2 capsules with meals, 1 capsule with snacks (not for children under 15 years)
Pancrease HL capsules	1–2 capsules with meals, 1 capsule with snacks (not for children under 15 years)

babies. Barrier creams will effectively prevent this.
- Rarely hypersensitivity reactions such as sneezing and skin rash may occur. Nurses may experience this when handling the preparations. Other side effects include nausea and vomiting and abdominal discomfort.
- High doses are associated with the development of bowel strictures in children with cystic fibrosis. Any new abdominal symptoms should be reported and reviewed.
- Patients with cystic fibrosis should take no more than 10 000 units of lipase per kg body weight daily.
- Ensure adequate fluid intake with high-dose preparations.
- These preparations are, to say the least, unpleasant. The nurse may play an important supportive role in encouraging the patient to persevere with this treatment.

Storage
- Preparations should be stored in a well-closed container in a cool place.
- Pancreatin is inactivated by heat.

P

PANCURONIUM (Pavulon)

Presentation
Injection – 4 mg in 2 ml

Actions and uses
Pancuronium is a muscle relaxant of the non-depolarizing type. Thus it reversibly paralyses skeletal muscle by competitive inhibition of acetylcholine, the transmitter substance released at the junction of the (motor) nerve and muscle fibre (motor endplate receptor). Drugs of this type are used to produce muscle relaxation during surgical anaesthesia.

Pancuronium has a long duration of action and is often used in intensive care patients where long-term mechanical ventilation is required.

Dosage
IV injection for use in surgery of long duration.

- Adult: for intubation, 50–100 microgram/kg, then 10–20 microgram/kg as required.
- Child: for intubation, 60–100 microgram/kg, then 10–20 microgram/kg as required.
- Neonate: for intubation, 30–40 microgram/kg, then 10–20 microgram/kg as required.

Intensive care: IV injection of 60 microgram/kg every 60–90 minutes.

Nursing implications
- All patients must have their respiration assisted or controlled.
- As mentioned above, muscle relaxants of this type are also used to produce paralysis in patients on assisted ventilation in ICUs.
- Side effects of pancuronium include tachycardia and hypertension.
- Overdosage with muscle relaxant drugs of this type may result in paralysis of the respiratory muscles. If this occurs, an anticholinesterase such as neostigmine (which potentiates acetylcholine by blocking its inactivation) must be administered.

Storage
Pancuronium injection is stored at 2–8°C protected from light.

PANTOPRAZOLE (Protium)

Presentation
Tablets (enteric coated) – 20 mg, 40 mg
Injection – 40 mg powder vial

Actions and uses
Like omeprazole, pantoprazole is a proton pump inhibitor, inhibiting gastric acid output. It is indicated for the treatment of benign gastric ulcer, gastrooesophageal reflux disease and duodenal ulcer. It is also used in

combination with antibiotics to eradicate *Helicobacter pylori*.

Dosage (adults only)
Oral.

- Benign gastric ulcer: 40 mg daily for 4 or 8 weeks.
- Gastrooesophageal reflux disease: 40 mg daily for 4 or 8 weeks, maintenance dose of 20–40 mg daily.
- Duodenal ulcer: 40 mg daily for 2 or 4 weeks.

Intravenous.

- Administer over 2–15 minutes (in 100 ml glucose 5% or 10% solution or sodium chloride 0.9% solution), 40 mg daily until oral route can be used. Indicated for duodenal or gastric ulcers and gastrooesophageal reflux.

Nursing implications
- Use with caution in liver disease, renal impairment, pregnancy and breastfeeding.
- Pantoprazole use may mask signs of gastric cancer.
- Adverse effects include gastrointestinal disturbances, headache and hypersensitivity, fever and liver enzyme changes.
- Reduced gastric acidity may increase the risk of gastrointestinal infections.

Storage
Pantoprazole preparations are stored at room temperature.

PAPAVERETUM
(Formerly Omnopon)

Presentation
Injection – 7.7 mg/ml (equivalent to 5 mg morphine/ml)
Injection – 15.4 mg/ml (equivalent to 10 mg morphine/ml)

Actions and uses
Papaveretum is a mixture of morphine, papaverine and codeine. In practice its analgesic activity is due to the morphine content. The actions and uses discussed under the Narcotic Analgesic Drugs (p. 238) apply to papaveretum. It is routinely used as a postoperative analgesic and as a premedication.

Dosage
Adults: intramuscular, subcutaneous or intravenous routes: 7.7–15.4 mg repeated 4–6 hourly as required.
Children:

- up to 1 month: 115.5 microgram/kg
- 1–12 months: 115.5–154 microgram/kg
- 1–12 years: 154–231 microgram/kg.

Nursing implications
- See the section on Narcotic Analgesic Drugs (p. 238).
- The IV dose should be 25–50% of the corresponding SC or IM dose.
- Papaveretum was recently reformulated, with noscapine being removed. It should be prescribed as 7.7 mg/ml or 15.4 mg/ml.
- Take care not to confuse with papaverine.

Storage
- The drug must be stored in a locked (Controlled Drug) cupboard.
- The drug is stored at room temperature.

PARACETAMOL
(e.g. Calpol, Disprol, Panadol)

Presentation
Tablets – 500 mg (plain and soluble), 120 mg soluble
Paediatric elixir – 120 mg/5 ml
Suspension – 120 mg/5 ml, 250 mg/5 ml

Actions and uses
Paracetamol has both analgesic (pain relieving) and antipyretic (temperature reducing) properties. It is used where mild analgesia is indicated for such common complaints as headache and musculoskeletal pain. It is particularly useful for the treatment of mild pain or pyrexia in groups of patients for whom salicylate therapy is

contraindicated, such as those with previous gastrointestinal bleeding, and also for the treatment of children under 12 years, who should not normally be given salicylates.

Dosage
Oral.

- Adults: 500 mg–1 g 4–6 hourly as required for pain. Maximum of 4 g/day.
- Children:
  - 2 months: 60 mg for postimmunization pyrexia only
  - 3 months–1 year: 60–120 mg, repeat every 4–6 hours, maximum of four times a day
  - 1–5 years: 120–250 mg repeat every 4–6 hours, maximum of four times a day
  - 6–12 years: 250–500 mg repeat every 4–6 hours, maximum of four times a day.

Rectal.

- Adult and child over 12 years: 0.5–1 g up to four times a day.
- Child 1–5 years: 125–250 mg up to four times a day.
- Child 6–12 years: 250–500 mg up to four times a day.

Nursing implications
- Few if any side effects are associated with the administration of this drug.
- Paracetamol is widely available for sale without prescription in Great Britain and although it is associated with negligible side effects when taken in normal dosage, it is extremely dangerous if taken as an overdose when severe and fatal liver damage may occur. A specific intravenous treatment regime with N-acetylcysteine is available but its efficacy depends on how quickly the patient receives it after taking the overdose. Thus any patient who has taken such an overdose must be referred to hospital with the utmost speed.
- As well as liver damage after overdosage, renal and cardiac damage may occur.

Storage
The drug is stored at room temperature. Do not store suppositories next to a heat source (e.g. radiator).

PAROXETINE (Seroxat)

Presentation
Tablets – 20 mg, 30 mg
Liquid – 20 mg in 10 ml

Actions and uses
Paroxetine is a selective serotonin reuptake inhibitor (SSRI) used in depression, obsessive-compulsive disorder, panic disorder and social phobia. It has more recently been licensed for the treatment of posttraumatic stress disorder. For the action and uses of paroxetine, see the section on Antidepressants (p. 31).

Dosage (adults only)
- Depression: 20 mg each morning, increase gradually if necessary to a maximum of 50 mg/day (maximum of 40 mg/day in the elderly).
- Obsessive-compulsive disorder: 20 mg each morning, increased gradually if necessary to 40 mg/day (maximum of 60 mg/day, elderly maximum of 40 mg/day).
- Panic disorder: 10 mg each morning, increased gradually if necessary to 40 mg/day (maximum 50 mg/day, elderly maximum 40 mg/day).
- Social phobia: 20 mg each morning. If no improvement after at least 2 weeks, increase in steps of 10 mg gradually to a maximum of 50 mg/day (elderly maximum 40 mg/day).

Nursing implications
- See the section on Antidepressants (p. 31).
- In the treatment of panic disorder, symptoms may worsen initially.
- Extrapyramidal reactions and withdrawal syndrome appear to be more common with paroxetine than other SSRIs.

Storage
Paroxetine is stored at room temperature.

PENICILLAMINE (Distamine)

Presentation
Tablets – 125 mg and 250 mg

Actions and uses
Penicillamine has two main actions.

1. It binds heavy metal ions by a process called 'chelation' and therefore may be used in the treatment of the following disorders:
   - lead poisoning, where it is thought to reduce the absorption of lead
   - Wilson's disease (hepatolenticular degeneration), where it increases the excretion of copper
   - mercury poisoning
   - cystinuria where it promotes the excretion of the more soluble form of cystine
   - chronic active hepatitis (rarely used).
2. It also reduces the inflammatory response in patients with severe rheumatoid arthritis. The reduction in the inflammatory response leads to a subsequent relief of symptoms. Expert advice required.

Dosage
Lead poisoning.

- Adults: 1–2 g daily in divided doses before food.
- Child: 20 mg/kg daily in divided doses before food.
- Continue until urinary lead concentration is stabilized.

Wilson's disease.

- Adult: 1.5–2 g daily in divided doses before food (maintenance 0.75–1 g daily).
- Elderly: 20 mg/kg/day in divided doses.
- Child: up to 20 mg/kg/day in divided doses (minimum 500 mg daily).

Cystinuria.

- Adult: 1–3 g daily in divided doses before food, prophylaxis, 0.5–1 g at night.
- Can be used for children and the elderly; in each case, adjust dose according to urinary cystine concentrations.

Severe rheumatoid arthritis.

- Adult: 125–250 mg daily before food. Increase only after 1 month by 125–250 mg each month to 500–750 mg daily in divided doses. Maximum 1.5 g/day.
- Elderly: initiate with 125 mg daily, maximum 1 g/day.
- Child: 15–20 mg/kg daily maintenance; start with a low dose increasing as above.

Nursing implications
- This drug should not be given to patients who are already receiving gold salts or antimalarial treatment such as chloroquine or hydroxychloroquine.
- Routine checks of white cell counts, platelet counts and urine tests for albumin should be performed at weekly intervals, at least initially, in patients on this treatment.
- Patients may be allergic to penicillamine. Patients who have already been found to be allergic to penicillin are particularly at risk from this.
- Adverse effects include sore throat, fever, skin rash, nausea, altered taste sensitivity, eosinophilia, leucopenia, agranulocytosis, thrombocytopenia, proteinuria and nephrotic syndrome.
- Patients who have already been found to be allergic to gold injections should never be given penicillamine.
- Discontinue treatment if no improvement after 1 year.
- Patients should be advised that it may take 6–12 weeks for any improvement to occur.
- Avoid use in pregnancy and renal impairment.

Storage
Penicillamine tablets are stored at room temperature.

PENICILLIN V

NB: Also referred to as phenoxymethylpenicillin. Several proprietary brands are available.

Presentation
Tablets – 250 mg
Oral solution – 125 mg in 5 ml, 250 mg in 5 ml

Actions and uses
Phenoxymethylpenicillin has a mode of action similar to that described for benzylpenicillin (p. 49). It is usually effective against Streptococcus and Pneumococcus and rarely effective against Staphylococcus. It is therefore indicated for the treatment of respiratory tract infection and tonsillitis and as prophylaxis against streptococcal infection following rheumatic fever and pneumococcal infections following splenectomy. Phenoxymethylpenicillin has an advantage over benzylpenicillin in that it is better absorbed and therefore is the drug of choice for oral penicillin treatment.

Dosage
Adults and children over 12 years: 500 mg (750 mg in severe infections) four times a day.
Children aged 6–12 years: 250 mg four times a day.
Children aged 1–5 years: 125 mg four times a day.
Children up to 1 year: 62.5 mg four times a day.
It is important to note that the drug should preferably be given 30 minutes to 1 hour before meals.

Nursing implications
- See the section on Benzylpenicillin (p. 49).

Storage
Tablets and powder for preparing oral liquid preparations are stored at room temperature. Syrup, suspension and elixir should be discarded 7 days after reconstitution, keep refrigerated.

PENTAZOCINE (Fortral)

Presentation
Tablets – 25 mg
Capsules – 50 mg
Injection – 30 mg in 1 ml, 60 mg in 2 ml
Suppositories – 50 mg

Actions and uses
Pentazocine is a derivative of the narcotic analgesic group of drugs but it has a much less potent analgesic effect when compared with morphine. It is, therefore, used in the management of moderate-to-severe pain.

Dosage
Oral.

- Adults: 25–100 mg 3–4 hourly after food.
- Child 6–12 years: 25 mg 3–4 hourly after food.

Subcutaneous, intramuscular or intravenous (adults).

- Moderate pain: 30 mg every 3–4 hours as required.
- Severe pain: 45–60 mg every 3–4 hours as required.

Child over 1 year.

- SC or IM up to 1 mg/kg as required.
- IV up to 500 microgram/kg as required.

Rectal.
Adults only: 50 mg up to four times a day.

Nursing implications
- See the section on Narcotic Analgesic Drugs (p. 238).
- Hallucinations and other behavioural abnormalities have been found to be a particular problem with this drug and occur in 10% of patients. The reason they have been reported only rarely is that they tend to be of a pleasant nature.
- Pentazocine is not subject to the safe custody requirements associated with Controlled Drugs, although prescription and handwriting requirements apply.

Storage
The drug is stored at room temperature.

PERGOLIDE (Celance)

Presentation
Tablets – 50 microgram, 250 microgram, 1 mg

Actions and uses

Pergolide is an ergot derivative used in the management of Parkinson's disease as it acts by stimulating dopamine receptors. It should only be used where levodopa alone is no longer adequate or is not tolerated.

Dosage

50 microgram daily for 2 days, then gradually increase by 100–150 microgram every third day over the next 12 days. Then increase by 250 microgram every third day to a usual maintenance of 3 mg daily. Take in divided doses.

Whilst titrating the pergolide dose, levodopa dosage can be gradually reduced.

Nursing implications

- Common side effects include abnormal involuntary movements and confusion, hallucinations and dizziness. Hypotension can also occur, particularly when treatment is commenced. Patients should be advised to exercise caution when driving or operating machinery.
- Use with caution in patients with heart disease and in pregnancy and breastfeeding.

Storage

Pergolide is stored at room temperature.

PERICYAZINE (Neulactil)

Presentation

Tablets – 2.5 mg, 10 mg
Syrup – 10 mg in 5 ml

Actions and uses

Pericyazine is a neuroleptic drug of the phenothiazine group which is used for its tranquillizing or calming effect in severely agitated patients with behavioural disorders such as schizophrenia, senile dementia and mental subnormality. When compared to other major tranquillizers such as chlorpromazine, pericyazine produces a marked sedative effect. Thus it is of particular use in disorders

characterized by aggressive or impulsive tendencies.

Dosage
Adults

Schizophrenia and other psychoses: start with 75 mg daily in divided doses, increase at weekly intervals by 25 mg according to response up to a maximum of 300 mg/day. Elderly patients should start on 15–30 mg daily. Short-term adjunctive management of severe anxiety, psychomotor agitation and violent or dangerously impulsive behaviour: start with 15–30 mg daily in two divided doses, adjust according to response. Elderly patients should start on 5–10 mg daily.

Children

Severe mental or behavioural disorders only: initially 500 microgram for a 10 kg child, increase dose by 1 mg for every additional 5 kg of body weight to a maximum total daily dose of 10 mg. Adjust according to response.

Nursing implications

- The nursing implications on Phenothiazines (p. 281) apply to pericyazine.
- It is important to note that pericyazine has a strong sedative action and may produce marked postural hypotension. It is for this reason that correspondingly low initial doses should be used for elderly subjects who are particularly susceptible to sudden fall in blood pressure and in whom fainting attacks and palpitation may occur.
- Children are similarly susceptible to the sedative and hypotensive actions of the drug.
- The unwanted effects of pericyazine may be less troublesome if the dosage is divided in such a way that the larger portion is administered at night.

Storage

Tablets and syrup preparations of pericyazine are stored at room temperature. Protect from light.

PERINDOPRIL (Coversyl)

Presentation
Tablets – 2 mg, 4 mg

Actions and uses
See section on ACE Inhibitors (p. 4).

Dosage
Range: 2–8 mg as a single daily dose.

Nursing implications
See section on ACE Inhibitors (p. 4).

Storage
Perindopril tablets are stored at room temperature.

PERPHENAZINE (Fentazin)

Presentation
Tablets – 2 mg, 4 mg

Actions and uses
Perphenazine is a phenothiazine and its actions and uses are described in the section on these drugs (p. 281). It is used predominantly for the treatment of severe anxiety and agitation associated with psychotic disorders but it is occasionally, in addition, used for the treatment of nausea and vomiting.

Dosage
- The usual oral adult dose is 4 mg three times daily increasing to a maximum of 24 mg per day if required. Elderly patients should receive one quarter to one half of the usual adult dose.
- Not recommended for children.

Nursing implications
See the section on Phenothiazine Drugs (p. 281).

Storage
Perphenazine tablets are stored at room temperature.

PETHIDINE

Presentation
Tablets – 50 mg

Injection – 50 mg in 1 ml, 50 mg in 5 ml, 100 mg in 2 ml, 100 mg in 10 ml

Actions and uses
The actions and uses of this drug are described in the section on Narcotic Analgesic Drugs (p. 238). Pethidine is less potent than morphine. It is fast acting but its effects are short lasting. It is useful in labour but it is not suitable for controlling severe continuing pain.

Dosage
Acute pain
Oral: adult, 50–150 mg every 4 hours as required; child, 0.5–2 mg/kg every 4 hours as required.
SC or IM: adult, 25–100 mg repeated after 4 hours; child, IM, 0.5–2 mg/kg.
Slow IV: adult only, 25–50 mg repeated after 4 hours.

Obstetric analgesia
SC or IM: 50–100 mg repeated 1–3 hours later if necessary. Maximum of 400 mg in 24 hours.

Premedication
IM: adult, 25–100 mg 1 hour before surgery; child, 0.5–2 mg/kg 1 hour before surgery.

Postop pain
SC or IM: adult, 25–100 mg 2–3 hourly as required; child, IM, 0.5–2 mg/kg.

Nursing implications
- The nursing implications for Narcotic Analgesic Drugs (p. 238) in general are described in the section on these drugs.
- It is worth noting that the side effects experienced with pethidine are particularly severe in the elderly.
- Pethidine is contraindicated in severe renal impairment.
- Convulsions can occur in overdose.

Storage
- The drug should be stored in a locked (Controlled Drug) cupboard.
- The drug is stored at room temperature.

PHENAZOCINE (Narphen)

Presentation
Tablets – 5 mg

Actions and uses
Phenazocine is a narcotic analgesic and its actions and uses are described in the section on these drugs (p. 238).

Dosage
For adults: 5–20 mg every 4–6 hours as required.

Nursing implications
- See the section on Narcotic Analgesic Drugs (p. 238).
- This drug may also be taken by the sublingual route in patients with swallowing difficulties or if nausea and vomiting is problematic.

Storage
- The drug should be stored in a locked (Controlled Drugs) cupboard.
- The drug is stored at room temperature.

PHENELZINE (Nardil)

Presentation
Tablets – 15 mg

Actions and uses
Phenelzine is a monoamine oxidase-inhibiting drug. Its actions and uses are described in the section on MAOIs (p. 228).

Dosage
15 mg three times daily or up to four times a day if necessary. Maximum dose of 30 mg three times a day in hospitalized patients.

Nursing implications
See the section on Monoamine Oxidase Inhibitors (p. 228).

Storage
Phenelzine tablets are stored at room temperature.

PHENINDIONE (Dindevan)

Presentation
Tablets – 10 mg, 25 mg and 50 mg

Actions and uses
Like warfarin, but rarely used, phenindione is an anticoagulant agent.

A number of the substances present in blood which play an important part in preventing bleeding by forming clots are produced by the liver from vitamin K. Phenindione inhibits the synthesis of these substances (known as clotting factors) and therefore reduces the ability of the blood to clot. Its principal uses are for the prevention and treatment of thromboembolic states such as deep venous thrombosis and pulmonary embolus. It is also used to prevent the formation of clot in cardiovascular disease, either on artificial heart valves or in the atria of patients who have atrial dysrhythmias.

Dosage
Adults.

- Loading dose: 200 mg on day 1, 100 mg on day 2. The dosage on day 3 should depend on the result of clotting studies.
- Maintenance dosage: depends on the results of blood clotting studies but usually lies within the range of 50–150 mg per day.

Nursing implications
- See Warfarin (p. 391).
- The daily maintenance dose of phenindione is, as noted above, determined by the results of clotting studies. As the effects of bleeding due to overcoagulation or thrombosis due to undercoagulation can be so rapidly catastrophic, strict adherence to the recommended dose is mandatory and the nurse may play an important role in ensuring that patients are aware of this.
- The effects of phenindione may be influenced by a number of factors listed below and the nurse may play an important role by identifying their

---

P

occurrence and alerting both the patient and medical staff. The following circumstances may lead to a requirement for alteration in dosage.

1. Acute illness such as chest infection or viral infection.
2. Sudden weight loss.
3. The concurrent administration of other drugs. A number of drugs may affect the patient's dosage requirements:
   - anticoagulant effect of phenindione may be enhanced by concomitant use of aspirin or other NSAIDs and antiplatelet drugs, e.g. clopidogrel
   - amiodarone inhibits the metabolism of phenindione
   - enhanced anticoagulant effect with fibrates, levothyroxine and testosterone
   - anticoagulant effect antagonized by oral contraceptives and vitamin K.

- The occurrence of haemorrhage in a patient on phenindione is an indication for immediate withdrawal of the drug and if the haemorrhage is at all serious or repetitive the patient should be immediately referred to hospital for further assessment and, if necessary, they may be given vitamin K which accelerates a return to normal clotting function.
- Phenindione is relatively contraindicated in patients with severe liver or kidney disease, haemorrhagic conditions or uncontrolled hypertension. It should also be used with great caution immediately after surgery or labour.
- Skin rash, fever, blood dyscrasia, diarrhoea, liver and kidney damage may all occur with this drug and because of these effects it is now less commonly used than warfarin.
- It is important for the nurse to note that metabolites of this drug may impart a pink or orange colour to the urine and this may be mistaken for haematuria. This is particularly important as haematuria is an indication for stopping drug therapy and urgently reassessing blood-clotting status.

Storage
The drug is stored at room temperature.

PHENOBARBITONE/ PHENOBARBITAL

Presentation
Tablets – 15 mg, 30 mg, 60 mg
Elixir – 15 mg in 5 ml
Injection – 200 mg in 1 ml

Actions and uses
Phenobarbitone is a member of the barbiturate group. Its major use in clinical practice is in the management of epilepsy, particularly grand mal, partial seizures and psychomotor seizures. It is additionally occasionally used as a sedative and hypnotic though this is a declining role for barbiturate drugs since safer alternatives exist.

Dosage
As an anticonvulsant
- Orally.
  - Adults: 60–180 mg daily taken as a single dose at night.
  - Children: 5–8 mg/kg body weight daily as a single dose or in two divided doses.
- By intramuscular injection.
  - Adults: 200 mg single dose, repeated after 6 hours if necessary.
  - Children: 15 mg/kg body weight as a single dose.

Status epilepticus
IV injection (dilute 1 in 10 with water for injection) 10 mg/kg to a maximum dose of 1 g. Inject at a rate no greater than 100 mg per minute.

Nursing implications
Barbiturates commonly produce over sedation and dependence.

Storage

Preparations containing phenobarbitone are stored at room temperature.

Chlorpromazine
Flupenthixol
Fluphenazine
Methotrimeprazine
  (levomepromazine)
Pericyazine
Perphenazine
Pipotiazine
Prochlorperazine
Promazine
Promethazine
Thioridazine
Trifluoperazine
Trimeprazine (alimemazine)
Zuclopenthixol

Actions and uses

Phenothiazines are primarily used for their antipsychotic properties. Some are also useful as antiemetics and in the management of diabetic neuropathy. Phenothiazine drugs can be divided into three main groups:

1. aliphatic derivatives, e.g. chlorpromazine
2. piperazine derivatives, e.g. fluphenazine
3. piperidine derivatives, e.g. pericyazine.

Piperazine phenothiazines are potent drugs and, of the three groups, are most likely to cause troublesome extrapyramidal side effects. The piperidine group have intermediate potency but cause marked antimuscarinic side effects. The aliphatic derivatives are least potent and cause pronounced sedative effects. All phenothiazines cause sedation, antimuscarinic and extrapyramidal side effects to some extent.
Phenothiazines act at many different receptor sites but it is by blocking dopamine receptors in the brain that they exert their antipsychotic effects. Choice of drug depends largely on each drug's predominant action, its side effect profile and the patient's susceptibility to these side effects. It is most important to use whichever drug gives the patient most benefit.

Dosage

See individual drugs.

Nursing implications

- The most troublesome side effects of these drugs are extrapyramidal symptoms which can be parkinsonian, dystonia, akathisia or tardive dyskinesia. They are unpredictable and largely depend on patient susceptibility, the type of drug and the dose.
- A common side effect of this group of drugs is postural hypotension. This is especially important in patients who are receiving other antihypertensive drugs and should always be borne in mind as a cause of symptoms of dizziness or faintness.
- Other common side effects include excessive sedation, gastrointestinal upset, photosensitivity and variation in body temperature, more often hypothermia but rarely hyperthermia may occur.
- Endocrine side effects of this drug include amenorrhoea, failure of ovulation, galactorrhoea and gynaecomastia.
- Phenothiazines may produce cholestatic jaundice and should be used with extreme caution in patients with liver disease.
- Occasionally phenothiazines may affect the production of white blood cells. This makes the patient more susceptible to infection. Any patient presenting with even simple symptoms such as a sore throat should have their white blood cell count checked.
- Neuroleptic malignant syndrome occurs rarely.

P

Storage
See individual drugs.

PHENOXYBENZAMINE (Dibenyline)

Presentation
Capsules – 10 mg
Injection – 100 mg in 2 ml

Actions and uses
Phenoxybenzamine is a powerful alpha-receptor blocker. It is used in clinical practice for its ability to block the alpha-receptors of the sympathetic nervous system, making it useful in the treatment of phaeochromocytoma (an adrenaline-secreting tumour).

The drug has been given by intravenous infusion to attempt to increase tissue perfusion in states of severe shock, now rarely used for this purpose.

Dosage
Orally, for phaeochromocytoma, 10 mg daily, increasing by 10 mg/day to 1–2 mg/kg daily in two divided doses.
IV infusion, in the intensive care setting as an adjunct in severe shock and phaechromocytoma, 1 mg/kg daily in 200 ml sodium chloride 0.9% solution. Give over at least 2 hours through a large vein and do not repeat within 24 hours.

Nursing implications
- The drug's vasodilator action may produce flushing of the skin of the head and neck, headache, dizziness, tachycardia and postural hypotension.
- The drug may occasionally cause slight gastrointestinal upset.
- Inhibition of ejaculation may occur.
- Other side effects include nasal congestion, dryness of the mouth and constricted pupils.
- Phenoxybenzamine is contraindicated in patients who have a history of cerebrovascular accident and in the 4 weeks after a myocardial infarction.
- Contact sensitization may occur so avoid skin contact. This includes nurses and medical staff.

Storage
The drug is stored at room temperature.

PHENTERMINE (Duromine, Ionamin)

Presentation
Capsules – 15 mg and 30 mg (both modified release)

Actions and uses
Anorexogenic drugs abolish hunger by a direct action on the central nervous system. They are thought to have a supplementary effect in that they increase the ability to perform mental and physical work without the need for increased food intake. It is licensed, although not recommended for use.

Dosage
For adults only: 15 or 30 mg daily at breakfast.

Nursing implications
- Note that this is now classified as a Controlled Drug as a result of recognition of its abuse potential.

Storage
The drug is subject to the storage conditions of other drugs controlled by the Misuse of Drugs Act. Store at room temperature.

PHENTOLAMINE (Rogitine)

Presentation
Injection – 10 mg in 1 ml

Actions and uses
This drug causes a reduction in blood pressure by dilating peripheral

vessels via an inhibitory effect on alpha-receptors of the sympathetic nervous system (i.e. it is an alpha-blocker). It is no longer used to treat hypertension but may still rarely be seen in use during the surgical removal of phaeochromocytomata, which are tumours associated with the production of excess catecholamines.

Dosage
Adults: 2–5 mg by intravenous injection. The drug is diluted in 50–100 ml sodium chloride 0.9% or glucose 5% and administered over 20–30 minutes.

Nursing implications
- Parenteral phentolamine frequently produces postural hypotension, flushing, dizziness, weakness and tachycardia.
- Contraindications include hypotension, history of myocardial infarction or evidence of coronary artery disease.
- Use with caution in asthmatics as sulphites in the ampoules may lead to hypersensitivity, bronchospasm and shock.

Storage
Solutions should be protected from light and stored in a cool place.

PHENYTOIN (Epanutin)

Presentation
Tablets – 50 mg, 100 mg
Capsules – 25 mg, 50 mg, 100 mg, 300 mg
Chewable tablets – 50 mg
Suspension – 30 mg in 5 ml
Injection – 250 mg in 5 ml

Actions and uses
Phenytoin inhibits the spread of abnormal electrical activity through the brain. It stabilizes the seizure threshold. Phenytoin may be given intravenously (or, more rarely, intramuscularly) to control status epilepticus and orally to prevent seizures, particularly tonic-clonic and partial seizures. It can also be used

as second-line therapy in trigeminal neuralgia.

Phenytoin has a narrow therapeutic index and there is a non-linear relationship between dose and plasma concentration. A small increase in dose can have a marked effect on plasma concentration, efficacy and incidence of side effects. Monitoring the concentration of phenytoin in the plasma is required to ensure patients are adequately treated yet not overdosed. The therapeutic concentration range is 10–20 mg/l or 40–80 micromol/l.

Dosage
Oral
Adult: initially 3–4 mg/kg (150–300 mg) daily, increasing gradually if necessary to a usual daily dose of 200–500 mg. It can be taken as a single daily dose or divided into two or three doses. Adjust dose according to plasma phenytoin concentration and clinical response.
Child: initially 5 mg/kg daily in two divided doses; adjust to a usual range of 4–8 mg/kg daily. Maximum 300 mg/day.

Intravenous
Status epilepticus, slow IV injection or infusion.

- Adult and child: 15 mg/kg loading dose at a rate no greater than 50 mg/min (neonates 1–3 mg/kg/min). Maintain with 100 mg every 6–8 hours with monitoring of plasma concentration.
- For injection, dilute in 50–100 ml of sodium chloride 0.9% solution (to a maximum concentration of 10 mg/ml) and use an in-line filter.

Nursing implications
- The nurse's principal role in the management of patients on these drugs is to contribute to the early detection of either effects of excess dosage or side effects of the drug. The effects of overdosage can be seen with too rapid intravenous injection, when cardiac arrhythmias may

arise. Patients receiving this drug should therefore have pulse, blood pressure and ECG monitoring. The clinical signs of excess dosage are ataxia, nystagmus, dysarthria and confusion.

- Side effects include nausea and vomiting, tenderness and hyperplasia of the gums, hirsutism, dizziness, headache, peripheral neuropathy and blood disorders, i.e. megaloblastic anaemia, low white cell counts, low platelet counts, pancytopenia and aplastic anaemia. Patients should be advised to recognize signs of blood or skin disorders, e.g. fever, sore throat and bruising, and report to their doctor immediately. Skin rashes, joint pains, fever and hepatitis can also occur.
- The nurse should be aware that patients receiving phenytoin may experience problems if other drugs that alter liver metabolism are added to their regime. One example of this is chloramphenicol, which reduces the metabolism of phenytoin in the liver and may produce toxicity with doses of phenytoin which previously had produced no unwanted effects. Other drugs which increase plasma phenytoin concentrations include NSAIDs, amiodarone, some antifungals, diltiazem, nifedipine and cimetidine. Phenytoin concentration is reduced by rifampicin. Phenytoin accelerates the metabolism of anticoagulants, cyclosporin, corticosteroids and oral contraceptives. There are many other possible interactions; nurses should consult product literature or contact their local pharmacy department for further information.
- Take with or after food.
- Phenytoin and phenytoin sodium preparations are not interchangeable.

- Phenytoin injection should be preceded and followed with a saline flush to avoid local venous irritation.

Storage
All preparations containing phenytoin may be stored at room temperature. Solutions of phenytoin should be protected from light.

PIMOZIDE (Orap)

Presentation
Tablets – 2 mg, 4 mg, 10 mg

Actions and uses
Pimozide is an antipsychotic drug which is used for its tranquillizing or calming effect in severely agitated patients with a range of behavioural disorders, including schizophrenia and paranoid psychosis. In this respect pimozide possesses many of the properties of the phenothiazines, particularly the piperazine group discussed in the section on Phenothiazines (p. 281).

Dosage
Adults: the dosage varies widely according to the nature and severity of the disorder under treatment. Initially 2–10 mg (increasing to up to 20 mg for acutely agitated patients) is administered. Thereafter the dose is gradually reduced to that which maintains the individual symptom free. Children: in children over 12 years, a dose of 1–3 mg daily has been used.

Nursing implications
- Adverse effects which are associated with the phenothiazine tranquillizers may also occur in patients treated with pimozide. The nursing implications on phenothiazines thus apply to this drug (p. 281).
- Extrapyramidal (parkinsonian) symptoms and tardive dyskinesia appear to be more common with pimozide than with the phenothiazines though the occurrence of unwanted sedation is less likely.

- Contraindications include a history of arrhythmias or congenital QT prolongation. ECG monitoring should be carried out before starting treatment with pimozide and annual ECG monitoring is recommended.
- Do not use with any other drug which can prolong the QT interval, e.g. antiarrhythmics or terfenadine. Also avoid concomitant use with clarithromycin, tricyclic antidepressants, antifungals, mefloquine and quinine and diuretics.

Storage
Pimozide tablets are stored at room temperature.

PINDOLOL (Visken)

Presentation
Tablets – 5 mg, 15 mg

Actions and uses
Pindolol is a non-selective beta-adrenoreceptor blocking drug. Its actions and uses are described under Beta-Adrenoreceptor Blocking Drugs (p. 51).

Dosage
The adult dosage regime for hypertension is usually a daily dose of 15 mg. Alternatively up to 45 mg may be given in two or three divided doses per day. In angina, use 2.5–5 mg up to three times a day.

Nursing implications
See the section on Beta-Adrenoreceptor Blocking Drugs (p. 51).

Storage
Pindolol tablets are stored at room temperature.

PIPERACILLIN (Pipril)

Presentation
Injection – 1 g, 2 g vials

Infusion – 4 g with 50 ml bottle of water for injection

Actions and uses
Piperacillin is an antipseudomonal penicillin with a broad spectrum of activity. It is active against many Gram-negative organisms, anaerobes and Gram-positive organisms including Streptococcus, Enterococci and *Staphylococcus aureus*. It has bactericidal properties. Piperacillin is active against many infections including bacterial septicaemia and endocarditis, urogenital tract infections, respiratory tract infections and skin and soft tissue infections. It is often administered as Tazocin® which contains tazobactam, rendering the combination active against beta-lactamase producing bacteria resistant to piperacillin alone.

Dosage
Adult

- Deep IM, IV injection over 3–5 minutes or IV infusion: 100–150 mg/kg/day in divided doses, increasing to 200–300 mg/kg/day in severe infections. Use at least 16 g per day in life-threatening infections. Any single dose greater than 2 g should be given IV.
- For adult surgical prophylaxis, piperacillin can be given by deep IM injection or IV injection over 3–5 minutes or by IV infusion, 2 g immediately prior to surgery. Then in the 24 hours following surgery, at least two doses of 2 g at 4- or 6-hour intervals.
- For acute gonorrhoea, 2 g should be given as a single dose by deep IM injection.

Child 1 month–12 years
Deep IM, IV injection over 3–5 minutes or IV infusion: 100–200 mg/kg/day in 3–4 divided doses, 200–300 mg/kg/day in severe infections.

Neonate

- IV injection over 3–5 minutes or IV infusion: age up to 7 days or over 7 days but weighing less than 2 kg, 150 mg/kg daily in three divided doses.

P

- Age greater than 7 days and weighing greater than 2 kg, 300 mg/kg daily in 3–4 divided doses.

Nursing implications
See Benzylpenicillin (p. 49).

Storage
Store piperacillin preparations at room temperature.

PIPERAZINE (Pripsen)

Presentation
Sachets – 4 g (each sachet contains 4 g of piperazine phosphate and standardized senna equivalent to 15.3 mg; total sennoside calculated as sennoside B)
Elixir – piperazine hydrate 750 mg in 5 ml

Actions and uses
This anthelmintic drug is effective in the treatment of threadworm (enterobiasis) and roundworm (ascariasis). In roundworm, the drug acts by producing a reversible muscle paralysis in the worm, allowing the worm to be dislodged from the gut wall and expelled in the faeces. Mode of action in threadworm infections is largely unknown.

Dosage
Elixir
Threadworms.

- Adult: 15 ml/day for 7 days
- Child under 2 on doctor's advice: 0.3–0.5 ml/kg/day for 7 days
- Child 2–3: 5 ml daily
- Child 4–6: 7.5 ml daily
- Child 7–12: 10 ml daily
- In all ages repeat the course after 1 week if necessary.

Roundworms.

- Adult: 30 ml single dose
- Child under 1 on doctor's advice: 0.8 ml/kg single dose
- Child 1–3: 10 ml
- Child 4–5: 15 ml
- Child 6–8: 20 ml
- Child 9–12: 25 ml
- In all ages repeat the dose after 2 weeks.

Oral powder (stir into a small glass of milk or water and drink immediately)
Threadworms.

- Adult and child over 6 years: 1 sachet
- Child 3 months – 1 year: on doctor's advice, 2.5 ml level spoonful
- Child 1–6 years: 5 ml level spoonful
- In all ages repeat after 14 days.

Roundworms.

- First dose as above. If there is a reinfection risk, the dose should be repeated every month for up to 3 months.

Nursing implications
- All members of the family must be treated.
- Use must be combined with hygienic measures; wash hands and scrub nails before each meal and after each visit to the toilet.
- Adverse effects include nausea and vomiting, colic, diarrhoea and allergy.
- Occasional neurological abnormalities including visual disturbance, dizziness and vertigo may occur.

Storage
The drug is stored at room temperature.

PIPERAZINE OESTRONE SULPHATE/ ESTROPIPATE (Harmogen)

Presentation
Tablets – 1.5 mg

Actions and uses
The actions and uses of oestrogenic substances in general are described in the section on these drugs (p. 257).
In clinical practice this drug is used for oestrogen replacement therapy and the relief of oestrogen deficiency symptoms at or after the menopause and following surgical or radiotherapeutic oophorectomy. It is also used in osteoporosis prophylaxis.

Dosage
1.5 mg daily continuously with a cyclical progestogen on 10–13 days of the cycle if the patient has an intact uterus. Up to 3 mg daily can be taken for vasomotor symptoms and menopausal vaginitis.

Nursing implications
See the section on Oestrogenic Hormones (p. 257).

Storage
The drug is stored at room temperature.

PIRACETAM (Nootropil)

Presentation
Tablets – 800 mg, 1.2 g
Oral solution – 333.3 mg in 1 ml

Actions and uses
Piracetam is licensed for adjunctive treatment of cortical myoclonus. It has an action on the CNS, protecting the cerebral cortex against hypoxia, and has been used in dementia and other cerebrocortical insufficiency disorders.

Dosage
For cortical myoclonus, adults only, the starting dose is 7.2 g daily, taken in divided doses. This can be increased according to response in increments of 4.8 g each day. Maximum recommended daily dose is 20 g.

Nursing implications
- Do not use in hepatic impairment or severe renal impairment. Avoid in pregnancy and breastfeeding.
- Adverse effects include diarrhoea and weight gain.
- The oral solution has a bitter taste so patients should be advised to follow each dose with a glass of water or soft drink.

Storage
Store at room temperature.

PIROXICAM (Brexidol, Feldene)

Presentation
Capsules – 10 mg, 20 mg
Tablets – 20 mg
Dispersible tablets – 10 mg, 20 mg
Dissolving tablets – 20 mg
Injection – 20 mg in 1 ml
Suppositories – 20 mg
Topical gel – 0.5%

Actions and uses
Piroxicam is an oxicam NSAID indicated for use in musculoskeletal conditions including rheumatoid arthritis, osteoarthritis and gout. See the section on Non-Steroidal Antiinflammatory Analgesic Drugs (p. 250).

Dosage
- The adult oral dose is 20 mg (10–30 mg maintenance) once per day. Double this dose may be taken for 48 hours following an acute skeletal muscle injury.
- Children over 6 years old can take piroxicam for juvenile arthritis: under 15 kg, 5 mg daily; 16–25 kg, 10 mg daily; 26–45 kg, 15 mg daily and greater than 46 kg, 20 mg daily.
- For acute gout 40 mg per day may be prescribed and taken for 4–6 days.
- Gel: apply to the affected area 3–4 times daily.
- Oral doses, above, may be administered by deep intramuscular injection in acute musculoskeletal injury or exacerbation of arthritis.
- The rectal dose is as for the oral route when compromised.

Nursing implications
- See the section on Non-Steroidal Antiinflammatory Analgesic Drugs (p. 250).
- Note that dispersible tablets and 'Melt' tablets (which very rapidly dissolve in the mouth) are oral alternatives for patients with swallowing difficulty, especially elderly people with dysphagia.

Storage
Piroxicam preparations are stored at room temperature.

PIZOTIFEN (Sanomigran)

Presentation
Tablets – 0.5 mg, 1.5 mg
Elixir – 0.25 mg in 5 ml

Actions and uses
Pizotifen inhibits the action of substances which are released within the blood vessels and which cause the vascular changes which lead to the symptoms of severe headache and migraine. It is an antihistamine and serotonin antagonist. In clinical practice it is used for the prophylaxis of migraine, vascular and cluster headaches.

Dosage
The dose ranges from 0.5 to 3 mg per day or up to 4.5 mg per day depending on individual patient response. Maximum single dose is 3 mg. Children can take up to 1.5 mg daily in divided doses with a single dose of 1 mg at night.

Nursing implications
- The nurse may play an important role in cautioning patients about the dangers of drowsiness associated with taking this drug, especially in relation to driving vehicles and operating machinery. Low doses should be used initially with gradual titration to higher doses as this helps to lessen any drowsiness.
- The drug should never be given to patients who have glaucoma or a predisposition to urinary retention. Use with caution in pregnancy and breastfeeding.
- Apart from drowsiness, common side effects include weight gain and increased appetite. Less frequently, dizziness and nausea have occurred.

Storage
The drug is stored at room temperature.

POLYTHIAZIDE (Nephril)

Presentation
Tablets – 1 mg

Actions and uses
See the section on Thiazide and Related Diuretics (p. 357). It is used for oedema and hypertension.

Dosage
The adult dose is 0.5–4 mg taken as a single daily dose. The diuretic action may last up to 48 hours.

Nursing implications
See the section on Thiazide and Related Diuretics (p. 357).

Storage
Polythiazide tablets are stored at room temperature.

POTASSIUM BICARBONATE

Presentation
Effervescent tablets – potassium bicarbonate 500 mg and potassium acid tartrate 300 mg equivalent to 6.5 mmol of potassium in each tablet

Actions and uses
Potassium bicarbonate is an alkalinizing agent used where sodium bicarbonate is less appropriate; for instance, when potassium deficiency has occurred in some renal tubular and gastrointestinal disorders giving rise to hyperchloraemic acidosis. This can be managed by replacing potassium with oral potassium bicarbonate or, in serious cases, with IV therapy.

Dosage
This will depend on the degree of acidosis and should be altered according to clinical response.

Nursing implications
- Nausea and vomiting can occur.
- Use with caution in cardiac disease and renal impairment. Do not use in hypochloraemia or hyperkalaemia (potassium concentration greater than 5 mmol/l).

Storage
Store at room temperature.

POTASSIUM CHLORIDE

Presentation
Syrup – 1 mmol in 1 ml
Effervescent tablets – two
preparations: 1. equivalent to
6.7 mmol of potassium and 6.7 mmol
of chloride; 2. equivalent to 12 mmol
of potassium and 8 mmol of chloride
Modified-release tablets – 600 mg,
equivalent to 8 mmol each of
potassium and chloride
Granules – each sachet equivalent to
20 mmol each of potassium and
chloride
IV preparations – potassium chloride
0.3% and glucose 5% intravenous
infusion; potassium chloride 0.3% and
sodium chloride 0.9% intravenous
infusion
Ampoules – 20 mmol potassium
in 10 ml

Actions and uses
Potassium chloride preparations
are used to replace potassium in
cases of potassium depletion
(hypokalaemia) with IV preparations
being used in cases of severe
depletion. Potassium loss can occur
for various reasons, but replacement
therapy is frequently required in the
following cases.

- Patients taking digoxin or other
antiarrhythmic drugs where
hypokalaemia can increase side
effects and induce arrhythmias.
- Secondary hyperaldosteronism.
- Excessive potassium loss in faeces,
e.g. chronic diarrhoea.
- Elderly patients with insufficient
dietary intake.
- Where drugs causing hypokalaemia
are taken, e.g. corticosteroids.

Dosage
- Depends primarily on plasma
potassium concentration.
- Prevention of hypokalaemia:
25–50 mmol/day orally with a
normal diet; use smaller doses if
renal impairment is present.
- Use larger oral doses where
mild–moderate depletion is already
present.
- Severe potassium depletion: IV
therapy is required, given by slow
intravenous infusion adjusted

according to plasma potassium
concentration.

Nursing implications
- The most important adverse
effects occur on rapid infusion of
the IV preparations. Potassium is
toxic to the heart and should be
infused at a rate not exceeding
20 mmol per hour (usually
20 mmol are given over at least
2–3 hours) and at a concentration
no greater than 40 mmol/l.
Specialist advice should be
sought before commencing
potassium infusions and ECG
monitoring is recommended in
serious cases.
- On preparation of infusions
always mix thoroughly, as
potassium can layer at the
bottom of infusion bags. Use
ready-prepared solutions
whenever possible.
- Potassium chloride ampoules
have on occasion been confused
with ampoules of water for
injection, with fatal
consequences. It is often
recommended that potassium
chloride ampoules are stored
separately from other injectable
drugs.
- Hyperkalaemia can occur,
especially in patients with renal
impairment. Use with caution in
elderly patients.
- Side effects of oral preparations
include nausea and vomiting.
- Use with caution in combination
with other drugs known to raise
plasma potassium concentrations,
e.g. ACE inhibitors, cyclosporin
and potassium-sparing diuretics.

Storage
Potassium chloride preparations are
stored at room temperature.

POTASSIUM CLORAZEPATE/ CLORAZEPATE DIPOTASSIUM (Tranxene)

Presentation
Capsules – 7.5 mg, 15 mg

Actions and uses

Potassium clorazepate is a member of the Benzodiazepine group (p. 47). Its principal use is in the treatment of anxiety.

Dosage

7.5–22.5 mg daily in two or three divided doses or 15 mg as a single dose at night. Not recommended for children. Elderly patients should use half the normal adult dose.

> ### Nursing implications
> See the section on Benzodiazepines (p. 47).

Storage

Capsules containing potassium clorazepate are stored at room temperature.

POTASSIUM PERCHLORATE

Presentation

Tablets – 200 mg

Actions and uses

Potassium perchlorate prevents the uptake of iodine by the thyroid gland and in this way inhibits the total amount of thyroxine produced by the gland. Its use in the treatment of thyrotoxicosis is limited by the occasional occurrence of severe side effects. It is also used in radiopharmacy for various tests, including thyroid function and brain visualization.

Dosage

Hyperthyroidism.

- Adults: 800 mg–1 g in divided doses daily with maintenance doses reduced to 200–500 mg daily.

Radiopharmacy (specialized brain scanning).

- Adults: 200–400 mg, 30–60 minutes prior to administration of radioisotope.
- Child 2–12 years: 200 mg as above.
- Child under 2 years: 100 mg as above.

> ### Nursing implications
> - Hypersensitivity reactions, including rashes and fever, have been reported.
> - The drug can produce gastrointestinal upset and nausea may be severe.
> - Serious adverse effects include aplastic anaemia, pancytopenia, leucopenia and nephrotic syndrome.
> - Some thyrotoxic patients receive a short course of potassium iodide prior to operation. Potassium perchlorate should never be given at the same time as it negates the action of potassium iodide in this situation.

Storage

Potassium perchlorate tablets are stored at room temperature. Protect from moisture.

PRAMIPEXOLE (Mirapexin)

Presentation

Tablets – 125 microgram (88 microgram base), 250 microgram (180 microgram base), 1 mg (700 microgram base)

Actions and uses

Pramipexole is a dopamine agonist used in combination with levodopa for patients with advanced Parkinson's disease.

Dosage

Confirm if dosage prescribed is for pramipexole base or salt.

Start with a dose of 88 microgram (base) three times a day; increase by doubling the dose every 5–7 days to 360 microgram (base) three times a day. The dose can be further increased if required by 540 microgram (base) daily at weekly intervals to a maximum of 3.3 mg each day. As pramipexole dose is increased, the levodopa dose can be decreased.

> ### Nursing implications
> - Side effects include nausea, constipation, drowsiness and

hallucinations. Dyskinesia can occur at the start of therapy, as can hypotension.
- Patients should be warned that drowsiness can affect driving or operation of machinery and should not undertake these tasks, especially as sudden onset of sleep can occur.
- Visual disorders can occur; ophthalmological testing is recommended.
- Use with caution in renal impairment, psychotic disorders and severe cardiovascular disease.
- Use with caution in pregnancy and do not use in breastfeeding.

Storage
Pramipexole preparations are stored at room temperature.

PRAVASTATIN (Lipostat)

Presentation
Tablets – 10 mg, 20 mg, 40 mg

Actions and uses
Pravastatin is one of a relatively new range of lipid-lowering drugs which are frequently described as HMG-CoA reductase inhibitors (which refers to their inhibitory action on cholesterol synthesis). Drugs of this type produce a marked and sustained fall in cholesterol (particularly low-density lipoprotein or LDL cholesterol) and triglyceride compared to that produced by other lipid-lowering agents and have consequently become very popular in recent years.

The drug may be used in patients with hypercholesterolaemia who are considered to be at risk of ischaemic heart disease and early cardiac death or hypertriglyceridaemia, in which case they are likely to develop peripheral vascular disease and pancreatitis. Usually such patients will have blood cholesterol levels well in excess of 7–8 mmol/litre or triglyceride levels above 3 mmol/litre. These may fall by up to 50% on treatment.

Statins are frequently prescribed for patients who have had coronary artery bypass surgery or angioplasty, have cerebrovascular disease or peripheral vascular disease. They are also used in the primary prevention of coronary events in at-risk patients such as those with not only high cholesterol but also smokers, hypertensives and diabetics.

Dosage
Adults: a single evening dose of 10–40 mg is given.

Nursing implications
- It should be noted that in many cases, elevated blood cholesterol is the result of obesity, inappropriate diet or alcohol excess and correction of these factors is more appropriate. It should be noted that treatment is lifelong and therefore very expensive.
- A few patients present with a familial hypercholesterolaemia and history of early cardiac death in the family. In these patients, life may be markedly prolonged by treatment. Patients with extensive cardiac disease, especially after coronary artery bypass grafting, should have their cholesterol maintained in the normal range.
- Side effects include headache and gastrointestinal effects but, most importantly, muscle effects such as myalgia, myositis and myopathy can occur. If myopathy occurs treatment should be discontinued. Patients must be advised to report to their doctor any unexplained muscle pain, tenderness or weakness.
- There is an increased risk of myopathy if pravastatin is taken concurrently with cyclosporin, fibrates or nicotinic acid.
- Use with caution in liver disease. Liver function tests should be carried out before starting treatment and regularly for the first month of treatment.
- Pravastatin is contraindicated in patients with active liver disease, in pregnancy and breastfeeding.

Storage

Pravastatin tablets are stored at room temperature. Protect from light and moisture.

PRAZOSIN (Hypovase)

Presentation

Tablets – 500 microgram, 1 mg, 2 mg, 5 mg

Actions and uses

Prazosin lowers the blood pressure by a direct action on the smooth muscle of blood vessels, described as selective alpha-1 blockade. It is used in the management of hypertension.

Prazosin also produces a secondary effect on the urethral sphincter, causing relaxation and thus permitting urine flow. This is of use in the treatment of dysuria associated with benign prostatic hyperplasia.

Dosage

A significant number of patients suffer from sudden collapse within 30–90 minutes of receiving their first dose of prazosin. For this reason all patients are commenced on low doses (500 microgram three times a day) and the dose is increased gradually until the required effect is obtained. The maximum dosage is 20 mg per day usually taken in divided doses.

For benign prostatic hyperplasia, lower doses are used, starting at 500 microgram twice daily and increasing to a maximum of 2 mg twice daily.

Nursing implications

- As noted above, sudden collapse may follow the initial dose of prazosin and therefore the initial dose must be small and is usually given on retiring to bed on the first night of treatment.
- Side effects include postural hypotension, drowsiness, headache, lethargy, weakness, palpitations and urinary frequency.
- Use with caution in renal impairment, pregnancy and breastfeeding.

Storage

Prazosin tablets are stored at room temperature.

PREDNISOLONE (Precortisyl, Prednesol, Predsol, Deltacortril)

Several other proprietary preparations containing prednisolone in many different formulations are also available.

Presentation

Tablets – 1 mg, 5 mg, 25 mg
Enteric coated – 2.5 mg and 5 mg
Soluble tablets – 5 mg
Injection (prednisolone acetate) – 25 mg in 1 ml
Eye/ear drops – 0.5%
Eye drops – 1%
Suppositories – 5 mg
Enema – 20 mg in 100 ml, 20 mg metered application in foam aerosol

Actions and uses

Prednisolone is a corticosteroid drug and has actions and uses similar to other Corticosteroids (p. 107).

Dosage

Dose ranges vary widely depending on the type of illness, the severity of the disease and the route of administration. It is therefore impossible to outline possible dosage regimes in this text.

Nursing implications

See the section on Corticosteroids (p. 107).

Storage

- Preparations containing prednisolone are stored at room temperature.
- In common with other eye drops, containers should not be used for more than 7 days for inpatients in a hospital ward or 4 weeks in the domestic situation as the risk of bacterial contamination becomes too great.

P

PRILOCAINE (Citanest)

Presentation
Injection – plain 0.5%, 1%, 2% and 4%; with felypressin 3%

Actions and uses
This drug is a local anaesthetic. Felypressin is a vasoconstrictor substance which prolongs the duration of its effects.

Dosage
There is considerable variation in the optimum dosage for individual use. It should be noted, however, that the maximum adult dose should not exceed 400 mg or 300 mg if used with felypressin.

Nursing implications
- At maximum dosage a chemical called methaemoglobin may be produced in the blood. This may lead to an appearance of cyanosis.

Storage
The drug is stored at room temperature.

PRIMIDONE (Mysoline)

Presentation
Tablets – 250 mg
Suspension – 250 mg in 5 ml

Actions and uses
Primidone is an anticonvulsant drug which is converted in the body to the active component phenobarbitone. It is used primarily for the treatment of grand mal epilepsy. In the past combinations of primidone and phenobarbitone were used to treat epilepsy but as they are in effect the same drug this practice is now discouraged.

Dosage
As individual doses are extremely variable, the following are simply guidelines for treatment and dosages should always be adjusted to individual requirements. It is recommended that initially 125 mg be given once daily late in the evening and every 3 days thereafter the dose should be increased by 125 mg until the daily dosage is 500 mg in two divided doses. Thereafter the dosage should be adjusted by 250 mg every 3 days until control is obtained or side effects occur up to a maximum of 1.5 g daily in divided doses. Average daily maintenance doses are as follows.

- Adults and children over 9 years: 750–1500 mg.
- Children: up to 2 years, 250–500 mg; 2–5 years, 500–750 mg; 6–9 years, 750–1000 mg.

It should be noted that although initial treatment is given once daily in the evening, by the time the dosage exceeds 250 mg in total it should be split into a twice-daily regime.

Nursing implications
- Primidone is converted in the body to phenobarbitone and therefore refer to this section.

Storage
The drug is stored at room temperature.

PROBENECID (Benemid)

Presentation
Tablets – 500 mg

Actions and uses
Probenecid acts directly on the kidney tubules to produce two main effects.

- It blocks the excretion of penicillin and some cephalosporin drugs from the renal tubules and may therefore be used to maintain high blood levels of these drugs.
- It promotes the excretion of uric acid and urate from the renal tubules and may therefore be used to reduce the blood urate concentration in hyperuricaemia and gout.

P

Dosage

- Hyperuricaemia and gout: adults usually receive 250 mg twice daily initially. The dose is increased after a week to 500 mg twice daily. Up to 2 g per day may be given in 2–4 divided doses where necessary.
- Adjunct therapy with penicillin and cephalosporins:
  - adults: 2 g daily in divided doses
  - children over 2 years old and weighing less than 50 kg: 25 mg/kg initially, then 10 mg/kg 6-hourly.
- Note that patients with renal impairment which is sufficient to retard the excretion of penicillin or cephalosporins must not receive probenecid.

- Probenecid must be used with caution in patients with a history of peptic ulcer disease.
- Probenecid must never be given to patients receiving methotrexate as it may induce methotrexate toxicity.
- Although probenecid reduces blood urate levels it may at the onset of treatment actually precipitate an acute attack of gout. It is common practice, therefore, to give concurrent therapy with an antiinflammatory drug, e.g. naproxen or colchicine, at the beginning of treatment.

Storage

Probenecid tablets are stored at room temperature.

PROCAINAMIDE (Pronestyl)

Presentation

Tablets – 250 mg
Injection – 1 g in 10 ml

Actions and uses

Procainamide is a class I antiarrhythmic agent. It has a depressant action on the heart and reduces contractility and excitability of heart muscle and conductivity of the electrical conducting tissues. It is therefore useful in the treatment of ventricular arrhythmias, particularly after myocardial infarction. Procainamide can also be used for atrial tachycardia. It may be given in an emergency either intravenously or intramuscularly and for long-term treatment it may be given orally.

Dosage

Adults only.

- Slow intravenous injection: 25–50 mg per minute up to a total of 1 g with continuous ECG and blood pressure monitoring.
- Intravenous infusion: 500–600 mg administered over 25–30 minutes with ECG monitoring. Maintain at a rate of 2–6 mg/min, starting oral treatment 3–4 hours after infusion.

Nursing implications

- The nurse may play a major role in preventing the occurrence of renal stone formation or renal colic in patients on this drug by continually monitoring their fluid intake and encouraging them to take an adequate amount of fluid each day as this reduces the incidence of such side effects.
- Aspirin blocks the effect of probenecid and as patients may frequently be taking this drug in addition to prescribed medication, the nurse may contribute to the management of such patients by ensuring that they know that they should never take aspirin when taking probenecid.
- Common side effects include anorexia, nausea, vomiting, headache and frequency of micturition.
- More rarely, allergic reactions may occur when patients are given this drug. They include anaphylactic shock, dermatitis, pruritus and fever.
- Rare serious side effects include nephrotic syndrome, liver damage and aplastic anaemia.

- Oral dosage: up to 50 mg/kg body weight daily is taken in divided doses at intervals ranging from 3 to 6-hourly. Higher doses may be required in atrial arrhythmias.
- A serum concentration of between 3 and 10 mg/l has been found to be effective.

Nursing implications
- The nurse will rarely see procainamide given intravenously outside the hospital setting. Rapid intravenous dosage of this drug can lead to hypotension, ventricular fibrillation and cardiac arrest. Constant monitoring of blood pressure and ECG monitoring are essential when the drug is given by the intravenous route.
- Side effects from procainamide occur most frequently after high dosage or in patients with heart failure or renal failure. The commonest side effects are anorexia, diarrhoea, nausea and vomiting.
- When patients have been on procainamide for a prolonged period of time, they may develop a syndrome similar to systemic lupus erythematosus with joint pains, skin lesions, pleuritic chest pain and the other features of this disease. The development of such symptoms in a patient on procainamide is an indication for blood tests to be carried out on the patient to detect LE cells and if these are present, the drug should be stopped and if necessary an alternative antidysrhythmic drug should be substituted. This syndrome characteristically resolves after withdrawal of the drug.
- Because procainamide depresses cardiac contractility, it may lead to the development of heart failure. The nurse should therefore monitor the patient for symptoms of heart failure such as breathlessness on exertion or on

lying flat in bed and ankle oedema.
- Use with caution in pregnancy and not at all in breastfeeding.

Storage
Procainamide tablets and solution for injection are stored at room temperature.

PROCARBAZINE

Presentation
Capsules – 50 mg

Actions and uses
The mode of action of procarbazine remains unclear but it would appear to prevent cell division by interfering with one of the basic biochemical steps necessary for this process. Its main use is in the treatment of Hodgkin's disease, although very rarely it may be indicated for the management of solid tumours.

Dosage
Adults: 50–300 mg orally divided in up to three doses daily. Maintenance dose, on remission, 50–150 mg daily to a cumulative total dose of at least 6 g.
Children (under expert advice): 50 mg daily for the first week, then maintain daily dose at 100 mg/m^2 body surface area until leucopenia or thrombocytopenia occurs or maximum response is obtained.

P

Nursing implications
- Nearly all patients suffer from anorexia, nausea and vomiting. These symptoms may become less troublesome as treatment continues.
- Bone marrow depression may produce thrombocytopenia and leucopenia. Regular blood counts are carried out during treatment to monitor this but should these effects arise, the patient would be at an increased risk of severe infection or haemorrhage.

- The drug should not be given to patients with severe liver or kidney disease.
- Procarbazine is derived from the hydrazines which is one group of monoamine oxidase inhibitors used in the treatment of depression.
- It should not be given concurrently with other monoamine oxidase inhibitors. Also avoid alcohol.
- Nurses should be aware of the risks posed by cytotoxic drugs. Some are irritant to the skin and mucous surfaces and care must be exercised when handling them. In particular, spillage or contamination of personnel or the environment must be avoided. If cytotoxic drugs are handled regularly, it is theoretically possible that repeated skin contact or inhalation may produce systemic toxic effects in nurses who have developed hypersensitivity to them. Most hospitals now operate a centralized (pharmacy-organized) additive service. While this reduces the risk of exposure to cytotoxic drugs, it is essential that nurses recognize and understand the local policy on their safe handling and disposal. The Health and Safety Executive has decreed that such a policy should be in place wherever cytotoxic drugs are administered. These should be adapted, wherever possible, to care of patients in the community.

P

Storage

Procarbazine capsules are stored at room temperature.

PROCHLORPERAZINE (Buccastem, Stemetil)

Presentation

Tablets – 5 mg, 25 mg
Buccal tablets – 3 mg
Syrup – 5 mg in 5 ml
Effervescent sachets – 5 mg/sachet
Injection – 12.5 mg in 1 ml
Suppositories – 5 mg, 25 mg

Actions and uses

Prochlorperazine is a member of the phenothiazine group and its actions and uses are described in the section on these drugs (p. 281). As this is a very widely used drug it is worth detailing its specific uses which are:

- for the treatment of severe anxiety states
- for the treatment of behavioural disorders in schizophrenia and other psychotic states
- for the treatment of nausea and vomiting, particularly when this is due to other drug therapy
- for the symptomatic relief of vertigo and vomiting in neurological disorders such as Menière's disease.

Dosage

Psychosis: 75–100 mg in total daily is given in 2–3 divided doses by the oral, rectal or intramuscular route. For severe anxiety, maximum daily dose is usually 40 mg. Not recommended for children.
Nausea and vomiting.

- The oral dose is 20 mg initially then 10 mg after 2 hours.
- Prevention: 5–10 mg orally 2–3 times a day.
- Child, over 10 kg only: 250 microgram/kg orally 2–3 times daily.
- Deep IM injection: 12.5 mg when required followed after 6 hours by oral dosing as above. Not recommended for children.
- Rectally: 25 mg when required followed after 6 hours by oral dosing as above. For nausea due to migraines, 5 mg three times a day. Not recommended for children.

For the treatment of vertigo and nausea associated with neurological disorders such as Menière's disease: 5 mg three times daily increased to 30 mg daily if required. Reduce after several weeks to 5–10 mg daily. Not recommended for children.

Nursing implications

The nursing implications of this drug are described under Phenothiazines (p. 281).

Storage

Preparations containing prochlorperazine are stored at room temperature but they should be protected from direct sunlight. Do not store suppositories next to a heat source (e.g. radiator).

PROCYCLIDINE (Arpicolin, Kemadrin)

Presentation

Tablets – 5 mg
Syrup – 2.5 mg in 5 ml, 5 mg in 5 ml
Injection – 10 mg in 2 ml

Actions and uses

The actions and uses of this drug are identical to those described for Benzhexol (p. 47).

Dosage

Adults.

- Orally: 2.5 mg three times a day initially, increasing if necessary to 30 mg daily (60 mg daily maximum).
- Parenterally (by intravenous or intramuscular injection): 5–10 mg repeated if necessary to a maximum of 20 mg daily.
- Use lower doses in the elderly.

Nursing implications

The nursing implications of benzhexol (p. 47) apply to this drug.

Storage

The drug is stored at room temperature.

PROGESTERONE (Crinone, Cyclogest, Gestone)

Presentation

Vaginal/rectal pessaries – 200 mg and 400 mg
Vaginal gel – 4%, 8%
Injection – 25 mg in 1 ml, 50 mg in 1 ml, 100 mg in 2 ml

Actions and uses

The actions and uses of progestational hormones are discussed under Progestogens (p. 297). See under dosage for some of progesterone's clinical indications.

Dosage

- For premenstrual syndrome (although not commonly recommended): 200–400 mg pessaries, rectally or vaginally once or twice daily from the 12th to 14th day of the menstrual cycle until menstruation recommences. Administer rectally if barrier methods of contraception are used, the patient has recently given birth or suffers from vaginal infection or recurrent cystitis.
- Progesterone deficiency: 1 applicatorful of 4% vaginal gel inserted on alternate days from day 15 to 25 of each cycle.
- Menopausal symptoms: 1 applicatorful of 4% vaginal gel inserted on alternate days for the last 12 days of eostrogen therapy in each cycle.
- Infertility due to inadequate luteal phase: 1 applicatorful of 8% vaginal gel inserted daily starting either after documented ovulation or on day 18–21 of cycle.
- *In vitro* fertilization: 1 applicatorful of 8% gel inserted daily for 30 days after laboratory evidence of pregnancy.
- Dysfunctional uterine bleeding: 5–10 mg by deep IM injection into the buttocks daily for 5–10 days until 2 days before expected onset of menstruation.

Nursing implications

See the section on Progestogens below.

Storage

The drug is stored at room temperature.

PROGESTOGENS

This group of drugs includes:
Allgloestrenol
Dydrogesterone
Hydroxyprogesterone
Medroxyprogesterone
Progesterone

Presentation

See individual drugs.

P

Actions and uses

The contribution of progesterone to oral contraceptive therapy is discussed in the section on Contraceptives (Oral) (p. 105).

Progestogens are used widely for a number of disorders.

- Obstetric problems:
  - habitual and threatened abortion
  - suppression of lactation
  - puerperal depression
- Gynaecological problems:
  - menstrual irregularities
  - functional uterine bleeding
  - endometriosis
  - menopausal symptoms
  - premenstrual tension
  - endometrial carcinoma
  - atrophic or senile vaginitis

Nursing implications

- The administration of progestogens can lead commonly to symptoms of gastrointestinal upset, headache, depression, urticaria, pruritus vulvae and change in menstrual function.
- Acne, weight gain and hypertension due to salt and water retention, gynaecomastia, vaginal candidiasis and vaginal discharge may occur when patients receive this drug.
- Less frequently, jaundice and liver damage have been produced.
- Progestogen drugs should be used with caution in patients with heart and kidney disease due to their salt- and water-retaining effects.
- Progestogens should not be given to pregnant women as they cause masculinization of the female fetus.
- The administration of progestogens to asthmatics and epileptics may lead to an exacerbation of their symptoms.

Storage

See specific drugs.

PROGUANIL (Paludrine)

Presentation

Tablets – 100 mg

Actions and uses

Proguanil is used for malaria prophylaxis and suppression. This drug is a folate antagonist, a dihydrofolate reductase inhibitor (with greater affinity for the plasmodial enzyme than human enzyme) which interferes with cell division, thus preventing malaria parasites from continuing to multiply in the body.

Proguanil is usually used with chloroquine for the prophylaxis of malaria. Used alone, it is not a treatment for malaria but can be used in combination with atovaquone for acute uncomplicated falciparum malaria.

Dosage

Adults: 200 mg
Child under 1 year: 25 mg
Child 1–4 years: 50 mg
Child 5–8 years: 100 mg
Child 9–14 years: 150 mg
All are daily doses which should be taken after food. Prophylactic therapy should start at least 24 hours before entering an infected area and continue for 4 weeks after leaving the area.

Nursing implications

- Always seek expert advice on recommendations for malaria prophylaxis as the regime used will depend on the country or region to be visited and any resistance to drug therapy in that area.
- Patients must be advised to take their tablets regularly and to continue for 4 weeks after leaving the infected area. They must also be advised of the importance of avoiding mosquito bites if at all possible.
- If a patient becomes ill within 1 year of return from an infected area, they must be advised to seek urgent medical advice.
- Side effects include gastrointestinal upsets, mouth ulcers and skin reactions.
- Use with caution in renal impairment and pregnancy (folate supplements required).
- Proguanil may enhance the anticoagulant effects of warfarin.

Storage

Proguanil tablets are stored at room temperature.

PROMETHAZINE (Phenergan, Avomine)

Presentation

Tablets – 10 mg, 25 mg (as hydrochloride), 25 mg (as teoclate)
Elixir – 5 mg in 5 ml
Injection – 25 mg in 1 ml

Actions and uses

Promethazine is a member of the phenothiazine group of drugs but is unusual in that it has little if any appreciable tranquillizing activity. It is, however, very useful for its antiemetic, sedative and antihistamine effects. It is particularly useful in the prevention and treatment of motion sickness and in the treatment of irradiation sickness, postoperative vomiting, the nausea and vomiting of pregnancy, drug-induced nausea and vomiting and for the symptomatic relief of nausea and vertigo in Menière's disease and other labyrinthine disturbances.

Dosage

For the treatment of nausea and vomiting.

- Adults, orally: 25–100 mg daily.
- Child 5–10 years, orally: 12.5–37.5 mg daily.

For motion sickness prevention.

- Adult, orally: 20–25 mg at night the evening before travel, repeat the dose the following morning if necessary.
- Child 2–5 years, orally: 5 mg at night the evening before travel and the following morning if necessary.
- Child 5–10 years, orally: 10–12.5 mg at night the evening before travel and the following morning if necessary.

For severe vomiting in pregnancy.

- 25 mg at bedtime, increased if required up to 100 mg daily.

For the treatment of allergy and anaphylactic reactions.

- Adult: orally, 25 mg at night or 25 mg twice daily or 10–20 mg

2–3 times a day. Deep IM injection: 25–50 mg, maximum 100 mg.
- Child 2–5 years: orally, 5–15 mg daily in divided doses.
- Child 5–10 years: orally, 10–25 mg daily in divided doses. Deep IM injection, 6.25–12.5 mg.

As a premedication.

- Adult: deep IM injection, 25–50 mg 1 hour before operation.
- Child 2–5 years: orally, 15–20 mg
- Child 5–10 years: orally, 20–25 mg, deep IM injection, 6.25–12.5 mg.

In emergencies.

- By slow IV injection, 25–50 mg given in water for injections at a concentration of 2.5 mg/ml. Maximum dose 100 mg.

Nursing implications

- Promethazine is a phenothiazine drug but in the dosages recommended and when used for the treatment of conditions described above, the problems encountered with phenothiazine drugs in general (p. 281) are rarely encountered.
- It is important to remember that sedation may commonly occur and patients must be warned about the dangers of taking this drug while operating heavy machinery or driving.
- Note IM injection may be painful.

Storage

Preparations containing promethazine are stored at room temperature.

PROPAFENONE (Arythmol)

Presentation

Tablets – 150 mg, 300 mg

Actions and uses

In order to understand the antiarrhythmic action of propafenone, a knowledge of cardiac conduction is required. Propafenone is a class 1C agent, so-called because of the nature of its action on the conducting tissues of the myocardium. It acts primarily on

P

the rapid depolarization phase of the cardiac action potential (i.e. it inhibits the fast inward sodium channel) and exerts a potent membrane-stabilizing effect. Conduction is slowed in the atria, at the atrioventricular node and, in particular, the His–Purkinje system. Changes which may be seen on the ECG include prolongation of the PR interval and QRS complex duration. In addition, propafenone possesses beta-blocking activity but is much less potent than recognized beta-blockers in this respect, e.g. only about 1/40th the potency of propranolol.

Propafenone is indicated for the prevention and management of ventricular arrhythmias and the prevention and management of paroxysmal supraventricular tachyarrhythmias where standard therapy has been ineffective or is contraindicated.

Dosage

Adults: initially 150 mg three times daily, increasing gradually to 300 mg twice daily and up to three times daily. Patients under 70 kg should have lower doses. It should be initiated under hospital supervision with ECG and blood pressure monitoring.

Nursing implications
- Patients may complain of a bitter taste.
- Common side effects of propafenone include dizziness, fatigue, nausea and vomiting, headache, constipation (and diarrhoea), allergic skin reactions, blurred vision and dry mouth.
- Propafenone is extensively metabolized in the liver and readily accumulates in patients with liver impairment. A suitable dosage reduction is frequently necessary.
- It should be avoided or administered with extreme caution in patients with marked hypotension, bradycardia, uncontrolled heart failure (unless related to the arrhythmia for which treatment is indicated)

and cardiogenic shock, severe obstructive airways disease and uncontrolled electrolyte disturbances.
- Patients with depression of the sinus node, atrial conduction and second- or third-degree atrioventricular block should be adequately paced before treatment is administered.
- Note that propafenone possesses beta-blocking activity, albeit weakly, and may precipitate heart failure in patients with poor cardiac reserve.
- Propafenone increases plasma levels of digoxin and warfarin and patients receiving such combinations should be carefully monitored for signs of digoxin intoxication or excessive anticoagulation.
- Raised levels of propranolol and metoprolol, but not of other beta-blockers, have also been noted and excessive beta-blockade may result.
- Plasma levels of propafenone may be increased by co-administration of cimetidine due to its inhibitory action on the metabolizing enzymes of the liver.
- There is an increased risk of ventricular arrhythmias if given concurrently with terfenadine.

Storage
Propafenone tablets are stored at room temperature.

PROPANTHELINE (Pro-Banthine)

Dosage
Tablets – 15 mg

Actions and uses
Propantheline is an antimuscarinic agent useful for the symptomatic relief of gastrointestinal disorders characterized by smooth muscle spasm. One of this drug's side effects is to produce urinary retention and for this reason it is used occasionally in the treatment of enuresis. Propantheline can also be used for gustatory sweating.

Dosage

Gastrointestinal disorders: 15 mg three times a day 1 hour before food and 30 mg at night. Maximum of 120 mg daily.
Adult enuresis: 15–30 mg 2–3 times daily 1 hour before food.

Nursing implications

The nursing implications of this drug are identical to those for Hyoscine Butylbromide (Buscopan) (p. 176).

Storage

Preparations containing propantheline are stored at room temperature.

PROPOFOL (Diprivan)

Presentation

Injection – 200 mg in 20 ml, 500 mg in 50 ml, 1 g in 100 ml, 1 g in 50 ml

Actions and uses

Propofol is an intravenous anaesthetic, commonly used because of its association with rapid recovery and negligible hangover effects. It has a rapid onset of action, having an effect within 30 seconds.

Dosage
Induction of anaesthesia by IV injection or infusion

- Adult: 1.5–2.5 mg/kg at a rate of 20–40 mg every 10 seconds.
- Child over 8 years: 2.5 mg/kg administered slowly until response. Can be given to younger children over 1 month of age (if 1% solution used; 2% solution can only be used for children over 3 years). Higher doses may be required. Administer slowly until response achieved.

Maintenance of anaesthesia

Adult.

- By IV injection: 25–50 mg repeated according to response.
- By IV infusion: 4–12 mg/kg/h

Child over 3 years.

- By IV injection or infusion: 9–15 mg/kg/h.

Sedation in intensive care

- Adult: IV infusion, 0.3–4 mg/kg/h.
- Not recommended for children under 16 years.

Sedation for surgical and diagnostic procedures (1% solution only)

- Adult: IV injection over 1–5 minutes, 0.5–1 mg/kg then IV infusion 1.5–4.5 mg/kg/h. If additional sedation is required, the dose can be topped up with 10–20 mg by IV injection.
- Not recommended for children.

Nursing implications

- Lower doses are generally required in patients over 55 years of age.
- Propofol is an oil-in-water emulsion so care must be taken if administered to patients with fat metabolism disorders and in those who may be receiving lipids through total parenteral nutrition.
- Delayed side effects can occur, especially convulsions, therefore special care must be taken when the drug is used in day surgery.
- Anaphylaxis has been reported and delayed recovery from anaesthesia. Bradycardia can occur but can be prevented by administration of an IV antimuscarinic.
- Like other general anaesthetics, propofol will cause increased hypotension if given concurrently with other blood pressure-lowering agents.

Storage

Propofol preparations are stored at room temperature.

PROPRANOLOL (Inderal)

Presentation

Tablets – 10 mg, 40 mg, 80 mg, 160 mg
Capsules (modified release) – 80 mg, 160 mg
Oral solution – 5 mg in 5 ml, 10 mg in 5 ml, 40 mg in 5 ml, 50 mg in 5 ml, 80 mg in 5 ml
Injection – 1 mg in 1 ml

Actions and uses

Propranolol is a non-selective beta-adrenoreceptor blocking drug. Its actions and uses are described under Beta-Adrenoreceptor Blocking Drugs (p. 51). It is used for hypertension, phaeochromocytoma, arrhythmias, anxiety, prophylaxis after myocardial infarction, migraine prophylaxis, essential tremor and thyrotoxicosis.

Dosage

- By intravenous injection in an emergency situation, up to 1 mg may be given over 1 minute. This can be repeated at 2-minute intervals to a maximum dose of 10 mg. Pulse, blood pressure and cardiac (ECG) monitoring must be continuous during the period of injection and injection must be stopped if profound bradycardia, hypotension or widening of the QRS complex occurs.
- Adult oral maintenance dosage ranges from 80 to 480 mg per day. In the treatment of hypertension, slow-release capsules are available and total dosage is given once daily. In the treatment of dysrhythmias and angina the dosage is usually divided and given twice, three or four times a day.

Nursing implications

See the section on Beta-Adrenoreceptor Blocking Drugs (p. 51).

Storage

Propranolol tablets, capsules and injection are stored at room temperature.

PROSTAGLANDIN E2
(Prostin E2, Dinoprostone)

Presentation

Tablets – 0.5 mg
Sterile solutions – 1 mg in 1 ml alcohol (0.75 ml ampoule), 10 mg in 1 ml alcohol (0.5 ml ampoule)

Actions and uses

Prostaglandin E2 has the capacity to induce contraction of the uterus.

It therefore has the following uses:

- the induction of labour
- termination of pregnancy
- the induction of labour in missed abortion
- treatment of hydatidiform mole.

Dosage

- For the induction of labour.
  - Orally: 0.5 mg initially and thereafter 1 mg at hourly intervals until an adequate uterine response has been achieved. Thereafter the dose may be reduced to 0.5 mg hourly.
  - Intravenously: 1 mg/ml solution in alcohol is diluted with 0.9% sodium chloride or 5% dextrose to produce a solution containing 1.5 microgram/ml. This is infused intravenously at a rate of 0.25 microgram/min for 30 minutes, the dose being subsequently maintained or increased according to patient response.
- For the termination of pregnancy or treatment of missed abortion or hydatidiform mole: a solution containing 5 microgram/ml is infused intravenously at a rate of 2.5 microgram/min for 30 minutes and then maintained or increased to 5 microgram/min. This higher concentration should be administered for at least 4 hours before further increases are made.
- For the termination of pregnancy: 1 ml of a solution containing 100 microgram/ml may be instilled extraamniotically through a suitable Foley catheter. Subsequent doses of 1 or 2 ml of the same concentration solution should be given at intervals usually of 2 hours according to uterine response.

Nursing implications
- Nausea, vomiting and diarrhoea occur commonly at doses required to terminate pregnancy by the intravenous route but are less common after the extra-amniotic route for termination. Such symptoms are rare when

the concentrations administered by the intravenous route for induction of labour are used.
- Transient cardiovascular symptoms have been noticed, including flushing, shivering, headache, dizziness.
- Very rarely convulsions and changes in the electro-encephalogram have occurred.
- Local tissue irritation or erythema may follow intravenous infusion. This will disappear within 2–5 hours of stopping the infusion.
- Infusion of this compound may occasionally lead to pyrexia.
- Uterine rupture has occurred only rarely with this substance.
- The drug should be used with caution in patients who have glaucoma or suffer from asthma.

Storage
- Prostaglandin preparations should be refrigerated.
- Once diluted, the solutions should be used within 24 hours.

PROTAMINE (Prosulf)

Presentation
Injection – 50 mg in 5 ml, 100 mg in 10 ml

Actions and uses
Protamine sulphate is a heparin antidote used to reverse the effects of heparin and restore the coagulation time of the blood in patients who are receiving heparin or have haemorrhaged due to an overdose of heparin. It acts by complexing with heparin sodium and heparin calcium, rendering the heparin inactive.

Dosage
1 mg neutralizes 80–100 units of heparin if given within 15 minutes of the heparin. Heparin is rapidly excreted, therefore lower doses of protamine are required the greater the time which has elapsed since heparin administration. Protamine should be administered by IV injection at a rate of 50 mg in approximately 10 minutes.

Nursing implications
- Side effects include nausea and vomiting, hypotension, bradycardia and dyspnoea. Hypersensitivity reactions have occurred.
- Ideally, the dosage used should be based on the patient's measured coagulation time.

Storage
Protamine injection is stored at room temperature.

PROTRIPTYLINE (Concordin)

Presentation
Tablets – 5 mg, 10 mg

Actions and uses
Protriptyline is a tricyclic antidepressant drug. Its actions and uses are described in the section on these drugs.

Dosage
For the treatment of depression in adults the total daily dose is 15–60 mg given in three divided doses.

Nursing implications
See the section on Antidepressant Drugs (p. 31).

Storage
Tablets containing protriptyline are stored at room temperature.

PYRAZINAMIDE (Zinamide)

Presentation
Tablets – 500 mg

Actions and uses
Pyrazinamide has been found to be effective against the organism *Mycobacterium tuberculosis* and is therefore used for the treatment of tuberculosis. Combination therapy is always used to treat tuberculosis and the choice of drugs used depends on a number of factors, including reducing the risk of resistance developing and patient compliance. Pyrazinamide is

commonly used in combination with isoniazid and rifampicin and is taken in the initial stages of treatment of tuberculosis. It is most effective against intracellular tuberculosis organisms.

Dosage

The recommended dosage is:

- adults, under 50 kg, 1.5 g daily; over 50 kg, 2 g daily
- child, 35 mg/kg daily.

Alternatively, pyrazinamide can be taken as part of an intermittent supervised regimen.

- Adults under 50 kg, 2 g three times a week; over 50 kg, 2.5 g three times a week.
- Child 50 mg/kg three times a week.

These doses are usually taken for the first 2 months of a 6-month treatment regimen.

Nursing implications

- Patients undergoing treatment for tuberculosis receive their drugs for considerable periods of time. The nurse may play an important role in reminding patients that their drug therapy must be taken regularly for as long as recommended by medical staff, whether or not they themselves feel that they have recovered.
- Common side effects experienced by patients on this drug include anorexia, nausea, vomiting, fever, tiredness, difficulty with micturition and arthralgia which may be due to gout (see below).
- Photosensitivity and skin rash may occur.
- The drug may affect concentration in the blood of uric acid and may precipitate attacks of joint pain due to gout.
- The main drawback to the drug's use is that it may cause serious disturbance of liver function. Patients should be advised of the signs of liver disorders, i.e. persistent nausea, malaise and jaundice, and report to their doctor immediately.

- The drug should be used with caution in patients with diabetes as loss of control has occurred when the drug has been introduced.
- The drug may occasionally cause some impairment of renal function.

Storage

The drug is stored at room temperature.

PYRIDOSTIGMINE (Mestinon)

Presentation

Tablets – 60 mg

Actions and uses

The actions of pyridostigmine are identical to those described for Neostigmine (p. 243). In clinical practice its principal use is in the management of myasthenia gravis, where it has the advantage over neostigmine of having a longer duration of action.

Dosage

For the treatment of myasthenia gravis.

- Adults: 30–120 mg 4–6 hourly according to individual response. Total daily dose usually 0.3–1.2 g, although doses above 720 mg daily are not advised.
- Neonates: 5–10 mg every 4 hours, 30–60 minutes before feeds.
- Child up to 6 years: start with 30 mg and titrate dose to response.
- Child 6–12 years: start with 60 mg and titrate dose to response.

Nursing implications

- The nursing implications of pyridostigmine are identical to those described for Neostigmine (p. 243).
- It is worth noting that in practice there are fewer problems with gastrointestinal upset with pyridostigmine as compared with neostigmine.

Storage

The drug is stored at room temperature.

PYRIMETHAMINE (Daraprim)

Presentation

Tablets – 25 mg

Actions and uses

Pyrimethamine is an antimalarial used, normally in combination with other drugs, in the prevention of malaria. In combination with sulfadoxine, it is not routinely used for the prophylaxis of malaria but rather for treating falciparum malaria, but in combination with chloroquine it is used for prophylaxis of malaria in areas of chloroquine-resistant falciparum malaria. It also possesses useful action against other parasitic organisms and is used in combination with a sulphonamide in the control of toxoplasmosis; this is an unlicensed use.

Dosage

For antimalarial prophylaxis (in combination with other drugs): seek expert advice on dosage schedules. Usual doses:

- adults and children over 10 years: 25 mg once a week
- children 5–10 years old: 12.5 mg each week
- child under 5 years: not recommended.

Nursing implications

- Always seek expert advice on recommendations for malaria prophylaxis as the regime used will depend on the country or region to be visited and any resistance to drug therapy in that area. Pyrimethamine is not considered to be a suitable prophylactic agent for travellers.
- Once-weekly administration for the suppression of malaria is not usually associated with side effects.
- Patients undergoing malaria prophylaxis must ensure that regular weekly doses are taken. It should be stressed that treatment must be continued for a period of 4 weeks after return from an area where malaria is endemic.
- With larger doses used in the treatment of toxoplasmosis, side effects may arise. These include megaloblastic anaemia, leucopenia, thrombocytopenia and aplastic anaemia. Very high doses have produced vomiting, convulsions and respiratory failure.

Storage

Tablets are stored at room temperature.

P

Q

QUETIAPINE (Seroquel)

Presentation
Tablets – 25 mg, 150 mg and 200 mg

Actions and uses
Quetiapine is an atypical antipsychotic agent used in the management of schizophrenia. It acts on several different receptors in the brain, having a high affinity for serotonin receptors, histamine receptors and alpha-1 adrenergic receptors.

Dosage
25 mg twice daily for 1 day, then 50 mg twice daily for 1 day, then 100 mg twice daily for 1 day, then 150 mg twice daily for 1 day then adjust dose according to response to a maximum of 750 mg daily in two divided doses. For elderly patients, start with 25 mg daily and increase by 25–50 mg daily.

Nursing implications
- Quetiapine may prolong the QT interval and therefore should be used with caution in patients with cardiovascular disease.
- Other side effects include headache, somnolence, dizziness, constipation, postural hypotension, and tachycardia. Occasionally neutropenia can occur.
- It should also be used with caution in pregnancy, epileptics and patients with Parkinson's disease.
- Quetiapine is contraindicated in breastfeeding.
- Phenytoin increases the metabolism of quetiapine.
- It should also be used with caution concurrently with other drugs which prolong the QT interval.

- Patients should be advised that drowsiness may occur so the ability to drive or operate machinery may be impaired.

Storage
Quetiapine tablets are stored at room temperature.

QUINAGOLIDE (Norprolac)

Presentation
Tablets – 25 microgram, 50 microgram, 75 microgram and 150 microgram

Actions and uses
Quinagolide is a dopamine D2 receptor agonist which inhibits the secretion of prolactin from the pituitary and is used to manage hyperprolactinaemia. It acts similarly to bromocriptine (p. 57) with similar contraindications and side effects.

Dosage
The daily dose should be taken at bedtime, starting with 25 microgram daily for 3 days. Increase the dose at intervals of 3 days by 25 microgram to a usual maintenance dose of 75–150 microgram daily.
It is not recommended for children.

Nursing implications
- Side effects with quinagolide are similar to those of bromocriptine (p. 57). Other side effects include syncope, anorexia, abdominal pain and diarrhoea.
- Hypotension can occur in the first few days of treatment; patients should be advised of this and recommended to take

precautions, especially when driving or operating machinery.
- If the patient is taking a hormonal contraceptive, she should be advised to use alternative non-hormonal precautions to avoid pregnancy.
- If pregnancy occurs during treatment, quinagolide should be discontinued.

Storage
Quinagolide tablets are stored at room temperature.

QUINALBARBITONE/ SECOBARBITAL (Seconal)

Presentation
Capsules – 50 mg, 100 mg

Actions and uses
Quinalbarbitone is a barbiturate drug which is taken at night as a hypnotic for patients already taking barbiturates.

Dosage
100 mg on retiring.

Nursing implications
Barbiturates are no longer favoured as hypnotics due to their abuse potential.

Storage
Quinalbarbitone capsules are stored at room temperature.

QUINAPRIL (Accupro)

Presentation
Tablets – 5 mg, 10 mg, 20 mg and 40 mg

Actions and uses
See section on ACE inhibitors (p. 4). Quinapril is used for essential hypertension and congestive heart failure.

Dosage
Hypertension: 2.5–80 mg daily; usual maintenance dose is 20–40 mg daily. Heart failure: 2.5–40 mg daily; usual maintenance dose is 10–20 mg daily.

Nursing implications
See section on ACE inhibitors (p. 4).

Storage
Quinapril tablets are stored at room temperature.

QUINIDINE (Kinidin)

Presentation
Tablets – 200 mg as sulphate
Modified-release tablets (Durules) containing 250 mg quinidine bisulphate

Actions and uses
Quinidine depresses heart function by reducing the excitability of the heart muscle and prolonging its refractory period. It is therefore useful in the treatment of cardiac dysrhythmias, particularly supraventricular and ventricular arrhythmias. It should only be used under specialist advice as quinidine itself can cause arrhythmias. Conventional tablets need to be taken in large and frequent dosage to maintain an effective blood level and it is therefore advantageous to use the sustained-release tablet to guarantee effectiveness of the drug.

Dosage
200–400 mg 3–4 times daily as conventional tablets or 500 mg to 1.25 g taken twice daily as modified-release tablets.
It should be noted that to avoid hypersensitivity all patients should be given a small test dose prior to commencement of the above regimes.

Nursing implications
- It is essential to give a small dose of quinidine to all patients prior to commencement of normal therapy to detect those who may be likely to suffer a hypersensitivity reaction. Symptoms which have been found to be associated with such hypersensitivity are as follows: tinnitus, vertigo, visual disturbance, headache, confusion, erythematous skin

Q

rashes, anorexia, nausea, vomiting, diarrhoea, chest pain, abdominal pain, fever, respiratory distress, cyanosis, hypotension and shock. Thrombocytopenic purpura has also occurred.
- Side effects which may occur in patients not hypersensitive to the drug include tinnitus, deafness, blurred vision, headache, dizziness and vomiting.
- Excess dosage of the drug may lead to cardiac arrhythmias including heart block, paroxysmal ventricular tachycardia, ventricular fibrillation and cardiac arrest. The nurse may play a vital role in their prevention by detecting such symptoms in patients on the drug and advising medical staff accordingly.
- There is an increased risk of arrhythmias if quinidine is taken concurrently with other antiarrhythmics, antidepressants, terfenadine, mefloquine and antipsychotics.
- If digoxin is given concurrently with quinidine, the digoxin dose should be halved.
- Verapamil and cimetidine increase plasma quinidine concentrations.
- Nifedipine decreases plasma quinidine concentrations.

Storage
Quinidine tablets are stored at room temperature.

QUININE

Presentation
Tablets (quinine sulphate) – 200 mg and 300 mg
Injection (quinine dihydrochloride) – 300 mg in 1 ml, 600 mg in 2 ml

Actions and uses
This drug is used for the treatment of falciparum malaria caused by *Plasmodium falciparum*. Once a second-choice drug for the treatment of malaria, it has returned to use as resistance to chloroquine has developed.
   It was noted that when quinine was used for malaria, it was effective in reducing painful night cramps suffered by a fair proportion of the older population. It continues to be used for this purpose.

Dosage
Malaria
Adults: orally, 600 mg (of quinine salt, hydrochloride, dihydrochloride or sulphate) every 8 hours for 7 days. By intravenous infusion in seriously ill patients, loading dose of 20 mg/kg (up to a maximum of 1.4 g) of quinine salt (as above) infused over 4 hours then, after 8–12 hours, maintenance dose of 10 mg/kg (up to a maximum of 700 mg) of quinine salt (as above) infused over 4 hours every 8–12 hours. Switch to oral treatment when the patient can take tablets.
Children: orally, 10 mg/kg (of quinine salt, hydrochloride, dihydrochloride or sulphate) every 8 hours for 7 days.

Night cramps
200–300 mg as a single dose on retiring.

Nursing implications
- Expert advice should be sought prior to administration of intravenous quinine.
- Certain individuals may prove hypersensitive to this drug and may suffer the following symptoms:
   - tinnitus, headache, visual disturbance and blindness
   - nausea and abdominal pain
   - skin rash
   - blood disorders including haemolytic anaemia and thrombocytopenia.
- It should be used with caution in atrial fibrillation, conduction defects, heart block and pregnancy.
- Quinine is contraindicated in haemoglobinuria and optic neuritis.
- There is an increased risk of ventricular arrhythmias if quinine is taken concurrently with amiodarone, terfenadine and pimozide.
- As quinine increases the plasma concentration of digoxin, the

digoxin dose may need to be decreased.

- Concurrent use with halofantrine should be avoided.
- Patients using quinine to treat leg cramps should be advised that it may take up to 4 weeks for any improvement to occur. Patients should be monitored for side effects during initiation of treatment and assessed every 3 months to determine if treatment should continue.

Storage

Quinine preparations are stored at room temperature.

Q

R

RABEPRAZOLE (Pariet)

Presentation
Tablets – 10 mg and 20 mg

Actions and uses
Like omeprazole, rabeprazole is a proton pump inhibitor, inhibiting gastric acid output. It is indicated for the treatment of benign gastric ulcer, gastrooesophageal reflux disease and duodenal ulcer.

Dosage
Adults only.

- Benign gastric ulcer: 20 mg daily in the morning for 6 or 12 weeks.
- Duodenal ulcer: 20 mg daily in the morning for 4 or 8 weeks.
- Gastrooesophageal reflux disease: 20 mg daily in the morning for 4–8 weeks continued at a maintenance dose of 10 mg or 20 mg daily if necessary.

Nursing implications
- Use with caution in liver disease, pregnancy and breastfeeding.
- Rabeprazole use may mask signs of gastric cancer.
- Adverse effects include gastrointestinal disturbances, headache and hypersensitivity.
- Reduced gastric acidity may increase the risk of gastrointestinal infections.

Storage
Rabeprazole tablets are stored at room temperature.

RALOXIFENE (Evista)

Presentation
Tablets – 60 mg

Actions and uses
Raloxifene is used for the prevention of vertebral fractures in post-menopausal women at increased risk of osteoporosis. This drug is a selective oestrogen receptor modulator (SERM) with a complex mode of action. It acts at oestrogen receptors throughout the body, affecting gene expression. Its principal action is to reduce bone resorption.

Dosage
60 mg daily

Nursing implications
- Side effects include venous thromboembolism, thrombo-phlebitis, hot flushes, leg cramps and peripheral oedema.
- Raloxifene is contraindicated in patients who have a history of venous thromboembolism. It should also not be used in patients with hepatic impairment, severe renal impairment, unexplained uterine bleeding or in patients who have endometrial or breast cancer, are pregnant or breastfeeding.
- Raloxifene does not reduce menopausal vasomotor symptoms.

Storage
Raloxifene tablets are stored at room temperature.

RALTITREXED (Tomudex)

Presentation
Injection – 2 mg powder in vial

Actions and uses
Raltitrexed is an antimetabolite. It is used for the palliative treatment of

advanced colorectal cancer for patients who have not tolerated, or where therapy was not appropriate with, 5-fluorouracil and folinic acid. This drug inhibits the action of the enzyme thymidylate synthase, thereby inhibiting the synthesis of thymidine triphosphate required for DNA synthesis. This action leads ultimately to cell death.

Dosage

Adults only, not recommended for children: 3 mg/m^2, IV given as an infusion in 50–250 ml of either sodium chloride 0.9% or dextrose 5% over 15 minutes. (Each 2 mg vial should be reconstituted with 4 ml of sterile water for injection prior to dilution with infusion fluid.) This dose should be repeated at intervals of 3 weeks depending on patient tolerance and toxicity.

Nursing implications

- Marked myelosuppression and gastrointestinal side effects can occur. Other side effects include altered liver function tests, rash, asthenia, fever and abdominal pain.
- Prior to each dose, patients must have a full blood count measured, liver transaminases, serum bilirubin and serum creatinine measurements performed. Dose reductions may be appropriate depending on the level of haematological and gastrointestinal toxicity. Seek expert advice.
- The dose should be reduced in renal impairment. Again, seek expert advice.
- Raltitrexed is contraindicated in severe renal impairment, pregnancy and breastfeeding.
- Do not give folinic acid or folic acid prior to or during treatment with raltitrexed.
- Nurses should be aware of the risks posed by cytotoxic drugs. Some are irritant to the skin and mucous surfaces and care must be exercised when handling them. In particular, spillage or contamination of personnel or the environment must be avoided. If cytotoxic drugs are handled regularly, it is theoretically possible that repeated skin contact or inhalation may produce systemic toxic effects in nurses who have developed hypersensitivity to them. Most hospitals now operate a centralized (pharmacy-organized) additive service. While this reduces the risk of exposure to cytotoxic drugs, it is essential that nurses recognize and understand the local policy on their safe handling and disposal. The Health and Safety Executive has decreed that such a policy should be in place wherever cytotoxic drugs are administered. These should be adapted, wherever possible, to care of patients in the community.

Storage

Unopened vials are stored at room temperature. Protect from light. Reconstituted vials should be stored in a refrigerator between 2 and 8°C. Discard 24 hours after reconstitution.

RAMIPRIL (Tritace)

Presentation

Tablets – 1.25 mg, 2.5 mg, 5 mg and 10 mg

Actions and uses

See section on ACE Inhibitors (p. 4). Ramipril is indicated for mild-to-moderate hypertension, congestive heart failure and following myocardial infarction in patients with heart failure.

Dosage

Range: 2.5–10 mg as a single daily dose or in two divided doses if being used as prophylaxis after myocardial infarction.

Nursing implications

See section on ACE Inhibitors (p. 4).

R

Storage

Ramipril tablets are stored at room temperature.

RANITIDINE (Zantac)

Presentation

Tablets – 75 mg, 150 mg, 300 mg (150 mg and 300 mg also available as effervescent tablets)
Syrup – 150 mg in 10 ml
Injection – 50 mg in 2 ml

Actions and uses

See Histamine H2-Receptor Antagonists (p. 169).

Dosage

Dosage for all indications is based on that used in the treatment of peptic ulceration, as follows.

Adults

- Oral, treatment: 300 mg daily, in two divided doses or as a single evening dose.
- Oral, maintenance: usually a single bedtime dose of 150 mg or 300 mg since it appears that overnight acid output is important in determining ulcer relapse rates.
- For Zollinger–Ellison syndrome higher doses are used, from 150 mg three times a day to as high as 6 g daily in divided doses.
- Injection: intramuscular therapy can be substituted for oral treatment when necessary, 50 mg every 6–8 hours. Intravenous bolus doses of 50 mg, diluted to 20 ml given over at least 2 minutes, repeated at intervals of 6–8 hours, or intravenous infusion in a dose of 50 mg given over 2 hours can be used in the acute stage. For the prophylaxis of stress ulceration, ranitidine can be given by slow IV injection of 50 mg (as above) followed by a continuous infusion of 125–250 microgram/kg/h until oral therapy can be started.
- For gastric acid reduction, in obstetrics, orally, 150 mg at onset of labour then every 6 hours; surgical procedures, slow IV (as above) or IM injection 50 mg, 45–60 minutes prior to induction of anaesthesia or orally, 150 mg 2 hours prior to induction of anaesthesia.

Children

Orally, 2–4 mg/kg twice daily up to a maximum daily dose of 300 mg.

Nursing implications

- The nursing implications described for Histamine H2-Receptor Antagonists apply (p. 169).
- Give intermittent ranitidine infusions in glucose 5%, sodium chloride 0.9% or compound sodium lactate.

Storage

Ranitidine preparations are stored at room temperature. The injection solution should be protected from light during storage.

RAZOXANE (Razoxin)

Presentation

Tablets – 125 mg

Actions and uses

Razoxane is a cytotoxic drug which prevents growth of malignant cells by interfering with the processes involved in cellular division. It can be used in the treatment of leukaemia, but is rarely used today.

Dosage

Acute leukaemia, 150–500 mg/m^2 for 3–5 days.

Nursing implications

- Common symptoms encountered with this drug include nausea, vomiting and diarrhoea.
- Skin rashes and alopecia may occur with this drug.
- When used in combination with radiotherapy, subcutaneous fibrosis, oesophagitis and pneumonitis may be produced.
- Nurses should be aware of the risks posed by cytotoxic drugs. Some are irritant to the skin and mucous surfaces and care must be exercised when handling them. In particular, spillage or contamination of personnel or the environment must be

avoided. If cytotoxic drugs are handled regularly, it is theoretically possible that repeated skin contact or inhalation may produce systemic toxic effects in nurses who have developed hypersensitivity to them. Most hospitals now operate a centralized (pharmacy-organized) additive service. While this reduces the risk of exposure to cytotoxic drugs, it is essential that nurses recognize and understand the local policy on their safe handling and disposal. The Health and Safety Executive has decreed that such a policy should be in place wherever cytotoxic drugs are administered. These should be adapted, wherever possible, to care of patients in the community.

Storage
Razoxane tablets are stored at room temperature. They should be protected from moisture and light.

REBOXETINE (Edronax)

Presentation
Tablets – 4 mg

Actions and uses
Reboxetine is a selective noradrenaline reuptake inhibitor indicated for the treatment of depression. See the section on Antidepressants (p. 31).

Dosage
4 mg twice daily increased if necessary after 3–4 weeks up to 10 mg daily in divided doses. Can be further increased to a maximum of 12 mg daily. Reboxetine is not recommended for children or elderly patients.

Nursing implications
- See the section on Antidepressants (p. 31).
- Side effects include dry mouth, constipation, insomnia, sweating, tachycardia, urinary hesitancy and retention and impotence.

- Reboxetine is contraindicated in pregnancy and breastfeeding.
- Use with caution in severe renal impairment, hepatic impairment, cardiovascular disease, epilepsy, bipolar disorder and glaucoma.
- Avoid concomitant use with macrolide antibiotics and imidazole and triazole antifungal agents.
- There is a risk of increased toxicity if reboxetine is taken concurrently with MAOIs. Do not start reboxetine until 2 weeks after stopping therapy with an MAOI and do not start an MAOI until 1 week after stopping reboxetine.

Storage
Reboxetine tablets are stored at room temperature.

REMIFENTANIL (Ultiva)

Presentation
Injection – 1 mg, 2 mg and 5 mg powders in vials

Actions and uses
Remifentanil is a narcotic analgesic indicated for use during induction and maintenance of general anaesthesia. For the action and uses of Narcotic Analgesics, see p. 238. Remifentanil differs from other narcotic agents in that it is not metabolized in the liver but by esterases in the blood and tissues. It has a short duration of action and can be given for prolonged periods at high doses without causing marked postoperative respiratory depression.

Dosage
Induction: IV infusion 0.5–1 microgram/kg/min (can be given as an initial bolus by IV injection of 20–250 microgram/ml solution, over not less than 30 seconds, at a dose of 1 microgram/kg).
Maintenance in ventilated patients: IV infusion 0.05–2 microgram/kg/min, adjusted according to response. Can be supplemented by IV injection every 2–5 minutes.

R

Maintenance in spontaneous respiration anaesthesia: IV infusion 40 nanogram/kg/min, adjusted according to response within range 25–100 nanogram/kg/min.
Not routinely recommended for use in children. Elderly patients (over 65 years) should initially receive half the normal adult dose, then titrate according to response.

Nursing implications
- See the section on Narcotic Analgesics (p. 238).
- Due to its short duration of action, a supplemental analgesic is required after stopping remifentanil infusions.
- Remifentanil can be reconstituted and diluted with: sterilized water for injection, 5% dextrose injection, 5% dextrose and sodium chloride 0.9% injection, 0.9% sodium chloride injection and 0.45% sodium chloride injection. For general anaesthesia, the recommended dilution is 50 microgram/ml.

Storage
Remifentanil vials are stored at room temperature.

REPAGLINIDE (Novonorm)

Presentation
Tablets – 500 microgram, 1 mg and 2 mg

Actions and uses
Repaglinide is a relatively new drug for the treatment of diabetes. It is a non-sulphonylurea hypoglycaemic agent which acts by stimulating insulin release from the pancreatic beta cells. It is indicated for non-insulin dependent diabetes which is uncontrolled by diet and exercise and can be given along with metformin if metformin alone has not controlled the diabetes.

Dosage
Start with a dose of 500 microgram 30 minutes before each main meal. Adjust dose at 1–2 weekly intervals, according to response, up to 4 mg as a single dose and to a maximum of

16 mg each day. Not recommended for children or adults over 75 years old.

Nursing implications
- Start with a dose of 1 mg before meals if switching from another hypoglycaemic agent.
- Repaglinide acts quickly and has a short duration, therefore timing of doses shortly before meals is important. If a meal is to be missed then the corresponding dose should be missed.
- Contraindications include diabetic ketoacidosis, severe renal or hepatic impairment, pregnancy and breastfeeding.
- Use with caution in mild-to-moderate renal impairment.
- Consider insulin therapy during concurrent illness or surgery.
- Side effects include gastrointestinal symptoms and hypersensitivity reactions.

Storage
Repaglinide tablets are stored at room temperature.

REPROTEROL (Bronchodil)

Presentation
Inhaler – 500 microgram per dose of metered aerosol

Actions and uses
This drug has a highly selective action on beta-2 receptors in bronchial smooth muscle, causing relaxation of muscle tone. It is used, therefore, for the treatment of reversible airways obstruction (bronchospasm) in asthma and other conditions such as bronchitis and emphysema.

Dosage
Adults and children over 6 years: one or two inhalations three times daily. More frequent, 3–6 hourly administration may be required to treat an acute attack.

Nursing implications
- Rarely, this drug may cause palpitation, tachycardia,

headache and fine muscle tremor.
- The drug should be used with caution in patients with heart disease manifest by rhythm disturbances, angina, hyper-thyroidism and hypertension.

Storage
- Reproterol preparations are stored at room temperature.
- Reproterol aerosols should never be punctured or incinerated after use.

RETEPLASE (Rapilysin)

Presentation
Injection – 10 units of powder per vial

Actions and uses
Reteplase is a fibrinolytic agent indicated for use in acute myocardial infarction. It acts by generating plasmin which degrades fibrin, the main component of thrombi, thus causing the breakdown of thrombi, i.e. dissolution of blood clots and removal of the blockage caused by the clot.

Dosage
IV injection of 10 units, administered over 2 minutes and repeated after 30 minutes. (Follow manufacturer's instructions on reconstitution.)

Nursing implications
- See the section on Alteplase (p. 20).
- Side effects include bleeding, nausea and vomiting.

Storage
Reteplase injection is stored at room temperature.

REVIPARIN (Clivarine)

Presentation
Injection – reviparin sodium 1432 IU anti-factor Xa activity per 0.25 ml

Actions and uses
Reviparin is a low molecular weight heparin licensed for the prevention of thrombosis and thromboembolism in patients undergoing surgery. For its actions and uses see the section on Dalteparin (p. 115).

Dosage
SC injection – 0.25 ml 2 hours prior to surgery, then 0.25 ml daily until the patient is fully mobile. It is usually given for 7 days.
Not recommended for children.

Nursing implications
- See the sections on Dalteparin and Heparin (p. 115).

RIFABUTIN (Mycobutin)

Presentation
Capsules – 150 mg

Actions and uses
This drug is a member of the rifamycin group and has the same actions and potential uses as those of rifampicin. In clinical practice rifabutin is most commonly indicated in the treatment of pulmonary tuberculosis and in other atypical mycobacterial infections. It has a special role in preventing MAC (*Mycobacterium avium/intracellulare* complex), a condition resembling Whipple's disease which causes extensive problems in AIDS patients and is very difficult to treat. Rifabutin prophylaxis may be commenced as soon as the CD4 lymphocyte count falls to below 0.2×10^9/litre.

Dosage
Adults (not recommended for children), treatment of pulmonary tuberculosis: 150–450 mg once daily administered in combination with other antituberculous therapy for at least 6 months.
Other non-tuberculous mycobacterial disease: 450–600 mg once daily in combination therapy for up to 6 months after negative cultures are obtained.
MAC prophylaxis in immunodeficiency: 300 mg once daily.

Nursing implications
The nursing implications on rifampicin (p. 316) also apply to this drug.

R

Storage

Rifabutin capsules are stored at room temperature.

RIFAMPICIN (Rifadin, Rimactane)

Rifampicin is also available in combination with isoniazid as Rifinah or Rimactazid.

Presentation

Capsules – 150 mg, 300 mg
Syrup – 100 mg in 5 ml
Injection – 600 mg powder in vial plus special solvent

Actions and uses

- Rifampicin is an antibacterial drug which is particularly effective against the tubercle bacillis (*Mycobacterium tuberculosis*). It has a bacteriostatic action, inhibiting further growth and replication of the organism at low dose, and a bactericidal action (killing the organisms) at high dosage. The drug is usually used in combination with other antituberculous agents for the prophylaxis and treatment of tuberculosis.
- The drug is used in combination with other antibiotics in the treatment of other infections including brucellosis, legionnaire's disease and serious staphylococcal infections.
- It is effective in the eradication of the organism *Neisseria meningitidis* (which causes bacterial meningitis) from the nasopharynx of carriers of the organism and it is also used to prevent the occurrence of meningococcal meningitis in patients who have been in close contact with a case or carrier.
- It is similarly used for prophylaxis of *Haemophilus influenzae* type B infection.

Dosage

Tuberculosis (in multiple drug regimen).

- Adults: 600 mg (450 mg if body weight under 50 kg) taken daily in a single dose. To ensure rapid and complete absorption, the drug should preferably be taken before meals.

- Children: 10 mg/kg as above.
- Taken for 6 months, combined with isoniazid and pyrazinamide and, if resistance suspected, with ethambutol and streptomycin.

Brucellosis, legionnaire's disease, staphyloccocal infection.

- Adults: orally or IV 600–1200 mg daily in two or four divided doses. (Rifampicin injection (used in severe infections) is first reconstituted with the solvent provided then further diluted in 250 ml (Rimactane) or 500 ml (Rifadin) sodium chloride 0.9% solution or glucose 5% or 10% solution and administered over 2–3 hours.)

Prophylaxis of meningococcal meningitis.

- Adults: 600 mg twice daily for 2 days.
- Children (over 3 months): 5 mg/kg (up to 1 year) or 10 mg/kg (1–12 years) twice daily for 2 days.

Haemophilus influenzae type B prophylaxis.

- Adults: 600 mg once daily for 4 days.
- Children 1–3 months: 10 mg/kg once daily for 4 days.
- Children over 3 months: 20 mg/kg once daily for 4 days (maximum 600 mg daily).

Nursing implications

- Patients undergoing treatment for tuberculosis receive their drugs for considerable periods of time. The nurse plays an important role in reminding patients that their drug therapy must be taken regularly for as long as recommended by medical staff, whether or not they themselves feel that they have recovered.
- As noted above, it is important that the drug should be administered prior to meals as it is rapidly and better absorbed if taken in this way.
- The drug is usually well tolerated but occasionally patients

experience gastrointestinal upset which may be manifest as anorexia, nausea, vomiting or diarrhoea.

- Rarely abnormal liver or kidney function may be detected in patients on this drug and regular blood tests are usually performed to detect the occurrence of this side effect.
- This drug may cause a reddish discolouration of urine, sputum and tears and to avoid potential worry and distress, patients should be warned to expect such an effect. In particular, patients should avoid use of soft contact lenses which might become permanently discoloured.
- Skin rashes and blood dyscrasias (leucopenia, thrombocytopenia or haemolytic anaemia) occasionally occur.
- Other rare side effects felt by the patient include dizziness, flushing, urticaria, oedema, muscle weakness and menstrual disturbance.
- Rifampicin is a potent inducer of the liver microsomal enzyme system, the consequence of which is the more rapid metabolism of certain drugs normally inactivated by the liver. Thus the actions of warfarin, theophylline, phenytoin, oral antidiabetic agents, antiarrhythmics and other drugs may be reduced in the presence of rifampicin.
- In particular, the action of the oral contraceptive pill can be impaired and breakthrough (mid-cycle) bleeding or even unexpected pregnancy may result. Patients should be advised on alternative contraception.
- There is no evidence that nursing meningitis patients increases the risk of infection to medical and nursing staff sufficient to warrant prophylaxis with rifampicin. This is reserved for family contacts.

Storage
The drug is stored at room temperature.

RILUZOLE (Rilutek)

Presentation
Tablets – 50 mg

Actions and uses
Riluzole should be used under specialist advice only in the management of motor neurone disease. It is used to extend life or the time to mechanical ventilation for patients with amyotrophic lateral sclerosis. The mode of action of this drug is unclear but it is thought that by its action on glutamate processes in the central nervous system, it helps to prevent cell death.

Dosage
50 mg twice daily in adults only.

Nursing implications
- Side effects include nausea and vomiting, asthenia, headache and abdominal pain.
- Riluzole is contraindicated in hepatic and renal impairment, pregnancy and breastfeeding.
- Neutropenia can occur; patients and their carers should be advised to seek immediate medical attention if signs of neutropenia arise, e.g. fever or sore throat.
- Dizziness or vertigo may affect ability to drive or carry out other skilled tasks so patients should be advised of this.

Storage
Riluzole tablets are stored at room temperature.

RISEDRONATE (Actonel)

Presentation
Tablets – 5 mg and 30 mg

Actions and uses
Risedronate is a bisphosphonate, indicated for the treatment of Paget's disease and established post-menopausal osteoporosis. It can also

R

be used for the prevention of osteoporosis in postmenopausal women with increased risk of osteoporosis and to maintain or increase bone mass in postmenopausal women undergoing long-term systemic corticosteroid therapy. It acts by inhibiting osteoclast activity, reducing bone resorption, increasing bone mass and reducing the fracture risk in osteoporosis. See also the section on Alendronate (p. 15).

Dosage

Paget's disease: 30 mg daily for 2 months.
Treatment and prevention of osteoporosis: 5 mg daily.
Not recommended for children.

Nursing implications
- See the section on Alendronate (p. 15).
- Oesophageal reactions have occurred in patients taking bisphosphonates so all patients should be advised to take their tablets whilst in an upright position, swallowed whole and followed with a full glass of water. Tablets should be taken at least 30 minutes before the first food of the day or at least 2 hours before or after food. If taken in the evening, take at least 30 minutes before going to bed.
- Side effects include gastrointestinal upsets, musculoskeletal pain, headache and rash.

Storage

Risedronate tablets are stored at room temperature.

RISPERIDONE (Risperdal)

Presentation

Tablets – 1 mg, 2 mg, 3 mg, 4 mg and 6 mg
Liquid – 1 mg in 1 ml

Actions and uses

Risperidone is an atypical antipsychotic agent licensed for acute and chronic psychoses. It is particularly useful in schizophrenia where positive and negative symptoms are present. It acts primarily at dopamine D2 receptors and at 5-hydroxytryptamine receptors.

Dosage

Commence with 2 mg in one or two divided doses on day 1, then 4 mg in one or two divided doses on day 2, with slower dose titration if necessary to a usual daily dose of 4–6 mg. Maximum daily dose is 16 mg, but doses above 10 mg daily are rarely used. For elderly patients or patients with impaired hepatic or renal function, commence with 500 microgram twice daily and increase in increments of 500 microgram twice daily to 1–2 mg twice daily. Not recommended for children under 15 years old.

Nursing implications
- Side effects include insomnia, agitation, anxiety and headache.
- Use with caution in cardiovascular disease, epilepsy and Parkinson's disease.
- Use lower doses in renal and hepatic impairment.
- Use with caution concurrently with drugs which prolong the QT interval.
- Carbamazepine can increase the metabolism of risperidone, reducing its plasma concentration.

Storage

Risperidone preparations are stored at room temperature. Once opened, the contents of the liquid bottle should be used within 3 months.

RITODRINE (Yutopar)

Presentation

Tablets – 10 mg
Injection – 10 mg in 1 ml

Actions and uses

Ritodrine is a beta-2 adrenoceptor agonist which has a direct action on the uterine smooth muscle, causing it to relax and therefore reducing contractions. It is used to prevent labour in the management of uncomplicated premature labour.

Dosage

For the treatment of uncomplicated premature labour, ritodrine is administered as soon as possible at the onset of labour as follows.

- Initially, 50 microgram/min by intravenous infusion in dextrose 5%. The infusion rate is increased gradually by 50 microgram/min every 10 minutes until the required response is obtained or the heart rate reaches 140 beats/min. This level of dosage is generally in the range 150–350 microgram/min. Intravenous infusions are continued for 12–48 hours after uterine contractions have ceased. If intravenous therapy is not possible, 10 mg ritodrine every 3–8 hours may be given by intramuscular injection and continued for 12–48 hours as above.
- Maintenance: oral ritodrine is started about 30 minutes before intravenous therapy is completed. Up to 10 mg every 2 hours is given for the initial 24 hours and reduced thereafter to 10–20 mg or less, 4–6 hourly depending upon response or the presence of troublesome side effects. The total oral dose must not exceed 120 mg/day. Oral therapy is continued for as long as it is required to prolong pregnancy, although it is not recommended, as prolonged therapy with ritodrine for more than 48 hours puts the mother at increased risk of side effects.

Nursing implications

- The drug may affect maternal pulse rate, leading to tachycardia and palpitations. The nurse may play an important role in titrating intravenous infusion dosage and preventing excess administration of the drug. It is important to note that a maternal tachycardia of up to 140 beats/min is generally acceptable in a healthy patient.

- Other side effects seen with this drug are flushing, sweating, tremor, nausea and vomiting.
- Extremely careful patient monitoring is essential in patients who have heart disease or for those who are receiving other drugs which may increase or reduce the response to ritodrine, e.g. monoamine oxidase inhibitors, tricyclic antidepressants and other drugs which stimulate the sympathetic nervous system and beta-adrenoreceptor blockers.
- It should be noted that the drug should be used with great care in patients on corticosteroid drugs as the risk of pulmonary oedema increases.
- The drug should be avoided or used with great caution in the following situations:
  - antepartum haemorrhage requiring immediate delivery
  - eclampsia and severe preeclampsia
  - intrauterine infection
  - intrauterine fetal death
  - maternal cardiac disease
  - cord compression
  - placenta praevia.
- It is important to note that the drug is much less effective if the membranes have been ruptured or if the cervix has dilated greater than 4 cm.

Storage

Ritodrine tablets and injection solution are stored at room temperature though they should be protected from light. Deterioration of the injection is evident if the solution is discoloured or if a precipitate has appeared in the solution. Solutions with any evidence of deterioration should be immediately discarded.

RITONAVIR (Norvir)

Presentation

Capsules – 100 mg
Oral solution – 400 mg in 5 ml

Actions and uses

Ritonavir is indicated for use in combination with other antiretroviral agents to treat patients with the HIV infection. It is a protease inhibitor, acting on the HIV protease enzyme to prevent the production of essential proteins.

Dosage

Adult: 600 mg every 12 hours. Child over 2 years: start with $250\,mg/m^2$ every 12 hours, increasing gradually by $50\,mg/m^2$ at intervals of 2–3 days to a dose of $350\,mg/m^2$ every 12 hours (maximum dose of 600 mg every 12 hours).

Nursing implications

- Treatment of HIV is expensive and the drugs can cause serious side effects, so they should be prescribed only under expert advice.
- The timing of commencement of therapy should be decided by those expert in the management of HIV and depends on symptoms, viral load and the CD4 count and should be weighed against drug toxicities and the likely development of drug resistance.
- Resistance to antiretroviral drugs is reduced by using combination therapy.
- Most antiretroviral agents are used in pregnancy although teratogenic effects are not yet fully understood. Mothers are advised not to breastfeed their infants as HIV can pass from mother to infant via the breast milk.
- Side effects include taste disturbances, nausea, diarrhoea and perioral tingling.
- Lipidodystrophy can be a problematic side effect; body fat redistribution can occur as can hyperlipidaemia, insulin resistance and diabetes mellitus.
- Do not use in severe hepatic impairment.
- Ritonavir interacts with a variety of drugs. In the liver, it is metabolized by the cytochrome P450 enzyme CYP3A and it also inhibits the action of this enzyme. Potentially hazardous interactions include an increase in the plasma concentration of amfebutamone, some opioid analgesics (e.g. dextropropoxyphene and pethidine) and some NSAIDS (e.g. piroxicam), amiodarone and other antiarrhythmics, rifabutin, clarithromycin, warfarin, ketoconazole, terfenadine, some anxiolytics (e.g. diazepam) and sildenafil.
- Ritonavir reduces the plasma concentration of theophylline and there is an increased risk of myopathy if ritonavir is taken concurrently with simvastatin.
- Importantly, ritonavir interacts with other antiretroviral agents; if used in combination with nelfinavir there may be an increased concentration of either drug. If used in combination with amprenavir, there may be an increased concentration of both drugs. Ritonavir increases the plasma concentration of indinavir and saquinavir and there is an increased risk of toxicity with efavirenz. Some of these interactions can be beneficial if prescribed appropriately.
- It is also important to advise women on the combined oral contraceptive pill that additional contraceptive measures should be taken as ritonavir may interfere with the pill's metabolism.

Storage

Ritonavir capsules are stored in a refrigerator. However, once dispensed, they can be stored at room temperature but must be used within 30 days of dispensing.

Ritonavir oral solution is stored at room temperature but again should be used within 30 days of dispensing. It must not be refrigerated. The solution should be shaken before use. If after shaking, particles or a precipitate are seen, a fresh supply should be obtained.

R

RITUXIMAB (Mabthera)

Presentation
Injection – 100 mg in 10 ml and 500 mg in 50 ml

Actions and uses
Rituximab is a monoclonal antibody indicated for relapsed or chemoresistant stage III–IV follicular lymphoma. It acts principally to cause lysis of B lymphocytes.

Dosage
Rituximab should only be administered in hospital under the supervision of experienced oncologists or haematologists. Product literature should be followed as regards administration.

Used as a single agent, the recommended adult dose is 375 mg/m^2 body surface area given as an IV infusion weekly for 4 weeks.

Nursing implications
- This drug should only be used under specialist advice and after fully consulting the product literature.
- Full resuscitation equipment must be at hand during the administration of this drug.
- Infusion-related side effects include cytokine release syndrome characterized by severe dyspnoea, bronchospasm and hypoxia. Other side effects include fever and chills, nausea and vomiting, allergic reactions including rash and angiooedema, flushing and tumour pain. These effects are common, particularly with the first infusion.
- Prior to each dose of rituximab, the patient should be given an analgesic, e.g. paracetamol, and an antihistamine, e.g. diphenhydramine, and use of a corticosteroid should be considered.
- Stop the infusion if adverse effects occur; these must be treated before the infusion is restarted.
- Use with caution in patients with a history of cardiovascular disease.
- Use with extreme caution in those with a high tumour burden or pulmonary insufficiency or infiltration as these patients are at increased risk of cytokine release syndrome.

Storage
Rituximab injection is stored in a refrigerator between 2 and 8°C. Protect from direct sunlight. Prepared infusion solutions are stable for 12 hours at room temperature or 24 hours if stored in a refrigerator.

RIVASTIGMINE (Exelon)

Presentation
Capsules – 1.5 mg, 3 mg, 4.5 mg and 6 mg

Actions and uses
Rivastigmine is an acetylcholinesterase inhibitor indicated for mild-to-moderate dementia in Alzheimer's disease. It acts by slowing down acetylcholine degradation, thereby facilitating cholinergic neurotransmission in the CNS, leading to enhanced cognition.

Dosage
Start with 1.5 mg twice daily, increase according to response and tolerability by 1.5 mg twice daily at intervals of at least 2 weeks. Usual dosage range is 3–6 mg twice daily with a maximum dose of 6 mg twice daily.

Nursing implications
- Side effects include weakness, anorexia, dizziness, nausea and vomiting and somnolence, with gastrointestinal effects occurring more commonly in women.
- Rivastigmine should be used with caution in renal and hepatic impairment, sick sinus syndrome and conduction abnormalities and in those with gastric or duodenal ulcers. Also use with caution in patients with asthma or obstructive pulmonary disease.

R

Storage

Rivastigmine capsules are stored at room temperature.

RIZATRIPTAN (Maxalt)

Presentation

Tablets – 5 mg and 10 mg
Wafers – 10 mg

Actions and uses

Rizatriptan is a 5-hydroxytryptamine (5-HT1) agonist, similar to sumatriptan. It is used in the treatment of acute migraine attacks. Acting at 5-HT1 receptors, it causes vascular contraction in intracranial blood vessels, reversing any dilatation or oedema in these vessels which is thought to cause migraine attacks.

Dosage

Adults only: 10 mg should be taken as soon as possible after the onset of an attack. A second dose can be taken 2 hours after the first, only if symptoms recur after an initial response. Maximum of 20 mg should be taken in 24 hours.

Nursing implications

- See Sumatriptan (p. 344).
- Halve the usual dose in patients who take propranolol and rizatriptan should not be taken within 2 hours of taking propranolol.
- Do not use for patients who have had previous cerebrovascular accidents or transient ischaemic attacks or in those who have peripheral vascular disease.

Storage

Rizatriptan preparations are stored at room temperature.

ROCURONIUM (Esmeron)

Presentation

Injection – 50 mg in 5 ml

Actions and uses

Rocuronium is a muscle relaxant of the non-depolarizing type. Thus it reversibly paralyses skeletal muscle by competitive inhibition of acetylcholine, the transmitter substance released at the junction of the (motor) nerve and muscle fibre (motor endplate receptor). Drugs of this type are used to produce muscle relaxation during surgical anaesthesia.

Rocuronium has an intermediate duration of action when compared with other drugs in its class but its onset of action is very fast, becoming effective within 2 minutes.

Dosage

Adults and children (not neonates).

- IV injection: for intubation, 600 microgram/kg, then 150 microgram/kg as maintenance.
- IV infusion: 300–600 microgram/kg/h after initial IV injection of 600 microgram/kg.

Nursing implications

- All patients must have their respiration assisted or controlled.
- Overdosage with muscle relaxant drugs of this type may result in paralysis of the respiratory muscles. If this occurs, an anticholinesterase such as neostigmine (which potentiates acetylcholine by blocking its inactivation) must be administered.

Storage

Rocuronium injection is stored at 2–8°C protected from light.

ROFECOXIB (Vioxx)

Presentation

Tablets – 12.5 mg and 25 mg
Suspension – 12.5 mg in 5 ml and 25 mg in 5 ml

Actions and uses

This drug is a NSAID indicated for the symptomatic relief of osteoarthritis. Unlike most other NSAIDs which inhibit the actions of cyclooxygenase-1 (COX-1) and COX-2, rofecoxib inhibits COX-2 only, at least at therapeutic doses. It does not inhibit the actions of COX-1 therefore the risks of gastrointestinal complications are reduced but not totally diminished. Gastrointestinal adverse effects can still occur and rofecoxib is contraindicated in patients at risk of gastrointestinal perforations, ulcers or bleeds. For further information on the actions and uses of NSAIDs, see the section on p. 250.

Dosage

Adults only: 12.5 mg daily, increased if necessary to 25 mg daily.

Nursing implications
- See the section on NSAIDs (p. 250).
- Side effects include mouth ulcers, chest pain, weight gain, sleep disturbance and depression.
- Do not use if creatinine clearance is less than 30 ml/min or in inflammatory bowel disease or severe congestive heart failure.

Storage

Rofecoxib preparations are stored at room temperature.

ROPINIROLE (Requip)

Presentation

Tablets – 250 microgram, 1 mg, 2 mg and 5 mg

Actions and uses

Ropinirole acts as an agonist at dopamine-D2 receptors and is indicated for use in Parkinson's disease as either monotherapy or in combination with levodopa.

Dosage

Start with 250 microgram three times a day. Increase at weekly intervals by increments of 750 microgram daily (i.e. week 2, 500 microgram three times a day, etc.) up to 3 mg daily. Thereafter adjust dose according to response, with increments of up to 3 mg daily, at weekly intervals. Maximum daily dose is 24 mg.

Nursing implications
- Side effects are similar to those seen with bromocriptine, but

---

also include leg oedema, abdominal pain and syncope. Drowsiness and sudden onset of sleep can occur. Patients should be advised of this and avoid operating machinery or driving.
- Do not use in hepatic or severe renal impairment, pregnancy or breastfeeding. Use with caution in severe cardiovascular disease and major psychotic disorders.
- When given concurrently with levodopa, the levodopa dose can be reduced by approximately 20%.
- There is the potential for certain drug interactions. Neuroleptics may reduce the effects of ropinirole. It is metabolized in the liver and may interact with other substrates of the cytochrome P450 enzyme CYP1A2, e.g. theophylline and ciprofloxacin. Oestrogens can increase plasma concentrations of ropinirole. Dosage adjustment may be required if HRT is started or stopped during treatment with ropinirole.

Storage

Ropinirole tablets are stored at room temperature. Protect from light.

ROPIVACAINE (Naropin)

Presentation

Injection ampoules – 20 mg in 10 ml, 75 mg in 10 ml, 100 mg in 10 ml
Infusion bags for epidural administration – 200 mg in 100 ml, 400 mg in 200 ml

Actions and uses

Ropivacaine is a local anaesthetic similar to lignocaine. It blocks local nerve pulses by reversibly reducing the membrane permeability of nerve fibres to sodium ions, increasing the excitability threshold of the nerve.

Dosage

Surgical anaesthesia.
Lumbar epidural: 15–20 ml of the 10 mg in 1 ml solution or 15–25 ml of the 7.5 mg in 1 ml solution

R

Caesarean section: 15–20 ml of the
7.5 mg in 1 ml solution
Thoracic epidural: 5–15 ml of the
7.5 mg in 1 ml solution
Major nerve block: 30–40 ml of the
7.5 mg in 1 ml solution
Field block: up to 30 ml of the 7.5 mg
in 1 ml solution

Acute pain.
Lumbar epidural: using the 2 mg in
1 ml solution, 10–20 ml followed by
10–15 ml at intervals of at least
30 minutes or 6–10 ml per hour as a
continuous infusion, given epidurally
for labour pain, or 6–14 ml per hour as
a continuous epidural infusion for
postoperative pain.
Thoracic epidural: continuous infusion
of 6–14 ml per hour of the 2 mg in
1 ml solution
Field block: up to 100 ml of the 2 mg
in 1 ml solution

Nursing implications
The nursing implications of
Bupivacaine (p. 60) apply to this
drug.

Storage
Ropivacaine preparations are stored at
room temperature.

ROSIGLITAZONE (Avandia)

Presentation
Tablets – 4 mg and 8 mg

Actions and uses
Rosiglitazone is a relatively new oral
antidiabetic agent. It is a
thiazolidinedione which acts by
reducing insulin resistance at adipose
tissue, skeletal muscle and in the liver.
Rosiglitazone is licensed for use in type II
diabetes in combination with other
oral hypoglycaemic agents. It can be
used with metformin in obese patients
or with a sulphonylurea in patients
with an intolerance or contraindication
to metformin. It is reserved for use
only when the diabetes is inadequately
controlled by maximal tolerated doses
of either metformin or sulphonylureas
alone.

Dosage
Adults only. Start with 4 mg daily in
one or two divided doses. Higher
doses are not used if it is taken in
combination with a sulphonylurea but
if it is taken in combination with
metformin, the daily dose can be
increased to 8 mg after 8 weeks
if required to improve glycaemic
control.

Nursing implications
- Side effects include anaemia,
  hypo- and hyperglycaemia,
  weight gain, headache,
  gastrointestinal upsets and
  fatigue.
- Do not use in hepatically impaired
  patients, those with severe renal
  impairment (use with caution
  in mild-to-moderate renal
  impairment) or a history of heart
  failure.
- Rosiglitazone should not be used
  in combination with insulin. It
  should also be used with caution
  in combination with paclitaxel, as
  metabolism of rosiglitazone may
  be impaired.
- Discontinue treatment if there are
  any signs of heart failure such as
  worsening fluid retention.
- Patients should have liver function
  tests performed before treatment
  commences, every 2 months
  during the first year of treatment
  and periodically thereafter.

Storage
Rosiglitazone tablets are stored at
room temperature.

S

SALBUTAMOL
(e.g. Ventolin, Volmax)

Presentation

Tablets – 2 mg, 4 mg
Modified-release tablets and
capsules – 4 mg, 8 mg
Oral solution – 2 mg in 5 ml
Injection – 500 microgram in 1 ml,
250 microgram in 5 ml, 5 mg in 50 ml,
5 mg in 5 ml (for intravenous infusion)
Metered dose inhaler – 100
microgram/metered inhalation
Autohaler – 100 microgram/
metered dose
Breath actuated inhaler – 100
microgram per dose
Dry powder for inhalation – 95
microgram/metered inhalation
(Clickhaler), disks containing 200
microgram or 400 microgram per
blister (Diskhaler); also Accuhaler
with disks containing 200 microgram
per blister
Rotacaps – 200 microgram, 400
microgram
Nebules – 2.5 mg in 2.5 ml, 5 mg in
2.5 ml
Respirator solution – 100 mg in 20 ml

Actions and uses

This drug stimulates receptors known
as beta-2 adrenergic receptors, the
effect of which is to relax bronchial
muscle and relieve bronchospasm.
Salbutamol is therefore used for the
acute and chronic relief of
bronchospasm in asthma and other
conditions such as chronic bronchitis,
where reversible airways obstruction
has been shown to exist.
It has an additional use in that it
may be given by intravenous infusion
for the management of premature
labour. In this case the beta-2
adrenergic stimulant action reduces
contraction of uterine muscle.

Dosage
For asthma and other conditions associated with reversible airways obstruction

Orally.

- Adult: 4 mg three or four times
  daily.
- Child under 2 years: 100
  microgram/kg four times a day
  (unlicensed).
- Child 2–6 years: 1–2 mg three or
  four times daily.
- Child 6–12 years: 2 mg three or
  four times daily.
- Child over 12 years: 2–4 mg three
  or four times daily.
- (Modified-release preparations are
  taken twice daily.)

Inhalation by aerosol.

- Adult: 100–200 microgram as
  required or for persistent
  symptoms, three or four times daily.
  For prophylaxis in exercise-induced
  bronchospasm, 200 microgram.
- Child: as above, but use 200
  microgram only when necessary
  and 100 microgram for prophylaxis.

Inhalation by powder.

- Adult: 200–400 microgram as
  required or three or four times daily
  for persistent symptoms. For
  prophylaxis in exercise-induced
  bronchospasm, 400 microgram.
- Child: as above using 200
  microgram. For prophylaxis in
  exercise-induced bronchospasm,
  200 microgram.

Inhalation by nebulized solution.

- The nebulized solution is used in
  severe acute asthma and where
  chronic bronchospasm has proved
  unresponsive to conventional
  therapy.

S

- Adults and children over 18 months: 2.5 mg up to four times a day, increased to 5 mg if required.

SC or IM injection.

- 500 microgram every 4 hours if required.

Slow IV injection.

- 250 microgram repeated if required.

IV infusion.

- Adult: start with 5 microgram/min, adjust according to response and heart rate to a normal range of 3–20 microgram/min.
- Child 1 month–12 years: 0.1–1 microgram/kg/min (unlicensed).
- For infusion, dilute in glucose 5% or sodium chloride 0.9%, 5 mg in 500 ml.

For the treatment of premature labour

An intravenous infusion is administered at a rate of 10–45 microgram/min and adjusted to control uterine contractions. It is usual to commence with a rate of 10 microgram/min and increase accordingly. Once uterine contractions have ceased the infusion rate should be maintained for 1 hour and then reduced by 50% decrements at 6-hourly intervals. (Dilute with glucose 5% to a concentration of 200 microgram/ml for use with a syringe pump or 20 microgram/ml for infusion by other methods.) Treatment may be continued orally with tablets, 4 mg given three or four times daily.

Nursing implications
- Common side effects include fine muscle tremor, palpitations, tachycardia, flushing and headache.
- Hypokalaemia can occur if salbutamol is taken in large doses. Extra caution is required when given with other drugs which can cause hypokalaemia, e.g. theophylline and corticosteroids.
- The drug should be used with caution in patients who have

heart disease manifest by rhythm disturbance or angina, hyperthyroidism and hypertension.
- Intramuscular use of the undiluted injection produces slight pain and stinging.
- In the management of premature labour intravenous infusion of salbutamol has occasionally caused nausea, vomiting and headache.

Storage
Preparations of salbutamol are stored at room temperature. Preparations should be protected from light. Aerosols should never be punctured or incinerated after use.

SALMETEROL (Serevent)

Presentation
Metered dose inhaler – 25 microgram/metered inhalation
Dry powder for inhalation – disks containing 50 microgram per blister (Diskhaler)
Breath-actuated inhaler – 50 microgram per dose (Accuhaler)

Actions and uses
Salmeterol is a long-acting beta-2 adrenoceptor stimulant with actions and uses similar to those of salbutamol. However, it is not indicated for the relief of an acute attack of asthma. It is inhaled twice daily by patients with reversible airways obstruction. Salmeterol is used along with regular antiinflammatory therapy, e.g. corticosteroids, and with a short-acting beta-2 adrenoceptor stimulant, e.g. salbutamol, inhaled as required.

Dosage
Adult: 50–100 microgram twice daily.
Child over 4 years: 50 microgram twice daily.

Nursing implications
- See Salbutamol above.
- Patients should be reminded that salmeterol is not for use in an acute attack.

- Patients should also be advised not to exceed the prescribed dose and if this proves to be inadequate, this should be reported to the doctor immediately.

Storage
Salmeterol preparations are stored at room temperature.

SAQUINAVIR (Fortovase, Invirase)

Presentation
Capsules – 200 mg

Actions and uses
Saquinavir is indicated for use in combination with other antiretroviral agents to treat patients with the HIV infection. It is a protease inhibitor, acting on the HIV protease enzyme to prevent the production of essential proteins.

Dosage
Adults and children over 16 years.

- Fortovase: 1.2 g every 8 hours.
- Invirase: 600 mg every 8 hours (used in combination with ritonavir).

Nursing implications
- Treatment of HIV is expensive and the drugs can cause serious side effects so they should be prescribed only under expert advice.
- The timing of commencement of therapy should be decided by those expert in the management of HIV and depends on symptoms, viral load and the CD4 count and should be weighed against drug toxicities and the likely development of drug resistance.
- Resistance to antiretroviral drugs is reduced by using combination therapy.
- Most antiretroviral agents are used in pregnancy although teratogenic effects are not yet fully understood. Mothers are advised not to breastfeed their infants as HIV can pass from mother to infant via the breast milk.
- Saquinavir must be taken within 2 hours after a meal.
- There are two different preparations of saquinavir and it is important that patients keep to the same preparation. Preparations should be prescribed by brand.
- The main side effects are nausea and diarrhoea; mouth ulcers and other gastrointestinal symptoms can also occur.
- Lipidodystrophy can be a problematic side effect; body fat redistribution can occur as can hyperlipidaemia, insulin resistance and diabetes mellitus.
- Do not use in severe liver impairment.
- Saquinavir has the potential to interact with several drugs, particularly as it inhibits a major enzyme involved in drug metabolism. Saquinavir itself is also metabolized by major enzymes in the liver. Use with caution with the following drugs: rifamycins, antiepileptics, terfenadine, pimozide, midazolam, dexamethasone, ergotamine and simvastatin. Importantly, saquinavir interacts with other antiretroviral agents; nevirapine and efavirenz reduce the plasma concentration of saquinavir, indinavir and ritonavir increase the plasma concentration of saquinavir and if saquinavir is used in combination with nelfinavir there may be an increased plasma concentration of either drug. Some of these interactions can be beneficial if prescribed appropriately.
- It is also important to advise women on the combined oral contraceptive pill that additional contraceptive measures should be taken as saquinavir may interfere with the pill's metabolism.

S

Storage
Saquinavir preparations are stored at room temperature.

SELEGILINE (Eldepryl, Zelapar)

Presentation
Tablets – 5 mg and 10 mg
Freeze-dried tablets – 1.25 mg
Syrup – 10 mg in 5 ml

Actions and uses
Selegiline, by complex actions in the brain, potentiates the action of levodopa (in Madopar and Sinemet) in the treatment of Parkinson's disease. It primarily acts by inhibiting the enzyme monoamine oxidase-B, thereby preventing the breakdown of dopamine. Selegiline is generally used in conjunction with levodopa, but can be used on its own in the early stages of Parkinson's disease.

Dosage
- Adults: initially 5 mg once daily, increased to 5 mg in the morning and at lunchtime if necessary.
- A 1.25 mg freeze-dried tablet is equivalent to 10 mg of conventional selegiline tablets. One 1.25 mg tablet is taken each morning before breakfast.

Nursing implications
- Selegiline is used in conjunction with Madopar or Sinemet (or levodopa alone) and it should be noted that a reduction in dosage of these drugs is often possible. The nurse must therefore be vigilant for the occurrence of levodopa side effects which indicate the need to reduce levodopa dosage.
- Selegiline should not be stopped abruptly as this may exacerbate symptoms.
- Lower starting doses are often used in the elderly to avoid initial confusion and agitation.
- Side effects include gastrointestinal symptoms, dry mouth, stomatitis, sore throat, hypotension and sleeping disorders.

- Avoid concomitant use with pethidine as hyperpyrexia and CNS toxicity can occur.
- Also use with caution concomitantly with antidepressants and follow manufacturer's guidelines.

Storage
Selegiline tablets are stored at room temperature.

SENNA (Senokot)

Presentation
Tablets – 7.5 mg
Granules – 15 mg in 5 ml
Syrup – 15 mg in 10 ml

Actions and uses
Senna, an anthraquinone, is a stimulant laxative having an irritant effect on the gut wall. It is used for the treatment of constipation, acting 8–12 hours after the dose is taken.

Dosage
Adults: 15–30 mg taken as a single dose at bedtime.
Children: 2–6 years, one-quarter of the adult dose; over 6 years, one half of the adult dose, under the advice of a doctor.

Nursing implications
- These preparations should be used with caution in pregnancy and with children.
- Patients should be advised to take senna with an adequate fluid intake and that such preparations will take effect within 8–12 hours.
- The granular form of this drug may be stirred into hot milk, sprinkled on food or eaten plain and as it is more acceptable to the patient, better compliance may be achieved.
- Because of its irritant effect on the bowel it may produce cramping abdominal pain. Avoid in intestinal obstruction.

S

Storage

Preparations containing senna are stored at room temperature. Liquid preparations are sensitive to light and should be kept in amber bottles. Granules should be kept in a closed, airtight container since they may absorb moisture from the air.

SERTRALINE (Lustral)

Presentation

Tablets – 50 mg and 100 mg

Actions and uses

Sertraline is a selective serotonin reuptake inhibitor used in the treatment and prevention of depression and any accompanying anxiety. It can also be used for obsessive-compulsive disorder. See the section on Antidepressants (p. 31) for further information on actions and uses.

Dosage

50 mg to 200 mg daily. Increase dose gradually over several weeks. Not recommended for children.

Nursing implications

- See the section on Antidepressants (p. 31).
- Side effects include gastrointestinal symptoms, anorexia, dyspepsia, tremor, dizziness, insomnia, somnolence, increased sweating, dry mouth, sexual dysfunction and menstrual irregularity.

Storage

Sertraline tablets are stored at room temperature.

SEVELAMER (Renagel)

Presentation

Capsule – 403 mg

Actions and uses

Sevelamer is a phosphate binder recently introduced for use where hyperphosphataemia occurs in haemodialysis patients.

Dosage

The dose used will depend on plasma phosphate concentrations but is generally in the range of 6–12 capsules daily in divided doses, taken with meals. It is not recommended for use in children.

Nursing implications

Do not use in bowel obstruction and avoid in pregnancy, breastfeeding and gastrointestinal disorders.

Storage

Sevelamer capsules are stored at room temperature.

SILDENAFIL (Viagra)

Presentation

Tablets – 25 mg, 50 mg and 100 mg

Actions and uses

Sildenafil has been recently introduced as the first oral preparation for use in erectile dysfunction. It works when the patient is already sexually stimulated. Sildenafil acts by inhibiting a specific phosphodiesterase enzyme (which breaks down cyclic guanosine monophosphate), enhancing the relaxant effects of nitric oxide, facilitating smooth muscle relaxation in the penis and an inflow of blood, thus restoring impaired erectile function.

Dosage

Sildenafil is taken as a single dose, initially 50 mg 1 hour before sexual activity. This dose can be adjusted according to response between 25 and 100 mg. Elderly patients should start on 25 mg. Only one dose should be taken a day with a maximum single dose of 100 mg.

Nursing implications

- Side effects include headache, flushing, dyspepsia and altered vision.
- The onset of sildenafil's therapeutic effect may be delayed if it is taken with food.

S

- Sildenafil is contraindicated in patients taking nitrates or in those where sexual activity would be inadvisable, e.g. recent stroke or myocardial infarction.
- Use with caution in those with cardiovascular disease, deformation of the penis or a predisposition to prolonged erection. Avoid use in severe hepatic impairment and use low dose in renal impairment and mild-to-moderate hepatic impairment.
- Do not use concomitantly with nitrates or nicorandil as their hypotensive effects are significantly enhanced.
- Do not use with ritonavir, as plasma sildenafil concentrations can be significantly increased. 25 mg should be used initially in patients taking other protease inhibitors.
- Nurses are advised to check local policies and current legislation regarding prescribing of sildenafil.

Storage

Sildenafil tablets are stored at room temperature.

SIMVASTATIN (Zocor)

Presentation

Tablets – 10 mg, 20 mg, 40 mg and 80 mg

Actions and uses

Simvastatin is one of a range of lipid-lowering drugs, which are frequently described as HMG-CoA reductase inhibitors (which refers to their inhibitory action on cholesterol synthesis). Drugs of this type produce a marked and sustained fall in cholesterol (particularly low-density lipoprotein or LDL cholesterol) and triglyceride compared to that produced by other lipid-lowering agents and have consequently become very popular in recent years.

The drug may be used in patients with hypercholesterolaemia, who are considered to be at risk of ischaemic heart disease and early cardiac death, or hypertriglyceridaemia in which case they are likely to develop peripheral vascular disease and pancreatitis. Usually such patients will have blood cholesterol levels well in excess of 7–8 mmol/l or triglyceride levels above 3 mmol/l. These may fall by up to 50% on treatment.

Statins are frequently prescribed for patients who have had coronary artery bypass surgery or angioplasty, have cerebrovascular disease or peripheral vascular disease. They are also used in the primary prevention of coronary events in at-risk patients such as those with not only high cholesterol but those who smoke, have hypertension or diabetes.

Dosage

- Primary hypercholesterolaemia, heterozygous familial hypercholesterolaemia and combined hyperlipidaemia, 10–80 mg at night.
- Homozygous familial hypercholesterolaemia, 40 mg at night or 80 mg daily in three divided doses with largest dose at night.
- Coronary heart disease, 20–80 mg at night.

Nursing implications

- It should be noted that in many cases, elevated blood cholesterol is the result of obesity, inappropriate diet or alcohol excess so nurses should pay particular attention to their role as health promoters and health educators.
- A few patients present with a familial hypercholesterolaemia and history of early cardiac death in the family. In these patients life may be markedly prolonged by treatment. Also, patients with extensive cardiac disease, especially after coronary artery bypass grafting, should have their cholesterol maintained in the normal range.
- Side effects include headache and gastrointestinal effects but,

most importantly, muscle effects such as myalgia, myositis and myopathy can occur. If myopathy occurs treatment should be discontinued. Patients must be advised to report to their doctor any unexplained muscle pain, tenderness or weakness.
- There is an increased risk of myopathy if simvastatin is taken concurrently with cyclosporin, fibrates or nicotinic acid, nefazodone, antifungals or protease inhibitors.
- Patients receiving warfarin should have their anticoagulant status carefully checked after starting simvastatin therapy. In the past, lipid-lowering drugs have been shown to increase the risk of bleeding in such patients.
- Use with caution in liver disease. Liver function tests should be carried out before starting treatment and regularly for the first month of treatment.
- Simvastatin is contraindicated in patients with active liver disease, in pregnancy and breastfeeding.

Storage
Simvastatin tablets are stored at room temperature and protected from light and moisture.

SODIUM AUROTHIOMALATE (Myocrisin)

Presentation
Injection – 0.5 ml ampoules containing 10 mg, 20 mg or 50 mg

Actions and uses
This drug is a gold salt and is used in the treatment of active progressive rheumatoid arthritis and juvenile arthritis which has not responded adequately to conventional antiinflammatory analgesic therapy. It is not in itself an analgesic but by modifying the autoimmune inflammatory process involved in the disease, it may lead to a reduction in pain. It should be administered under expert advice.

Dosage
- Adults: a course of deep intramuscular injections, each of 50 mg, is usually given at weekly intervals until there is evidence of a response. If there is no response after a total of 1 g has been given, stop therapy. For the first few weeks less than 50 mg may be given so that any severe side effects may be detected before patients have received large doses. Once the patient shows a response the interval between injections can be increased to 4 weeks and decreased again if a relapse occurs.
- Children: as above using doses of 1 mg/kg to a maximum of 50 mg weekly with a test dose of one tenth to one-fifth of the calculated dose.

Nursing implications
- Early side effects from this drug may precede the more serious life-threatening side effects. The nurse has an important role in identifying early side effects which include skin rashes, pruritus, a metallic taste in the mouth, a painful throat or tongue, mouth ulcers, bruising, bleeding gums, menorrhagia, nose bleeds, dry cough or progressive breathlessness.
- Serious side effects include skin eruptions, pulmonary fibrosis, renal toxicity, blood dyscrasia such as agranulocytosis, thrombocytopenia and aplastic anaemia.
- The drug should never be given to patients with severe liver or kidney disease, blood dyscrasias or exfoliative dermatitis, systemic lupus erythematosus, necrotizing enterocolitis, pulmonary fibrosis, porphyria or in pregnancy and breastfeeding.
- Laboratory tests such as blood counts, urine tests for protein and chest X-rays are carried out regularly during a course of treatment. Nurses should advise patients that these tests are essential.

- During treatment the details of the course of treatment and laboratory results are usually recorded together on a pre-designed 'gold card'. The nurse should ensure such cards are accurately completed.

Storage

Sodium aurothiomalate injection is stored at room temperature. Protect from light.

SODIUM CLODRONATE (Bonefos, Loron)

Presentation

Capsules – 400 mg
Tablets – 800 mg, 520 mg
Injection – 300 mg in 5 ml, 300 mg in 10 ml

Actions and uses

Sodium clodronate is a bisphosphonate used in hyper-calcaemia of malignancy and in the management of osteolytic lesions, hypercalcaemia and bone pain associated with skeletal metastases in patients with carcinoma of the breast or multiple myeloma. It acts by inhibiting the formation and dissolution of calcium phosphate and it inhibits bone resorption, thereby lowering plasma calcium concentrations.

Dosage

- Osteolytic lesions, hypercalcaemia and bone pain associated with skeletal metastases in patients with carcinoma of the breast or multiple myeloma: orally, 1.6 g daily as a single dose or in two divided doses. This can be increased if necessary to a maximum of 3.2 g per day. NB: Each 520 mg Loron® tablet is equivalent to two 400 mg Loron® capsules.
- Hypercalcaemia of malignancy: slow IV infusion of 300 mg daily for a maximum of 7–10 days or a single dose infusion of 1.5 g. Give 300 mg in 500 ml of sodium chloride 0.9% solution over at least 2 hours or 1.5 g in 500 ml of

sodium chloride 0.9% solution over at least 4 hours.

Nursing implications

- Patients should be counselled regarding timing of dose in relation to food intake as any food, particularly calcium-rich products, taken 1 hour before or after sodium clodronate can impair absorption. Patients should also avoid antacids, iron and mineral supplements during this time period.
- An adequate fluid intake should be maintained.
- Side effects include gastrointestinal disturbances and skin reactions.
- Do not use in moderate to severe renal impairment, pregnancy or breastfeeding.

Storage

Sodium clodronate preparations are stored at room temperature.

SODIUM CROMOGLYCATE (Intal, Nalcrom, Opticrom, Rynacrom, Vividrin)

Presentation

Spincaps for inhalation – 20 mg
Metered dose inhaler – 5 mg/metered inhalation
Capsules – 100 mg
Nasal spray – 2%
Aqueous nasal spray – 4%
Nebulizer solution – 20 mg in 2 ml
Eye drops – 2%

Actions and uses

This drug binds to cells present in the airways which under certain conditions would normally release chemicals which increase muscle tone in the airways, causing bronchospasm manifest as dyspnoea and wheezing. It is therefore useful for the prophylactic treatment of conditions associated with bronchospasm. When rhinitis and conjunctivitis are caused by an allergic reaction, the cells which release the chemicals causing the symptoms may be prevented from releasing these chemicals by the

S

application of this drug directly to the nasal or conjunctival surfaces. Sodium cromoglycate may also be useful in food allergy, used along with dietary avoidance.

Dosage

For the treatment of bronchospasm.

- By aerosol inhalation: adult and child, 10 mg four times daily increasing to 6–8 times daily in severe cases.
- By inhalation of nebulized solution: adult and child, 20 mg four times a day increasing to six times a day in severe cases.
- By inhalation of powder: adult and child, the normal dose is 1 spincap (contents of each capsule are inhaled through a spinhaler) at intervals ranging from 3 to 6 hours.

For the treatment of food allergy.

- Adults: 200 mg orally four times a day before meals.
- Children (over 2 years): up to 100 mg orally four times daily before meals.

For the treatment of allergic rhinitis.

- 4% aqueous nasal spray, one squeeze into each nostril 2–4 times daily.
- 2% nasal spray, one spray into each nostril 4–6 times daily.

For conjunctivitis, one or two drops into the eye four times daily using 2% eye drops.

Nursing implications

- It is essential to advise patients that this drug should only be used for the prevention of attacks of bronchospasm and is ineffective in the management of an acute attack. Inhaled doses may be taken before exercise.
- A special whistle-type spinhaler is available to encourage proper use of spincaps in young children.
- In the initial stages of treatment it is essential that patients are aware that the drug does not produce immediate effect. The nurse plays an important role in educating the patient on the benefits of continuing with treatment.
- Bronchospasm can result from inhalation of sodium cromoglycate. This can be prevented by previous inhalation of selective beta-2 adrenoceptor stimulant.
- When the drug is taken orally for the management of food allergy it may be either swallowed whole or taken in a solution. It is worth noting that when food allergy is being treated, administration in a solution is preferred.
- As with other eye drops, the drug itself may produce slight irritation to the eyes.
- It should be clearly understood that the spincaps are for inhalation and should not be swallowed.

Storage

- Preparations containing sodium cromoglycate are stored at room temperature.
- Capsules and solutions should be stored in moisture-proof containers and protected from light.
- Eye drops should be discarded 4 weeks after opening.

SODIUM FEREDETATE (Sytron)

Presentation

Elixir – 55 mg of elemental iron in 10 ml

Actions and uses

See the section on Iron (Oral) (p. 186). It is indicated for the treatment of iron deficiency anaemia.

Dosage

Adults: 5 ml three times a day increasing gradually to 10 ml three times a day.
Infant and premature infants: 2.5 ml twice a day; use smaller doses initially.
Child 1–5 years: 2.5 ml three times daily.

Child 6–12 years: 5 ml three times daily.

Nursing implications
See the section on Iron (Oral) (p. 186).

Storage
The drug is stored at room temperature.

SODIUM NITROPRUSSIDE (Nipride)

Presentation
Injection – 50 mg in 5 ml

Actions and uses
Sodium nitroprusside has a direct action on blood vessels, causing peripheral vasodilatation and a reduction in peripheral resistance. It is therefore useful in the management of hypertension. It is available for intravenous infusion only and has been found useful in the treatment of hypertensive crises.

Dosage
- Hypertensive crisis: the drug is usually given by continuous infusion in dextrose 5% 50 mg diluted in 250–1000 ml. The initial rate is between 0.5 and 1.5 microgram/kg body weight per minute, then adjusted by increments of 0.5 microgram/kg/min within the range 0.5–8 microgram/kg/min. Maintenance dosage depends on the control obtained but 3 microgram/kg/min has been found to be the average infusion required to maintain the blood pressure at 30–40% below the pretreatment blood pressure.
- Maintenance of blood pressure at 30–40% lower than pretreatment diastolic blood pressure: 20–400 microgram/min IV infusion.
- Controlled hypotension in surgery: maximum of 1.5 microgram/kg/min by IV infusion.
- Heart failure: 10–15 microgram/min initially by IV infusion, increased every 5–10 minutes if required within the range of 10–200

microgram/min for a maximum of 3 days.

Nursing implications
- The injection solution is prepared by first mixing with dextrose 5% in the vials provided, then the required amount is added to dextrose 5% for infusion. Once sodium nitroprusside has been diluted in dextrose for infusion, it will deteriorate if exposed to sunlight. Some of the products of deterioration are harmful and therefore it is essential that the nurse ensures that the infusion bottle and as much of the infusion apparatus as possible is completely shielded from exposure to light.
- During the initial period of treatment the blood pressure must be monitored on an almost continuous basis.
- Patients on other antihypertensives may require lower doses.
- Sodium nitroprusside has a very short duration of action and therefore infusions must be constantly monitored to ensure that accidental reduction or increase in infusion rate does not occur as drastic effects may ensue.
- Prolonged therapy may be associated with cyanide intoxication. This is characterized by tachycardia, sweating, hyperventilation, cardiac dysrhythmia and metabolic acidosis.
- Common side effects with this drug include nausea, vomiting, anorexia, abdominal pain, apprehension, restlessness, muscle twitching, retrosternal chest pain, palpitations and dizziness.

Storage
Sodium nitroprusside vials are stored at room temperature. Protect from light and moisture.

SODIUM PICOSULFATE (Laxoberal)

Presentation
Elixir – 5 mg in 5 ml

Actions and uses
Sodium picosulfate is a laxative converted by bacterial action into an active substance in the gut. It acts by stimulating the mucosa in the large intestine, causing peristalsis, and by stimulating the mucosa in the rectum it causes a feeling of fullness and enhances motility. It tends to produce bowel evacuation 10–14 hours after administration. Sodium picosulfate is used for constipation and bowel evacuation before abdominal radiological procedures, endoscopy and surgery.

Dosage
Adults: 5–10 ml at night.
Child under 4 years: 0.25 ml/kg at night.
Child 4–10 years: 2.5–5 ml at night.
Child over 10 years: 5–10 ml at night.

Nursing implications
- In common with most laxatives, excessive doses may produce abdominal discomfort.
- As the drug requires the presence of gut bacteria to convert it to its active component its effectiveness may be lost in patients who are taking broad-spectrum antibiotics.
- It can be diluted with purified water to aid compliance.

Storage
Sodium picosulfate is stored at room temperature. It should be protected from light.

SODIUM VALPROATE (Epilim)

Presentation
Tablets – 200 mg and 500 mg (enteric coated), 100 mg (crushable tablets)
Modified-release tablets – 200 mg, 300 mg and 500 mg
Oral solution – 200 mg in 5 ml
Injection – 400 mg vial

Actions and uses
This drug is an anticonvulsant used in the treatment of epilepsy. Sodium valproate's mode of action is not fully understood, but it is thought to act by potentiating the inhibitory effects of gamma aminobutyric acid (GABA) in the CNS. It is indicated for use in all forms of epilepsy, but is of particular value in primary generalized epilepsy.

Dosage
NB: Individual dosage requirements vary greatly. The following doses are given as a guideline only.

Oral
- Adults: an initial dose of 600 mg daily in two divided doses is given. This is increased every 3 days until an optimum response is achieved. The usual dose range is 1–2 g per day.
- Children:
  - over 20 kg body weight: 400 mg daily initially increasing to maintenance doses usually in the range 20–30 mg/kg body weight per day in total
  - under 20 kg body weight: 20 mg/kg daily initially increased to an appropriate maintenance dose provided plasma concentrations are monitored.

Injection
- Adults: 400–800 mg by slow intravenous injection (over 3–5 minutes) or intravenous infusion, up to a maximum of 2.5 g total dose daily.
- Children: 20–30 mg/kg body weight daily by slow intravenous injection or intravenous infusion. Dose may be increased further provided plasma concentrations are monitored.

Nursing implications
- This drug should preferably be taken with or immediately after food in order to minimize the common side effect of gastrointestinal irritation. Enteric-coated tablets may have to be used if gastric upset still occurs.
- Metabolites of sodium valproate are excreted in the urine and may give false-positive results for ketones. It is especially

S

important that this effect be recognized in diabetic patients where the presence of ketonuria usually leads to hospital referral.

- As this drug may reduce the number of platelets circulating in the blood, unexplained bruising or haemorrhage should always be taken as an indication to check the patient's blood and if thrombocytopenia has been produced, the drug should be stopped.
- Liver damage may occasionally occur and the drug is contraindicated in active liver disease or if there is a family history of severe hepatic dysfunction.
- Hair loss may occur in some patients.
- When the drug is used in high dosage tremor may be a problem.
- If doses greater than 40 mg/kg daily are administered to children, they should have their clinical chemistry and haematological parameters monitored.
- Sodium valproate interacts with antidepressants, chloroquine, mefloquine and antipsychotics, each antagonizing the anticonvulsant effect of the drug.
- On infusion, reconstitute the contents of the vial with the water provided, then dilute with either glucose 5% or sodium chloride 0.9%.

Storage

The drug is stored at room temperature.

SOTALOL (Beta-Cardone, Sotacor)

Presentation

Tablets – 40 mg, 80 mg, 160 mg, 200 mg
Injection – 40 mg in 4 ml

Actions and uses

Sotalol is a non-selective beta-adrenoreceptor blocking drug. Its actions are described in the section on these drugs (p. 51). Sotalol is now only indicated for ventricular arrhythmias or prophylaxis of supraventricular arrhythmias and use should be accompanied by ECG monitoring.

Dosage

It may be given intravenously in emergency situations for cardiac dysrhythmias in a dosage of 20–120 mg. This is usually given over 10 minutes and is repeated as necessary with 6-hour intervals between doses. Careful monitoring of pulse, blood pressure and electrocardiogram is necessary during administration.

The oral daily adult maintenance dose range is 120–640 mg and it may be given as a single dose or in two divided doses, particularly at higher doses. Doses of 480 mg daily and higher are used for life-threatening ventricular arrhythmias under specialist supervision.

Nursing implications

- See the section on Beta-Adrenoreceptor Blocking Drugs (p. 51).
- Sotalol can itself cause arrhythmias, particularly torsade de pointes, potentially fatal in susceptible patients.

Storage

Sotalol tablets and injection are stored at room temperature.

SPIRONOLACTONE (Aldactone)

Presentation

Tablets – 25 mg, 50 mg and 100 mg
Oral suspensions – 5 mg in 5 ml, 10 mg in 5 ml, 25 mg in 5 ml, 50 mg in 5 ml and 100 mg in 5 ml

Actions and uses

Spironolactone inhibits the adrenal hormone aldosterone, increasing excretion of sodium while conserving potassium, and thus is a 'potassium-sparing' diuretic which prevents excessive potassium loss. It is usually given together with other diuretics to prevent the development of hypokalaemia (excessive blood potassium loss) which often occurs in patients treated with diuretic drugs. Spironolactone is of particular value in the treatment of oedema occurring in patients with liver cirrhosis and it has more recently become employed in the treatment of patients with severe heart failure.

It is usually unnecessary for patients treated with spironolactone to be given potassium supplement tablets such as Slow K or Sando K.

Dosage
Adults: 100–200 mg daily increased to a maximum of 400 mg daily if required. For heart failure the dose is usually 25 mg daily.
Child: 3 mg/kg daily in divided doses, increased if required.

Nursing implications
- Patients receiving spironolactone should be observed for the occasional occurrence of excessive potassium retention. This is particularly important in patients with renal failure and manifests as confusion, drowsiness, anorexia, nausea, vomiting and other features of uraemia.
- Less common side effects include breast enlargement in the male, milk secretion in the female and skin rashes.
- It should not be used in hyperkalaemia, hyponatraemia, pregnancy, breastfeeding or Addison's disease.

Storage
Spironolactone preparations are stored at room temperature.

STANOZOLOL (Stromba)

Presentation
Tablets – 5 mg

Actions and uses
Stanozolol is an anabolic steroid. This group of drugs is usually associated with increased protein synthesis, enhanced muscle development and weight gain. However, stanozolol has fibrinolytic properties which make it particularly useful in treating vascular symptoms of Behçet's disease and in angiooedema.

Dosage
Behçet's disease: 10 mg daily
Hereditary angiooedema: adult, 2.5–10 mg daily to control attacks, then reduced to, e.g. 2.5 mg three times a week. Child, 1–6 years, 2.5 mg daily initially; 6–12 years, 2.5–5 mg daily initially, reduce dose for maintenance.

Nursing implications
- Side effects include mild androgenic effects, e.g. acne, hirsutism and amenorrhoea.
- It is contraindicated in pregnancy, breastfeeding, liver disease, prostate cancer and IDDM.
- It is not indicated for the treatment of loss of appetite, unexplained weight loss or failure to thrive in children.
- Stanozolol is sometimes abused by athletes; it is not to be used as a tonic or body builder.
- Stanozolol may enhance the effects of oral anticoagulants.

Storage
The drug is stored at room temperature.

STAVUDINE (Zerit)

Presentation
Capsules – 15 mg, 20 mg, 30 mg and 40 mg
Oral solution for reconstitution – 1 mg in 1 ml

Actions and uses
Stavudine is a nucleoside reverse transcriptase inhibitor with actions and uses similar to those of zidovudine. It is indicated for use in HIV infection when used in combination with other antiretroviral drugs.

Dosage
Adult under 60 kg: 30 mg twice a day.
Adult over 60 kg: 40 mg twice a day.

S

Child over 3 months, under 30 kg:
1 mg/kg twice a day.
Child over 3 months, over 30 kg:
adult dose.

Nursing implications

- Drugs used in the treatment of HIV can cause serious side effects. They should be prescribed only under expert advice.
- The timing of commencement of therapy should be decided by those expert in the management of HIV and depends on symptoms, viral load and the CD4 count and should be weighed against drug toxicities and the likely development of drug resistance.
- Resistance to antiretroviral drugs is reduced by using combination therapy.
- Most antiretroviral agents are used in pregnancy although teratogenic effects are not yet fully understood. Mothers are advised not to breastfeed their infants as HIV can pass from mother to infant via the breastmilk.
- Stavudine should be taken at least 1 hour before food.
- The main side effect with stavudine is peripheral neuropathy. The drug should be discontinued if signs of peripheral neuropathy develop, e.g. numbness and impaired touch sensation, but it may be restarted at half the dose if symptoms resolve.
- Use with caution in liver disease. Treatment should be suspended or discontinued if there are abnormal liver function tests, hepatic steatosis occurs, there is progressive hepatomegaly or unexplained lactic acidosis.
- Use with caution in patients with a history of pancreatitis and avoid concomitant use with drugs that can cause pancreatitis or peripheral neuropathy.
- Note that zidovudine may inhibit intracellular activation of stavudine.

Storage

Stavudine preparations are stored at room temperature.

STILBOESTROL
(now Diethylstilbestrol)

Presentation

Tablets – 1 mg and 5 mg
Pessaries – 500 microgram with lactic acid 5%

Actions and uses

Diethylstilbestrol is an oestrogenic substance which is used in clinical practice for breast cancer in postmenopausal women, prostate cancer (rarely) and as a topical treatment for vaginal atrophy.

Dosage

Breast cancer: 10–20 mg daily.
Prostate cancer: 1–3 mg daily.
Vaginal atrophy: 2 pessaries inserted at night for 2–3 weeks only

Nursing implications

See the section on Oestrogens (p. 257).

Storage

The drug is stored at room temperature.

STREPTOKINASE
(Kabikinase, Streptase)

Presentation

Injection – 250 000 and 750 000-unit vials for reconstitution and 1.5 million-unit vials for reconstitution

Actions and uses

Streptokinase is a fibrinolytic agent with several important uses including the treatment of life-threatening deep vein thrombosis and pulmonary embolism and acute myocardial infarction. It can be used for other thrombotic conditions, e.g. thrombosed arteriovenous shunts. Streptokinase acts by generating plasmin, which degrades fibrin, the main component of thrombi, thus causing the breakdown of thrombi, i.e. dissolution of blood clots and removal of the blockage caused by the clot. See also the section on Alteplase (p. 20).

Dosage

- Deep vein thrombosis, pulmonary embolism, acute arterial thromboembolism, central retinal venous or arterial thrombosis: IV infusion of 250 000 units over 30 minutes followed by 100 000 units every hour for up to 12–72 hours with monitoring of clotting factors. (Follow manufacturer's instructions for administration.)
- Myocardial infarction: IV infusion of 1.5 million units over 60 minutes administered within 12 hours of the MI, preferably within 1 hour if possible.

Nursing implications

- See the section on Alteplase (p. 20).
- There is an increased risk of haemorrhage in patients who are receiving, or who have recently received, other anticoagulant drugs.
- Side effects of the drug include nausea, vomiting, bleeding, headache, back pain and allergic anaphylactic reactions with flushing and dyspnoea. Allergic reactions can be largely avoided by giving the intravenous dose slowly. Corticosteroids can also be given prophylactically.
- Patients should be given a card which states that they have received streptokinase therapy.

Storage

Streptokinase is stored at room temperature.

STREPTOKINASE/ STREPTODORNASE (Varidase Topical)

Presentation

Vials containing streptokinase 100 000 units and streptodornase 25 000 units

Actions and uses

The combination of these two enzymes in solution is suitable for use by local application to help in the dissolution of clotted blood and fibrinous or purulent accumulations. This preparation can also be used as a desloughing agent to cleanse necrotic, infected and sloughy wounds. Streptokinase activates a fibrinolytic enzyme in serum, ultimately causing dissolution of blood clots and dissolution of any fibrinous material in wound exudates. Streptodornase liquefies the viscous products of dead cells and pus.

Dosage

Consult product literature for alternative methods of application but in general, each vial is reconstituted with 20 ml of either sodium chloride 0.9% solution or water for injection and the resulting solution is used to soak gauze which is applied to the wound once or twice daily. The wound should then be covered by a semiocclusive dressing.

Nursing implications

- It is essential to note that vials of Varidase powder are for local application only and should never be administered parenterally.
- Nurses should avoid excessive shaking of the vials as this may inactivate the enzymes and cause frothing.
- The vials do not contain a preservative and therefore are not intended for multidose use.
- Occasional allergic skin reactions may occur.

Storage

Varidase Topical is kept in its original pack in a refrigerator. Once reconstituted, solutions are stable for 1 day if refrigerated.

STREPTOMYCIN

Presentation

Injection – 1 g powder for reconstitution

Actions and uses

This aminoglycoside (see Gentamicin – p. 158) antibiotic is reserved for the treatment of tuberculosis when used in combination with other antituberculosis agents. It is rarely used nowadays except in cases where resistant organisms are present. It is also used in combination with doxycycline in brucellosis.

Dosage

- Tuberculosis: deep IM injection of 15 mg/kg daily to a maximum of 1 g/day.
- Reduce dose in patients under 50 kg, over 40 years old and in renal impairment.
- Brucellosis: seek expert advice.

Nursing implications

- See the section on Gentamicin (p. 158).
- The most important toxic effect of this drug is damage to the auditory nerve with resultant deafness and loss of balance. The risk of this increases with high dosage, prolonged duration of treatment or when the patient is over 40 years of age. Recovery may occur over weeks or months but is often incomplete. The development of any symptoms suggestive of damage to the auditory nerve is an indication immediately to stop treatment.
- Plasma drug concentrations should be monitored in patients with renal impairment.
- Allergic reactions may occur, including rash and fever.
- Vague feelings of paraesthesia of the lips, headache, lassitude and dizziness may occur after each injection. They are less common if the patient is kept at rest after an injection. This is because with muscular activity, absorption from the intramuscular injection site is increased and high plasma concentrations may occur.
- The nurse should note that these injections are particularly painful.

- It is essential that the nurse notes that streptomycin is a potent skin sensitizer and severe skin reactions may occur in nurses who handle the drug if they are sensitive to it. The wearing of protective gloves during handling of the drug is therefore advised.

Storage

Streptomycin preparations are stored at room temperature.

SUCRALFATE (Antepsin)

Presentation

Tablets – 1 g
Suspension – 1 g in 5 ml

Actions and uses

Sucralfate is used in the treatment of gastric and duodenal ulcer and chronic gastritis and for the prophylaxis of gastrointestinal haemorrhage from stress ulceration in very ill patients. It exerts an action which is similar to that of tri-potassium di-citrato bismuthate (De-Nol). Briefly, the drug binds to protein in the ulcer crater, thereby forming a protective layer of a chemically complex substance which resists further digestion of the ulcer by gastric acid and pepsin and therefore aids healing.

Dosage

- Benign gastric and duodenal ulcer and chronic gastritis: 1 g four times a day or 2 g twice a day. Take for 4–6 weeks or up to 12 weeks in resistant cases.
- Prophylaxis of stress ulceration: 1 g six times a day of the suspension.
- Not recommended for children.

Nursing implications

- Patients should be instructed to take each dose 1 hour before meals with a single dose at bedtime.
- The absorption of tetracycline, quinolones, warfarin and phenytoin may be impaired by

S

the presence of sucralfate and such combinations should be avoided or, if necessary, doses of these drugs should not be given within 2 hours of sucralfate administration.
- The drug should be used with caution in patients with kidney impairment due to the possibility of aluminium retention. However, it is interesting to note that sucralfate has been administered to a patient with renal failure in an attempt to bind phosphate in the gut and so reduce hyperphosphataemia.
- Side effects include constipation and other gastrointestinal symptoms.

Storage
Sucralfate preparations are stored at room temperature.

SULFASALAZINE (Salazopyrin)

Presentation
Tablets – 500 mg plain and enteric coated
Suspension – 250 mg in 5 ml
Suppositories – 500 mg
Enema – 3 g in 100 ml

Actions and uses
Sulfasalazine is a combination of two drugs, an antiinflammatory salicylic acid derivative (5-aminosalicylic acid or 5-ASA) and an antiinfective sulphonamide derivative, sulfapyridine. The sulfapyridine acts only as a carrier, delivering the 5-ASA to its site of action in the colon.
It is used for the treatment of and maintenance of remission of ulcerative colitis and the treatment of active Crohn's disease and it is further used as a disease-modifying drug in the treatment of rheumatoid arthritis.

Dosage
- Adults: 1–2 g four times per day initially orally. Once remission of the disease has been obtained lower daily dosages, i.e. 1.5–2 g in total per day, may be sufficient. In

rheumatoid arthritis, under expert advice: the required dose is gradually adjusted to the individual starting with 500 mg daily, then twice daily, three times daily, etc. up to a total daily dose, if necessary, of 3 g. Enteric-coated tablets are used for this indication.
- Children over 2 years: 40–60 mg/kg body weight daily initially, reducing to a maintenance dose of 20–30 mg/kg body weight daily. Not recommended in juvenile arthritis.
- The drug may also be given for a local effect via suppositories. These should be given morning and night after defecation. An alternative local treatment is one enema given daily, usually at bedtime.

Nursing implications
- It is important to note that sulfasalazine is a combination of a salicylate and sulphonamide and therefore is contraindicated in patients with a history of allergy to sulphonamide drugs or salicylates.
- The salicylate component may give any of the side effects described in the section on non-steroidal antiinflammatory analgesic drug (p. 250). Aminosalicylates can cause serious blood disorders so patients should be advised to report any signs or symptoms of this, including unexplained bleeding, bruising, sore throat or fever.
- Avoid in moderate or severe renal impairment.
- The sulphonamide component of sulfasalazine can produce any of the side effects associated with sulphonamides (p. 343).

Storage
Preparations containing sulfasalazine are stored at room temperature.

S

SULFINPYRAZONE (Anturan)

Presentation
Tablets – 100 mg, 200 mg

Actions and uses
Sulfinpyrazone is a uricosuric agent. It increases the urinary excretion of uric acid and urate and is therefore useful for the treatment of hyperuricaemia and gout. It has no analgesic properties and is therefore only useful for reducing blood urate in the long term.

Dosage
The initial dose of sulfinpyrazone is 100–200 mg daily taken with meals or milk. The dosage is gradually increased over 2–3 weeks until the daily dosage of 600 mg is reached. After the blood urate concentration has been controlled the maintenance dose may be reduced to as low as 200 mg daily.

Nursing implications
- The nurse may play an important role in helping to prevent the serious side effect of urate stone formation by monitoring carefully patients' fluid intake and encouraging them to drink large quantities of fluid daily.
- As aspirin antagonizes the uricosuric action of this drug, the nurse may play an important role in educating all patients to avoid taking aspirin at the same time as sulfinpyrazone.
- The drug may occasionally produce gastrointestinal upset and gastric bleeding and therefore must be used with caution in patients with a history of peptic ulcer disease. Patients should be advised to take this medication with food or milk.
- Rare side effects for which withdrawal of treatment is necessary include skin rashes and blood dyscrasias (aplastic anaemia, leucopenia and thrombocytopenia).
- Interactions include enhanced anticoagulant effect of warfarin and acenocoumarol, enhanced antidiabetic effect of sulphonylureas and increased plasma concentration of phenytoin.

Storage
Sulfinpyrazone tablets are stored at room temperature.

SULINDAC (Clinoril)

Presentation
Tablets – 100 mg, 200 mg

Actions and uses
See the section on non-steroidal antiinflammatory analgesic drugs (p. 250). Sulindac is used in rheumatic disease, other musculoskeletal disorders and acute gout.

Dosage
The usual adult dose is 100–200 mg twice daily, usually taken with fluids at mealtimes.

Nursing implications
See the section on non-steroidal antiinflammatory analgesic drugs (p. 250).

Storage
Sulindac tablets are stored at room temperature.

SULPHONAMIDES

Presentation
See individual compounds.

Actions and uses
The sulphonamide group of drugs, although chemically unrelated to antibiotics, were once widely used for the prevention and treatment of a wide variety of diseases due to bacterial infection. They are in fact the forerunner to the modern antibiotics which have now largely replaced them in clinical use. The following sulphonamides are, however, still used: sulfamethoxazole (in co-trimoxazole), sulfasalazine (which contains sulfapyridine).

All bacteria require folic acid in order to be able to grow and multiply. This folic acid is usually synthesized by bacteria themselves within cells. Sulphonamides act by preventing the production of folic acid in bacterial cells. The sulphonamides have a bacteriostatic rather than bactericidal action. The former term means that they prevent further growth and reduplication of cells whereas the latter term implies that the drug actually kills cells already present in the body. In practice, many organisms are found to be resistant to sulphonamides. This is because these organisms have developed alternative means of synthesizing folic acid to the pathway of synthesis that is blocked by the drug. Sulphonamides have a wide range of action against both Gram-positive and Gram-negative organisms. They are used to treat a wide range of infections including bacterial diarrhoea, urinary infection, chest infection, bacterial meningitis, venereal disease and various dermatological infections.

Dosage
See individual drugs.

Nursing implications
- Unless a high fluid intake and urine output is achieved there is a danger that patients receiving these drugs may suffer kidney damage due to crystallization of the drug in the renal tract. However, this is now rarely a real concern given the disappearance of many drugs from the group. Nevertheless, the nurse may play an important role in both encouraging a high fluid intake and in monitoring urine output so that early warning of inadequate fluid intake may be obtained.
- There are two important instances in which sulphonamides may affect the action of other drugs concurrently being administered to patients.
  - In diabetic patients on oral antidiabetic drugs, the sulphonamides may precipitate hypoglycaemia with dizziness, sweating, tachycardia, fainting and eventually coma. Such patients should be carefully observed and warned of the dangers of this potential complication.
  - In patients receiving the drug warfarin for the purpose of anticoagulation, the coincident administration of sulphonamides may lead to an increase in warfarin's action with the resultant danger of severe haemorrhage. Regular checks on clotting function should therefore be made when sulphonamides are instituted in such cases.
- Hypersensitivity reactions to sulphonamides may occur and these include skin rash, fever, joint pains and the more severe erythema multiforme and Stevens–Johnson syndrome.
- As well as the danger of the drug precipitating into the kidney substance when fluid intake is poor, sulphonamides may have a direct damaging action on the kidney.
- Sulphonamides may exert a wide range of toxic effects on the blood and bone marrow leading to megaloblastic anaemia, haemolytic anaemia, thrombocytopenia and aplastic anaemia. More rarely, agranulocytosis (complete absence of white cells) with resultant risk of overwhelming infection may occur. As a result they are now rarely used in the elderly.
- Liver damage and jaundice may occasionally occur. Jaundice is specially likely to occur in very young children and may be dangerous. Such patients should not, therefore, receive sulphonamides.

S

SULPIRIDE
(Dolmatil, Sulparex, Sulpitil)

Presentation
Tablets – 200 mg

Actions and uses
Sulpiride has actions and uses similar to those described for the phenothiazines although it has major chemical differences to drugs such as chlorpromazine. It is an antipsychotic used in the management of schizophrenia.

Dosage
Adults: 200–400 mg twice daily with a maximum of 800 mg daily where negative symptoms are predominant and a maximum of 2.4 g daily where positive symptoms are predominant. In elderly patients, start with lower doses and increase gradually.

Not recommended for children under 14 years.

Nursing implications
The nursing implications described for the phenothiazines (p. 281) also apply to this drug.

Storage
Sulpiride tablets are stored at room temperature.

SUMATRIPTAN (Imigran)

Presentation
Tablets – 50 mg and 100 mg
Injection – 6 mg in 0.5 ml prefilled syringe
Nasal spray – 20 mg in 0.1 ml unit dose

Actions and uses
This drug stimulates 5-HT1 receptors which are specific target sites for the naturally occurring neurotransmitter 5-hydroxytryptamine (serotonin). Stimulation of these receptors, which are found in abundance in the cranial blood vessels, results in constriction of the carotid arterial circulation and a consequent reduction in blood flow through the intracranial and extracranial vessels which are dilated during a migraine attack. Thus sumatriptan rapidly aborts migraine attacks and cluster headaches, within 10–15 minutes by subcutaneous injection and nasal spray or 30–40 minutes after oral administration. It is ineffective for migraine prophylaxis.

Dosage
Adults only.

- Oral: 50 mg (or 100 mg if required) should be taken as soon as possible after the onset of an attack. A second dose can be taken only if symptoms recur after an initial response. Maximum of 300 mg should be taken in 24 hours.
- Subcutaneous injection: 6 mg should be injected as soon as possible after the onset of an attack. A second dose can be injected after not less than 1 hour, only if symptoms recur after an initial response. Maximum of 12 mg should be injected in 24 hours.
- Intranasally: 20 mg (one spray) should be sprayed into one nostril as soon as possible after the onset of an attack. A second dose can be taken after not less than 2 hours, only if symptoms recur after an initial response. Maximum of 40 mg should be taken in 24 hours.

Nursing implications
- Where there is no response to the first dose of sumatriptan, a second dose is not advised. However, patients may take one further dose to abort a subsequent attack within any 24-hour period.
- Subcutaneous injections are administered by the patients themselves using a special 'Auto-Injector' device, which is also available on prescription. Tablets should be swallowed whole with water.
- As a result of the possible widespread vasoconstrictor action of sumatriptan at other receptor sites, patients with angina or a history of ischaemic heart disease, previous myocardial infarction or coronary

vasospasm or uncontrolled hypertension should not receive this drug. It is also contraindicated in patients who have had previous cerebrovascular accidents or transient ischaemic attacks and in those with peripheral vascular disease.

- Ergotamine, another widely used drug in migraine attacks, must not be taken concurrently. The combined vasoconstrictor action of the two drugs may produce severe vasospasm.
- Also patients with depression who are treated with monoamine oxidase inhibitors or newer selective serotonin reuptake inhibitors (fluoxetine, fluvoxamine, paroxetine and sertraline) should not take sumatriptan since a potentially serious 'serotonin syndrome' may result.
- Reported side effects include ischaemic pain and tingling sensations which indicate developing ischaemia often affecting the chest and throat; flushing, dizziness, paraesthesia and weakness. Nausea and vomiting and altered liver function has also been reported.

Storage

Sumatriptan preparations are stored at room temperature and protected from light.

SUXAMETHONIUM (Anectine)

Presentation

Injection – 100 mg in 2 ml

Actions and uses

Suxamethonium is a depolarizing muscle relaxant acting by mimicking acetylcholine at the neuromuscular junction. It is broken down slowly compared to the breakdown of acetylcholine and therefore causes prolonged muscle relaxation. It is important to note that

the action of suxamethonium cannot be reversed. It has a rapid onset of action and its effect deteriorates quickly so it is useful in situations where a brief duration of action is desirable, e.g. tracheal intubation.

Dosage
IV injection

Adults: 1 mg/kg (or in the range 0.3–1.1 mg/kg, 20–100 mg) to a maximum of 500 mg/h
Infant under 1 year: 2 mg/kg
Child 1–12 years: 1–2 mg/kg

IV infusion

Adults and children: 2–5 mg/min (up to 500 mg/h) using a solution of 1–2 mg/ml in glucose 5% or sodium chloride 0.9%

IM injection

Infant: up to 4–5 mg/kg
Child: up to 4 mg/kg to a maximum of 150 mg

Nursing implications

- Suxamethonium should be administered after anaesthesia as painful muscle fasciculations can occur.
- Tachycardia occurs after single use, while bradycardia may occur if several doses are given to adults or after the first dose in children. Atropine given as premed can help reduce any bradycardia.
- It should not be used in patients with a family history of malignant hyperthermia (as suxamethonium can cause hyperthermia) or in those with low plasma cholinesterase activity or in hyperkalaemia.
- Note that prolonged paralysis may occur with high or repeated doses of suxamethonium and assisted ventilation will be required until muscle function returns.

Storage

Suxamethonium injection is stored in a refrigerator protected from light.

S

SYNTOMETRINE
(Combination of Ergometrine and Oxytocin)

Presentation

Syntometrine is available as a parenteral solution containing 500 microgram of ergometrine maleate and 5 units of oxytocin in 1 ml.

Actions and uses

The combination of these two drugs is effective by intramuscular injection in the stimulation of uterine contraction. In clinical practice it is used mainly to stimulate uterine contraction in labour and it may also be given to prevent or treat postpartum haemorrhage.

Dosage

- To stimulate uterine contraction and cessation of bleeding after birth of the placenta: an intramuscular injection of 1 ml is usually administered.
- When used for the other reasons described above, dosage varies according to the clinical practice of the centre concerned and the nurse is advised to seek advice from her local obstetric unit.

Nursing implications

- High doses may cause excessive uterine contraction and dosage should therefore be carefully monitored to prevent the potentially disastrous occurrence of a ruptured uterus.
- When high doses of syntometrine are given with large volumes of electrolyte-free fluid, water intoxication may occur. Initially headache, anorexia, nausea, vomiting and abdominal pain may be the presenting features and this progresses to lethargy, drowsiness, unconsciousness and grand mal-type seizures. The concentration of blood electrolytes may be markedly disturbed.

Storage

Over long periods, the drug should be stored in a refrigerator and protected from light. However, if it is stored at room temperature (up to 25°C) it is stable for 2 months.

S

T

TACROLIMUS (Prograf)

Presentation
Capsules – 500 microgram, 1 mg and 5 mg
Injection – 5 mg in 1 ml for dilution for intravenous infusion

Actions and uses
Tacrolimus, like cyclosporin, is a calcineurin inhibitor used as an immunosuppressant agent in patients with liver and kidney transplants. It works by inhibiting the formation of cytotoxic lymphocytes by suppressing T-cell activation and T-helper cell dependent B-cell proliferation. It also inhibits lymphokine formation. By inhibiting these immunological processes, tacrolimus facilitates graft acceptance and successful organ transplantation. It can be used as a primary immunosuppressant in liver and kidney allograft recipients and in the management of allograft rejection which has been resistant to other immunosuppressive regimens.

Dosage
Liver transplantation; start dose within 6 hours of transplant.

- Adult: orally, 100–200 microgram/kg/day in two divided doses; IV infusion 10–50 microgram/kg over 24 hours.
- Child: orally, 300 microgram/kg/day in two divided doses; IV infusion 50 microgram/kg over 24 hours.

Renal transplantation; start dose within 24 hours of transplant.

- Adult: orally, 150–300 microgram/kg/day in two divided doses; IV infusion 50–100 microgram/kg over 24 hours.
- Child: orally, 300 microgram/kg/day in two divided doses; IV infusion 100 microgram/kg over 24 hours.

Maintenance doses are adjusted according to response.

Nursing implications
- Glucose 5% or sodium chloride 0.9% are used as infusion fluids with the final concentration being 4–100 microgram/ml and total volume of 20–250 ml.
- Tacrolimus infusion is incompatible with PVC. Once reconstituted, use within 24 hours.
- Capsules should be swallowed whole with a glass of water and taken on an empty stomach, an hour before food.
- Patients should be advised that tacrolimus may affect their performance of skilled tasks including driving.
- Side effects include neurotoxicity, nephrotoxicity, altered glucose metabolism and cardiomyopathy. Cardiomyopathy has been reported in children.
- The CSM advises that patients have ECG monitoring and their dose reduced or tacrolimus stopped if abnormalities occur.
- Other side effects include gastrointestinal upsets, hypertension, tremor, headache, insomnia, perception disorder and visual disorders, hypercalcaemia, hypophosphataemia and leucocytosis.
- Tacrolimus must not be used in pregnancy and non-hormonal methods of contraception should be used while taking tacrolimus.
- It must not be used in breastfeeding or concurrently with cyclosporin.

T

- Tacrolimus is subject to other drug interactions including an increased risk of nephrotoxicity with NSAIDs and amphotericin, increased plasma tacrolimus concentrations with clarithromycin, erythromycin, quinupristin/dalfopristin, nefazodone, imidazoles, nifedipine and diltiazem and an increased risk of hyperkalaemia with potassium-sparing diuretics and potassium salts.

Storage
Tacrolimus preparations are stored at room temperature. Protect the injection from light.

TAMOXIFEN (Nolvadex, Soltamox, Tamofen)

Presentation
Tablets – 10 mg, 20 mg, 40 mg
Oral solution – 10 mg in 5 ml

Actions and uses
Tamoxifen is an oestrogen receptor antagonist which has two major uses. It is used in the treatment of breast cancer (when the primary tumour is oestrogen receptor positive) where it acts by preventing oestrogen from binding to its receptors, thereby inhibiting oestrogen's stimulation of nucleic acid synthesis. Use of tamoxifen will increase survival and delay the growth of metastases. It can also be used for oestrogen receptor-positive metastatic breast cancer.
The second use of tamoxifen is in the stimulation of ovulation in patients suffering from infertility. Tamoxifen occupies oestrogen receptors in the hypothalamus, induces gonadotrophin release and interferes with feedback mechanisms.

Dosage
- For the treatment of breast cancer: 20 mg daily.
- For the treatment of anovulatory infertility: 20 mg daily on the second, third, fourth and fifth days of the menstrual cycles if patients are menstruating regularly. The dose may be increased to 40 mg or 80 mg

in subsequent courses. In women who are not menstruating regularly the initial course may begin on any day with subsequent courses starting 45 days later or on day 2 of cycle if menstruation occurs.

Nursing implications
- Because of its oestrogen antagonist action, it frequently produces hot flushing, vaginal bleeding and pruritus vulvae. Suppression of menstruation commonly occurs in premenstrual women.
- Gastrointestinal upset, light-headedness and fluid retention may occur.
- Thrombocytopenia has been rarely reported.
- When used for the treatment of breast cancer patients with bony metastases may experience an exacerbation of pain; this is sometimes associated with hypercalcaemia.
- As there is a small risk of endometrial cancer, patients should be advised to report any symptoms such as abnormal vaginal bleeding, vaginal discharge and pelvic pain.
- Do not use tamoxifen in pregnancy or breastfeeding.
- Tamoxifen can enhance the anticoagulant effect of acenocoumarol and warfarin.

Storage
Tamoxifen tablets are stored at room temperature.

TAMSULOSIN (Flomax)

Presentation
Capsules (modified release) – 400 microgram

Actions and uses
Tamsulosin is a selective alpha-blocker which acts on the urethral sphincter, causing relaxation and thus permitting urine flow. This is of use in the treatment of dysuria associated with benign prostatic hyperplasia.

Dosage
400 microgram daily, taken after breakfast

Nursing implications
- Side effects include postural hypotension, drowsiness, headache, lethargy, weakness and palpitations.
- Patients should be advised that the performance of skilled tasks such as driving may be affected.
- Tamsulosin should not be used in severe liver impairment, postural hypotension or micturition syncope.

Storage
Tamsulosin capsules are stored at room temperature.

TEICOPLANIN (Targocid)

Presentation
Injection – 200 mg and 400 mg powders for reconstitution

Actions and uses
Teicoplanin is a glycopeptide antibiotic with similar actions and uses to vancomycin. It has a longer duration of action than vancomycin, allowing it to be administered once daily. Teicoplanin is often used where patients have not tolerated vancomycin, particularly if they have developed nephrotoxicity or ototoxicity. Teicoplanin should still be used with caution in those patients sensitive to vancomycin.

Dosage
Adults.

- IM injection, IV injection or IV infusion 400 mg initially, then 200 mg daily or in severe infections (by the IV route) 400 mg 12-hourly for three doses then 200 mg or 400 mg daily. Higher doses still may be required in patients over 85 kg, in severe burns or endocarditis.

Child over 2 months.

- IV injection or IV infusion 10 mg/kg initially 12-hourly for three doses,

then 6 mg/kg daily or in severe infections or neutropenia 10 mg/kg daily. After the initial doses, the IM route can be used but IV is preferred in children.

Neonate.

- IV infusion, a single dose of 16 mg/kg then 8 mg/kg daily.

Orthopaedic surgery prophylaxis.

- 400 mg IV injection at induction of anaesthesia.

Nursing implications
- Side effects include gastro-intestinal upsets, rash, pruritus, fever, bronchospasm, rigors, urticaria, angiooedema and anaphylaxis.
- It should be used with caution in patients sensitive to vancomycin. The dose should be reduced in patients with renal impairment and renal and auditory function monitored with prolonged administration or if given concurrently with other nephrotoxic or neurotoxic drugs.
- Teicoplanin infusion can be administered in glucose 5%, sodium chloride 0.9% or compound sodium lactate solutions after reconstitution with the water for injection provided. Infuse over 30 minutes.

Storage
Teicoplanin injection is stored at room temperature. Use immediately after reconstitution.

TELMISARTAN (Micardis)

Presentation
Tablets – 20 mg, 40 mg and 80 mg

Actions and uses
Telmisartan is an angiotensin II (AT1 receptor) antagonist, similar to Losartan. It is indicated for the treatment of hypertension.

Dosage
20–40 mg daily increased if necessary to 80 mg daily.

Nursing implications

- Drugs of this type have few side-effects.
- Telmisartan is contraindicated in severe renal impairment, biliary obstruction and breastfeeding.

Storage

Telmisartan tablets are stored at room temperature.

TEMAZEPAM

Presentation

Tablets – 10 mg, 20 mg
Gel-filled capsules – 10 mg, 15 mg, 20 mg and 30 mg
Oral solution – 10 mg in 5 ml

Actions and uses

Temazepam is a benzodiazepine drug (p. 47). It has a marked sedative effect and is therefore taken at night as a hypnotic. It is particularly interesting to note that this drug has a very short action. It therefore tends to produce less hangover effect the following day and is particularly useful in treating insomnia in elderly patients where daytime confusion can be avoided. Temazepam is also used for preanaesthetic medication because of its sedative and anxiolytic properties.

Dosage

- As a hypnotic, adults only: 10–40 mg taken on retiring. It is recommended that as low a dose as possible be used for elderly patients.
- For premedication: adult 20–40 mg single dose, child 1 mg/kg (up to a maximum of 30 mg) single dose, both taken 30 minutes to 1 hour before the surgical procedure.

Nursing implications

- See the section on Benzodiazepines (p. 47).
- Note that the gel-filled capsules are not prescribable on the NHS; they are particularly subject to abuse. The contents of these capsules are injected by drug abusers and gangrene can occur as a result.

Storage

Preparations containing temazepam are stored at room temperature.

TENOXICAM (Mobiflex)

Presentation

Tablets – 20 mg
Injection – 20 mg powder for reconstitution

Actions and uses

Tenoxicam is an oxicam NSAID indicated for use in musculoskeletal conditions, including rheumatoid arthritis.

Dosage

Adults only.

- Orally: rheumatic disease, 20 mg daily; acute musculoskeletal disorders, 20 mg daily for 7–14 days.
- IV or IM injection: dose as for oral administration for the first 1–2 days of therapy.

Nursing implications

- See the section on Non-Steroidal Antiinflammatory Analgesic Drugs (p. 250).

Storage

Tenoxicam preparations are stored at room temperature.

TERAZOSIN (Hytrin)

Presentation

Tablets – 2 mg, 5 mg, 10 mg

Actions and uses

Terazosin is a selective alpha-1 blocking drug which is chemically related to prazosin and has the actions and uses described for that drug.

Dosage

- Hypertension: 2–10 mg taken as a single daily dose.
- Benign prostatic hypertrophy: 1 mg initially increasing until symptoms are controlled. Up to 10 mg daily may be required.

Nursing implications

- As with prazosin, patients may experience an early rapid fall in blood pressure and care is required when introducing therapy in those with a history of syncope. 1 mg should be prescribed initially and the dose taken at bedtime.
- Dizziness and postural hypotension are therefore possible side effects.
- Some patients may experience lethargy and the vasodilator action may result in development of peripheral oedema.
- Terazosin should not be used in postural hypotension or micturition syncope.

Storage

Terazosin tablets are stored at room temperature.

TERBINAFINE (Lamisil)

Presentation

Tablets – 250 mg
Cream – 1%

Actions and uses

Terbinafine is an antifungal drug used specifically in the treatment of dermatophytic skin and nail infections including ringworm: tinea pedis, tinea cruris and tinea corporis. It acts by interfering with fungal sterol production, causing a deficiency in ergosterol, an accumulation of squalene and ultimately fungal cell death.

Dosage

Adults only.

- Oral: when topical therapy is ineffective, 250 mg once daily for up to 4 weeks (tinea cruris); up to 6 weeks (tinea pedis); and for 4 weeks (tinea corporis). Nail infections require treatment for up to 3 months.
- Topical: for more easily treated dermatophyte and yeast infections cream is rubbed well into the skin once or twice daily for periods of 1–2 weeks.

Nursing implications

- Patients may complain of gastrointestinal upsets and, in particular, disturbances of taste.
- Other side effects include allergic skin reactions, headaches, arthralgia and myalgia. In the event of altered liver function the drug must be immediately discontinued.
- Avoid use in established liver disease and the concurrent use with drugs which may also cause changes in liver enzyme levels.

Storage

Terbinafine preparations are stored at room temperature.

TERBUTALINE (Bricanyl)

Presentation

Tablets – 5 mg and 7.5 mg sustained release
Syrup – 1.5 mg in 5 ml
Inhalation – 250 microgram/dose of metered aerosol or 'spacer' inhaler
Turbohaler – dry powder inhaler, 500 microgram/inhalation
Respirator solution – 10 mg in 1 ml (20 ml bottle)
'Respules' unit dose – 5 mg in 2 ml
Injection – 500 microgram in 1 ml

Actions and uses

This drug stimulates beta-2 adrenergic receptors in the smooth muscle of the airways, with the result that the airways dilate. It is used in clinical practice for the prevention and treatment of conditions such as asthma and chronic bronchitis which produce bronchospasm. Terbutaline may also be administered to reduce uterine contraction in the management of premature labour.

Dosage
For the treatment of bronchospasm

- By inhalation:
  - metered aerosol: adult and child, 250–500 microgram, three or four times a day

T

- inhalation of powder (Turbohaler): 500 microgram up to four times a day
- for acute severe conditions respirator solution is administered via a suitable nebulizer. Adult: 5–10 mg 2–4 times daily with additional doses if required. Child: up to 3 years 2 mg, 3–6 years 3 mg, 6–8 years 4 mg, over 8 years 5 mg, 2–4 times daily.
- Orally: 2.5 mg three times a day increasing after 1–2 weeks to 5 mg three times daily for adults. Children: 75 microgram/kg three times per day. Children 7–15 years, 2.5 mg 2–3 times a day.
- Parenteral, when a rapid therapeutic response is required:
  - by subcutaneous, intramuscular and slow intravenous injection: 250–500 microgram up to four times daily for adults. Children 2–15 years 10 microgram/kg to a maximum of 300 microgram total
  - by intravenous infusion: 1.5–5 microgram/min for 8–10 hours, using a solution containing 3–5 microgram/ml, i.e. dilute 1.5–2.5 mg with 500 ml glucose 5% (or sodium chloride 0.9%).

For the management of premature labour

If syringe pump available, 100 microgram/ml solution in glucose 5%. If syringe pump not available, 10 microgram/ml solution in glucose 5%. Start with 5 microgram/min for 20 minutes, then increase every 20 minutes by 2.5 microgram/min until contractions stop (do not exceed 20 microgram/min). Continue for 1 hour then decrease by 2.5 microgram/min every 20 minutes until a dose is reached which maintains suppression of contractions. Continue with this infusion rate for 12 hours, then switch to oral therapy with 5 mg every 8 hours (or SC injection 250 microgram every 6 hours for a few days before switching to oral) for desired period of time.

Nursing implications
- Common side effects produced are muscle tremor, palpitation, tachycardia, flushing and headache.
- The drug should be used with great caution in patients who have heart disease manifest by rhythm disturbance or angina, thyrotoxicosis and hypertension.
- Hypokalaemia can occur if terbutaline is taken in large doses. Extra caution is required when given with other drugs which can cause hypokalaemia, e.g. theophylline and corticosteroids.
- For use in premature labour, see nursing implications for Ritodrine (p. 318).

Storage
- Preparations are stored at room temperature.
- Aerosols must not be punctured or incinerated after use.

TERFENADINE

Presentation
Tablets – 60 mg

Actions and uses
Terfenadine is an antihistamine. The actions and uses of antihistamines in general are described in the Antihistamine section (p. 33). Terfenadine is used for symptomatic relief of allergy, e.g. allergic rhinitis and urticaria.

Dosage
For adults and children over 50 kg.

- Allergic rhinitis and conjunctivitis: 60 mg once or twice daily or 120 mg once a day.
- Allergic skin reactions: 120 mg daily in single or two divided doses.

Nursing implications
- See the section on Antihistamines (p. 33).
- Studies with this drug indicate that sedation is less of a problem than with other antihistamines.
- During 1992 the Committee on Safety of Medicines drew attention to the possibility that serious cardiac dysrhythmias

may arise in patients who receive excessive doses or in whom plasma concentrations are otherwise likely to be raised. The latter may arise if erythromycin or clarithromycin are co-prescribed with terfenadine or if the patient consumes grapefruit juice. Other drugs which should not be co-prescribed with terfenadine include tricyclic anti-depressants, citalopram, fluoxetine, fluvoxamine, nefazodone, some antifungals, quinine, some antivirals and pentamidine. The drug is best avoided in patients with heart disease who may be predisposed to ventricular rhythm disturbances.

- Avoid the use of terfenadine in hepatic impairment and hypokalaemia and stop therapy if syncope occurs and investigate for arrhythmias.

Storage

The drug is stored at room temperature.

TERLIPRESSIN (Glypressin)

Presentation

Injection – 1 mg vial with 5 ml diluent

Actions and uses

Terlipressin is chemically related to vasopressin and is used for its ability to constrict blood vessels in the hepatic portal circulation, thereby reducing blood flow. It is administered in the treatment of bleeding associated with portal hypertension and oesophageal varices. Unlike vasopressin, terlipressin can be administered as bolus intravenous injections and the risk of reduction in coronary blood flow (producing angina and even infarction) is minimized.

Dosage

Adults: 2 mg by IV bolus injection followed by 1–2 mg repeat doses every 4–6 hours until bleeding is controlled.

Nursing implications

- Although terlipressin is less likely than vasopressin to produce coronary artery constriction and hypertension, patients with cardiovascular disease must nevertheless be carefully monitored during treatment.
- Terlipressin may produce abdominal cramping, blanching and headache due to its action on gut smooth muscle and surface and cerebral blood vessels.
- Failure to achieve rapid control of variceal haemorrhage is an indication for surgical intervention.

Storage

Terlipressin injection is stored at room temperature.

TESTOSTERONE (Andropatch, Sustanon, Testoderm, Virormone)

Presentation

Capsules – Restandol contains 40 mg testosterone undecanoate
Injection:

- testosterone enantate (non-proprietary) 250 mg in 1 ml oily injection
- Sustanon 100 contains testosterone proprionate 20 mg, testosterone phenylproprionate 40 mg and testosterone isocaproate 40 mg, all in 1 ml oily injection
- Sustanon 250 contains testosterone proprionate 30 mg, testosterone phenylproprionate 60 mg, testosterone isocaproate 60 mg and testosterone decanoate 100 mg, all in 1 ml oily injection
- Virormone contains testosterone proprionate 100 mg in 2 ml injection.

Subcutaneous implants – testosterone 100 mg and 200 mg
Transdermal preparations:

- Andropatch patches releasing testosterone 2.5 mg in 24 hours or 5 mg in 24 hours
- Testoderm scrotal patches releasing testosterone 6 mg in 24 hours

T

- Virormone patches releasing testosterone 5 mg in 24 hours.

Actions and uses

Testosterone is a natural androgen produced in the adrenal cortex, the testis in men and in small amounts in the ovaries of women. It has many effects including involvement in the development of secondary sexual characteristics in males and causing an increase in muscular strength, physical vigour and libido. It is indicated for use in androgenic deficiency states, delayed puberty, breast cancer (where administration of testosterone can manipulate other hormones sufficiently to cause tumour regression) and in HRT for women.

Dosage
Oral

Androgen deficiency: 120–160 mg daily for 2–3 weeks reducing to a maintenance dose of 40–120 mg daily.

IM injection

- Testosterone enantate (non-proprietary): slow IM injection for hypogonadism, 250 mg every 2–3 weeks reducing to a maintenance dose of 250 mg every 3–6 weeks; for breast cancer, 250 mg every 2–3 weeks.
- Sustanon 100: deep IM injection for androgen deficiency, 1 ml every 2 weeks.
- Sustanon 250: deep IM injection for androgen deficiency, 1 ml every 3 weeks.
- Virormone: IM injection for androgen deficiency, 50 mg 2–3 times a week; for delayed puberty, 50 mg weekly; for breast cancer, 100 mg 2–3 times a week.

Implant

- Male hypogonadism: 100–600 mg. 600 mg is usually sufficient to maintain plasma testosterone concentrations within the normal range for 4–5 months.
- Menopausal women sometimes receive testosterone implants along with HRT at doses of 50–100 mg every 4–8 months.

Transdermal preparations

- Andropatch, for androgen deficiency in men associated with primary or secondary hypogonadism. Apply patches to clean, dry, unbroken skin on the back, abdomen, upper arm or thigh. Replace patch every 24 hours, applying it to a different area of skin. Start with the 5 mg patch applied at night, then adjust dose to between 2.5 mg and 7.5 mg daily.
- Testoderm, for testosterone deficiency. Apply to clean, dry, shaved scrotal skin each morning. NB: Patches should not be worn in the bath, shower or while swimming, but they can be removed for up to 2 hours and then replaced.
- Virormone patches, for testosterone deficiency. Apply patches to clean, dry, unbroken skin on the back, arms or upper buttocks. Replace every 24 hours preferably each morning. Two patches can be worn if required. NB: Patches should not be worn in the bath or shower, while swimming or during vigorous exercise, but they can be removed for up to 2 hours and then replaced.

Nursing implications

- All patients receiving testosterone may experience an increase in weight, an increase in muscle bulk and salt and water retention with resultant hypertension and oedema.
- When it is given to female patients, testosterone suppresses menstrual function and virilization may occur characterized by deepening of the voice, hirsutism and atrophy of the breasts. Increased libido is a further feature.
- Prolonged treatment with testosterone has been noted to cause an increased incidence of tumours of the liver.
- Testosterone should never be given to patients with prostate cancer as it may stimulate tumour growth. It is also

contraindicated in breast cancer in men, patients with a history of primary liver tumour, hypercalcaemia, pregnancy, breastfeeding and nephrosis.
- Testosterone should be used with caution in patients with cardiac failure, renal failure or liver impairment as it may lead to worsening of the patient's condition.
- Use also with caution in patients with epilepsy as an increased frequency of seizures may be precipitated.
- Testosterone may aggravate the symptoms of migraine so use with caution in migraine sufferers.

Storage
Preparations are stored at room temperature, protected from light.

TETRACYCLINE (Achromycin)

Presentation
Tablets – 250 mg
Capsules – 250 mg
Topical solution – powder for reconstitution, tetracycline 2.2 mg in 1 ml
Ointment – 3%

Actions and uses
For general notes on actions and uses see Tetracyclines (below).
The drug is effective against local infections caused by both Gram-positive and Gram-negative organisms including streptococci, staphylococci and coliform organisms.

Dosage
Oral
- Exacerbations of bronchitis, brucellosis: 1–2 g daily in total taken in four divided doses half an hour before meals.
- Acne: 500 mg twice a day. (If no improvement after 3 months tetracycline should be stopped and a different antibiotic used. Maximum improvement is usually seen after 4–6 months of treatment,

but treatment can be continued for 2 years or longer in severe cases.)
- Rosacea: 500 mg twice a day.
- Primary, secondary or early latent syphilis: 500 mg every 6 hours for 2 weeks.
- Non-gonococcal urethritis: 500 mg every 6 hours for 1–3 weeks.
- Diabetic diarrhoea: two or three doses of 250 mg.

Topical
- 3% ointment: apply 1–3 times daily in susceptible bacterial skin infections.
- Topical solution: apply twice daily for acne.

Local application
Tetracycline can be used as a mouthwash in the management of severe recurrent aphthous ulceration and oral herpes. The contents of a 250 mg capsule should be stirred into a small amount of water and the solution used as a mouthwash, held in the mouth for 2–3 minutes and repeated 3–4 times a day. Do not swallow. Note this is an unlicensed indication.

Nursing implications
- See the section on Tetracyclines (below).
- Patients should be advised to swallow the oral preparations whole, with plenty of fluid, while sitting or standing.
- Patients should also note that they should not take milk, indigestion remedies or medicines containing iron or zinc at the same time of day as this medicine.

Storage
The drug is stored at room temperature.

TETRACYCLINES

This group of antibiotics includes:
Chlortetracycline
Demeclocycline
Doxycycline
Lymecycline

Minocycline
Oxytetracycline
Tetracycline

Actions and uses

The tetracycline group of antibiotics are bacteriostatic, i.e. they prevent further growth and multiplication of bacteria but do not kill them. The mechanism of action is by interfering with the synthesis of proteins necessary for growth and division of bacterial cells.

Tetracyclines have a broad spectrum of activity against both Gram-positive and Gram-negative organisms. It is important to note that infections due to Proteus and *Pseudomonas aeruginosa* are usually not sensitive to tetracyclines. They are used for the following conditions.

- They are frequently used to treat acute exacerbations of chronic bronchitis and upper and lower respiratory tract infections.
- They are effective in the treatment of the following specific infections:
  - brucellosis
  - Q-fever
  - infections due to rickettsia (typhus)
  - non-specific urethritis
  - sinusitis
  - pustular acne vulgaris
  - pneumonia due to mycoplasma and psittacosis
  - trachoma.

Topical applications for skin, eye and ear infections due to staphylococcal, streptococcal and coliform organisms are available.

Bacterial resistance to the tetracyclines is increasing so their use is declining.

Dosage

See specific drugs.

Nursing implications

- Gastrointestinal upsets including heartburn, anorexia, nausea and vomiting commonly occur with this drug. It is important to note that if the drug is given with milk or food to try to reduce these symptoms, the actual concentration absorbed may be reduced and therefore the treatment may be rendered ineffective. The nurse may play an important role in discouraging the patient from taking the tablets with milk or especially antacids.
- Diarrhoea may sometimes occur. This may be due to a change in the flora of the gut caused by tetracyclines but it may also be due to superinfection with Proteus, Pseudomonas or Staphylococcus or *Clostridium difficile* (the latter organism causing pseudomembranous enterocolitis). It is therefore recommended that the drug be discontinued if patients develop severe and persistent diarrhoea.
- If the drug is taken during late pregnancy or administered to young children (less than 12 years of age), permanent staining of the teeth and bones may occur. This is because tetracyclines have been found to be taken up by growing bones and teeth. This group of drugs is therefore, for this reason, contraindicated in pregnant women, breastfeeding and young children.
- Patients with impaired renal function should not be given tetracyclines as they may worsen the degree of renal failure by inhibiting body protein synthesis.
- Other adverse effects include photosensitivity reactions and hypersensitivity producing urticaria, asthma, dyspnoea, itching, oedema and hypotension.
- Tetracyclines affect blood-clotting function and therefore if they are given to patients already on anticoagulants, the anticoagulant dose may have to be altered.
- The coincident administration of antacids, iron tablets and milk will all reduce the amount of tetracycline absorbed from the gut and may render its administration ineffective.

- Superinfection with fungi, i.e. oral candidiasis, or Proteus, Pseudomonas and Staphylococcus may occur.

Storage
See specific drugs.

THEOPHYLLINE (Nuelin, Slo-Phyllin, Theo-Dur, Uniphyllin)

Presentation
Tablets – 125 mg
Modified-release tablets – 175 mg, 200 mg, 250 mg, 300 mg, 400 mg
Modified-release capsules – 60 mg, 125 mg, 250 mg
Liquid – 60 mg in 5 ml

Actions and uses
Theophylline has the actions and uses described for aminophylline though it is not itself water soluble and cannot therefore be produced in an injectable form.

Dosage
Adults: 125–250 mg (conventional tablets) taken three or four times daily. In most cases, modified-release tablets or capsules are taken twice daily; the usual dose is one or two modified-release tablets or capsules.
Children: initially a dose of up to 5 mg/kg body weight is given followed by maintenance doses of 2.5 mg/kg or more every 6 hours. Children aged 3–5 years or more should if possible take slow-release preparations, e.g. one or two tablets or capsules twice daily. For this purpose Slo-phyllin capsules may be preferred since they can be opened and taken as small pellets to facilitate administration.

Nursing implications
- See the section on Aminophylline (p. 23).
- Note that different slow-release preparations may produce different plasma concentration profiles (i.e. are not necessarily bioequivalent). Patients should ideally continue to receive a given brand whether in hospital or the community.

- The individual dosage is determined by the plasma theophylline concentration. The target range is 55–110 micromol/litre (10–20 mg/litre).

Storage
Theophylline preparations are stored at room temperature.

THIAZIDE AND RELATED DIURETICS

This group of drugs includes:
Bendrofluazide/bendroflumethiazide
Chlorthalidone/chlortalidone
Cyclopenthiazide
Hydrochlorothiazide
Indapamide
Metolazone
Polythiazide
Xipamide

Actions and uses
Most of the plasma passing through the kidney is reabsorbed at various sites along the tubules of the kidney. Thiazide diuretics decrease the ability of the kidney to reabsorb sodium and water in the distal part of the tubules, thus increasing urine output. They are therefore useful in diseases where fluid accumulates in the form of oedema, i.e. heart failure, nephrotic syndrome and liver cell failure. In addition, they have a direct action on blood vessel walls which leads to a reduction in blood pressure and they may therefore be used in the treatment of hypertension.

Onset of action is within 1–2 hours and duration of action tends to be for some hours. They therefore produce a more gentle and long-lasting diuresis than 'loop' diuretics, such as frusemide.

Dosage
See individual drugs.

Nursing implications
- This group of drugs can cause important side effects which must be detected as early as possible to prevent their potentially serious consequences.

T

- Hypokalaemia: the patient may become apathetic and confused and may develop muscle weakness or abdominal distension. If these signs are noticed more serious effects of hypokalaemia, such as potentially fatal cardiac arrhythmias in patients on digoxin or coma in patients with liver cell failure, may be prevented. (In patients on digoxin or with liver cell failure coincident administration of potassium supplements or a potassium-sparing diuretic such as spironolactone may be useful.)
- Dehydration may occur, causing postural hypotension and collapse.
- An increase in blood urate may occur, causing gout. Joint pains in patients on these drugs should always make the nurse suspect this complication.
- The drugs may alter glucose metabolism, leading to hyperglycaemia and glycosuria. Thus any diabetic patient receiving these drugs should be followed up closely in case change in treatment is required.
- Thrombocytopenia may occur very rarely. This may be detected initially by observing small haemorrhages or bruises in the skin and if confirmed by checking the platelet count, the drug should be stopped.
- Thiazides should not be used in patients with hypokalaemia, hyponatraemia, hypercalcaemia, severe renal or hepatic impairment, symptomatic hyperuricaemia or Addison's disease.

Storage
    See individual drugs.

THIOGUANINE/TIOGUANINE (Lanvis)

Presentation
    Tablets – 40 mg

Actions and uses
    Thioguanine is a cytotoxic drug which is used for the treatment of acute leukaemia, e.g. acute myelogenous leukaemia and acute lymphoblastic leukaemia.

Dosage
    Adults and children: a single oral daily dose of 2–2.5 mg/kg body weight is usually given. Treatment courses may last from 5 to 20 days.

Nursing implications
- Bone marrow suppression with resultant increased risk of haemorrhage, anaemia and infection is the most serious adverse effect from this drug. Frequent blood counts are usually performed during treatment courses.
- Symptoms commonly produced include diarrhoea, nausea, vomiting and anorexia.
- Stomatitis and jaundice due to altered liver function may occur with this drug.
- Hyperuricaemia, occasionally resulting in gout and impairment of renal function, may be produced.

Storage
    Thioguanine tablets are stored at room temperature.

THIOPENTAL/THIOPENTONE (Intraval)

Presentation
    Injection – 500 mg vials for preparation of a 2.5% solution

Actions and uses
    Thiopental sodium is a barbiturate drug. It has no analgesic properties, but it is used as an intravenous anaesthetic. It has a rapid onset and short duration of action.

Dosage
    For induction of anaesthesia: 2.5% (25 mg in 1 ml) solution is used and injected very slowly into a superficial vein. The total dosage administered

is that required to induce anaesthesia and in general is not likely to be more than 4 mg/kg. Initially 100–150 mg is given over 10–15 seconds, followed by a further dose after 30–60 seconds if required. Doses in excess of 500 mg may be associated with an unnecessarily prolonged recovery time and other complications.

For induction of anaesthesia in children, use 2–7 mg/kg.

Nursing implications
- The injection solution is highly alkaline and will cause irritation if injected outside the vein.
- Patients may still be drowsy up to 24 hours after the injection.
- As solutions are strongly alkaline they should not be mixed with other drugs in the same syringe.

Storage
Vials containing thiopental sodium as dry powder are stored at room temperature. When reconstituted, however, solutions readily break down, producing cloudiness and precipitation or crystallization. Solutions are therefore not suitable for prolonged storage and should be discarded immediately after use.

THIORIDAZINE (Melleril)

Presentation
Tablets – 10 mg, 25 mg, 50 mg, 100 mg
Syrup/suspension – 25 mg in 5 ml, 100 mg in 5 ml

Actions and uses
Thioridazine is a member of the phenothiazine group of drugs and its actions are described in the section dealing with these drugs (p. 281) Thioridazine is associated with cardiotoxicity due to its ability to cause QT-interval prolongation. It should now only be used under specialist supervision as second-line treatment of schizophrenia.

Dosage
Adults: 50–300 mg daily in divided doses, up to a maximum of 600 mg daily in hospitalized patients.
Not recommended for use in children.

Nursing implications
- See the section on Phenothiazines (p. 281).
- Use is contraindicated in patients with:
  - significant cardiac disease, e.g. angina, bradycardia or heart failure
  - a history of ventricular arrhythmias
  - QT-interval prolongation or a family history of QT-interval prolongation
  - uncorrected hypokalaemia or hypomagnesaemia
  - concurrent use with other drugs known to cause QT-interval prolongation
  - reduced cytochrome P450 2D6 liver enzyme activity
  - concurrent use with other drugs that inhibit or are metabolized by cytochrome P450 2D6.
- Patients on thioridazine should have baseline ECG screening and their electrolytes monitored and these tests repeated after each dose change and every 6 months.

Storage
Thioridazine is stored at room temperature, protected from direct sunlight.

THROMBOLYTIC DRUGS

Presentation
See the individual sections for streptokinase, alteplase and reteplase.

Actions and uses
All three of the above drugs are indicated for the acute treatment of myocardial infarction. They act by dissolving clots in coronary arteries, thus allowing reperfusion of cardiac muscle and reduction in infarct size and a diminution in mortality.

Streptokinase is additionally indicated for the intravascular dissolution of thrombi and emboli in extensive deep venous thrombosis, pulmonary embolism, acute or subacute occlusion of peripheral arteries and central retinal venous or arterial thrombosis.

Dosage
See individual drugs.

Nursing implications
- In the treatment of myocardial infarction it has been demonstrated that the earlier the drug is given, the better the effect. This holds for all three treatments.
- The nurse may play an important role in identifying contraindications to treatment; these are as follows.
  - History of cerebrovascular disease.
  - Uncontrolled hypertension.
  - Known bleeding diathesis.
  - Recent severe internal bleeding, major surgery or trauma or puncture of major non-compressible blood vessels.
  - Active peptic ulceration.
  - Other known contraindications to fibrinolytic therapy, e.g. acute pancreatitis, bacterial endocarditis.
  - Severe liver disease including hepatic failure, sclerosis, portal hypertension and active hepatitis. Active pancreatitis and oesophageal varices.
  - Recent prolonged or traumatic resuscitation.
  - Coagulation defects.
  - Aortic dissection.
  - Coma.
  - Heavy vaginal bleeding.
  - Active pulmonary disease with cavitation.
- The commonest and most serious complication after administration of these drugs is bleeding. Careful control by pressure on the site where the drug or other intravenous therapy may be administered is essential.
- Side effects specific to each of the three therapies are listed under the individual drugs.

Storage
See specific drugs.

THYROXINE/LEVOTHYROXINE (Eltroxin)

Presentation
Tablets – 25 microgram, 50 microgram and 100 microgram

Actions and uses
Thyroxine is the hormone released by the thyroid gland which is essential for maintaining a normal metabolic rate. Deficiency leads to obesity, coarse skin and hair, hoarseness, constipation, impairment of intellect, an inability to tolerate cold temperatures and in severe cases it may lead to psychosis or coma. Thyroxine's primary use is in the treatment of disorders associated with underproduction of thyroid hormone.

Dosage
- Replacement therapy may be taken orally once daily in the morning. It is not essential to take the drug any more than once a day as it takes a particularly long time for it to be metabolized and multiple daily dosages are of no benefit.
- The actual dose necessary for patients is variable and is usually adjusted by observing clinical improvement and measuring thyroid hormone in the blood. Normal adult replacement doses vary between 50 and 200 microgram per day.
- It is essential that replacement therapy should be commenced at very low dosages and very cautiously in elderly patients and patients with ischaemic heart disease (see below).
- For congenital hypothyroidism and juvenile myxoedema: child up to 1 month, initially 5–10 microgram/kg/day; over 1 month, initially 5 microgram/kg/day then adjust in steps of 25 microgram every 2–4 weeks until there are signs of mild toxic effects, then reduce the dose slightly.

Nursing implications

- Any patient receiving thyroxine is likely to be on this drug for life. As the effects of stopping the drug take some time to manifest themselves, patients may come to believe that the drug is unnecessary. As hypothyroidism has many effects on physical and mental function and in the long term may lead to death due to ischaemic heart disease, it is essential that all patients be encouraged to take replacement dosage regularly.
- Thyroxine has no adverse effects when given in appropriate dosage. However, if too much is given too quickly, especially to elderly patients or patients with angina, severe angina or myocardial infarction may be precipitated. Such patients should receive initially doses as low as 25 microgram on alternate days for the first 1–2 months followed by cautious increases in dose over the next 6 months or so to a full replacement regime.
- Excessive dosage may produce anginal pain, cardiac dysrhythmias, palpitations, cramps, tachycardia, diarrhoea, restlessness, excitability, headache, flushing, sweating, weight loss and muscle weakness.
- Any patients who have hypothyroidism due to inadequate pituitary function (hypopituitarism) should always have steroid replacement treatment commenced before thyroxine is commenced. Failure to do this may lead to death.

Storage
Tablets containing thyroxine are stored at room temperature. The tablets should be protected from light.

TIAGABINE (Gabitril)

Presentation
Tablets – 5 mg, 10 mg and 15 mg

Actions and uses
Tiagabine is a relatively new anticonvulsant used as adjunctive treatment for partial seizures with or without secondary generalization which are not satisfactorily controlled with other antiepileptics. Tiagabine acts by inhibiting GABA uptake, increasing its inhibitory actions in the brain.

Dosage
- With enzyme-inducing drugs (e.g. phenytoin and phenobarbitone): 5 mg twice a day for 1 week, then increase in increments of 5–10 mg at weekly intervals to a dose of 30–45 mg daily. Daily doses above 30 mg should be taken in three divided doses.
- With non-enzyme inducing drugs: start with 15–30 mg daily and adjust as required.
- Not recommended for children under 12.

Nursing implications

- Side effects include diarrhoea, tiredness, dizziness, nervousness, tremor, concentration difficulties, depressed mood, emotional lability and speech impairment.
- Use with caution in liver impairment.

Storage
Tiagabine tablets are stored at room temperature.

TIAPROFENIC ACID (Surgam)

Presentation
Tablets – 200 mg, 300 mg
Modified-release capsules – 300 mg

Actions and uses
Tiaprofenic acid is a member of the propionic acid group of non-steroidal antiinflammatory drugs. It therefore has the actions and uses described under NSAIDS (p. 250).

Dosage

Adults: 600 mg daily in divided doses.

Nursing implications

- The nursing implications for NSAIDS apply to this drug (p. 250).
- Severe cystitis has occurred with tiaprofenic acid. It should not be prescribed for patients with urinary tract disorders and should be stopped if any urinary tract symptoms occur. Patients should be advised to seek medical advice if symptoms such as increased urinary frequency or pain on urination occur, and to stop the medication.

Storage

Tiaprofenic acid preparations are stored at room temperature.

TIMENTIN

Timentin is a combination of ticarcillin and clavulanic acid.

Presentation

Injection – 3.2 g powder for reconstitution, ticarcillin 3 g and clavulanic acid 200 mg

Actions and uses

Ticarcillin, a carboxypenicillin, is a derivative of the penicillin group of antibiotics. It has a wider spectrum of activity than the parent drug benzylpenicillin and is effective against many Gram-positive and Gram-negative organisms. Its mode of action is identical to that described for benzylpenicillin. The indications for its use are for the treatment of infection at any site in the body caused by an organism sensitive to ticarcillin. It is of particular interest to note that ticarcillin is often effective in the treatment of serious infections due to Pseudomonas species which are commonly resistant to other antibiotics.

By adding clavulanic acid, the spectrum of activity of ticarcillin may be broadened as clavulanic acid prevents the breakdown and therefore the inactivation of ticarcillin by penicillinase (beta-lactamase). This substance is produced by a number of bacteria and effectively renders them penicillin resistant. Some bacteria, therefore, resistant to ticarcillin alone, may be effectively treated by timentin. In practice, this may prove particularly important in the treatment of urinary tract infections due to *E. coli* and Pseudomonas spp., skin and soft tissue infections due to *Staphylococcus aureus* and general systemic and respiratory infections due to Gram-negative microorganisms.

Dosage

Adults: usually 3.2 g (as timentin) by intravenous injection at intervals of 4, 6 or 8 hours depending upon severity of infection and susceptibility of the pathogen involved.

Children: usually based on a dose of 80 mg/kg timentin (i.e. 75 mg timentin + 5 mg clavulanic acid) by intravenous injection at 8-hourly intervals or 12-hourly intervals in neonates.

Nursing implications

- Timentin is administered by rapid intravenous infusion in 50–100 ml minibags containing glucose 5% over 30–40 minutes.
- Lower doses, e.g. adult doses of 1.6 mg 8–12 hourly, are used for patients with moderate to severe renal impairment.
- Timentin should not be administered by direct intravenous bolus or intramuscular injection.
- Note that heat is produced when powder is dissolved and also that the resulting solution has a straw-coloured appearance.
- Timentin is often prescribed together with gentamicin or a related aminoglycoside antibiotic and while such combinations are useful, these drugs must not be mixed in solution.
- For other nursing implications see Co-amoxiclav p. 103.

Storage

Timentin injection is stored at room temperature. Solutions should be prepared immediately before use.

TIMOLOL (Betim, Blocadren, Timoptol)

Presentation

Tablets – 10 mg
Eye drops – 0.25%, 0.5%
Long-acting eye drops – 0.25%, 0.5%

Actions and uses

Timolol is a non-selective beta-adrenoreceptor blocking drug and its actions are described in the section on these drugs (p. 51).

In addition, it is applied to the eye in the treatment of glaucoma (ocular hypertension). In this condition it lowers intraocular pressure by reducing aqueous humor production.

Dosage

The adult oral range is 15–60 mg daily in two or three divided doses.

- Hypertension: start with 10 mg daily in one or two divided doses increased gradually to a maximum of 60 mg daily if required. Give in divided doses above 20 mg daily.
- Angina: 10–45 mg daily in 2–3 divided doses.
- Prophylaxis after MI: 5 mg twice a day for 2 days, then 10 mg twice a day. Start 7–28 days after the MI.
- Migraine prophylaxis: 10–20 mg daily.
- Glaucoma: one drop instilled in the eye twice daily, starting with the lower strength and increasing to 0.5% if required. The long-acting preparations are instilled once daily.

Nursing implications

See the section on Beta-Adrenoreceptor Blocking Drugs (p. 51).

Storage

Timolol tablets are stored at room temperature. Note that eye drops, after opening, should be used within 7 days for hospitalized patients and 4 weeks for others, due to the risk of bacterial contamination.

TINIDAZOLE (Fasigyn)

Presentation

Tablets – 500 mg

Actions and uses

This drug is a member of the nitromidazole group of which metronidazole is the forerunner. It therefore has the actions and uses of metronidazole but its action is more prolonged so that once or twice daily dosing is possible. In practice, its uses include prophylaxis and treatment of anaerobic infections and treatment of bacterial vaginosis and acute ulcerative gingivitis.

Dosage

- Anaerobic infections: initially 2 g followed by doses of 1 g daily or 500 mg twice daily for 5–6 days.
- Bacterial vaginosis/acute ulcerative gingivitis: a single 2 g dose is used.
- Prophylaxis prior to abdominal surgery: a single 2 g dose 12 hours before surgery.
- Intestinal amoebiasis: 2 g daily for 2–3 days; child 50–60 mg/kg daily for 3 days.
- Amoebic involvement of liver: 1.5–2 g daily for 3–6 days; child, 50–60 mg/kg daily for 5 days.
- Urogenital trichomoniasis and giardiasis: single 2 g dose; child single dose of 50–75 mg/kg, repeat once if necessary.

Nursing implications

The nursing implications section under Metronidazole (p. 222) applies to this drug.

Storage

Tinidazole tablets are stored at room temperature.

TINZAPARIN (Innohep)

Presentation

Injection – 2500 units in 0.25 ml syringe, 3500 units in 0.35 ml syringe, 4500 units in 0.45 ml syringe, 10 000 units in 0.5 ml syringe, 14 000 units in 0.7 ml syringe, 18 000 units in 0.9 ml syringe, 20 000 units in 2 ml vial, 40 000 units in 2 ml vial

Actions and uses

Tinzaparin is a low molecular weight heparin licensed for the prevention of thrombosis and thromboembolism in patients undergoing surgery. It is also used in the treatment of deep vein thrombosis and pulmonary embolism. For its actions and uses see the section on Dalteparin (p. 115).

Dosage
Prophylaxis of deep vein thrombosis by SC injection

- General surgery: 3500 units 2 hours prior to surgery, then 3500 units every 24 hours for 7–10 days.
- Orthopaedic surgery, high-risk patients: 50 units/kg 2 hours prior to surgery, then 50 units/kg every 24 hours for 7–10 days or 4500 units 12 hours prior to surgery, then 4500 units every 24 hours for 7–10 days.

Treatment of deep vein thrombosis and pulmonary embolism by SC injection

175 units/kg daily for at least 6 days and until adequate oral anticoagulation is achieved.

> ## Nursing implications
> - See the sections on Dalteparin (p. 115) and Heparin (p. 167).
> - Tizaparin preparations contain sulphites which may cause hypersensitivity reactions, particularly in asthmatics.

Storage

Tinzaparin injection is stored at room temperature.

TIZANIDINE (Zanaflex)

Presentation

Tablets – 2 mg and 4 mg

Actions and uses

Tizanidine is an alpha-2 adrenoceptor agonist, used in the management of spasticity associated with multiple sclerosis or spinal cord injury. It acts in the central nervous system, reducing pathologically induced increased muscle tone.

Dosage

Start with 2 mg daily increased gradually in steps of 2 mg up to 24 mg daily or a maximum of 36 mg daily. Not recommended for children.

> ## Nursing implications
> - Side effects include drowsiness, fatigue, insomnia, dizziness, dry mouth, nausea, gastrointestinal disturbances and reduced blood pressure.
> - Patients should be advised of drowsiness and to expect impaired performance of skilled tasks.
> - Do not use in severe liver impairment and use with caution in the elderly and those with renal impairment.

Storage

Tizanidine tablets are stored at room temperature.

TOBRAMYCIN (Nebcin, Tobi)

Presentation

Injection – 40 mg in 1 ml, 20 mg in 2 ml, 80 mg in 2 ml
Nebulizer solution – 300 mg in 5 ml

Actions and uses

Tobramycin is an aminoglycoside antibiotic similar to gentamicin. Its actions and uses are described in the section on this drug (p. 158). It may occasionally be effective for the treatment of microorganisms resistant to gentamicin. It can be used, nebulized, for the treatment of pulmonary *Pseudomonas aeruginosa* infection in cystic fibrosis.

Dosage

- IM slow IV injection or IV infusion: adult, 3 mg/kg daily in three divided doses. Increase to 5 mg/kg daily in 3–4 divided doses in severe infections. Child over 1 week,

2–2.5 mg/kg every 8 hours.
Neonate 2 mg/kg every 12 hours.
- IM injection for urinary tract infection: 2–3 mg/kg daily as a single dose.
- Treatment of chronic pulmonary *Pseudomonas aeruginosa* infection in cystic fibrosis: adults and children over 6 years, inhalation of nebulized solution, 300 mg every 12 hours for 28 days, repeat after 28-day interval.

Nursing implications
- The nursing implications on gentamicin (p. 158) apply to this drug.
- When given by intravenous infusion the drug is diluted with 50–100 ml of normal saline or 5% dextrose in adults, and appropriately lower volumes in children. The infusion is administered over a period of 20–60 minutes.
- If serum concentrations are measured, the 1-hour peak should not exceed 10 mg/l and the predose trough should be less than 2 mg/l.

Storage
The drug is stored at room temperature.

TOLBUTAMIDE

Presentation
Tablets – 500 mg

Actions and uses
Tolbutamide is an oral hypoglycaemic agent used in type 2 diabetes mellitus. For its actions and uses see the section on Gliclazide (p. 160).

Dosage
500 mg to 2 g daily in 2–3 divided doses is recommended.

Nursing implications
See the section on Gliclazide (p. 160).

Storage
Tablets are stored at room temperature.

TOLFENAMIC ACID (Clotam)

Presentation
Tablets – 200 mg

Actions and uses
Tolfenamic acid is a non-steroidal antiinflammatory drug used in the treatment of acute migraine attacks. See the section on NSAIDs (p. 250).

Dosage
200 mg at the onset of migraine attack. The dose can be repeated after 1–2 hours if required.

Nursing implications
- See the section on NSAIDs (p. 250).
- To minimize gastric irritation, patients should be advised to take the medication with food or milk.
- When dysuria is present, patients should be advised to increase fluid intake.
- If the patient is also experiencing nausea and vomiting, an antiemetic may be taken.

Storage
Tolfenamic acid tablets are stored at room temperature.

TOLTERODINE (Detrusitol)

Presentation
Tablets – 1 mg and 2 mg

Actions and uses
Tolterodine is an antimuscarinic drug indicated for use in urinary frequency, urgency and incontinence with actions and uses similar to those of oxybutynin.

Dosage
2 mg twice a day, reduced to 1 mg twice a day if required to reduce side effects.
Not recommended for children.

T

Nursing implications
- Adverse effects include typical antimuscarinic effects, e.g. dry mouth and constipation.
- Do not use in urinary retention, uncontrolled angle closure glaucoma, myasthenia gravis, severe ulcerative colitis or toxic megacolon, pregnancy or breastfeeding.

Storage
Tolterodine tablets are stored at room temperature.

TOPIRAMATE (Topamax)

Presentation
Tablets – 25 mg, 50 mg, 100 mg and 200 mg
Sprinkle capsules – 15 mg, 25 mg and 50 mg

Actions and uses
Topiramate is an anticonvulsant used as adjunctive treatment for partial seizures with or without secondary generalization not satisfactorily controlled with other antiepileptics. It can also be used for seizures associated with Lennox–Gastaut syndrome and for primary generalized tonic-clonic seizures. Topiramate has several modes of action, reducing the frequency of action potential generation in certain neurones, enhancing the activity of GABA and increasing its inhibitory actions in the brain and it acts as a weak antagonist at one of the glutamate receptors in the brain, inhibiting excitatory activity.

Dosage
Adults: start with 25 mg a day for 1 week, then increase in increments of 25–50 mg daily at intervals of 1–2 weeks to a usual dose of 200–400 mg daily in two divided doses. Maximum of 800 mg daily.
Child: 2–16 years, start with 25 mg a night for 1 week, then increase in increments of 1–3 mg/kg daily at intervals of 1–2 weeks to a usual dose of 5–9 mg/kg daily in two divided doses.

Nursing implications
- Side effects include abdominal pain, ataxia, anorexia, asthenia, confusion, nausea and weight loss.
- The dose of topiramate should be titrated gradually. It may be necessary to use smaller dose increases or longer intervals than described above.
- The sprinkle capsules can be swallowed whole or opened and the contents sprinkled on soft food.

Storage
Topiramate preparations are stored at room temperature.

TOPOTECAN (Hycamtin)

Presentation
Injection for intravenous infusion – powder for reconstitution, 4 mg vial

Actions and uses
Topotecan is a topoisomerase I inhibitor used in the treatment of ovarian cancer where first-line or subsequent therapy has failed. It acts by inhibiting the topoisomerase enzyme which is involved in DNA replication.

Dosage
IV infusion over 30 minutes: 1.5 mg/m^2 daily for 5 consecutive days. Repeat course at least four times at intervals of 3 weeks.

Nursing implications
- Side effects include neutropenia, thrombocytopenia, anaemia, alopecia, nausea, gastrointestinal upset, stomatitis, abdominal pain, fatigue and asthenia.
- Patients should report any symptoms of infection such as fever, sore throat, chest infection. Febrile neutropenia requires hospitalization for intravenous antibiotic therapy.
- Blood counts must be monitored regularly and doses adjusted accordingly.
- Doses should be reduced in moderate renal impairment.

T

- Topotecan should not be used in severe renal or severe hepatic impairment.
- Do not use where severe myelosuppression is already present or in pregnancy or breastfeeding.
- Patients should be given contraceptive advice to avoid pregnancy during treatment and for at least 3 months following treatment.
- Treatment toxicity can result in hair loss.
- Nurses should be aware of the risks posed by cytotoxic drugs. Some are irritant to the skin and mucous surfaces and care must be exercised when handling them. In particular, spillage or contamination of personnel or the environment must be avoided. If cytotoxic drugs are handled regularly, it is theoretically possible that repeated skin contact or inhalation may produce systemic toxic effects in nurses who have developed hypersensitivity to them. Most hospitals now operate a centralized (pharmacy-organized) additive service. While this reduces the risk of exposure to cytotoxic drugs, it is essential that nurses recognize and understand the local policy on their safe handling and disposal. The Health and Safety Executive has decreed that such a policy should be in place wherever cytotoxic drugs are administered. These should be adapted, wherever possible, to care of patients in the community.

Storage
Topotecan preparations are stored at room temperature. Protect from light. Use immediately after reconstitution.

TORASEMIDE (Torem)

Presentation
Tablets – 2.5 mg, 5 mg, 10 mg

Actions and uses
Torasemide is a loop diuretic with actions and uses similar to those of furosemide/frusemide and bumetanide. It is used in oedema and hypertension.

Dosage
Oedema: 5 mg each morning, increased if required to 20 mg each morning or to a maximum of 40 mg daily.
Hypertension: 2.5 mg daily increased if required to 5 mg daily.

Nursing implications
See the section on Frusemide (p. 154).

Storage
Torasemide tablets are stored at room temperature.

TRAMADOL (Dromadol, Tramake, Zamadol, Zydol)

Presentation
Capsules – 50 mg
Sachets – effervescent powder, 50 mg and 100 mg
Soluble tablets – 50 mg
Modified-release tablets – 75 mg, 100 mg, 150 mg, 200 mg, 300 mg and 400 mg
Modified-release capsules – 50 mg, 100 mg, 150 mg and 200 mg
Injection – 100 mg in 2 ml

Actions and uses
Tramadol is a narcotic analgesic with actions and uses as described in the section on Narcotic Analgesics (p. 238). It is used for moderate-to-severe pain.

Dosage
- Orally: 50–100 mg a maximum of every 4 hours; doses higher than 400 mg daily are seldom required.
- IM injection, IV injection or infusion: 50–100 mg every 4–6 hours and for postoperative pain, 100 mg initially, then 50 mg every 10–20 minutes if required to a total of 250 mg including initial dose, in the first hour, then 50–100 mg every 4–6 hours to a maximum of 600 mg daily.
- Tramadol is not recommended for children.

T

> **Nursing implications**
> The nursing implications of Narcotic Analgesics (p. 238) apply to tramadol.

Storage
Tramadol preparations are stored at room temperature.

TRANDOLAPRIL (Gopten, Odrik)

Presentation
Capsules – 500 microgram, 1 mg, 2 mg

Actions and uses
See the section on ACE Inhibitors (p. 4). Trandolapril is indicated for use in mild-to-moderate hypertension and following myocardial infarction in patients with left ventricular dysfunction.

Dosage
Range: 1–4 mg as a single daily dose.

> **Nursing implications**
> See section on ACE Inhibitors (p. 4).

Storage
Trandolapril capsules are stored at room temperature.

TRANEXAMIC ACID (Cyklokapron)

Presentation
Tablets – 500 mg
Injection – 500 mg in 5 ml

Actions and uses
Tranexamic acid is an antifibrinolytic agent. It impairs fibrin dissolution, inhibits fibrinolysis and prevents bleeding in situations such as dental extraction and menorrhagia.

Dosage
Orally:

- local fibrinolysis: 15–25 mg/kg two or three times per day.
- menorrhagia: 1–1.5 g three or four times per day for 3–4 days.

- hereditary angiooedema: 1–1.5 g two or three times per day.

Slow IV injection, local fibrinolysis: 0.5–1 g three times per day.

> **Nursing implications**
> - Common side effects include gastrointestinal upset (nausea, vomiting and diarrhoea), postural hypotension and dizziness.
> - There is an increased incidence of thrombosis with this drug.
> - The risk of thrombosis is markedly increased if patients have reduced renal function or are concurrently receiving oral contraceptive medication.

Storage
The drug is stored at room temperature.

TRANYLCYPROMINE (Parnate)

Presentation
Tablets – 10 mg

Actions and uses
Tranylcypromine is a monoamine oxidase-inhibiting drug. Its actions and uses are described in the section on these drugs (p. 228).

Dosage
10 mg two or three times daily.

> **Nursing implications**
> See the section on Monoamine Oxidase-Inhibiting Drugs (p. 228).

Storage
Tranylcypromine tablets are stored at room temperature.

TRAZODONE (Molipaxin)

Presentation
Tablets – 150 mg
Capsules – 50 mg and 100 mg
Liquid – 50 mg in 5 ml

Actions and uses

Trazodone is an antidepressant drug which is derived from and is closely related chemically to tricyclic antidepressants. Its actions and uses are similar to those described for Tricyclic Antidepressants (p. 31).

Dosage

Adults: 150–600 mg in total per day administered in two or three divided doses. Larger doses should be administered in hospital only. Not recommended for children.

Nursing implications

- See the section on Antidepressant Drugs (p. 228).
- This drug in particular is associated with priapism in males. This occurs rarely but if it does, trazodone should be discontinued immediately.

Storage

Trazodone preparations are stored at room temperature.

TRIAMCINOLONE (Adcortyl, Kenalog, Lederspan)

Presentation

Deep intramuscular injection – 40 mg in 1 ml, 80 mg in 2 ml
Intraarticular/intradermal injection – 10 mg in 1 ml, 50 mg in 5 ml, 40 mg in 1 ml
Cream, ointment and dental paste – 0.1%
Aqueous nasal spray – 55 microgram/metered spray

Actions and uses

Triamcinolone is a corticosteroid drug and has actions and uses as described in the section on these drugs (p. 107). It is used by a number of routes for conditions as follows.

- It is administered topically for the management of inflammatory skin conditions.
- It may be given orally as a dental paste.
- It may be administered by deep intramuscular injection for suppression of inflammatory and allergic disorders such as hay fever or asthma.
- Direct intraarticular injection may be given where appropriate for such conditions as arthritis, bursitis and tendonitis.

Dosage

- Topical applications are applied two to four times daily sparingly.
- Dental paste is applied two to four times daily.
- Nasal spray: adults and children over 12 years, 110 microgram into each nostril once a day, reducing to 55 microgram when control of allergic rhinitis has been achieved. Children 6–12 years, 55 microgram into each nostril once a day.
- For intraarticular injection or intrasynovial injection: 2.5–80 mg is given according to joint size.
- For intradermal injection: 2–3 mg (maximum 5 mg) at any one site. Total maximum of 30 mg.
- Deep IM injection into gluteal muscle: 40 mg of triamcinolone acetonide for depot effect, repeat according to patient response. Maximum single dose of 100 mg.

Nursing implications

See the section on Corticosteroid Drugs (p. 107).

Storage

Preparations containing triamcinolone are stored at room temperature.

TRIAMTERENE (Dytac)

Presentation

Capsules – 50 mg
Also combined with thiazide diuretics in Dyazide and Dytide.

Actions and uses

Triamterene has a very mild diuretic action. It achieves this by inhibition of sodium excretion in the distal tubules with resultant sodium and water loss in the urine. As a diuretic alone it is of little use. However, it has an action on the renal tubule which reduces potassium excretion and it may

T

therefore be used in combination with thiazide diuretics to prevent the common dangerous side effect of hypokalaemia encountered when thiazide diuretics are given alone. Hypokalaemia is particularly serious in patients who are on digoxin treatment or in those with serious hepatic dysfunction such as cirrhosis.

Dosage

- The daily dose is 150–250 mg initially, reduced to alternate days after 1 week.
- The daily dose is usually divided with doses taken after breakfast and lunch.
- Triamterene produces maximum effect after 8 hours and its actions may continue for 2–3 days after therapy is withdrawn.

Nursing implications

- By far the most important problem which may arise in patients on triamterene is the development of hyperkalaemia which is especially likely to occur if patients have impaired renal function. Hyperkalaemia is difficult to detect clinically and is extremely danger-ous because of the possibility of precipitation of cardiac arrest.
- Side effects are infrequent but nausea, vomiting, leg cramps and dizziness may occur.
- In common with other diuretics, triamterene may alter blood glucose levels and therefore treatment requirement in patients with diabetes mellitus may be altered.
- Triamterene may colour the urine so patients should be advised of this.

Storage

Triamterene capsules are stored at room temperature.

TRIBAVIRIN/RIBAVIRIN (Rebetol, Virazole)

Presentation

Nasal aerosol – 6 g
Capsules – 200 mg

Actions and uses

Ribavarin is an antiviral agent which is active against a range of viruses including influenza A and B viruses and parainfluenza. It is used in the treatment of infections due to respiratory syncytial virus (RSV), a common cause of chronic recurring lower respiratory infections in the first few years of life. In infants and children with established cardiorespiratory disease, RSV infection may present a special hazard: in otherwise healthy children it produces only mild symptoms. The precise mechanism whereby ribavarin prevents viral replication is unknown. Ribavirin is also used, under specialist advice, in combination with interferon alfa-2b for chronic hepatitis C.

Dosage

Bronchiolitis: the drug is delivered by aerosol or nebulization as a 20 mg/ml solution for 12 hours or longer daily over 3–7 days.

Chronic hepatitis C: orally, adults over 18 years of age, 75 kg or less, 400 mg in the morning and 600 mg in the evening; over 75 kg, 600 mg in the morning and 600 mg in the evening.

Nursing implications

- Ribavarin solution may be delivered via an oxygen mask or in a tent or hood. It is administered via a special small particle aerosol generator. Patients must be monitored closely for signs of worsening respiratory function and fluid levels and electrolytes should be monitored.
- Ribavirin is contraindicated in pregnancy and breastfeeding. Pregnancy must be excluded before treatment with the oral preparation and effective contraception used during treatment and for 4 months after treatment in women and for 7 months after treatment in men. If a male patient's partner is pregnant, condoms must be used. Routine monthly preg-nancy tests are recommended during treatment. Pregnant

women, including nurses, should avoid exposure to the aerosol.

- The oral preparation should be used with caution in cardiac disease and gout and not used at all in severe cardiac disease, haemoglobinopathies, renal impairment or severe hepatic impairment, autoimmune disease, any history of severe psychiatric disease or uncontrolled thyroid disease.
- Prior to commencing treatment with the oral preparation and in weeks 2 and 4 of treatment, the patient should have a full blood count, platelets, electrolytes, serum creatinine, liver function and uric acid measured and measured thereafter if clinically indicated.
- Side effects of the inhaled preparation include worsening respiration and bacterial pneumonia.
- Side effects of the oral preparation include haemolytic anaemia and reticulocytosis.

Storage

Ribavarin preparations are stored at room temperature. The solution is prepared with water for injection and should be used within 24 hours of reconstitution.

TRICYCLIC ANTIDEPRESSANTS

This group of drugs includes:
Amitriptyline
Amoxapine
Clomipramine
Dosulepin/dothiepin
Doxepin
Imipramine
Lofepramine
Nortriptyline
Trimipramine

Actions and uses

These drugs are used for the treatment of depression caused by either psychotic disturbance (endogenous depression) or as a reaction to a precipitating factor such as the death of a close relative (reactive depression).

The precise mechanism of action of tricyclic antidepressants is not clearly understood.

Some tricyclic antidepressants have marked sedative properties and are therefore very effective in treating depressed patients who also have features of agitation or anxiety. Conversely, other drugs in the group tend to be stimulant and are particularly useful when depression is accompanied by marked retardation.

This group of drugs has been used in other situations as follows:

- they have been used successfully in the treatment of enuresis in childhood
- trimipramine has been used in the treatment of peptic ulcer disease.

See also the section on Antidepressant Drugs in general (p. 31).

Dosage

See individual drugs.

Nursing implications

- See the section on Antidepressant Drugs in general (p. 31).
- Perhaps the most important point to make about tricyclic drugs is that they take a number of weeks to exert their antidepressant effect. As the effect is delayed and as depressed patients may be particularly likely to fail to comply with treatment, the nurse may play an important role in ensuring that the patient does take the prescription.
- Tricyclic drugs lower the seizure threshold and therefore increase the frequency of fitting in epileptic patients. They should therefore be avoided in epileptic patients if at all possible.
- The total daily dose may be taken once in the evening if a sedative effect during the day is not required. This has the added benefit of helping patients get to sleep.
- Tricyclic drugs have anticholinergic or 'atropine-like' effects, which are particularly likely to

T

occur during the early period of treatment and may be particularly troublesome in elderly patients. These effects include dry mouth, blurred vision, constipation, urinary retention and tachycardia.
  - Constipation may lead to paralytic ileus.
  - Blurred vision is due to pupillary dilatation and these drugs should be used with caution in patients with glaucoma.
  - Urinary retention may be particularly troublesome in patients with symptoms of prostatism.
- Other side effects include gastrointestinal upset such as gastric pain, anorexia, nausea and vomiting, fatigue, malaise, dizziness, confusion, cardiac conduction defects and hypotension. The latter two effects indicate that the drug should be used with caution in patients with a history of heart disease.
- It is recommended that patients receiving tricyclic antidepressants should not concurrently receive a monoamine oxidase inhibitor antidepressant.
- Large doses of tricyclic antidepressants have caused hyperpyrexia, convulsions, circulatory failure, cardiac arrest, respiratory failure, cyanosis, coma and death.
- Deaths have also occurred from agranulocytosis and jaundice.

Storage
See individual drugs.

TRIFLUOPERAZINE (Stelazine)

Presentation
Tablets – 1 mg, 5 mg
Modified-release capsules – 2 mg, 10 mg, 15 mg
Syrup – 1 mg in 5 ml
Oral solution – 5 mg in 5 ml

Actions and uses
Trifluoperazine is a member of the phenothiazine group of drugs and its actions and uses are described in the section on these drugs (p. 281).

Dosage
Schizophrenia and other psychoses.

- Adults, initially, 5 mg twice a day or 10 mg daily if the modified-release preparation is used. Increase by 5 mg after 1 week. The dose can be further increased at intervals of 3 days according to response.
- Children up to 12 years, initially up to 5 mg daily in divided doses. Adjust dose according to patient response, weight and age.

Short-term adjunctive management of severe anxiety and for severe nausea and vomiting.

- Adults, 2–4 mg daily in divided doses or as a single daily dose; if the modified-release preparation is used, increase to a maximum of 6 mg daily if required.
- Children 3–5 years, up to 1 mg daily, 6–12 years, up to 4 mg daily.

Nursing implications
See the section on Phenothiazines (p. 281).

Storage
The drug is stored at room temperature. Liquid preparations should be protected from direct sunlight.

TRILOSTANE (Modrenal)

Presentation
Capsules – 60 mg, 120 mg

Actions and uses
Trilostane inhibits steroid synthesis by an action on the adrenal cortex, reducing levels of both hydrocortisone (cortisol) and aldosterone. It is of use in conditions associated with overproduction of these steroids, i.e. Cushing's syndrome and primary hyperaldosteronism. Trilostane can also be used for postmenopausal breast cancer, if taken along with glucocorticoid replacement therapy. It is used for patients who have relapsed after initial oestrogen receptor antagonist therapy.

Dosage
The dose must be carefully adjusted in the individual but usually lies in the range 120–480 mg daily or more, taken in up to four divided doses. For breast cancer the maintenance dose is 960 mg daily or 720 mg daily if the higher dose is not tolerated.

Nursing implications
- Trilostane must not be used for the treatment of pregnant patients or women who are breastfeeding.
- Some patients may experience flushing, some nausea and nasal stuffiness.
- It is important to avoid co-administration of trilostane and potassium-conserving diuretics (amiloride, spironolactone and triamterene) which may produce a marked retention of potassium. Patients who receive such combinations must be carefully monitored for developing hyperkalaemia.

Storage
Trilostane capsules are stored at room temperature.

TRIMEPRAZINE/ALIMEMAZINE (Vallergan)

Presentation
Tablets – 10 mg
Syrup – 7.5 mg in 5 ml, 30 mg in 5 ml

Actions and uses
Trimeprazine, an antihistamine, is a member of the phenothiazine group of drugs which is particularly valuable as an antipruritic drug for the treatment of itch associated with dermatological conditions such as urticaria. It is also used for the preoperative medication of children.

Dosage
For the treatment of pruritus.
- Adults: 10 mg, 2–3 times a day up to a maximum of 100 mg daily in severe cases.
- Elderly: 10 mg once or twice a day.

- Children over 2 years: 2.5–5 mg 3–4 times a day.

For preoperative medication of children: 2–7 years, up to 2 mg/kg 1–2 hours before surgery.

Nursing implications
- Apart from unwanted drowsiness or sedation trimeprazine does not cause any of the many problems caused by other Phenothiazines (p. 281).

Storage
The drug is stored at room temperature. Liquid preparations should be protected from direct sunlight.

TRIMETHOPRIM (Monotrim, Trimopan)

Presentation
Tablets – 100 mg, 200 mg
Suspension – 50 mg in 5 ml
Injection – 100 mg in 5 ml

Actions and uses
Trimethoprim is an antibacterial agent which prevents the growth of bacteria by inhibiting the synthesis of the cellular constituent folinic acid within the cell. This substance is essential for growth and division of bacteria. The drug has various indications including the treatment of urinary tract infections and acute and chronic bronchitis.

Dosage
Oral treatment of acute infections.
- Adults: 200 mg twice daily.
- Child age 6 weeks to 5 months: 25 mg twice daily.
- Child age 6 months to 5 years: 50 mg twice daily.
- Child age 6–12 years: 100 mg twice daily.

Oral treatment of chronic infections and prophylaxis.
- Adults: 100 mg at night.
- Child: 1–2 mg/kg at night.

Slow IV injection or infusion for the treatment of acute infections.
- Adult: 150–250 mg twice daily.

- Child under 12 years: 6–9 mg/kg daily in divided doses.

Nursing implications
- If taken in short courses, very few problems are encountered with this drug. Occasionally nausea and vomiting occur and, more rarely, megaloblastic anaemia. This latter effect may be prevented by concurrent administration of folinic acid.
- Because of its potential to interfere with the metabolism of folic acid in cells, the drug is not recommended for use during pregnancy nor for administration to very young children. There is an increased risk of an antifolate effect if taken concurrently with pyrimethamine and methotrexate and a risk of haematological toxicity with azathioprine and mercaptopurine.
- Do not use in severe renal impairment or where dyscrasias are present.

Storage
The drug is stored at room temperature.

TRIMIPRAMINE (Surmontil)

Presentation
Tablets – 10 mg, 25 mg
Capsules – 50 mg

Actions and uses
Trimipramine is a tricyclic antidepressant drug. Its actions and uses in general are described in the section on these drugs (p. 371). It should be noted that trimipramine has a marked sedative action and is particularly useful where depression is associated with sleep disturbance, anxiety or agitation.

Dosage
For the treatment of depression in adults 50–300 mg is given at night 2 hours before retiring or in divided doses, e.g. morning and night. Lower doses should be used in elderly patients.

Nursing implications
- See the nursing implications in the section on Tricyclic Antidepressant Drugs (p. 371).
- As this drug has a marked sedative action it should only be given during the day if it is felt that the sedative action would be advantageous, i.e. if patients are particularly anxious or agitated.

Storage
Trimipramine preparations are stored at room temperature.

TRI-POTASSIUM DI-CITRATO BISMUTHATE (De-Noltab)

Presentation
Tablets – 120 mg

Actions and uses
When this drug is exposed to the acid in the stomach it forms a complex which is thought to coat the surface of the ulcer bed, preventing further acid from reaching it and therefore reducing further damage to that area. It is effective in the treatment of both gastric and duodenal ulcers.

Tri-potassium di-citrato bismuthate can be used in combination with a proton pump inhibitor and two antibacterials (for 2 weeks) in the eradication of resistant cases of *Helicobacter pylori* infection. This pathogen is found in the mucosa of a large proportion of patients with peptic ulcer disease which does not readily respond to conventional therapy. Bismuth chelate appears to have a bactericidal action against this bacterium.

Dosage
Two tablets twice a day or one tablet four times a day for 28 days, repeated if necessary.

Nursing implications
- It is important to note that the drug causes a dark staining of the tongue and tends to blacken the colour of the stool.

Patients may find this distressing, especially if they have not been warned of the possibility of these effects occurring prior to starting the drug.

- Patients should be advised to take each dose with half a glass of water 30 minutes before food and if taking the tablets four times a day, the last dose should be taken 2 hours after the evening meal. Avoid milk during the treatment and do not take at the same time as antacids.
- Difficulties with compliance are often experienced because the drug has a foul taste and ammoniacal odour.
- Apart from the inconvenient effects mentioned above, the drug is not associated with any major side effects.

Storage
Tri-potassium di-citrato bismuthate tablets are stored at room temperature.

TROPISETRON (Navoban)

Presentation
Capsules – 5 mg
Injection – 2 mg in 2 ml and 5 mg in 5 ml

Actions and uses
Tropisetron is a member of the group of drugs including ondansetron and granisetron which selectively inhibit the effects of 5-hydroxytryptamine (5-HT, serotonin) at specific binding sites called 5-HT1 receptors. Stimulation of these receptors in the gastrointestinal tract and chemoreceptor trigger zone induces nausea and triggers the vomiting reflex. Drugs of this type are therefore used to prevent and treat nausea and vomiting in patients who are exposed to various emetogenic stimuli including anticancer drugs and radiotherapy. More recently, they have been shown to be similarly effective in the control of postoperative nausea and vomiting.

Dosage
Prevention of nausea and vomiting induced by cytotoxic chemotherapy.

- Adult: 5 mg by slow IV injection or infusion just prior to chemotherapy, then orally, 5 mg every morning, 1 hour before food, for 5 days.
- Child over 2 years: 200 microgram/kg (to a maximum of 5 mg) by slow IV injection (over at least 1 minute) or infusion just prior to chemotherapy, then, 200 microgram/kg daily for 4 days.
- Child over 25 kg: 5 mg by slow IV injection (over at least 1 minute) or infusion just prior to chemotherapy, then orally if possible (or by slow IV injection, over at least 1 minute, or infusion), 5 mg every morning for 5 days.

Postoperative nausea and vomiting.

- By slow IV injection or infusion, for prevention, give 2 mg just prior to induction of anaesthesia or for treatment, give 2 mg within 2 hours of the end of anaesthesia.

Nursing implications
- The nursing implication aspects for Ondansetron (p. 261) also apply to this drug.
- Side effects include constipation, diarrhoea and abdominal pain.
- The drug may be injected slowly via the drip tubing of a running infusion fluid or added to 100 ml sodium chloride 0.9% or glucose 5% injection and administered over 30 minutes.

Storage
Tropisetron capsules and injection are stored at room temperature but must be protected from light during storage.

T

U

UROFOLLITROPIN (Metrodin)

Presentation
Injection – 75 units and 150 units of powder for reconstitution

Actions and uses
Urofollitropin is a preparation of follicle-stimulating hormone which has been extracted from the urine of postmenopausal women. It is used in the treatment of infertility for women who have hypopituitarism or in women who have not responded to clomifene. Urofollitropin can also be used in superovulation treatment for assisted conception. In men it can be used for the stimulation of spermatogenesis in cases of congenital or acquired hypogonadotrophic hypogonadism.

Dosage
Urofollitropin is administered by subcutaneous or intramuscular injection. The dose used depends largely on patient response. This can be assessed by measuring follicle size or oestrogen secretion. In men the dose used is generally 150 units three times a week.

Nursing implications
- Side effects include headache, ovarian hyperstimulation, multiple pregnancy and local reactions at the injection site.
- Use with caution in patients who have ovarian cysts, adrenal or thyroid disorders, hyper-prolactinoma or pituitary tumour.
- Up to five ampoules of the injection can be dissolved in 1 ml of diluent, thus avoiding large-volume injections.

Storage
Urofollitropin injection is stored at room temperature. Protect from light.

URSODEOXYCHOLIC ACID (Destolit, Urdox, Ursofalk, Ursogal)

Presentation
Tablets – 150 mg, 250 mg and 300 mg
Capsules – 250 mg
Suspension – 250 mg in 5 ml

Actions and uses
Ursodeoxycholic acid is a bile acid used for the dissolution of gallstones and to treat primary biliary cirrhosis. It increases the bile acid pool and thus the amount of dissolved cholesterol and it has a protective effect on the liver. It prevents precipitation of cholesterol from solution and therefore prevents the formation of cholesterol gallstones; existing cholesterol stones will gradually redissolve, possibly obviating the need for surgical removal. Advances in laparoscopic cholecystectomy and endoscopic biliary techniques now limit the use of this drug.

Dosage (adults)
Dissolution of gallstones: the effective range is 8–12 mg/kg body weight daily, taken as a single dose at bedtime or in two divided doses. Treatment should not extend beyond 2 years and should continue for 3–4 months after radiological disappearance of the gallstones. Primary biliary cirrhosis: 10–15 mg/kg body weight daily in 2–4 divided doses.

Nursing implications
- Side effects include nausea, vomiting and diarrhoea. Gallstone calcification can occur.

- It is important to note that ursodeoxycholic acid therapy is not a suitable treatment for all patients with gallstones and that the nature and size of the stones are important. Those for whom treatment is unsuitable are:
    - patients with radioopaque stones
    - those with non-functioning gallbladders
    - pregnant patients or females contemplating pregnancy (non-hormonal contraceptive measures must be taken in women of child-bearing age)
    - patients with chronic liver disease or inflammatory bowel disease
    - patients with peptic ulcers.
- Patients should be given advice regarding their diet, i.e. avoid excessive cholesterol and calories.

Storage

Ursodeoxycholic acid preparations are stored at room temperature.

U

V

VALACICLOVIR (Valtrex)

Presentation
Tablets – 500 mg

Actions and uses
Valaciclovir is a pro-drug of aciclovir (see the section on Aciclovor, p. 8) licensed for use in the treatment of herpes zoster and herpes simplex infections of the skin and mucous membranes. It can be used for the treatment of genital herpes.

Dosage (Adults only)
Herpes zoster: 1 g three times a day for 7 days.
Herpes simplex, first episode: 500 mg twice daily for 5 days or 10 days if it is a severe infection.
Herpes simplex, recurrent infection: 500 mg twice daily for 5 days.
Herpes simplex, suppression: 500 mg daily in one or two divided doses or 500 mg twice daily for immunocompromised patients.

Nursing implications
- See the section on Aciclovir (p. 8).
- Side effects include gastrointestinal upsets, headache, rash, dizziness, confusion and hallucinations.
- Use with caution in renal impairment.

Storage
Valaciclovir tablets are stored at room temperature.

VALPROIC ACID (Convulex)

Presentation
Capsules – 150 mg, 300 mg and 500 mg

Actions and uses
This drug is an anticonvulsant with the actions and uses described under sodium valproate (p. 335), of which this is its acidic form. Sodium valproate and valproic acid are interchangeable on a dose-for-dose basis but there may be differences in bioavailability and close serum level monitoring is recommended if transferring from one drug to the other.

Dosage
Adults and children: initially a dose of 15 mg/kg daily is administered and carefully adjusted upwards by increments of 5–10 mg/kg daily until seizure control is obtained or a maximum of 30 mg/kg is reached. This drug is administered twice, three times or four times daily.

Nursing implications
The nursing implications section under sodium valproate (p. 335) also applies to this drug.

Storage
Valproic acid capsules are stored at room temperature.

VALSARTAN (Diovan)

Presentation
Capsules – 40 mg, 80 mg and 160 mg

Actions and uses
Valsartan is an angiotensin II (AT1 receptor) antagonist, similar to Losartan. It is indicated for the treatment of hypertension.

Dosage
80 mg daily, increasing to 160 mg daily after at least 4 weeks if required. Start with 40 mg daily in the elderly,

patients with mild-to-moderate hepatic impairment, moderate-to-severe renal impairment or intravascular volume depletion.

Nursing implications
- Drugs of this type are generally well tolerated.
- Valsartan is contraindicated in severe hepatic impairment, cirrhosis and biliary obstruction.

Storage
Valsartan capsules are stored at room temperature.

VANCOMYCIN (Vancocin)

Presentation
Capsules – 125 mg, 250 mg
Injection – 500 mg vial and 1 g vial

Actions and uses
This antibiotic has a bactericidal action and is effective against a wide range of aerobic and anaerobic Gram-positive bacteria including multi-resistant staphylococci. It is thought to act by binding to bacterial cell walls, inhibiting cell wall synthesis and damaging the cytoplasmic membrane. Its use is limited to situations where other less toxic antibiotics such as penicillins or cephalosporins have been shown to be ineffective or where patients with severe infection are known to be allergic to penicillin or cephalosporins. Vancomycin is commonly used for MRSA infections, empiric therapy in febrile neutropenic patients who have not responded to first-line therapy and endocarditis. Unfortunately, vancomycin-resistant enterococci infections are becoming more frequent.

Vancomycin is not sufficiently well absorbed after oral administration and this route is used exclusively for the treatment of gastrointestinal infections, notably pseudomembranous colitis due to the anaerobic organism *Clostridium difficile*. This may develop in patients who receive broad-spectrum antibiotics when it manifests as intense bloody diarrhoea.

Dosage
The dose frequently varies from those stated below depending on measured plasma concentrations and the type of infection being treated.

- Oral: the adult oral dosage for *Clostridium difficile* infection is 125 mg four times daily for 7–10 days. Children over 5 years old should receive half the adult dose. Children under 5 years old should receive 5 mg/kg every 6 hours.
- Intravenous infusion:
  - adults: 500 mg 6-hourly or 1 g 12-hourly
  - babies less than 1 week: 15 mg/kg as a single loading dose, then 10 mg/kg 12-hourly; babies 1–4 weeks old: 15 mg/kg as a single loading dose, then 10 mg/kg every 8 hours
  - older children should receive 10 mg/kg every 6 hours.

Nursing implications
- As noted above, vancomycin is a highly toxic drug and its use should be restricted to the situations described above.
- The intravenous administration of vancomycin leads to frequent toxic effects including local irritation and/or thrombophlebitis and generalized hypersensitivity which includes the 'red man syndrome' where flushing and an erythematous rash affects the face, neck and upper torso.
- Severe hypotension can occur after too rapid an infusion. It is essential to use appropriate dilutions of the injection and adhere by infusion rates. 500 mg must be administered over at least 60 minutes and diluted in at least 100 ml of infusion fluid, either glucose 5% or sodium chloride 0.9%.
- In high doses the drug is toxic to the auditory nerve (producing deafness) and the kidney. It is therefore used with caution in patients with renal impairment and should be avoided in patients with a history of deafness.

- Lower doses are often required in elderly patients.
- Other side effects include blood disorders, nausea, chills, fever and anaphylaxis.
- There is an increased risk of ototoxicity if administered with aminoglycosides or loop diuretics and an increased risk of nephrotoxicity with aminoglycosides.
- The oral drug is less well absorbed and produces less severe toxic effects.

Storage

The drug is stored at room temperature.

VECURONIUM (Norcuron)

Presentation

Injection – 10 mg vial

Actions and uses

Vecuronium is a muscle relaxant of the non-depolarizing type. Thus it reversibly paralyses skeletal muscle by competitive inhibition of acetylcholine, the transmitter substance released at the junction of the (motor) nerve and muscle fibre (motor endplate receptor). Drugs of this type are used to produce muscle relaxation during surgical anaesthesia.

Dosage

- Intravenous injection, adults and children over 5 months: initially 80–100 microgram/kg followed by 20–30 microgram/kg as required.
- For neonates and children up to 4 months: initially 10–20 microgram/kg then increase dose according to response.
- Intravenous infusion, given after initial intravenous injection: 0.8–1.4 microgram/kg/min.

Nursing implications

- All patients must have their respiration assisted or controlled.
- Muscle relaxants of this type are also used to produce paralysis in patients on assisted ventilation in ICUs.
- Overdosage with muscle relaxant drugs of this type may result in paralysis of the respiratory muscles. If this occurs, an anticholinesterase such as neostigmine (which potentiates acetylcholine by blocking its inactivation) must be administered.

Storage

Vecuronium injection is stored at room temperature, protected from light.

VENLAFAXINE (Efexor)

Presentation

Tablets – 37.5 mg, 50 mg and 75 mg
Modified-release capsules – 75 mg and 150 mg

Actions and uses

Venlafaxine is an antidepressant drug which inhibits the reuptake of 5-hydroxytryptamine (serotonin) and noradrenaline. For further information, see the section on Antidepressants (p. 31).

Dosage (adults only)

Initially 75 mg daily in two divided doses, increasing to 150 mg daily in two divided doses if required. In severely depressed or hospitalized patients, 150 mg daily can be given as a starting dose, increasing gradually in increments of up to 75 mg every 2–3 days to a maximum of 375 mg daily. Modified-release preparations are taken once daily.

Nursing implications

- See the section on Antidepressants (p. 31).
- Do not use in severe hepatic or renal impairment, pregnancy or breastfeeding. Use half doses in moderate hepatic and renal impairment.
- Use with caution in heart disease and epilepsy and monitor blood pressure when using doses above 200 mg daily.

- Side effects include nausea, headache, insomnia, somnolence, dry mouth, dizziness, constipation, asthenia, sweating and nervousness. If any type of allergic reaction occurs such as a rash or urticaria, patients should report to their doctor.
- Venlafaxine does interact with MAOIs and therefore should not be started until at least 2 weeks after stopping an MAOI and an MAOI should not be started until at least 1 week after stopping venlafaxine.

Storage

Venlafaxine preparations are stored at room temperature.

VERAPAMIL (Cordilox, Securon, Univer)

Presentation

Tablets – 40 mg, 80 mg, 120 mg, 160 mg
Tablets (modified release) – 120 mg and 240 mg
Capsules (modified release) – 120 mg, 180 mg and 240 mg
Oral solution – 40 mg in 5 ml
Injection – 5 mg in 2 ml

Actions and uses

Verapamil is a Calcium Antagonist (p. 67). Verapamil decreases the oxygen requirement of the heart muscle and also reduces peripheral resistance. These two actions make it useful in the treatment of angina pectoris. It has also been found to be useful for the abolition of supraventricular dysrhythmias. It is thought that the drug acts by influencing the movement of calcium ions across cell membranes. Peripheral vasodilatation is associated with a fall in blood pressure so it is also used in the treatment of hypertension.

Dosage

Adults.

- Intravenously for cardiac dysrhythmias: 5 mg, given over 2–3 minutes, repeated after 5–10 minutes if

required. Orally for supraventricular arrhythmias, 40–120 mg three times daily.
- The oral maintenance dose for the prophylaxis of angina is 80–120 mg three times a day.
- The oral antihypertensive dose is 240–480 mg daily in 2–3 divided doses.
- Single daily doses may be taken as slow-release preparations.

Children: the intravenous dose for cardiac dysrhythmias is as follows.

- Neonates: 0.75–1 mg,
- Infants: 0.75–2 mg; 1–5 years: 2–3 mg; 6–15 years: 2.5–5 mg.
- Alternatively, children 0–1 year, 0.1–0.2 mg/kg body weight, 1–15 years, 0.1–0.3 mg/kg body weight.

Nursing implications

- See the section on Calcium Antagonists (p. 67).
- The most important point to remember with this drug is that it should never be given intravenously (and with great caution orally) to patients who are already receiving or have in the immediate past received beta-adrenergic blocking drugs as the combination of these two can lead to hypotension and asystole.
- As verapamil can produce hypotension when given intravenously, patients should be placed in the supine position prior to receiving such therapy.
- The oral preparation of the drug is associated with few side effects of which constipation, nausea and vomiting are the most common.
- Grapefruit juice may affect the metabolism of verapamil.
- Verapamil is subject to several drug interactions, including the interaction with antiarrhythmics mentioned in the section on calcium antagonists. Verapamil can enhance the effects of carbamazepine and increase the plasma concentration of digoxin, cyclosporin and theophylline.

Storage

Verapamil tablets, capsules and injection are stored at room temperature.

VIGABATRIN (Sabril)

Presentation

Tablets – 500 mg
Sachets – 500 mg

Actions and uses

Vigabatrin is an anticonvulsant drug. It is chemically related to gamma-aminobutyric acid (GABA), a substance which is produced naturally in the brain and a deficiency of which is associated with epilepsy. After conversion to its active form, vigabatrin produces an irreversible inhibition of the enzyme responsible for inactivation of GABA, thereby enhancing brain GABA levels. It has been used in the treatment of epilepsy associated with partial and generalized seizures, when resistant to established anticonvulsant drugs.

Dosage

- Adults: initially, a dose of 1 g daily is given in addition to existing anticonvulsant therapy and increased by increments of 500 mg until control of epilepsy is achieved. The usual upper dose limit is 3 g daily. Tablets may be taken as a single daily dose or in two divided daily doses.
- Children: initially, 40 mg/kg daily, then the dose is adjusted according to body weight. 10–15 kg: 0.5–1 g daily, 15–30 kg: 1–1.5 g daily, 30–50 kg: 1.5–3 g daily, over 50 kg: 2–3 g daily.
- Vigabatrin can also be used for infantile spasms in West's syndrome; as monotherapy, a dose of 50 mg/kg daily is used, then adjusted according to response up to 150 mg/kg daily.

Nursing implications

- Vigabatrin is contraindicated in patients with visual field defects as it is associated with causing this condition in about one-third of those treated with this drug. Visual field testing should be carried out prior to treatment commencing and every 6 months thereafter. Patients must be advised to report any new visual symptoms.
- Changes in mood, confusion and other behavioural disturbances may arise. Children in particular may appear excited or agitated.
- Other side effects include drowsiness, fatigue, dizziness and nervousness.
- Vigabatrin is excreted unchanged by the kidney and patients with renal impairment require lower doses.
- When given in combination with phenytoin, a reduction of up to 20% in blood phenytoin levels has been reported. The mechanism for this interaction is unclear and adjustment of phenytoin dosage may be necessary. Vigabatrin sometimes also lowers the plasma concentration of phenobarbital and primidone.
- In common with other anticonvulsant therapy, patients must be warned against sudden discontinuation of therapy, which might precipitate serious convulsions.

Storage

Vigabatrin preparations are stored at room temperature.

VINBLASTINE (Velbe)

Presentation

Injection – 10 mg vials

Actions and uses

Vinblastine's actions are similar to those described for Vincristine (p. 383). It has been found to be of most value in the management of Hodgkin's disease and non-Hodgkin's lymphomas. It has also been used in combination with other drugs in the treatment of a variety of solid tumours including breast cancer, testicular cancer and resistant choriocarcinoma.

Dosage

The drug is given by intravenous injection usually at weekly intervals at a dose of 6 mg/m^2 but this varies with the type of condition treated and the state of the patient. It must **not** be administered intrathecally. It is given by intravenous injection either directly or via the drip tubing of a running 0.9% sodium chloride infusion.

Nursing implications

- For intravenous injection only. Vinblastine is not for intrathecal injection; this causes severe neurotoxicity which is usually fatal.
- Vinblastine more commonly affects the bone marrow than vincristine and therefore patients receiving this drug are at increased risk of severe infection and haemorrhage.
- Vinblastine may cause slight neurotoxicity but this effect is not as severe as that seen with vincristine.
- Gastrointestinal effects include blistering in the mouth, anorexia, nausea, vomiting, constipation, paralytic ileus, abdominal pain, pharyngitis and bleeding from healed peptic ulcer sites.
- Other adverse effects include hair loss, malaise, weakness, dizziness and pain at the tumour site.
- Leakage from intravenous injection sites produces severe irritation, cellulitis and phlebitis.
- The drug is contraindicated in pregnancy.
- Nurses should be aware of the risks posed by cytotoxic drugs. Some are irritant to the skin and mucous surfaces and care must be exercised when handling them. In particular, spillage or contamination of personnel or the environment must be avoided. If cytotoxic drugs are handled regularly, it is theoretically possible that repeated skin contact or inhalation may produce systemic toxic effects in nurses who have developed hypersensitivity to them. Most hospitals now operate a centralized (pharmacy-organized) additive service. While this reduces the risk of exposure to cytotoxic drugs, it is essential that nurses recognize and understand the local policy on their safe handling and disposal. The Health and Safety Executive has decreed that such a policy should be in place wherever cytotoxic drugs are administered. These should be adapted, wherever possible, to care of patients in the community.

Storage

Vinblastine vials are stored in a refrigerator. Reconstituted solutions may be stored in a refrigerator for up to 28 days if the special diluent (containing a bactericide) is used. Alternatively reconstituted solution should not be used after 24 hours.

VINCRISTINE (Oncovin)

Presentation

Injection – 1 mg in 1 ml, 2 mg in 2 ml, 5 mg in 5 ml

Actions and uses

Vincristine is a cytotoxic drug, the action of which is incompletely understood. Basically vincristine acts during cell division, preventing completion of the process. It also inhibits cellular activities such as phagocytosis (engulfment of bacteria or particles) and chemotaxis (cell movement in response to a chemical stimuli).

Vincristine has been found to be particularly valuable in the treatment of leukaemias, including acute and chronic lymphocytic leukaemia, and in the management of advanced Hodgkin's disease and other lymphomas. Other malignancies which have been shown to respond to treatment with this drug include breast cancer, head and neck cancers, neuroblastoma, Wilms' tumour (kidney tumour occurring mainly in children) and rhabdomyosarcoma (a tumour affecting skeletal muscles).

Dosage

Vincristine is given by intravenous injection. It must **not** be administered intrathecally.

Generally, the dose used is 1.4–1.5 mg/m² up to a **maximum of 2 mg** given at weekly intervals. The dose should be adjusted for each individual as required to achieve therapeutic levels while avoiding toxicity. For children, up to 2 mg/m² weekly is given. If the child weighs 10 kg or less, start with 0.05 mg/kg.

It is given by intravenous injection either directly or via the drip tubing of a running 0.9% sodium chloride or glucose in water infusion.

Nursing implications

- For intravenous injection only. Vincristine is not for intrathecal injection; this causes severe neurotoxicity which is usually fatal.
- Bone marrow suppression is less common with this drug than with many other cytotoxics but if it occurs the patient will be at risk of serious infection and haemorrhage.
- The most important side effect of vincristine is neurotoxicity which most frequently presents as peripheral neuropathy, either sensory, motor or mixed. Initial symptoms may be slight and patients may complain of tingling or numbness in the fingers and toes. Subsequently tendon reflexes may disappear. If the early signs of neurotoxicity are ignored, damage may progress and be irreversible. Thus patients must be closely questioned about the development of these symptoms and if present, the drug should be immediately stopped.
- Gastrointestinal effects may occur and include anorexia, nausea, vomiting, constipation or diarrhoea. Oral ulceration and abdominal cramps are also known to occur. Constipation may be particularly severe in the elderly and may give rise to intestinal obstruction.
- Other side effects include diplopia, malaise, depression, headache and psychotic reactions. Alopecia, weight loss and fluid retention or low serum sodium due to inappropriate secretion of antidiuretic hormone have been known to occur.
- Leakage into surrounding tissues after intravenous injection causes severe irritation. If administered via the drip tubing of a running 0.9% sodium chloride infusion, it is important to check first whether the infusion is working correctly and to look for signs of local leakage before administering the drug.
- The drug is contraindicated in pregnancy.
- Nurses should be aware of the risks posed by cytotoxic drugs. Some are irritant to the skin and mucous surfaces and care must be exercised when handling them. In particular, spillage or contamination of personnel or the environment must be avoided. If cytotoxic drugs are handled regularly, it is theoretically possible that repeated skin contact or inhalation may produce systemic toxic effects in nurses who have developed hypersensitivity to them. Most hospitals now operate a centralized (pharmacy-organized) additive service. While this reduces the risk of exposure to cytotoxic drugs, it is essential that nurses recognize and understand the local policy on their safe handling and disposal. The Health and Safety Executive has decreed that such a policy should be in place wherever cytotoxic drugs are administered. These should be adapted, wherever possible, to care of patients in the community.

Storage

Vincristine is stored in a refrigerator. Protect from light.

VINDESINE (Eldisine)

Presentation
Injection – 5 mg powder in vials

Actions and uses
Vindesine's actions are similar to those described for vincristine (above). It is used in the treatment of acute lymphoblastic leukaemia in childhood which is resistant to standard treatments, in blast crisis phases of chronic myeloid leukaemia and in malignant melanoma resistant to standard treatments. Vindesine can also be used in breast cancer.

Dosage
Vindesine is given by intravenous injection. It must **not** be administered intrathecally.

Usually 3–4 mg/m^2 body surface area (or up to 5 mg/m^2 in children) is given by bolus intravenous injection at weekly intervals. It is given by intravenous injection either directly or via the drip tubing of a running 0.9% sodium chloride infusion or dextrose 5% infusion.

Nursing implications
- See the section on Vincristine (above).
- Vindesine can cause severe myelosuppression so patients receiving this drug are at increased risk of severe infection and haemorrhage.
- Nurses should be aware of the risks posed by cytotoxic drugs. Some are irritant to the skin and mucous surfaces and care must be exercised when handling them. In particular, spillage or contamination of personnel or the environment must be avoided. If cytotoxic drugs are handled regularly, it is theoretically possible that repeated skin contact or inhalation may produce systemic toxic effects in nurses who have developed hypersensitivity to them. Most hospitals now operate a centralized (pharmacy-organized) additive service. While this reduces the risk of exposure to cytotoxic drugs, it is essential that nurses recognize and understand the local policy on their safe handling and disposal. The Health and Safety Executive has decreed that such a policy should be in place wherever cytotoxic drugs are administered. These should be adapted, wherever possible, to care of patients in the community.

Storage
Vindesine preparations are stored in a refrigerator. Reconstituted solutions may be stored in a refrigerator for up to 28 days if the special diluent (containing a bactericide) is used. Alternatively reconstituted solution should not be used after 24 hours.

VINORELBINE (Navelbine)

Presentation
Injection – 10 mg in 1 ml, 40 mg in 4 ml and 50 mg in 5 ml all for dilution

Actions and uses
Vinorelbine, like vincristine, is a vinca alkaloid relatively recently introduced for the treatment of advanced breast cancer resistant to anthracycline regimens and for advanced non-small cell lung cancer.

Dosage
Vinorelbine is given by intravenous injection. It must **not** be administered intrathecally.

The usual dose is 25–30 mg/m^2 (to a maximum of 60 mg) administered intravenously at weekly intervals. It must be diluted before use with either 20–50 ml of sodium chloride 0.9% solution prior to slow bolus injection over 5–10 minutes, or with 125 ml sodium chloride 0.9% solution prior to short infusion over 20–30 minutes. 5% dextrose can also be used as a diluent.

Not recommended for use in children.

Nursing implications

- See the section on Vincristine (p. 383).
- Vinorelbine can cause severe myelosuppression so patients receiving this drug are at increased risk of severe infection and haemorrhage.
- Nurses should be aware of the risks posed by cytotoxic drugs. Some are irritant to the skin and mucous surfaces and care must be exercised when handling them. In particular, spillage or contamination of personnel or the environment must be avoided. If cytotoxic drugs are handled regularly, it is theoretically possible that repeated skin contact or inhalation may produce systemic toxic effects in nurses who have developed hypersensitivity to them. Most hospitals now operate a centralized (pharmacy-organized) additive service. While this reduces the risk of exposure to cytotoxic drugs, it is essential that nurses recognize and understand the local policy on their safe handling and disposal. The Health and Safety Executive has decreed that such a policy should be in place wherever cytotoxic drugs are administered. These should be adapted, wherever possible, to care of patients in the community.

Storage

Vinorelbine injection is stored in a refrigerator and protected from light. The reconstituted solution can be kept for 24 hours in a refrigerator.

VITAMIN A (Retinol)

Presentation

Vitamin A is available in a preparation of fish liver oil in doses expressed in terms of international units. It is also available in compound preparations containing other vitamins.

Injection – vitamin A palmitate, 100 000 units in 2 ml

Actions and uses

In the normal body, vitamin A is produced from precursors in the diet and is essential for maintenance of healthy mucus-secreting epithelial surfaces and for the maintenance of normal vision via the production of a retinal pigment known as rhodopsin. In clinical practice, vitamin A is indicated only for the treatment of deficiency states, which are very rare in this country. Symptoms of deficiency states include night blindness, drying and change in the microscopic make-up of skin and other body surfaces and drying and degeneration of the superficial layers of the eye.

Vitamin A can be given in combination with vitamins C and D to pregnant women or nursing mothers and children.

Dosage

- Orally, usually, 700 units daily for pregnant women, nursing mothers and children aged 1 month to 5 years (use in babies is determined by the volume of formula milk consumed each day).
- Deep IM injection in deficiency states, 100 000 units monthly or weekly in acute deficiency states. For liver disease, 100 000 units every 2–4 months. For infants and children use half the adult dose.

Nursing implications

- Excessive doses of vitamin A may be toxic and can cause rough skin, dry hair and an enlarged liver. Massive overdose can also cause a raised erythrocyte sedimentation rate and raised serum calcium and alkaline phosphatase concentrations.
- If taken in large quantities, vitamin A can cause birth defects. Supplements of vitamin A should not be taken in pregnancy or by women planning a pregnancy unless advised by a doctor.

Storage

Vitamin A preparations are stored at room temperature.

VITAMIN B COMPLEX

Presentation
Vitamin B complex is available either as preparations of its components (see below) or in multivitamin preparations. Vitamin B complex comprises B1 (thiamine), B2 (riboflavin), B6 (pyridoxine) and nicotinamide. There are other substances classed as members of the vitamin B group but their efficacy has not been confirmed.

Actions and uses
Vitamin B complex is indicated for the treatment of deficiency disorders of components of the complex. Symptoms of deficiency disorders are as follows.

- Thiamine deficiency may present as:
  - beri-beri characterized by anorexia, emaciation, cardiac arrhythmias and, in the 'wet' form of the disease, oedema
  - neurological symptoms due to thiamine deficiency which are known as Wernicke's encephalopathy and Korsakoff's psychosis, seen in chronic alcoholism. Symptoms include agitation, behavioural disturbance, loss of memory and confusion and usually require parenteral administration of vitamins.
- Riboflavine deficiency: causes a rough scaly skin on the face, red swollen cracked lips, stomatitis and a swollen red tongue. Congestion of conjunctival blood vessels may also be seen.
- Nicotinamide deficiency produces diarrhoea, dermatitis and dementia.
- Pyridoxine deficiency may produce peripheral neuritis, roughening of the skin or anaemia. Deficiency can occur during treatment with isoniazid.

Dosage
- See under multivitamins (p. 231) for administration and dosage of parenteral vitamin B.
- Thiamine, orally: 10–25 mg daily for mild chronic deficiency or 200–300 mg daily for severe deficiency.
- Pyridoxine, orally: 20–50 mg up to three times daily for deficiency

states. For isoniazid neuropathy prophylaxis, 10 mg daily or 50 mg three times a day for treatment. For idiopathic sideroblastic anaemia, 100–400 mg daily in divided doses and for premenstrual syndrome, 50–100 mg daily.
- Vitamin B compound tablets are used for the prophylaxis of vitamin B deficiency and are taken in a dose of one or two tablets daily. Vitamin B compound strong tablets are used to treat vitamin B deficiency and are taken in a dose of one or two tablets three times daily.

Nursing implications
- Side effects are rare with these preparations but concern has been raised regarding toxicity occurring after prolonged use of high-dose pyridoxine. Nurses should follow local policy on this matter.
- Serious allergic reactions including anaphylaxis can occur when vitamin B is administered parenterally. Use should be restricted to patients in whom parenteral treatment is essential. Administer IV injections slowly and have facilities available to treat anaphylaxis.
- It should be noted that there is not a 10 mg preparation of pyridoxine readily available. Nurses should again follow local policies on dosage recommendations.

Storage
Vitamin B preparations are stored at room temperature.

VITAMIN C (Ascorbic Acid)

Presentation
Vitamin C is available in many preparations either singly or in combinations of multivitamins.

Actions and uses
Vitamin C is essential for the maintenance of normal body function. Its sole real indication in clinical practice is for the treatment of vitamin C

deficiency, known commonly as scurvy. The clinical features of this are weakness, tiredness, lassitude, bleeding and diseased gums, haemorrhage around the hairs of the legs, peripheral oedema and sudden cardiac failure. In addition, wounds heal very poorly and bones may be affected by osteoporosis. Anaemia may also occur.

Dosage
Prophylaxis: 25–75 mg daily.
Treatment of scurvy: not less than 250 mg daily in divided doses.

Nursing implications
There are no problems associated with the administration of this drug.

Storage
Vitamin C preparations are stored at room temperature.

VITAMIN D

Alfacalcidol (1alpha-hydroxychole-calciferol)
Calcitriol (1,25-dihydroxychole-calciferol)
Colecalciferol (cholecalciferol or vitamin D3)
Dihydrotachysterol
Ergocalciferol (calciferol or vitamin D2)

Presentation
See individual drugs

Actions and uses
The drugs listed above are all prepara-tions of various forms of vitamin D.

- Vitamin D is essential for the normal growth of bones and teeth. Calcium and phosphate homeostasis is controlled by vitamin D substances and parathyroid hormone. It should only be used in clinical practice if vitamin D deficiency has been clearly demonstrated. Vitamin D deficiency causes rickets in children and osteomalacia in adults. The commonest cause in European communities is steatorrhoea. In immigrants inadequate intake in the diet and poor exposure to sun (which stimulates the production of vitamin D in the body) may be contributory features. Asians who consume unleavened bread and elderly patients with poor nutrition may also suffer from vitamin D deficiency.
- Vitamin D deficiency can also arise as the result of intestinal malabsorption or chronic liver disease.
- Vitamin D may also be used to treat the rare condition of hypoparathyroidism.
- In chronic renal disease the body is incapable of producing the active derivatives of vitamin D necessary to maintain normal healthy bones so where therapy is required, alfacalcidol or calcitriol should be prescribed.
- Calcitriol is licensed for use in postmenopausal osteoporosis.

Dosage
See individual drugs.

Nursing implications
- An excess of vitamin D causes high blood calcium. This may cause anorexia, nausea, vomiting, constipation, abdominal pain and increased urine output and subsequently renal stones and renal failure. Patients receiving pharmacological doses of vitamin D should have their plasma calcium concentration checked at regular intervals.
- Nursing mothers who are taking vitamin D excrete the vitamin in their breast milk which can cause hypercalcaemia in the infant.
- Vitamin D is contraindicated in hypercalcaemia and metastatic calcification.

Storage
Preparations of vitamin D are stored at room temperature.

VITAMIN E (Tocopherols)

Presentation
Suspension (alpha tocopheryl acetate) – 500 mg in 5 ml
Tablets (tocopheryl acetate) – 50 mg and 200 mg

NB: Vitamin E is also available in a number of proprietary multivitamin preparations.

Actions and uses

The actual function of vitamin E has not yet been identified. Oral supplements do not appear to be essential in adults and in children with congenital cholestasis, parenteral vitamin E is required to treat abnormally low levels of the vitamin associated with neuromuscular abnormalities. Vitamin E has not been shown to be of value in any other condition for which it has been tried.

Dosage

The dosage for vitamin E has not been clearly defined but the doses recommended with the suspension are:

- malabsorption in cystic fibrosis: adult, 100–200 mg daily; child under 1 year, 50 mg daily; child over 1 year, 100 mg daily
- malabsorption in abetalipoproteinaemia: adult and child, 50–100 mg/kg daily
- malabsorption in chronic cholestasis: infant, 150–200 mg/kg daily.

Nursing implications

Vitamin E can cause diarrhoea and abdominal pain if doses greater than 1 g per day are taken.

Storage

Vitamin E preparations are stored at room temperature.

VITAMIN K (Konakion, Synkovit)

Presentation

Tablets – phytomenadione 10 mg (Konakion)
Injection – phytomenadione 1 mg in 0.5 ml, 2 mg in 0.2 ml and 10 mg in 1 ml

NB: Menadiol sodium phosphate is a synthetic water-soluble form of vitamin K available as 10 mg tablets.

Actions and uses

Vitamin K is a naturally occurring fat-soluble vitamin, essential for the synthesis of clotting factor (prothrombin, factor VII, factor IX and factor X).

It is indicated for:

- the treatment of vitamin K deficiency which is usually manifest as an increased bleeding tendency. The commonest cause of vitamin K deficiency is malabsorption
- reversing the effects of warfarin
- premature infants who may have a relative deficiency of vitamin K. They are often given therapeutic vitamin K to avoid the development of bleeding complications.

Menadiol sodium phosphate is a water-soluble analogue of vitamin K which is better absorbed from the gut in fat malabsorption syndrome which commonly occurs in biliary obstruction and liver disease.

Dosage

- To treat vitamin K deficiency due to malabsorption: 10 mg is given by intramuscular injection until clotting studies have been shown to be normalized.
- To prevent vitamin K deficiency in malabsorption syndromes, menadiol sodium phosphate, orally, 10 mg daily.
- As an antidote to anticoagulant drugs, the British Society of Haematology guidelines should be followed. The main points are, for patients on warfarin who have a major bleed, the warfarin should be stopped and 5 mg of vitamin K administered by slow IV injection accompanied by prothrombin complex concentrate or fresh frozen plasma, and if a patient's INR is >8.0 and they have risk factors for bleeding, 0.5 mg of vitamin K should be administered by slow IV injection or 5 mg orally. Refer to guidelines for further information.
- For the prophylactic treatment of newborn infants: 1 mg should be administered by intramuscular injection. Vitamin K can also be administered orally, using the mixed micelle preparation (Konakion MM Paediatric) with two doses of 2 mg given in the first week of life and a third dose of 2 mg to breastfed babies at 1 month of age. This mixed micelle preparation can also be used intravenously to treat haemorrhagic disease of the newborn.

Nursing implications
- The too rapid intravenous administration of vitamin K has caused reactions including facial flushing, sweating, a sense of chest constriction, cyanosis and peripheral vascular collapse.
- There are several preparations of vitamin K injection. Nurses should ensure that the correct preparation is used for the intended indication and consult product literature for dosage and administration.

Storage

Vitamin K preparations are stored at room temperature. Tablets should be stored in a well-closed container, protected from light.

V

W

WARFARIN (Marevan)

Presentation
Tablets – 0.5 mg, 1 mg, 3 mg, 5 mg

Actions and uses
A number of the substances in the blood which play an important part in preventing bleeding by forming clots are produced by the liver from vitamin K. Warfarin inhibits the synthesis of these substances (known as clotting factors) and therefore reduces the ability of the blood to clot. Its principal uses are for the prevention and treatment of thromboembolic states such as deep vein thrombosis and pulmonary embolus. It is also used to prevent the formation of clot in cardiovascular disease either on artificial heart valves or in the atria of patients who have atrial dysrhythmias.

Dosage
The general principle is to give a loading dose over 48 hours and subsequently adjust the dosage to the patient's individual requirements as gauged on the results of clotting tests such as prothrombin time and INR.

Loading dose: 10 mg on the first day and second day (lower doses are used in patients with abnormal liver function, cardiac failure, those receiving parenteral nutrition, those who have a low body weight or are elderly). The dosage on the third day should depend on the result of the clotting test used.
Maintenance: this depends on results of clotting tests, but is usually 3–9 mg daily.

Nursing implications
- The daily maintenance dose of warfarin is, as noted above, determined by the results of clotting studies. As the effects of bleeding due to over anticoagulation or thrombosis due to under anticoagulation can be so rapidly catastrophic, strict adherence to the recommended dose is mandatory and the nurse may play an important role in ensuring that patients are aware of this.
- The effects of warfarin may be influenced by a number of factors listed below and the nurse may play an important role by identifying their occurrence and alerting both the patient and medical staff. The following circumstances may lead to a requirement for alteration in dosage.
  - Acute illness such as chest infection or viral infection.
  - Sudden weight loss.
  - The concurrent administration of other drugs. A number of drugs may affect the patient's dosage requirements. Where drugs are known to interfere with anticoagulant control, this has been noted in the nursing implications sections of this book.
- The occurrence of haemorrhage in a patient on warfarin is an indication for immediate withdrawal of the drug and if the haemorrhage is at all serious or repetitive the patient should be immediately referred to hospital for further assessment and if necessary they may be given vitamin K which accelerates a return normal clotting function.
- Warfarin is relatively contraindicated in patients with

severe liver or kidney disease, haemorrhagic conditions or uncontrolled hypertension. It should also be used with great caution immediately after surgery or labour.
- Hair loss, skin rash and diarrhoea may rarely occur.

Storage

The drug may be stored at room temperature.

W

XAMOTEROL (Corwin)

Presentation
Tablets – 200 mg

Actions and uses
Xamoterol is a beta-blocker and the section under beta-adrenoreceptor blocking drugs (p. 51) should be consulted for a general account of these compounds. However, xamoterol is notably different from other beta-blockers so far, in that it also possesses marked beta-stimulant properties and can actually stimulate resting heart rate and contractility. Thus the beta-blocking properties on the heart are only manifest when there is excessive sympathetic drive (i.e. when the heart is stressed) while the problem of resting bradycardia and hypotension commonly seen with other beta-blockers is much less likely to occur.

Xamoterol is occasionally used for the treatment of mild heart failure (deterioration would occur in patients with moderate or severe heart failure). Its beta-stimulant properties support resting cardiac function while its beta-blocking properties protect the heart from sympathetic overactivity.

Dosage
Adults: initially 200 mg daily (under hospitalization) for 1 week increasing to 200 mg twice daily thereafter.

Nursing implications
- The Committee on Safety of Medicines has stressed that xamoterol is only indicated in the treatment of mild heart failure. Early experience in more severe heart failure was associated with an increase in mortality.

- It is contraindicated in various situations which include:
  - patients who are short of breath or fatigued at rest or on limited or minimal exercise
  - patients with a resting tachycardia, hypotension, peripheral oedema or a history of acute pulmonary oedema
  - any patient on 40 mg or more of frusemide a day or any patient who requires ACE inhibitor treatment.
- For the above reason, xamoterol therapy is only initiated in hospitals where the facility for close monitoring exists.
- Other side effects include gastrointestinal disturbances, headaches, dizziness and bronchospasm. Palpitations, hypotension and chest pain have also been reported.

Storage
Xamoterol tablets are stored at room temperature.

XIPAMIDE (Diurexan)

Presentation
Tablets – 20 mg

Actions and uses
Xipamide is a drug which has both a useful diuretic and hypotensive action. It may therefore be used in the treatment of hypertension and also in the management of heart failure (see Thiazide Diuretics section, Actions and uses, p. 357).

Dosage
The usual daily adult dose is 20–40 mg taken once daily in the morning.

Up to 80 mg daily may be required in the management of oedema.

> **Nursing implications**
> - See the nursing implications for Thiazide Diuretics (p. 357).
> - This drug may also produce gastrointestinal upset and dizziness.

Storage

Xipamide tablets are stored at room temperature.

Z

ZAFIRLUKAST (Accolate)

Presentation
Tablets – 20 mg

Actions and uses
Zafirlukast, like montelukast, is a leukotriene receptor antagonist. It is indicated for use in the prophylaxis of asthma.

Dosage
Adults and children over 12 years: 20 mg twice daily.

Nursing implications
- See the section on Montelukast (p. 230).
- It is contraindicated in liver impairment and breastfeeding.
- Side effects include gastro-intestinal disturbances, headache and hypersensitivity reactions.

Storage
Zafirlukast tablets are stored at room temperature.

ZALCITABINE (Hivid)

Presentation
Tablets – 375 microgram and 750 microgram

Actions and uses
Zalcitabine is a nucleoside reverse transcriptase inhibitor with actions and uses similar to those of zidovudine. It is indicated for use in HIV infection when used in combination with other antiretroviral drugs.

Dosage
Adult: 750 microgram every 8 hours. Not recommended for children under 13 years.

Nursing implications
- Zalcitabine can cause serious side effects and should be prescribed only under expert advice.
- The timing of commencement of therapy should be decided by those with specialist expertise in the management of HIV and depends on symptoms, viral load and the CD4 count and should be weighed against drug toxicities and the likely development of drug resistance.
- Resistance to antiretroviral drugs is reduced by using combination therapy.
- Most antiretroviral agents are used in pregnancy although teratogenic effects are not yet fully understood. Mothers are advised not to breastfeed their infants as HIV can pass from mother to infant via the breast milk.
- The main side effects with zalcitabine are peripheral neuropathy and mouth ulceration. The drug should be discontinued immediately if signs of peripheral neuropathy develop, e.g. numbness and impaired touch sensation. Other side effects include gastrointestinal effects, pharyngitis, headache and dizziness. Pancreatitis can also occur; if it does the drug should be permanently discontinued. The drug should be suspended if signs of impending pancreatitis occur. If another drug known to cause pancreatitis is to be prescribed, temporarily suspend zalcitabine.
- Use with caution in liver disease. Treatment should be suspended or discontinued if there are

abnormal liver function tests, hepatic steatosis occurs, there is progressive hepatomegaly or unexplained lactic acidosis.
- Interactions – avoid concomitant use with drugs that can cause pancreatitis or peripheral neuropathy.

Storage
Zalcitabine tablets are stored at room temperature.

ZANAMIVIR (Relenza)

Presentation
Powder for inhalation – 5 mg per blister in a Diskhaler

Actions and uses
Zanamivir has been recently introduced for the treatment of influenza A and B in patients who have symptoms where influenza is present in the community. It inhibits neuraminidase, an enzyme on the surface of the influenza virus, which is essential to the virus, allowing it to replicate in the respiratory tract. To be effective, treatment with zanamivir must be started within 48 hours of the onset of symptoms.

Dosage
Adults and children over 12 years: 10 mg inhaled twice daily for 5 days.

Nursing implications
- Side effects include gastro-intestinal upsets and occasionally bronchospasm, respiratory impairment and rash.
- Use with caution in the elderly, patients with pulmonary disease including asthma, immuno-compromised patients and in those with uncontrolled chronic illness.
- If patients use other inhalers, these should be used before zanamivir.

Storage
Zanamivir is stored at room temperature.

ZIDOVUDINE (Retrovir)

Presentation
Capsules – 100 mg, 250 mg
Tablets – 300 mg
Syrup – 50 mg in 5 ml
Infusion – 200 mg in 20 ml

Actions and uses
Zidovudine is an antiretroviral agent, i.e. it is active against retroviruses of which the human immunodeficiency virus (HIV or AIDS virus) is perhaps the best known. It is a nucleoside reverse transcriptase inhibitor with a complex mode of action so the following is a simplified version only.

Zidovudine is a chemical analogue of thymidine which, on entering human (normal and viral-infected) cells, is converted by intracellular enzymes to zidovudine triphosphate via a series of phosphorylation reactions. Zidovudine triphosphate in turn inhibits the formation of pro-viral DNA (which is essential for viral proliferation) by competitive inhibition of the enzyme viral reverse transcriptase.

Zidovudine was the first effective antiretroviral agent for the treatment of HIV infection. However, several newer reverse transcriptase inhibitors (and other antiretroviral agents) have since been developed and are used in combinations with zidovudine.

Zidovudine is indicated for HIV infection in combination with other antiretroviral drugs and as monotherapy for the prevention of maternal–fetal HIV transmission.

Dosage
Oral
- Adult: 500–600 mg daily in 2–3 divided doses depending on preparation used.
- Child over 3 months: 360–480 mg/m^2 daily in 3–4 divided doses to a maximum of 200 mg every 6 hours. Taking zidovudine after food limits any nausea.
- NB: higher doses can be used to treat or prevent HIV-associated neurological dysfunction.

Intravenous
Infusions are administered in glucose 5%, diluted to a concentration of 2 mg/ml or 4 mg/ml and given over

1 hour. This route is generally only used when the oral route is temporarily compromised. Adults should receive 1–2 mg/kg every 4 hours and children 80–160 mg/m² every 6 hours.

Prevention of maternal–fetal HIV transmission

Women should start treatment when they reach 14 weeks gestation with 100 mg orally, five times a day until the beginning of labour. During labour and delivery, the intravenous infusion is used at a dose of 2 mg/kg over 1 hour, then 1 mg/kg/h until the umbilical cord is clamped. Newborn infants should then receive 2 mg/kg orally 6-hourly, starting within 12 hours of birth and continuing for 6 weeks. If the oral route is compromised, the infant should receive 1.5 mg/kg intravenously every 6 hours.

Nursing implications

- Drugs used in the treatment of HIV can cause serious side effects and should be prescribed only under expert advice.
- The timing of commencement of therapy should be decided by those with specialist expertise in the management of HIV and depends on symptoms, viral load and the CD4 count and should be weighed against drug toxicities and the likely development of drug resistance.
- Resistance to antiretroviral drugs is reduced by using combination therapy.
- Most antiretroviral agents are used in pregnancy although teratogenic effects are not yet fully understood. Mothers are advised not to breastfeed their infants as HIV can pass from mother to infant via the breast milk.
- Anaemia, leucopenia and neutropenia are the most common severe adverse reactions to zidovudine. Occasionally transfusions are required for severely anaemic patients. Zidovudine should not be used in patients with abnormally low neutrophil or haemoglobin levels.

- Other commonly reported side effects are anorexia, nausea, vomiting and abdominal pain, fever, myopathy, headache and paraesthesia. A variety of other effects have been attributed to zidovudine including taste disturbance, diarrhoea, chest pain, lack of concentration, breathlessness, urinary frequency, pruritus and flu-like symptoms. Severe neurological toxicity has resulted in convulsions. As well as the need for proper evaluation of the effectiveness of this drug, it is equally important to establish a true picture of its toxic potential, a role for which the nurse is well placed.
- Use with caution in liver disease. Treatment should be suspended or discontinued if there are abnormal liver function tests, hepatic steatosis occurs, there is progressive hepatomegaly or unexplained lactic acidosis.
- Due to the possibility of serious haematological toxicity the administration of other drugs which are potentially toxic to the bone marrow should be avoided. Profound myelosuppression can occur with ganciclovir.
- Accumulation of zidovudine is likely to occur in patients with kidney impairment and dosage adjustment may become necessary.

Storage

Zidovudine preparations are stored at room temperature, protected from light.

ZINC SULPHATE (Solvazinc)

Presentation

Eye drops – 0.25%
Tablets – 125 mg effervescent

Various topical preparations in combination with other products.

Actions and uses

- Topical: zinc sulphate possesses a soothing (astringent) action and

Z

aids granulation which renders it useful when applied locally in inflammatory conditions, e.g. applied to indolent ulcers and to the cornea in conjunctivitis.

- Oral: oral tablets or capsules are used to correct zinc deficiency (zinc is an essential trace element in the diet), to aid wound healing and in the treatment of acrodermatitis enteropathica.

Dosage
- Topical: apply to inflammatory lesions twice daily. Eye drops: apply up to four times daily.
- Oral: adults and children over 30 kg, 125 mg in water 1–3 times daily. Child under 10 kg, 62.5 mg daily, child 10–30 kg, 62.5 mg 1–3 times daily.

Nursing implications
- The only side effect of note is the production of gastrointestinal upsets which are reduced if dosages are taken immediately after meals.
- Melaena and anaemia following haemorrhagic gastric erosion have been reported.
- It is important to note that zinc sulphate was formerly used as an emetic but this indication is no longer valid.

Storage
Preparations containing zinc sulphate are stored at room temperature.

ZOLMITRIPTAN (Zomig)

Presentation
Tablets – 2.5 mg

Actions and uses
Zolmitriptan is a 5-HT1 (5-hydroxy-tryptamine) agonist, similar to sumatriptan. It is used in the treatment of acute migraine attacks. Acting at 5-HT1 receptors, it causes vascular contraction in intracranial blood vessels, reversing any dilatation or oedema in these vessels which is thought to cause migraine attacks.

Dosage
Adults only: 2.5 mg should be taken as soon as possible after the onset of an attack. A second dose can be taken 2 hours after the first if the migraine persists or recurs. A 5 mg dose can be taken in subsequent attacks if 2.5 mg has not proved satisfactory. Maximum of 15 mg should be taken in 24 hours.

Nursing implications
- See Sumatriptan (p. 344).
- Additionally contraindicated in Wolff–Parkinson–White syndrome or arrhythmias associated with accessory cardiac conduction pathways.
- Additional side effects include drowsiness and transient hypertension.

Storage
Zolmitriptan preparations are stored at room temperature.

ZOLPIDEM (Stilnoct)

Presentation
Tablets – 5 mg and 10 mg

Actions and uses
Zolpidem is an imidazopyridine hypnotic used for the short-term treatment of insomnia. It is not a benzodiazepine, but acts at the same receptors as benzodiazepines at the GABA receptor complex. Zolpidem preferentially binds to one of the receptor subtypes, modulating the chloride ion channel and leading to its sedative effect. The effects of zolpidem, like the benzodiazepines, can be reversed with flumazenil.

Dosage
10 mg (or 5 mg in the elderly) taken at bedtime.

Nursing implications
- In view of problems of dependency with benzodiazepines in the past it must be stressed that all hypnotics should be prescribed for short-term use only.

Z

- Patients taking courses of hypnotics may experience rebound insomnia when these are stopped and careful counselling to reduce concern is often required.
- Zolpidem has a short duration of action compared with some of the benzodiazepines. A hangover effect is unlikely but patients should still be advised that drowsiness may persist to the next day and may affect their ability to drive or perform skilled tasks.
- Zolpidem will enhance the effects of alcohol.
- Zolpidem is contraindicated in obstructive sleep apnoea, acute pulmonary insufficiency, respiratory depression, myasthenia gravis, severe hepatic impairment, psychotic illness, pregnancy and breastfeeding.
- It should be used with caution in patients with depression, a history of drug or alcohol abuse or hepatic or renal impairment.
- Ritonavir interacts with zolpidem, increasing the plasma concentration of zolpidem, so concomitant use should be avoided as extreme sedation and respiratory depression can occur.
- Side effects include gastrointestinal upsets, headache, drowsiness and asthenia.

Storage

Zolpidem preparations are stored at room temperature.

ZOPICLONE (Zimovane)

Presentation

Tablets – 3.75 mg and 7.5 mg

Actions and uses

Zopiclone is a cyclopyrrolone type of hypnotic which induces and maintains sleep of about 6 hours duration without producing sedation or 'hangover' into the next day. Zopiclone is not itself a benzodiazepine but it acts at the same receptors as benzodiazepines at the GABA receptor complex. The effects of zopiclone, like the benzodiazepines, can be reversed with flumazenil.

Dosage

Adults: a single dose of 7.5 mg is taken on retiring. Maximum treatment period of 4 weeks.

Nursing implications

- In view of problems of dependency with benzodiazepines in the past it must be stressed that all hypnotics should be prescribed for short-term use only.
- Patients taking courses of hypnotics may experience rebound insomnia when these are stopped and careful counselling to reduce concern is often required.
- Although a hangover effect is unlikely, patients should still be advised that drowsiness may persist to the next day and may affect their ability to drive or perform skilled tasks.
- Lower doses, e.g. 3.75 mg, may be more appropriate in elderly people, who are very sensitive to sedative drugs.
- Patients with liver impairment may also be very sensitive to zopiclone and require reduced dosage. Use with caution also in renal impairment and in those with a history of drug abuse or psychiatric illness.
- Since there is no evidence that zopiclone is safe in pregnancy it should be avoided in this situation. Also it is excreted in breast milk and should not be given to nursing mothers.
- Zopiclone is contraindicated in myasthenia gravis, respiratory failure, severe sleep apnoea syndrome and severe hepatic impairment.
- Zopiclone interacts with erythromycin and quinupristin/dalfaprostin, with the metabolism of zopiclone being inhibited.
- Gastrointestinal upsets have been reported and some patients have complained of a 'metallic' taste during treatment.

Z

Storage
Zopiclone tablets are stored at room temperature.

ZOTEPINE (Zoleptil)

Presentation
Tablets – 25 mg, 50 mg and 100 mg

Actions and uses
Zotepine is an atypical antipsychotic agent indicated for use in schizophrenia. It acts by reducing CNS dopamine function, acting as an antagonist at dopamine receptors. It also has an effect at other receptors: 5-HT (hydroxytryptamine), alpha-1 adrenoceptors and histamine-1 receptors.

Dosage
Start with 25 mg three times a day, increasing according to response at intervals of 4 days to a maximum of 100 mg three times a day. Elderly patients should start on a lower dose of 25 mg twice daily and increase as required to a maximum of 75 mg twice daily.

Not recommended for children.

Nursing implications
- Side effects include weight gain, dizziness, hypotension and tachycardia, extrapyramidal symptoms, constipation, dyspepsia and liver enzyme abnormalities.
- Use with caution in cardiovascular disease, epilepsy and Parkinson's disease.
- Zotepine should not be used concomitantly with high doses of other antipsychotics. It should not be used in acute gout or in patients with a history of kidney stones.
- Fluoxetine and diazepam increase the plasma concentration of zotepine so use together with caution. Use with caution concurrently with other CNS depressants, hypotensive agents and anaesthetics.

Storage
Zotepine tablets are stored at room temperature.

APPENDICES

Appendix 1: Nurse Prescribers' Formulary

ALMOND OIL EAR DROPS

Contains almond oil as sole ingredient. A pale yellow oil having a characteristic odour and a bland 'nutty' taste.

Actions and uses
Almond oil has demulcent (soothing) properties and in this form acts as a wax solvent or softener to facilitate removal of ear wax. Ear wax is a normal body secretion which provides essential protection of the sensitive lining of the ear but which on occasion accumulates and dries out so causing deafness or impairing visual inspection of the ear drum. The demulcent properties are of additional benefit if irritation or inflammation is also present.

Dosage
Apply ear drops generously 3–4 times daily prior to ear syringing.

Nursing implications
- Patients should apply the ear drops for several days and up to 1 week prior to ear syringing. Preferably lie with the treated ear uppermost for 5–10 minutes after application.
- Syringing should be avoided or medical advice sought if patients have a history of recurrent infections of the outer ear (otitis externa), have had past ear surgery or perforation of the ear drum. This is also important if hearing is confined to one ear only since the risk of damage to the ear, however remote, is nonetheless unacceptable.

Storage
Store at room temperature. Protect from light and avoid storage next to a heat source (radiator, etc.).

AQUEOUS CREAM

Contains Hydrated Emulsifying Ointment preserved with chlorocresol.

Actions and uses
Aqueous Cream is a hydrated form of Emulsifying Ointment. Unlike Emulsifying Ointment, however, it is not used as a soap substitute but rather it is applied directly to the skin surface. Aqueous Cream is an emollient which creates a soothing, protective film when applied to dry skin. It is used in various associated dermatological conditions.

Dosage
Apply as required to maintain adequate hydration of the skin surface.

Nursing implications
- Note that Aqueous Cream is miscible with water and can be readily washed off. Reapplication after washing is therefore necessary.

Storage
Store at room temperature.

ARACHIS OIL ENEMA

Contains arachis oil as sole ingredient. A colourless or pale yellow oil being odourless or having a faint 'nutty' odour and a bland 'nutty' taste.

Actions and uses
Arachis oil is a local lubricant and faecal softener used to treat hard

impacted faeces in patients with severe constipation particularly if untreated or unresponsive to standard laxative therapy. The latter often arises if laxatives have been overlooked for patients receiving prolonged regular analgesia with opioid analgesics which uniformly produce chronic constipation. Arachis oil administered per rectum is a rapid and usually effective means of evacuating the bowel and should be tried before manual evacuation is attempted.

Dosage
A single dose of 100 ml or more is instilled in the rectum. Proportionately smaller volumes are used in children and can be calculated on 2 ml/kg body weight basis.

Nursing implications
- NB: Arachis Oil contains Peanut Oil. It can invoke serious allergic reactions including anaphylaxis in any individual with peanut allergy.
- The enema should be warmed before use by placing the pack in warm (not hot) water for 5–10 minutes.
- To use, remove the cap and lubricate the delivery tube. Insert into rectum and squeeze container gently until the contents or an estimated proportion thereof is dispelled. Discard any unused portion.
- Arachis oil enema is *not recommended* for children under 3 years of age.

Storage
Store at room temperature. Protect from light and avoid storage next to a heat source (radiator, etc.).

ASPIRIN TABLETS, DISPERSIBLE

Tablets containing 300 mg acetylsalicylic acid.

Actions and uses
Aspirin or acetylsalicylic acid possesses analgesic, antiinflammatory and antipyretic activity and is used in the treatment of mild pain and also to lower elevated body temperature in febrile conditions. A further use for aspirin arises as a result of its inhibitory effects on platelet aggregation but lower doses may be required and it is unlikely that nurses will be required to prescribe aspirin for this indication.

Dosage
The usual adult analgesic and antipyretic dose is 600–900 mg administered 4–6 hourly as required to a maximum of 4 g daily. Higher doses, previously used in the treatment of inflammatory disease, are now rarely used since more effective and better tolerated NSAIDs exist.

Children over 12 years should receive doses of the order 300–600 mg but note caution associated with Reye's syndrome, below.

Nursing implications
- Aspirin *should not be prescribed* for children under the age of 12 years (unless specifically indicated and under medical supervision). This follows the recognition many years ago that aspirin may be associated with the development of Reye's syndrome, a potentially fatal CNS condition, in young children.
- Aspirin dispersible tablets are mixed with 20–30 ml water before administration.
- Aspirin causes notable gastrointestinal upsets in a proportion of patients associated with dyspepsia of varying severity, nausea, vomiting, diarrhoea and gastric bleeding. It should be administered with caution or indeed avoided in those with active or recent peptic ulceration or a history of gastrotoxicity related to aspirin administration. Paracetamol is a suitable alternative in such cases.
- A proportion of asthmatics, perhaps as much as 10%, are at risk from development of bronchospasm when aspirin is administered. It should therefore be used with caution in asthmatics and discontinued if wheeze or breathlessness occurs.

- Skin rashes in patients with aspirin hypersensitivity are occasionally reported.
- Aspirin is *very* toxic to young children in overdosage and given its availability in many households it is particularly important that it be stored out of reach of children.

Storage

Store at room temperature in a *dry* place (*not* the bathroom cabinet). Aspirin readily hydrolyses in the presence of moisture to yield acetic acid or vinegar. A strong vinegary smell indicates the breakdown of aspirin tablets.

BISACODYL SUPPOSITORIES
BISACODYL TABLETS

Suppositories containing 5 mg and 10 mg bisacodyl. Tablets are enteric-coated and contain 5 mg bisacodyl.

Actions and uses

Bisacodyl is a laxative of the stimulant type resembling senna and danthron in its action. It produces a marked increase in bowel motility and subsequent evacuation of faecal contents. Stimulant laxatives are only indicated where constipation is related to poor bowel motility or where rapid and complete bowel evacuation is required prior to endoscopic or radiological examination or before bowel surgery. Suppositories of bisacodyl act rapidly, within 30 minutes to 1 hour of administration, while tablets are taken at night to promote bowel emptying the following morning i.e. around 8 hours later.

Dosage

Adults require 10 mg at night and up to 30 mg if complete bowel evacuation is sought. Alternatively, 10 mg administered as a rectal suppository.
Children require 5 mg and up to 10 mg by mouth or 5–10 mg rectally depending upon age.

Nursing implications

- Bisacodyl is a stimulant laxative and as such can cause excessive bowel motility associated with griping or cramping pain or discomfort.

Storage

Store at room temperature in a *dry* place (*not* the bathroom cabinet). Aspirin readily hydrolyses in the presence of moisture to yield acetic acid or vinegar. A strong vinegary smell indicates the breakdown of aspirin tablets.

CADEXOMER-IODINE OINTMENT
CADEXOMER-IODINE PASTE
CADEXOMER-IODINE POWDER

Iodosorb ointment (10 g, 20 g), and powder (3 g sachet) and Iodoflex paste with gauze backing (5 g, 10 g, 17 g) containing a cadexomer microbead-iodine carrier system providing iodine 0.9%.

Actions and uses

Cadexomer-iodine like povidone-iodine is an iodophore – a compound consisting of iodine in association with a carrier from which free iodine is gradually released. It has absorbent and antiseptic properties which are of specific benefit in the treatment of chronic wounds and ulcers including venous ulcers and pressure sores. Note however the reluctance to routinely use antiseptics including iodine-based products in modern wound care.

Dosage

Ointment: apply to wound to a depth of around 3 mm and cover with a retaining dressing. Renew dressing as required i.e. once saturated with exudate. Normally used thrice weekly.
Paste: apply to wound surface, remove gauze backing and cover with a secondary dressing. Renew when saturated, approximately 3 times per week.
Powder: apply to depth 3 mm and cover with sterile gauze dressing. Change when saturated approximately 3 times per week.

Nursing implications

- Note the reluctance to routinely use iodine-based antiseptics in the treatment of chronic wounds and ulcers.
- Cadexomer-iodine is intended for the treatment of *moist* wounds only.
- Systemic absorption of iodine is possible, especially if large surfaces are treated. Do not use in patients with thyroid disease, those on concurrent lithium therapy or in pregnancy or if breastfeeding.
- Do not apply more than 150 g ointment or paste per week.

Storage
Store at room temperature.

CALAMINE CREAM
CALAMINE LOTION
CALAMINE LOTION, OILY

Contains Calamine (which is Zinc Carbonate coloured with a small amount of Ferric Oxide), Zinc Oxide, Bentonite, Sodium Citrate, Liquified Phenol, Glycerol in purified water or cream or oily base.

Actions and uses
Calamine preparations are used for relief of symptoms of mild sunburn, pruritis, insect bites and stings and other minor skin irritation when its cooling (soothing) effect may be beneficial. It may be applied as aqueous lotion or as an oily lotion or cream depending upon ease of application, requirement for prolonged contact or based on its cosmetic acceptability.

Dosage
Apply to the skin surface as required.

Nursing implications
- Calamine preparations should be applied gently to affected skin, using a cotton wool ball if necessary.

Storage
Store at room temperature.

EMULSIFYING OINTMENT BP

Contains Emulsifying Wax (a soapy substance) mixed with White Soft paraffin and Liquid Paraffin.

Actions and uses
Emulsifying Ointment is used mainly as a soap substitute by patients with various, notably dry, skin conditions including psoriasis. It is also applied to dry skin, most often in its hydrated form (i.e. as Aqueous Cream). It may also be preferred to commercial soaps for those who are hypersensitive to various detergents, perfumes, colourings, etc. After use, Emulsifying Ointment leaves a soothing, protective film over the skin surface on which it promotes hydration. This is described as an emollient action.

Dosage
Use frequently in place of soap.

Nursing implications

- A small scoop of Emulsifying Ointment is mixed with warm water and applied to the skin as required.
- It may also be used as a bath emollient in which case several scoops are held under a running tap and allowed to disperse in the bathwater. Note that Emulsifying Ointment may render the bath slippery and great care should be taken to prevent accidents when bathing patients.

Storage
Store at room temperature.

CATHETER MAINTENANCE
SOLUTION, CHLORHEXIDINE

Uro-Tainer containing Chlorhexidine 0.02% in 100 ml with applicator attached.

Actions and uses
The Uro-Tainer system has been available for over 10 years in the UK. It has been widely adopted as a convenient method for maintaining urethral catheters in place of the traditional bladder washout pack and

syringe routine which is both cumbersome and time consuming. Without proper maintenance, the retention of urinary catheters is associated with encrustation and leakage and discomfort for the patient frequently necessitating catheter change. The Uro-Tainer Chlorhexidine is used as frequently as necessary from twice daily to once weekly to prevent or reduce bacterial growth in the bladder. It may be used where there is recurrent infections of the lower urinary tract (perhaps requiring systemic antibiotic therapy) with common bowel organisms such as *Escherichia coli*.

Dosage

Use varies from twice daily to once weekly depending upon risk of contamination.

Nursing implications

Use of the Uro-Tainer system:

- Uro-Tainer is a one piece system that connects directly to the drainage funnel of the Foley catheter.
- Step 1. Remove the protective cover around the Uro-Tainer tip.
- Step 2. Clamp off the Uro-Tainer tubing using the plastic clamp provided.
- Step 3. Swab the Foley catheter drainage funnel at the connection point.
- Step 4. Connect the Uro-Tainer to the catheter funnel and unclamp the tubing.
- Step 5. The solution is now instilled by gravitational force with the Uro-Tainer bag raised to a level above the urinary bladder.
- Step 6. Instil for 10–20 minutes then drain by allowing solution to return to the Uro-Tainer bag after repositioning it at a level below the urinary bladder.

Pharmaceutical considerations

- Store in a cool place.
- Inspect for damage (e.g. moisture accumulating in the outer bag) prior to use.
  NB: Not for intravenous infusion.

CATHETER MAINTENANCE SOLUTION, MANDELIC ACID

Uro-Tainer containing Mandelic Acid 1% in 100 ml aqueous solution with applicator attached.

Actions and uses

The Uro-Tainer system has been available for over 10 years in the UK. It has been widely adopted as a convenient method for maintaining urethral catheters in place of the traditional bladder washout pack and syringe routine which is both cumbersome and time consuming. Without proper maintenance, the retention of urinary catheters is associated with encrustation and leakage and discomfort for the patient frequently necessitating catheter change. The Uro-Tainer Mandelic Acid is used specifically to prevent bladder infection due to bacteria which produce the urea splitting 'urease' enzyme of which *Proteus* and *Pseudomonas* are common examples.

Dosage

Use once or twice daily according to risk of infection.

Nursing implications

Use of the Uro-Tainer system:

- Uro-Tainer is a one piece system that connects directly to the drainage funnel of the Foley catheter.
- Step 1. Remove the protective cover around the Uro-Tainer tip.
- Step 2. Clamp off the Uro-Tainer tubing using the plastic clamp provided.
- Step 3. Swab the Foley catheter drainage funnel at the connection point.
- Step 4. Connect the Uro-Tainer to the catheter funnel and unclamp the tubing.
- Step 5. The solution is now instilled by gravitational force with the Uro-Tainer bag raised to a level above the urinary bladder.
- Step 6. Instil for 10–20 minutes then drain by allowing solution to return to the Uro-Tainer bag after repositioning it at a level below the urinary bladder.

Pharmaceutical considerations
- Store in a cool place.
- Inspect for damage (e.g. moisture accumulating in the outer bag) prior to use.

NB: Not for intravenous infusion.

CATHETER MAINTENANCE SOLUTION, SODIUM CHLORIDE

Uro-Tainer containing Sodium Chloride 0.9% (*normal saline*) in 100 ml with applicator attached.

Actions and uses
The Uro-Tainer system has been available for over 10 years in the UK. It has been widely adopted as a convenient method for maintaining urethral catheters in place of the traditional bladder washout pack and syringe routine which is both cumbersome and time consuming. Without proper maintenance, the retention of urinary catheters is associated with encrustation and leakage and discomfort for the patient frequently necessitating catheter change. The Uro-Tainer Sodium Chloride 0.9% is used for routine cleansing and mechanical wash out of cell debris and small blood clots which might otherwise accumulate and lead to blockage.

Dosage
Use daily as required.

Nursing implications
Use of the Uro-Tainer system:

- Uro-Tainer is a one piece system that connects directly to the drainage funnel of the Foley catheter.
- Step 1. Remove the protective cover around the Uro-Tainer tip.
- Step 2. Clamp off the Uro-Tainer tubing using the plastic clamp provided.
- Step 3. Swab the Foley catheter drainage funnel at the connection point.
- Step 4. Connect the Uro-Tainer to the catheter funnel and unclamp the tubing.
- Step 5. The solution is now instilled by gravitational force

with the Uro-Tainer bag raised to a level above the urinary bladder.
- Step 6. Instil for 10–20 minutes then drain by allowing solution to return to the Uro-Tainer bag after repositioning it at a level below the urinary bladder.

Pharmaceutical considerations
- Store in a cool place.
- Inspect for damage (e.g. moisture accumulating in the outer bag) prior to use.

NB: Not for intravenous infusion.

CATHETER MAINTENANCE SOLUTION, SOLUTION G

Uro-Tainer containing Citric Acid 3.23% in 100 ml aqueous solution with applicator attached.

Actions and uses
The Uro-Tainer system has been available for over 10 years in the UK. It has been widely adopted as a convenient method for maintaining urethral catheters in place of the traditional bladder washout pack and syringe routine which is both cumbersome and time consuming. Without proper maintenance, the retention of urinary catheters is associated with encrustation and leakage and discomfort for the patient frequently necessitating catheter change. The Uro-Tainer Suby G contains citric acid and is used to dissolve crystals which become formed in the bladder and catheter. Uro-Tainer Solution R should be used if the problem persists and complete blockage results or to aid removal of the catheter in this situation.

Dosage
Use from twice daily to once weekly according to severity of the problem.

Nursing implications
Use of the Uro-Tainer system:

- Uro-Tainer is a one piece system that connects directly to the drainage funnel of the Foley catheter.

- Step 1. Remove the protective cover around the Uro-Tainer tip.
- Step 2. Clamp off the Uro-Tainer tubing using the plastic clamp provided.
- Step 3. Swab the Foley catheter drainage funnel at the connection point.
- Step 4. Connect the Uro-Tainer to the catheter funnel and unclamp the tubing.
- Step 5. The solution is now instilled by gravitational force with the Uro-Tainer bag raised to a level above the urinary bladder.
- Step 6. Instil for 10–20 minutes then drain by allowing solution to return to the Uro-Tainer bag after repositioning it at a level below the urinary bladder.

Pharmaceutical considerations

- Store in a cool place.
- Inspect for damage (e.g. moisture accumulating in the outer bag) prior to use.
  NB: Not for intravenous infusion.

CATHETER MAINTENANCE SOLUTION, SOLUTION R

Uro-Tainer containing Citric Acid 6% in 100 ml aqueous solution with applicator attached.

Actions and uses

The Uro-Tainer system has been available for over 10 years in the UK. It has been widely adopted as a convenient method for maintaining urethral catheters in place of the traditional bladder washout pack and syringe routine which is both cumbersome and time consuming. Without proper maintenance, the retention of urinary catheters is associated with encrustation and leakage and discomfort for the patient frequently necessitating catheter change. The Uro-Tainer Solution R is used to dissolve persistent crystallization in the catheter or bladder (despite use of Suby G solution) and to unblock an already encrusted catheter or aid its removal.

Dosage

Use between twice daily and once weekly according to severity of the problem.

Nursing implications

Use of the Uro-Tainer system:

- Uro-Tainer is a one piece system that connects directly to the drainage funnel of the Foley catheter.
- Step 1. Remove the protective cover around the Uro-Tainer tip.
- Step 2. Clamp off the Uro-Tainer tubing using the plastic clamp provided.
- Step 3. Swab the Foley catheter drainage funnel at the connection point.
- Step 4. Connect the Uro-Tainer to the catheter funnel and unclamp the tubing.
- Step 5. The solution is now instilled by gravitational force with the Uro-Tainer bag raised to a level above the urinary bladder.
- Step 6. Instil for 20–30 minutes then drain by allowing solution to return to the Uro-Tainer bag after repositioning it at a level below the urinary bladder.

Pharmaceutical considerations

- Store in a cool place.
- Inspect for damage (e.g. moisture accumulating in the outer bag) prior to use.
  NB: Not for intravenous infusion.

CLOTRIMAZOLE CREAM 1%

Contains Clotrimazole 1% in a preserved cream base.

Actions and uses

Clotrimazole is a broad spectrum antifungal agent which is applied topically in the treatment of skin infections due to dermatophytes (fungi which are parasitic on the skin). Common among these are *Trichophyton* species, yeasts such as *Candida*, and various moulds and other fungi which cause common conditions including ringworm (Tinea), athlete's foot, paronychia, pityriasis versicolor, erythrasma and intertrigo.

Dosage
Apply 2–3 times daily.

Nursing implications
- The cream should be applied evenly and thinly to the affected area and gently rubbed in.
- It is important to continue to treat the area for 2 weeks to 1 month after resolution of the skin lesion in order to prevent the risk of relapse.
- If applied for treatment of athlete's foot, the feet should be first washed and dried (especially between the toes) before application of Clotrimazole Cream.
- Aerosol spray, liquid and dry powder preparations also exist and may be more suitable for some lesions.

Storage
Store at room temperature.

CO-DANTHRAMER CAPSULES

Contains Danthron 25 mg and Polaxamer 200 mg in each capsule.

Actions and uses
Co-danthramer is the name given to a combination of the stimulant laxative, danthron (which directly increases lower bowel motility and colonic clearance) plus the lubricant, polaxamer (which promotes liquification of the faecal mass so aiding evacuation). This combination is now confined to palliative care to prevent or treat constipation in patients receiving regular opioid analgesia (e.g. morphine).
The laxative effect of co-danthramer is evident within 6–12 hours of dosing.

Dosage
Adults usually require 1–2 capsules at bedtime.
The children's dose is based on half the adult dose.

Nursing implications
- In common with other stimulant laxatives, this medicine should not

---

be used in acute or painful abdominal conditions associated with intestinal inflammation or obstruction.
- Danthron may cause discolouration of the urine and impart a reddish/pink colour to the perianal skin.
- Staining of the buttocks can occur in incontinent and/or bedridden patients leading to superficial skin irritation. Such preparations should not therefore be used in infants who are wearing nappies or adults using incontinence pads.
- Laxatives of this type should be avoided in pregnancy. Further, danthron is excreted in breast milk and may affect the breastfeeding infant if taken regularly or in high dosage.

Storage
Store at room temperature and protect from light.

CO-DANTHRAMER CAPSULES, STRONG

Contains Danthron 37.5 mg and Polaxamer 500 mg in each capsule.

Actions and uses
Co-danthramer is the name given to a combination of the stimulant laxative, danthron (which directly increases lower bowel motility and colonic clearance) plus the lubricant, polaxamer (which promotes liquification of the faecal mass so aiding evacuation). This combination is now confined to palliative care to prevent or treat constipation in patients receiving regular opioid analgesia (e.g. morphine).
The laxative effect of co-danthramer is evident within 6–12 hours of dosing.

Dosage
Adults usually require 1–2 capsules at bedtime.
Standard strength capsules are preferred for use in children.

Nursing implications
- In common with other stimulant laxatives, this medicine should not

be used in acute or painful abdominal conditions associated with intestinal inflammation or obstruction.

- Danthron may cause discolouration of the urine and impart a reddish/pink colour to the perianal skin.
- Staining of the buttocks can occur in incontinent and/or bedridden patients leading to superficial skin irritation. Such preparations should not therefore be used in infants who are wearing nappies or adults using incontinence pads.
- Laxatives of this type should be avoided in pregnancy. Further, danthron is excreted in breast milk and may affect the breastfeeding infant if taken regularly or in high dosage.

Storage
Store at room temperature and protect from light.

CO-DANTHRAMER ORAL SUSPENSION

Contains Danthron 25 mg and Polaxamer 200 mg in each 5 ml.

Actions and uses
Co-danthramer is the name given to a combination of the stimulant laxative, danthron (which directly increases lower bowel motility and colonic clearance) plus the lubricant, polaxamer (which promotes liquification of the faecal mass so aiding evacuation). This combination is now confined to palliative care to prevent or treat constipation in patients receiving regular opioid analgesia (e.g. morphine).

The laxative effect of co-danthramer is evident within 6–12 hours of dosing.

Dosage
Adults usually require one or two 5 ml spoonfuls at bedtime.
The children's dose is based on half the adult dose.

Nursing implications
- In common with other stimulant laxatives, this medicine should not be used in acute or painful abdominal conditions associated with intestinal inflammation or obstruction.
- Danthron may cause discolouration of the urine and impart a reddish/pink colour to the perianal skin.
- Staining of the buttocks can occur in incontinent and/or bedridden patients leading to superficial skin irritation. Such preparations should not therefore be used in infants who are wearing nappies or adults using incontinence pads.
- Laxatives of this type should be avoided in pregnancy. Further, danthron is excreted in breast milk and may affect the breastfeeding infant if taken regularly or in high dosage.

Storage
Store at room temperature and protect from light.

CO-DANTHRAMER ORAL SUSPENSION, STRONG

Contains Danthron 75 mg and Polaxamer 1000 mg in each capsule.

Actions and uses
Co-danthramer is the name given to a combination of the stimulant laxative, danthron (which directly increases lower bowel motility and colonic clearance) plus the lubricant, polaxamer (which promotes liquification of the faecal mass so aiding evacuation). This combination is now confined to palliative care to prevent or treat constipation in patients receiving regular opioid analgesia (e.g. morphine).

The laxative effect of co-danthramer is evident within 6–12 hours of dosing.

Dosage
Adults usually require one 5 ml spoonful at bedtime.
Use standard strength liquid for children.

Nursing implications

- In common with other stimulant laxatives, this medicine should not be used in acute or painful abdominal conditions associated with intestinal inflammation or obstruction.
- Danthron may cause discolouration of the urine and impart a reddish/pink colour to the perianal skin.
- Staining of the buttocks can occur in incontinent and/or bedridden patients leading to superficial skin irritation. Such preparations should not therefore be used in infants who are wearing nappies or adults using incontinence pads.
- Laxatives of this type should be avoided in pregnancy. Further, danthron is excreted in breast milk and may affect the breast-feeding infant if taken regularly or in high dosage.

Storage

Store at room temperature and protect from light.

CO-DANTHRUSATE CAPSULES

Contains Danthron 50 mg and Docusate sodium 60 mg in each capsule.

Actions and uses

Co-danthrusate is the name given to a combination of the stimulant laxative, danthron (which directly increases lower bowel motility and colonic clearance) plus the lubricant, docusate sodium (which promotes liquification of the faecal mass so aiding evacuation). This combination is now confined to palliative care to prevent or treat constipation in patients receiving regular opioid analgesia (e.g. morphine).

The laxative effect of co-danthrusate is evident within 6–12 hours of dosing.

Dosage

Adults usually require 1–3 capsules at bedtime.
The children's dose is based on half the adult dose.

Nursing implications

- In common with other stimulant laxatives, this medicine should not be used in acute or painful abdominal conditions associated with intestinal inflammation or obstruction.
- Danthron may cause discolouration of the urine and impart a reddish/pink colour to the perianal skin.
- Staining of the buttocks can occur in incontinent and/or bedridden patients leading to superficial skin irritation. Such preparations should not therefore be used in infants who are wearing nappies or adults using incontinence pads.
- Laxatives of this type should be avoided in pregnancy. Further, danthron is excreted in breast milk and may affect the breastfeeding infant if taken regularly or in high dosage.

Storage

Store at room temperature and protect from light.

CO-DANTHRUSATE ORAL SUSPENSION

Contains Danthron 50 mg and Docusate sodium 60 mg in each 5 ml.

Actions and uses

Co-danthrusate is the name given to a combination of the stimulant laxative, danthron (which directly increases lower bowel motility and colonic clearance) plus the lubricant, docusate sodium (which promotes liquification of the faecal mass so aiding evacuation). This combination is now confined to palliative care to prevent or treat constipation in patients receiving regular opioid analgesia (e.g. morphine).

The laxative effect of co-danthrusate is evident within 6–12 hours of dosing.

Dosage

Adults usually require one to three 5 ml spoonfuls at bedtime.
The children's dose is based on half the adult dose.

Nursing implications
- In common with other stimulant laxatives, this medicine should not be used in acute or painful abdominal conditions associated with intestinal inflammation or obstruction.
- Danthron may cause discolouration of the urine and impart a reddish/pink colour to the perianal skin.
- Staining of the buttocks can occur in incontinent and/or bedridden patients leading to superficial skin irritation. Such preparations should not therefore be used in infants who are wearing nappies or adults using incontinence pads.
- Laxatives of this type should be avoided in pregnancy. Further, danthron is excreted in breast milk and may affect the breastfeeding infant if taken regularly or in high dosage.

Storage
Store at room temperature and protect from light.

CROTAMITON LOTION

Eurax Lotion containing Crotamiton 10%.

Actions and uses
Crotamiton relieves persistent itching for 6–10 hours after application to the skin surface and is used in the treatment of pruritis. It is occasionally used to treat scabies but other preparations are generally preferred for this purpose.

Dosage
Pruritis – apply to the affected area 2–3 times daily.
Scabies – after bathing and thorough drying, apply to the entire body with the exception of the face and scalp. Repeat once daily for 3–5 days.

Nursing implications
- When applied in the treatment of scabies the lotion should be rubbed in well until no traces remain on the skin surface.
- Crotamiton is irritant – do not apply to areas around the eyes or on broken or weeping skin.

Storage
Store at room temperature.

CROTAMITON CREAM

Eurax Lotion containing Crotamiton 10%.

Actions and uses
Crotamiton relieves persistent itching for 6–10 hours after application to the skin surface and is used in the treatment of pruritis. It is occasionally used to treat scabies but other preparations are generally preferred for this purpose.

Dosage
Pruritis – apply to the affected area 2–3 times daily.
Scabies – after bathing and thorough drying, apply to the entire body with the exception of the face and scalp. Repeat once daily for 3–5 days.

Nursing implications
- When applied in the treatment of scabies the cream should be rubbed in well until no traces remain on the skin surface.
- Crotamiton is irritant – do not apply to areas around the eyes or on broken or weeping skin.

Storage
Store at room temperature.

DEXTRANOMER BEADS

Contains microspherical 'beads' of dextranomer in 60 g dispenser.

Actions and uses
Dextranomer a member of the hydrogel group of dressings. It is a highly hydrophilic (water attracting) dextran polymer prepared as microspherical 'beads' and used for debridement (i.e. removal of dead or

infected tissue) of moist wounds, venous ulcers, burns, etc. The presterilized beads are sprinkled over the wound and left in place to absorb exudate and prevent crust formation. Dextranomer beads are estimated to absorb up to four times their weight of exudate. Debris and bacteria are carried away from the wound surface by capillary action and local oedema is reduced.

Dosage
Beads are sprinkled over the moist wound and covered by a suitable secondary dressing. They are washed out and replaced before full saturation occurs, usually once or twice daily.

Nursing implications
- DO NOT use on dry wounds.
- Dextranomer's capacity to absorb exudate is relatively limited and it is of little use in heavily exudating wounds. Other preparations may be preferred for all but only minor burns.
- Do not leave on a low exudating wound for longer than 24 hours. A dry crust may form which is difficult and painful to remove.
- Use one canister for treatment of a single patient for one day in order to limit risk of cross-infection.
- Caution: avoid spilling beads on the floor. They render the surface very slippery and increase the risk of a fall. Injuries have been reported among staff and patients.

Storage
Dextranomer beads are stored in their well sealed containers under dry conditions and at room temperature.

DEXTRANOMER PASTE

Contains dextranomer 6.4 g in 10 g paste consisting also of polyethylene glycol and water.

Actions and uses
Dextranomer is a member of the hydrogel group of dressings. It is a highly hydrophilic (water attracting)

dextran polymer which in paste form is suitable for application to exudative and infected wounds and ulcers. The paste is used to absorb wound exudate and prevent crust formation, as for dextranomer beads but is more suitable for application to shallow wounds.

Dosage
Apply using a spatula to a depth of at least 3 mm. The wound is covered by a suitable secondary dressing and the dressing changed before full saturation occurs, usually from twice daily to alternate days.

Nursing implications
- DO NOT use on dry wounds.
- Dextranomer's capacity to absorb exudate is relatively limited and it is of little use in heavily exudating wounds. Other preparations may be preferred for all but only minor burns.
- To reduce likelihood of pain on application, prior wetting of the wound using normal saline is recommended.
- Avoid contact with the eye.
- Application to deep fistulae and flask-shaped wounds with narrow opening should be avoided as the paste may be difficult to remove.

Storage
Dextranomer paste foil packed pouches are stored at room temperature.

DIMETHICONE BARRIER CREAM

A cream preparation containing at least 10% dimethicone (e.g. Conotrane Cream containing 22% dimethicone 350 and Siopel containing 10% dimethicone 1000, both with preservative).

Actions and uses
Dimethicone is a silicone oil consisting of dimethylsiloxane polymers of varying viscosities hence the descriptions (350 and 1000) in the above examples. It is used for its water-resistant properties to provide a protective barrier for the skin surface when exposed to aqueous irritant

substances. A typical example is in the prevention of napkin dermatitis caused by prolonged contact of urine with the skin surface. An antiseptic (e.g. benzalkonium chloride, cetrimide) is usually added to reduce the risk of co-existing infection.

Dosage
Apply to clean dry intact skin several times daily or as often as necessary. In the case of napkin dermatitis, this usually means at every nappy change.

Nursing implications
- DO NOT apply to broken skin or to acutely inflamed or weeping skin surfaces.
- Silicone fluids such as dimethicone are chemically and pharmacologically inert. There is no absorption across the skin surface.
- Hypersensitivity (e.g. allergic contact dermatitis) may follow exposure to the antiseptic contained in proprietary creams.

Storage
Store at room temperature.

DOCUSATE CAPSULES

Dioctyl capsules each containing Docusate Sodium 100 mg.

Actions and uses
Docusate sodium is a stool softener by virtue of its surfactant properties. Its action on dry impacted faeces results in the increased uptake of water and fats into the faecal mass so improving mobility and bowel emptying. It may be used alone where chronic constipation is associated with faecal impaction but is used most often in combination with a stimulant laxative such as danthron (co-danthrusate) or as part of a laxative cocktail in difficult constipation such as that encountered in conjunction with chronic pain control using opioid analgesics.

Dosage
Commence treatment with a high dose (up to 500 mg daily) reduced thereafter once a response is achieved.

Usual adult dose is 100 mg three times daily.

Nursing implications
- Paediatric dosing is with liquid preparation.
- DO NOT use in children <6 months of age.
- DO NOT use in the presence of GI obstruction.

Storage
Store at room temperature.

DOCUSATE ENEMA

Norgalax Micro-enema containing Docusate Sodium 120 mg in 10 g single use pack.

Actions and uses
Docusate sodium is a stool softener by virtue of its surfactant properties. Its action on dry impacted faeces results in the increased uptake of water and fats into the faecal mass so improving mobility and bowel emptying. The enema may be used at any time in the treatment of constipation associated with faecal impaction but is most likely to be required in an acute situation or as part of the bowel preparation prior to surgery or GI tract investigation.

Dosage
A single dose is usually sufficient. The amount instilled may be scaled down if required for a child.

Nursing implications
- The enema nozzle is inserted in the rectum and the contents delivered by squeezing gently on the pack.
- Local docusate sodium enema is effective within a few minutes and up to 20 minutes of administration.
- Avoid using in intestinal obstruction.

Storage
Store at room temperature.

DOCUSATE ENEMA COMPOUND

Fletcher's Enemette containing Docusate Sodium 90 mg plus Glycerol 3.78 g in each 5 ml mini-enema.

Actions and uses

Docusate sodium is a stool softener by virtue of its surfactant properties. Its action on dry impacted faeces results in the increased uptake of water and fats into the faecal mass so improving mobility and bowel emptying. The enema may be used at any time in the treatment of constipation associated with faecal impaction but is most likely to be required in an acute situation or as part of the bowel preparation prior to surgery or GI tract investigation. When combined with glycerol, the local irritant properties have a further mild stimulant effect.

Dosage

A single dose is usually sufficient. The amount instilled may be scaled down if required for a child.

Nursing implications

- The enema nozzle is inserted in the rectum and the contents delivered by squeezing gently on the pack.
- Local docusate sodium enema is effective within a few minutes and up to 20 minutes of administration.
- Avoid using in intestinal obstruction.

Storage

Store at room temperature.

DOCUSATE ORAL SOLUTION

Docusol liquid containing Docusate Sodium 50 mg in 5 ml in sugar-free vehicle.

Actions and uses

Docusate sodium is a stool softener by virtue of its surfactant properties. Its action on dry impacted faeces results in the increased uptake of water and fats into the faecal mass so improving mobility and bowel emptying. It may be used alone where chronic constipation is associated with faecal impaction but is used most often in combination with a stimulant laxative such as danthron (co-danthrusate) or as part of a laxative cocktail in difficult constipation such as that encountered in conjunction with chronic pain control using opioid analgesics.

Dosage

Commence treatment with a high dose (up to 500 mg daily) reduced thereafter once a response is achieved. Usual adult dose is 100 mg three times daily.

Nursing implications

- DO NOT use in children <6 months of age. See Docusate Oral Liquid, Paediatric.
- DO NOT use in the presence of GI obstruction.

Storage

Store at room temperature.

DOCUSATE ORAL SOLUTION, PAEDIATRIC

Docusol liquid containing Docusate Sodium 12.5 mg in 5 ml in sugar-free vehicle.

Actions and uses

Docusate sodium is a stool softener by virtue of its surfactant properties. Its action on dry impacted faeces results in the increased uptake of water and fats into the faecal mass so improving mobility and bowel emptying. It may be used alone where chronic constipation is associated with faecal impaction but is used most often in combination with a stimulant laxative such as danthron (co-danthrusate) or as part of a laxative cocktail in difficult constipation such as that encountered in conjunction with chronic pain control using opioid analgesics.

Dosage

Children >6 months – 12.5 mg three times daily.
Children 2–12 years – 12.5–25 mg three times daily.

Nursing implications
- DO NOT use in children <6 months of age.
- DO NOT use in the presence of GI obstruction.

Storage
Store at room temperature.

ECONAZOLE CREAM 1%

Ecostatin Cream and Pevaryl Cream for application to the skin
Gyno-Pevaryl Cream for application in the vagina.

Actions and uses
Econazole is an antifungal drug for topical application in the treatment of fungal infections of the skin due to dermatophytes. It is of particular use in ringworm (tinea) infection but also infection associated with yeasts, moulds and other fungi, including athlete's foot and infected napkin rash. A specific formulation for application in the vagina is also available to treat vaginal candidiasis or thrush and in the treatment of candida balanitis.

Dosage
- Skin infection – Apply with gentle rubbing to the skin twice daily, morning and evening.
- Vaginal candidiasis – Instil one applicatorful high into the vagina twice daily for 7 days or once in the evening for 14 days.

Nursing implications
- Application to skin should be continued for 2–3 days after signs of infection have cleared.
- Application in vaginal candidiasis must continue for the duration of the course even if symptoms such as itching and burning have resolved.
- Fungal nail infections (tinea unguium) are very resistant to local treatment and a course of systemic therapy (e.g. itraconazole, terbinafine tablets) may be necessary.

- Allergic contact dermatitis may occur in patients who are sensitized to any component of the cream.

Storage
Store at room temperature.

EMOLLIENT PREPARATIONS

In addition to Aqueous Cream, Emulsifying Ointment and Hydrous Ointment (Oily Cream), a wide range of proprietary emollient products, which can be prescribed by Brand Name, exist. These are as follows:

Alcoderm Cream	Keri Therapeutic
Alcoderm Lotion	Lotion
Dermamist	LactiCare
Diprobase Cream	Lipobase
Diprobase Ointment	Neutrogena Cream
E45 Cream	Oilatum Cream
Epaderm	Ultrabase
Humiderm Cream	Unguentum M
Hydromol Cream	

Actions and uses
Emollients are topical preparations which are designed to soothe, smooth and hydrate the skin in dermatological conditions associated with a dry, scaly or itchy skin surface. They may therefore be applied to a dry skin in any eczematous disorder and in psoriasis.

Dosage
See individual product package inserts. Most are used when required and often at least once or twice daily.

Nursing implications
- See individual product package inserts for details on use.
- Emollients have a purely physical action on the skin and are not associated with systemic toxicity.
- Proprietary products do however contain a range of chemical substances including preservatives which can, on occasion, cause an allergic contact dermatitis in a sensitized patient.

Storage

See individual proprietary products. All are stored at room temperature.

EMOLLIENT BATH ADDITIVES

Apart from Emulsifying Ointment, a range of commercial products exist which are intended for addition to the bath and which can be prescribed by Brand Name. These are as follows:

Alpha Keri Bath Oil
Balneum
Diprobath
Emmolate Bath Oil
Hydromol Emollient
Oilatum Emollient
Oilatum Gel

Actions and uses

Emollients are preparations which are designed to soothe, smooth and hydrate the skin in dermatological conditions associated with a dry, scaly or itchy skin surface. Bath emollients are intended for addition to the bath water. Upon bathing their residual effect on the skin surface is of value when used in conjunction with topical emollient preparations.

Dosage

See individual package inserts for information on addition to the bath water.

Nursing implications

- To obtain an optimum residual effect on the skin surface, avoid excessive rinsing or rubbing with a towel.
- Caution – these products will make the bath very slippery and accidents have been reported. Children and the elderly in particular should be supervised during bathing.
- Allergic contact dermatitis may occur in a patient who is sensitized to any of the ingredients in these products.

Storage

See individual products.

FOLIC ACID PREPARATIONS

Includes:
Folic acid solution 400 microgram in 5 ml
Folic acid tablets 400 microgram

Actions and uses

Folic acid preparations of this strength are intended for use during pregnancy when the folate requirement is increased and as a consequence the risk of folate deficiency megaloblastic anaemia arises. Although this was in the past considered controversial, given a reasonably healthy diet, folic acid supplements are now used routinely prior to and during early pregnancy. This follows acknowledgement of a link between folate deficiency in pregnancy and neural tube defects. An Expert Advisory Group, on behalf of the Department of Health, has issued advice in recent years on folate supplementation to prevent *first occurrence* of neural tube defect. It is recommended that women who are *planning* a pregnancy take folic acid 400 microgram daily *before* conception and during the first 12 weeks of pregnancy once it occurs. Women who fail to do so should commence treatment *as soon as pregnancy is suspected* and continue until the 12th week of pregnancy.

Dosage

400 microgram taken daily prior to a planned pregnancy and for the first 12 weeks of pregnancy.

Nursing implications

- Note that high risk groups (including diabetics, pregnancies where neural tube defects have previously arisen, and men or women with spina bifida themselves who contemplate pregnancy) require to take a much higher dose of folic acid – currently 5 mg daily (or 4 mg daily when tablets of this strength become available).

Storage

Store at room temperature.

GLYCEROL SUPPOSITORIES

(Note that glycerol was formerly known as glycerin)

Actions and uses

Once glycerol is inserted into the rectum its osmotic (fluid retaining) effect and mild stimulant action results in the passage of a moist, lubricated stool within about 15–30 minutes. Glycerol suppositories are therefore used to achieve rapid bowel evacuation prior to bowel examination, investigation or surgery or as a relatively simple method of reversing prolonged constipation unresponsive to dietary change or oral laxative therapy.

Dosage

Insert one suppository, moistened with water before use.

Nursing implications

- Glycerol 4 g suppositories are for adults. Suppositories of 2 g and 1 g are also available for use in infants and children respectively.
- The only side effect of any note is local, usually mild, irritation but this, in part, explains glycerol's laxative action.

Storage

Store in a cool, dry place. Overheating may melt the suppository and the hygroscopic (water retaining) nature of glycerol may result in its liquification.

Note that 1 g and 2 g suppositories are also available for use in infants and children respectively.

ISPAGHULA HUSK PREPARATIONS

Includes:
Ispaghula Husk Granules (Fybogel 3.5 g, Regulan 3.4 g) Sachet (Orange/Lemon/Lime Flavours) in packs of 30 Sachets
Ispaghula Husk Granules, Effervescent (Fybozest Orange) 265 g Container with measure
Ispaghula Husk Powder (Konsyl Micronized Powder 6 g, 12 g) Sachet in packs of 60

Actions and uses

Ispaghula husk powder and granules are made from the dried ripe seeds of a plant (*Plantago* spp.). It is thus a form of natural fibre which is formulated in the above preparations into a (relatively) palatable medicinal fibre product. The various preparations are used mainly in the treatment of constipation, particularly if associated with poor dietary fibre intake. The action is purely physical in that fibre remains in the bowel to add to the stool bulk and water content (may absorb up to 40 times its weight of water) and hence improve stool consistency. Ispaghula husk is safe and effective in managing and maintaining bowel function in pregnancy. It may also be used to regulate stool formation in patients with an ileostomy, colostomy, diverticular disease, irritable bowel syndrome and ulcerative colitis. A further, but only occasional, use is to regulate the serum cholesterol in patients with hypercholesterolaemia. This is based on the known cholesterol lowering effect of high fibre diets rich in fruit and vegetables.

Dosage

A single sachet or scoopful is taken twice daily. Infants and children may receive doses based on one-half to one level 5 ml spoonful (or 1–2 teaspoonsful).

Nursing implications

- It is important that constipation in children be investigated if it persists and a medical referral may eventually be necessary.
- The dose is stirred into a glass of water and taken immediately. A generous fluid intake should be maintained in conjunction with any dietary fibre product.
- An alternative is to administer unflavoured granules/powder with food provided the food itself has a high fluid content.
- DO NOT use if there is bowel obstruction or if constipation is associated with hard impacted faeces.

- The only side effect of note is the occurrence of flatulence and bloating in the early treatment period.

Storage
Store at room temperature. Keep dry.

LACTITOL POWDER

A white crystalline, slightly sweet-tasting powder with no additives in 10 g sachets in packs of 10 sachets.

Actions and uses
Lactitol consists of two disaccharides (sugars), galactose and sorbitol, neither of which are broken down in the gut or absorbed to a significant extent so that they appear in the colon in large quantity. Once there, the action of colonic bacteria converts the sugars to short chain fatty acids (acetic, propionic and butyric acids) with the following consequences.

- It has a laxative effect as a result of an increase in osmotic pressure within the colon with retention of water, and an increase in the water content of the stool and hence stool volume.
- The pH falls (i.e. the colon becomes more acidic) so that the absorption of ammonia, produced by colonic bacteria, is reduced. This has the effect of greatly reducing the risk of hepatic encephalopathy in patients with liver disease.

Dosage
Constipation in adults: 10–20 g (1–2 sachets) are taken once daily with the morning or evening meal.
Constipation in children: dose is based on 250 mg/kg body weight.
Portal systemic encephalopathy: Administer 0.5–0.7 mg/kg/day according to response. Divide into 3 daily doses.

Nursing implications
- Treatment may be associated with abdominal discomfort with cramping pain, flatulence and bloating.

- DO NOT use in patients with GI obstruction.
- The initial doses may take up to 48 hours to act in constipation.
- Advise patients to maintain a generous fluid intake in order to ensure the maximum laxative effect.
- The dose can be adjusted eventually to obtain one soft stool daily or two soft stools daily if treating hepatic disease.
- If required to be administered via the NG tube, premixing with warm water 10 ml to each 10 g sachet then further dilution to obtain a 40% solution is recommended.

Storage
Store at room temperature.

LACTULOSE POWDER

Consists of 'Duphalac Dry' – a dry powder containing 95% lactulose in each 10 g unit dose sachet.

Actions and uses
As for Lactulose Solution, see below.

Dosage
Adults: for treatment of constipation, 1 sachet (10 g) is taken twice a day. Note that much higher doses are prescribed under medical supervision for the treatment of hepatic encephalopathy. For example, 20–30 g three times daily increased as required to produce 2–3 soft stools daily.
Children: 5–10 years, contents of ½ sachet (5 g) twice daily.
Children <5 years, Lactulose Solution is preferred.

Nursing implications
- The dose is taken from a spoon, tipped onto the tongue then swallowed with water or other suitable drink. Alternatively, it may be sprinkled over food or mixed with water or fruit juice beforehand.
- Treatment may be associated with abdominal discomfort with cramping pain, flatulence and bloating.
- DO NOT use in patients with GI obstruction.

- The initial doses may take up to 48 hours to act in constipation.
- Advise patients to maintain a generous fluid intake in order to ensure the maximum laxative effect.
- The dose can be adjusted eventually to obtain one soft stool daily or two soft stools daily if treating hepatic disease.
- If required to be administered via the NG tube, premixing with warm water 10 ml to each 10 g sachet then further dilution to obtain a 40% solution is recommended.

Storage
Store at room temperature.

LACTULOSE SOLUTION

Pale yellow liquid containing 3.35 g in each 5 ml, equivalent to 67% solution.

Actions and uses
Lactulose is a synthetic disaccharide which is not broken down in the small intestine so that it appears in the colon in large quantity. Once there, the action of colonic bacteria converts it to short chain fatty acids (acetic, propionic and butyric acids) with the following consequences.

- It has a laxative effect as a result of an increase in osmotic pressure within the colon with retention of water, and an increase in the water content of the stool and hence stool volume.
- The pH falls (i.e. the colon becomes more acidic) so that the absorption of ammonia, produced by colonic bacteria, is reduced. This has the effect of greatly reducing the risk of hepatic encephalopathy in patients with liver disease.

Dosage
Constipation in adults: 15–20 ml taken twice daily with the morning or evening meal.
Constipation in children: <5 years, 5 ml twice daily, or 5–10 years 10 ml twice daily. Babies, <1 year, 2.5 ml twice daily.

Portal systemic encephalopathy: Administer 30–50ml three times daily then adjust to produce 2–3 soft stools daily.

Nursing implications
- Treatment may be associated with abdominal discomfort with cramping pain, flatulence and bloating.
- DO NOT use in patients with GI obstruction.
- The initial doses may take up to 48 hours to act in constipation.
- Advise patients to maintain a generous fluid intake in order to ensure the maximum laxative effect.
- The dose can be adjusted eventually to obtain one soft stool daily or two soft stools daily if treating hepatic disease.

Storage
Store at room temperature.

LIGNOCAINE GEL BP

15 ml tubes containing Lignocaine HCl 2% in a hydroxyethylcellulose-derived, water miscible lubricant base. Also 20 ml 'concertina' packs.

Actions and uses
Lignocaine is a rapid onset, short acting local anaesthetic which in lubricant base is used to produce surface anaesthesia as an aid to relevant urological, endotracheal and rectal examination or surgical manipulation. Such procedures include (i) application to the urethra during cystoscopy and catheterization, (ii) application to the naso-pharynx during endoscopy, bronchoscopy or intubation and (iii) application to the rectal mucosa during proctoscopy. Lignocaine Gel 2% is also used to alleviate pain associated with cystitis and urethritis. It may also be applied to painful lesions in the mouth or other mucous surfaces.

Dosage
Apply sufficient gel to the relevant surface and/or instrument or tubing. For urethral anaesthesia, adult males

will require 10–20 ml gel (200–400 mg lignocaine) or more depending upon the level of anaesthesia required. Females require administration of 5–10 ml portions to fill the entire urethra. 10–20 ml is usually adequate for endoscopy or 5 ml applied to the surface of the tube prior to insertion in endotracheal intubation.

Nursing implications
- Surface anaesthesia commences within 5 minutes of application and persists for about 20–30 minutes thereafter. For painful procedures, it may be necessary to wait for about 10 minutes before introducing any instrument to the anaesthetized surface.
- Lignocaine is readily absorbed from mucous surfaces and the application of excessive amounts is to be discouraged. High systemic levels of lignocaine can impair cardiac conduction and induce convulsions, especially in patients with liver impairment. Avoid accidental introduction of lignocaine into the lumen of tube or catheter.
- Note that any lignocaine introduced into the oropharynx may interfere with the swallowing reflex and increase the risk of aspiration as a result.
- A few individuals may develop contact and systemic allergic reactions to lignocaine. Anaphylaxis has been rarely reported.

Storage
Lignocaine Gel is stored at room temperature. Each tube is intended for single use only.

LIGNOCAINE OINTMENT

Water soluble topical anaesthetic containing 50 mg lignocaine in each 1 g, i.e. 5% lignocaine w/w. The ointment base contains carbowaxes (which melt rapidly and spread evenly) and propylene glycol (a preservative). The ointment is readily miscible with water and easily washed off therefore.

Actions and uses
Lignocaine is a rapid onset, short acting local anaesthetic which produces surface anaesthesia. Lignocaine ointment is used in the following conditions.

- Treatment of difficult pruritis and painful burns and skin abrasions including insect bites, sunburn, herpes zoster neuralgia, sore nipples, etc.
- Treatment of discomfort and itch associated with haemorrhoids/anal fissures.
- Surface anaesthesia of the gums in dentistry prior to local anaesthetic injections.
- To reduce pain and discomfort associated with urological, endotracheal and rectal examination or surgical manipulation. Such procedures include (i) application to the urethra during cystoscopy and catheterization, (ii) application to the naso-pharynx during endoscopy, bronchoscopy or intubation and (iii) application to the rectal mucosa during proctoscopy.

Dosage
Apply a thin layer to the affected surface. May also be applied on a gauze pad.

Apply to the tube prior to endo-tracheal intubation.

Not more than 35 g ointment should be applied in any 24 hour period.

Nursing implications
- Surface anaesthesia commences within 5 minutes of application and persists for about 20–30 minutes thereafter. For painful procedures, it may be necessary to wait for about 10 minutes before introducing any instrument to the anaesthetized surface.
- Lignocaine is readily absorbed from mucous surfaces and the application of excessive amounts is to be discouraged. High systemic levels of lignocaine can impair cardiac conduction and induce convulsions, especially in patients with liver impairment. Avoid accidental introduction of

lignocaine into the lumen of tube or catheter.

- Note that any lignocaine introduced into the oropharynx may interfere with the swallowing reflex and increase the risk of aspiration as a result.
- A few individuals may develop contact and systemic allergic reactions to lignocaine. Anaphylaxis has been rarely reported.

Storage
Store at room temperature.

LIGNOCAINE AND CHLORHEXIDINE GEL

Instillagel containing Lignocaine HCl 2% + Chlorhexidine gluconate 0.25% in a preserved, sterile hydroxyethylcellulose/propylene glycol gel base, 11 ml syringe.

Actions and uses
Instillagel is used for instillation along the urethra prior to bladder catheterization. It aids catheterization as a result of its lubricant and local anaesthetic properties and the risk of local infection is reduced by the presence of Chlorhexidine within the gel base.

Dosage
Instil as required to completely fill the urethra with a gel (mucous) cast.

Nursing implications
Instil as follows:

1. Wear sterile disposable gloves.
2. Clean the glans and/or urethral orifice with a standard disinfectant e.g. chlorhexidine + cetrimide sachet.
3. Hold the penis by the glans and stretch gently.
4. Fill the urethral lumen by applying gentle pressure to the syringe plunger.
5. Apply the penile clamp to prevent leakage back out from the urethra.

6. The catheter can then be passed after about 5 minutes once the local anaesthetic effect has fully developed.

Storage
Store in the external medicines cupboard.
NB: Not for injection.

MACROGOL ORAL POWDER, COMPOUND

Includes:
Movicol sachets each containing 13.125 g Macrogol 3350 + 178.5 g sodium bicarbonate + 350.7 g sodium chloride + 46.6 g potassium chloride
Klean-Prep sachets each containing 59 g Macrogol 3350 + 5.685 g sodium sulphite + 1.685 g sodium bicarbonate + 1.465 g sodium chloride + 743 mg potassium chloride

Actions and uses
Macrogols are large complex substances widely used in the formulation of medicines. Macrogol 3350 is a powerful osmotic laxative which taken orally is unabsorbed from the gastrointestinal tract within which it exerts a strongly hydrophilic (water-loving) action. This results in the attraction and accumulation of fluid within the bowel, the production of moist and mobile stools and a rapid laxative effect. Compound macrogol oral powder is an effective laxative in the management of chronic constipation and dry faecal impaction. It is also used to promote effective bowel cleansing prior to bowel surgery, radiological examination or colonoscopy. The compound powder includes a balanced amount of sodium and potassium salts aimed at reducing the risk of excessive fluid and electrolyte loss and electrolyte disturbance as a result of its action in the bowel.

Dosage
Movicol – in chronic constipation, one sachet is administered 2 or 3 times daily. In faecal impaction,

up to 8 sachets daily are administered for a maximum of 3 days.

Klean-Prep – contents of 4 sachets are taken prior to the specific procedure, the previous day or split half the day before and the remainder on the appointed morning.

Nursing implications
- The sachets include a precise description of their reconstitution.
- Drinking large volumes of macrogol based liquid before investigative or surgical procedures may cause nausea which can be reduced by prior treatment with an antiemetic such as domperidone.

Storage
Store in a cool dry place.

MAGNESIUM HYDROXIDE MIXTURE

Consists of an aqueous suspension of hydrated magnesium oxide and contains the equivalent of 8% w/w magnesium hydroxide approximately. Suspension also contains magnesium sulphate and sodium hydroxide and is made up in chloroform water.

Actions and uses
Magnesium hydroxide is both an antacid and osmotic laxative but Magnesium Hydroxide Mixture is almost exclusively used as the latter. It owes its laxative action to its continued presence in the bowel (there is little systemic absorption) and its ability to attract and retain fluid by osmotic attraction. Thus a very fluid stool is produced and passed within 6–8 hours of oral dosing. Magnesium Hydroxide Mixture is a useful agent when early evacuation of the bowel is required using the oral route. It is particularly useful where dry impacted faeces render the stool difficult to pass and when excessive straining must be avoided.

As an antacid, magnesium hydroxide is usually included in combination with other antacids e.g. aluminium hydroxide in Maalox and Mucogel.

This is especially helpful since aluminium salts tend to constipate if taken on their own.

Dosage
The laxative dose varies from 25 to 50 ml taken twice daily. Much lower doses are used in antacid mixtures.

Nursing implications
- Magnesium Hydroxide is a suspension. The bottle must be shaken well before use.
- There are no side effects of note with this preparation except when used over-zealously. Some patients may complain of the chalky taste of the mixture however.
- Although little absorption of magnesium occurs, frequent or regular use of Magnesium Hydroxide Mixture should be discouraged in those with renal impairment in whom accumulation of magnesium (hypermagnesaemia) may occur.
- In practice, many elderly patients are actually hypomagnesaemic and the absorption and accumulation of magnesium in this group may indeed be advantageous.

Storage
Store at room temperature. Preferably used within 1 month of opening.

MAGNESIUM SULPHATE PASTE

Contains: Dried Magnesium sulphate with phenol and glycerol mixed to a paste-like constituency.

Actions and uses
Magnesium sulphate paste is thought to prevent bacterial growth and accumulation when applied to boils or similar heavily contaminated skin lesions. It exerts a strong osmotic action which evacuates the lesion by a mechanism which has been described as a 'drawing effect'. It is most effective for early cleansing of heavily infected lesions.

Dosage
Apply as a thick layer. Replace when it becomes too fluid as a result of over-dilution with exudate.

Nursing implications

- For short term use only. Once a healthy granulating wound base has formed, application of Magnesium sulphate paste should be discontinued.
- Apply liberally to infected area and cover with gauze dressing.

Storage

Store in a cool place. The paste will readily absorb moisture from the atmosphere. Discard if too runny. Stir well before use.

MALATHION LOTION

Contains: Malathion 0.5% in aqueous or alcohol base.

Actions and uses

Malathion is a pediculicide indicated for the treatment of head lice and pubic lice.

Dosage

Use alcohol based lotion, if possible. This contains substances called terpenes which are themselves also effective pedulicides. It may however be necessary to use aqueous lotion for patients with scalp eczema which is irritated by alcoholic solutions or for some asthmatics who may develop wheeze.
Head lice: Apply 30–50 ml lotion to DRY HAIR protecting the shoulders with a towel. See below for details.
Pubic lice: Apply liberally to the pubic hair and hair between the legs and around the anus.

Nursing implications

- To ensure complete eradication of lice, one further treatment after 7 days is recommended.
- Wear disposable gloves at all times during administration of treatments.
- Make a small parting in the hair along which a few drops of lotion are poured (Note they are HEAD lice not HAIR lice) and massage into the surrounding scalp and hair.

- Make another parting a little way away and apply more lotion and repeat. Continue until the whole scalp has been covered.
- The lotion must remain on the scalp for **about 12 hours** or overnight for maximum effect.
- Allow to dry naturally on the scalp. Do not use a hairdryer, which can reduce the chemical stability of malathion.
- The hair may then be washed on the following morning with a normal shampoo. Note that prior hair washing can render subsequent treatment ineffective.
- Do not use head lice shampoos – these are ineffective. Also, do not use head lice preparations to prevent infestation – this only promotes resistance to available pediculicides.

Storage

Store in a cool dry place, in the external medicines cupboard.
Note that alcoholic lotions are flammable.

MEBENDAZOLE PREPARATIONS

Includes:
Mebendazole Oral Suspension – Vermox Suspension containing 100 mg mebendazole in each 5 ml
Mebendazole Tablets – Pripsen Mebendazole or Vermox Tablets each containing 100 mg mebendazole

Actions and uses

Mebendazole is an anthelmintic or antihelminth. The Helminths in question include threadworms, roundworms, whipworms and hookworms all of which infest the gastrointestinal tract. Mebendazole kills the worms by blocking the uptake of nutrient glucose by both the larval and adult forms which subsequently fail to thrive and develop normally.

Dosage

Administered to all ages over 2 years:
Threadworms – 100 mg with a second dose necessary after 2–3 weeks if reinfestation occurs.

Whipworms, roundworms and hookworms – 100 mg twice daily for 3 days.

Nursing implications
- Mebendazole is not licensed for children under 2 years. Seek medical advice on treatment of younger children.
- Avoid in pregnancy, piperazine (Pripsen) may be preferred.
- It is not known if mebendazole is excreted to any extent in breast milk.
- Abdominal pain and diarrhoea may occasionally follow oral dosing. Skin rashes and urticaria have developed in patients with hypersensitivity.
- Preparations contain a number of inactive ingredients (excipients) which may rarely cause allergic reactions in sensitized individuals.
- Vermox suspension must be well shaken before use.

Storage
Store at room temperature.

METHYLCELLULOSE TABLETS

Celevac tablets containing 500 mg methylcellulose.

Actions and uses
Methylcellulose is a hydrophilic substance. It readily attracts and absorbs water in the GI tract and in doing so swells substantially to form a bulky moist gel-like mass which stimulates bowel function and promotes bowel emptying. The tablets are a simple means of treating constipation but are also used to regulate bowel emptying (establish continence) in patients with colostomies, ileostomies, diverticular disease and secretory diarrhoea. Finally, because of the bulk forming action and its association with a feeling of fullness methylcellulose products are sometimes used to reduce appetite in weight management programmes.

Dosage
The daily adult dose is in the range 6–12 tablets taken in two divided doses. To control appetite, 3 tablets are mixed in a tumblerful of warm water or fruit juice and taken before meals and when hunger pangs are otherwise present.

Nursing implications
- The action of methylcellulose is entirely local and no systemic toxicity results.
- It is important to establish the cause of constipation or diarrhoea beforehand to ensure that such treatment is appropriate.

Storage
Methycellulose tablets are stored in a cool dry place.

MICONAZOLE PREPARATIONS

Includes:
Miconazole Oral Gel – Daktarin 15 g and 80 g tubes containing 2% miconazole in white, orange flavoured gel.
Miconazole Cream – Daktarin Cream containing miconazole 2% in an aqueous base which includes macragol stearate, glycol stearate, unsaturated polyglycolized glycerides, liquid paraffin, benzoic acid and butylated hydroxyanisole.

Actions and uses
Miconazole is an imidazole antifungal agent i.e. belonging to the family which includes clotrimazole, ketoconazole, and econazole. It has a broad spectrum of activity against common pathogenic fungi (including yeasts and dermatophytes) and is also active against gram-positive bacteria such as Staphylococcus and Streptococcus.

- The gel formulation is for oral treatment of fungal infections of the mouth (e.g. oral candidiasis) and superinfection with gram-positive bacteria.
- The cream is for topical treatment of fungal infections and bacterial superinfections of the skin such as athlete's foot, intertrigo, napkin rash, erythrasma, and pityriasis versicolor. It is not particularly effective in nail infections.

Dosage

Gel: Adults require 1–2 × 5 ml spoonfuls of gel in the mouth four times a day. Children over 6 years require 1 × 5 ml spoonful of gel in the mouth four times a day. Children aged 2–6 years require 1 × 5 ml spoonful of gel in the mouth twice a day. Younger children require $\frac{1}{2}$ × 5 ml spoonful of gel in the mouth twice a day.
Cream: Adults and children should apply cream to the affected area twice daily.

Nursing implications
- To prevent relapse of skin infections, treatment should be continued for 10 days after all lesions have resolved.
- Occasionally, local application is associated with irritation and rarely allergic contact dermatitis.
- Oral gel may be associated with nausea and vomiting and diarrhoea.

Storage

Store at room temperature.

MOUTHWASH SOLUTION TABLETS

Contain thymol plus colouring and flavouring.

Actions and uses

Mouthwash solution tablets provide a convenient way of preparing the mouthwash in solution. Thymol has antiseptic, antifungal and deodorizing properties. The tablets are used for routine mouth disinfection and cleansing and mouth freshening.

Dosage

Dissolve one tablet in a tumblerful of warm water prior to uses. Use as often as appropriate.

Nursing implications
Rinse the mouth thoroughly then spit out. The solution may cause nausea and vomiting if swallowed in large quantities.

Storage

Store in a cool dry place in well sealed containers.

NYSTATIN PREPARATIONS

Includes:
Nystatin Oral Suspension – contains ready-mixed liquid of strength 100 000 unit nystatin in 1 ml. Also present: ethanol, flavourings, glycerin, methyl parahydroxybenzoate, propyl parahydroxybenzoate, sodium carboxymethylcellulose, sodium phosphate and sucrose. Specifically formulated to adhere to the buccal mucosa and so persist in the mouth after oral administration.
Nystatin Pastilles – aniseed flavoured pastilles each containing 100 000 unit nystatin.

Actions and uses

Nystatin is an antifungal agent active against *Candida albicans* and used in the treatment of oral candidiasis or thrush. This frequently arises in patients receiving cytotoxic chemotherapy and corticosteroids, including high dose steroid inhalers. Those with marked immunodeficiency and extensive oropharyngeal candidiasis usually require systemic therapy in addition to local nystatin.

Dosage

Usually 1 ml (100 000 unit) placed in the mouth or one pastille sucked four times a day after meals. For extensive oral candidiasis in adults, 5 ml oral suspension used as a mouthwash four times daily may be appropriate.

Nursing implications
- Nystatin is not absorbed after oral administration so that patients should be instructed to swallow without risk of systemic effects.
- Nystatin oral preparations are generally well tolerated. Occasionally oral irritation or allergic reactions do occur or diarrhoea follows if large quantities are swallowed.
- Denture wearers should be advised to add 2–5 ml nystatin suspension to denture soaks overnight. This might reduce the possibility of reinfection.

Storage

Store at room temperature. DO NOT dilute oral suspension – this interferes with its adhesive properties.

OLIVE OIL EAR DROPS

Contains olive oil only in a suitable dropper bottle.

Actions and uses

Olive oil has demulcent (soothing) properties and in this form acts as a wax solvent or softener to facilitate removal of ear wax. Ear wax is a normal body secretion which provides essential protection of the sensitive lining of the ear but which on occasion accumulates and dries out so causing deafness or impairing visual inspection of the ear drum. The demulcent properties are of additional benefit if irritation or inflammation is also present.

Dosage

Apply ear drops generously 3–4 times daily prior to ear syringing.

Nursing implications

- Patients should apply the ear drops for several days and up to 1 week prior to ear syringing. Preferably lie with the treated ear uppermost for 5–10 minutes after application.
- Syringing should be avoided or medical advice sought if patients have a history of recurrent infections of the outer ear (otitis externa), have had past ear surgery or perforation of the ear drum. This is also important if hearing is confined to one ear only since the risk of damage to the ear, however remote, is nonetheless unacceptable.

Storage

Store at room temperature. Protect from light and avoid storage next to a heat source (radiator, etc.).

PARACETAMOL PREPARATIONS

Includes:
- Paracetamol Tablets BP containing 500 mg per Tablet
- Paracetamol Tablets, Soluble BP containing 500 mg per Tablet
- Paracetamol Oral suspension containing 120 mg in 5 ml, 250 mg in 5 ml (also sugar-free versions available)

Actions and uses

Paracetamol is a simple analgesic for the treatment of mild to moderate pain. It acts by blocking pain transmission in the spinal cord but it does not possess antiinflammatory action in addition. A non-steroidal antiinflammatory drug (NSAID) such as naproxen, ibuprofen or diclofenac may therefore be more appropriate to treat pain associated with joint and soft tissue injury or for postoperative pain control. Paracetamol also possesses antipyretic properties and is used to control elevated temperatures associated with acute infections, notably in children at risk from febrile convulsions. It is also administered as a single dose to prevent pyrexia in children aged 2 months following routine immunizations.

Dosage

- The usual adult dose is 1 g every 4–6 hours taken for pain as required. It is advised, however, that the total daily dose should not exceed 4 g or 8 tablets.
- Children's doses are 60–120 mg (3 months–1 year); 120–250 mg (1–5 years); 250–500 mg (6–12 years). Repeat every 4–6 hours as required but up to a maximum of 4 daily doses.
- Postimmunization prophylaxis (2 months old): 60 mg single dose.

Nursing implications

- In the case of children under 3 months (except for postimmunization pyrexia), paracetamol should only be prescribed by or used on the instructions of a doctor.

- Apart from its well known and serious hepatotoxicity in overdosage, there is a risk of chronic liver injury when paracetamol is taken by adults on a regular basis in a daily dose exceeding 4 g or 8 tablets. Note that paracetamol is often contained in proprietary over the counter medicines and patients may, in fact, be unaware that they are taking it.
- Paracetamol poisoning is relatively common. Any adult who is suspected of ingesting as little as 15 g in a single dose requires urgent treatment to prevent potentially life-threatening liver failure.
- Young children are less susceptible than adults to the liver injury produced by acute overdosage since they do not convert paracetamol to its toxic metabolite to the extent. Nevertheless hepatotoxicity is still a major risk and the frequency of daily dosing is limited to 4 occasions in children.
- Paracetamol is otherwise very well tolerated. Other side effects are rarely reported.
- If pain is not controlled by daily doses up to 4 g, rather than to persist with increasing dosage, it may be appropriate to consider a more potent analgesic or the addition of a NSAID, or both. In such cases the doctor should be informed immediately.
- Although paracetamol does not possess antiinflammatory activity, it might still suffice for the treatment of joint pain in the elderly. Such patients often experience severe and potentially serious gastrointestinal pain, ulceration and bleeding when treated with a NSAID.

Storage

Store at room temperature.

PERMETHRIN PREPARATIONS

Includes:
Permethrin Cream – Lyclear Dermal Cream containing

Permethrin Cream Rinse – Lyclear Crème Rinse containing permethrin 1% and isopropanol 20% in an orange cream rinse base.

Actions and uses

Permethrin is one of the pyrethroid insecticides/pediculocides which has been developed from a natural plant source (pyrethrum). The important point is that it is not an organo-phosphorous chemical agent and it has little, if any, toxicity in humans/other mammals. Permethrin is rapidly absorbed by the insect to produce fatal electrophysiological disturbances within its excitable nerve tissue (i.e. it is an insect neurotoxin). In practice Permethrin Cream is used in the treatment of scabies (*Sarcoptes scabiei*) and Permethrin Cream Rinse in head lice (*Pediculus capitis*) infestation.

Dosage

Permethrin Cream – Apply over the whole body then wash off after 8–12 hours.
Permethrin Cream Rinse – Apply to clean damp hair then rinse and dry off after 10 minutes.

Nursing implications

- Permethrin Cream is not normally recommended for application to the head and neck except in the case of children when the scalp, face, ears and neck should be treated. This is also appropriate for the elderly, the immunocompromised and in the event of treatment failure.
- Reapply the cream to hands if hands are washed within 8 hours of initial application.
- A single 30 g tube of Permethrin Cream should suffice for all but the largest patient.
- Cream Rinse is applied to washed hair while still damp. Although the period of application is short (10 minutes), a residual effect remains.
- Postapplication itch, redness and stinging may occur but is short-lived. Rarely allergic skin rashes have been reported.

- Other restrictions such as a ban on swimming within a few days of application DO NOT apply in the case of permethrin.

Storage

Store at room temperature but not in the vicinity of a direct heat source such as a radiator. Protect from light.

PHENOTHRIN PREPARATIONS

Includes:

Phenothrin Alcoholic Lotion – Full Marks Lotion containing phenothrin 0.2% in isopropanol.

Phenothrin Aqueous Lotion – Full Marks Liquid containing 0.5% in an aqueous base.

Phenothrin Foam Application – Full Marks Mousse containing phenothrin 0.5%.

Note that the presence of isopropanol in the alcoholic lotion increases the killing efficacy of phenothrin so that a lower concentration is sufficient in this product.

Actions and uses

Phenothrin is one of the pyrethroid insecticides/pediculocides which has been developed from a natural plant source (pyrethrum). The important point is that it is not an organophosphorous chemical agent and it has little, if any, toxicity in humans/other mammals. Phenothrin is rapidly absorbed by the insect to produce fatal electrophysiological disturbances within its excitable nerve tissue (i.e. it is an insect neurotoxin). In practice Phenothrin Aqueous Lotion and Foam Application is used in the treatment of head lice (*Pediculus capitis*) infestation and Alcoholic Lotion in head lice and pubic (crab) lice (*Pthirus pubis*).

Dosage

All products, apply according to the package instructions.

Nursing implications

- Apply Full Marks Lotion to DRY HAIR. Sprinkle onto hair and rub gently over the scalp ensuring that the entire surface is moistened. Pay particular attention to the back of the neck and behind the ears. Allow to dry naturally. DO NOT apply heat. Wash hair with the usual shampoo 2 hours after application.
- To treat pubic lice – apply Full Marks Lotion to the pubic hair and hair between the legs and around the anus. Allow to dry as above.
- Apply Full Marks Liquid to the hair and rub in until the entire scalp is thoroughly moistened. Let hair dry naturally in a warm, well ventilated room. Shampoo the hair after 12 hours or, if preferred, the next day. Remove dead lice and discarded shells (nits) using a fine toothed comb.
- Apply Full Marks Mousse to dry hair after first shaking the canister. Apply at various points across the scalp then gently rub in until the entire scalp is treated. Pay particular attention to the temples and the crown of the head. Leave on for 30 minutes. DO NOT use a hair dryer. Wash off with the usual shampoo. While hair is still damp, comb thoroughly with a fine toothed comb to remove dead lice and nits.

Storage

Store at room temperature but not in the vicinity of a direct heat source such as a radiator. Protect from light.

PHOSPHATES ENEMA

Fletchers' Phosphate Enema contains: Sodium acid phosphate 12.8 g and Sodium phosphate 10.24 g in purified water 128 ml. Standard and long tube varieties are available.

Fleet Enema contains: Sodium acid phosphate 21.4 g and Sodium phosphate 9.4 g in purified water 133 ml. Standard tube.

Actions and uses

Rectal administration of Sodium acid phosphate/Sodium phosphate produces a rapid and extensive watery bowel clearance as a result of an osmotic (water retaining) action. Phosphates enema is used to achieve bowel evacuation prior to bowel investigations (radiological or endoscopic) and bowel surgery. It is also used to reverse acute or chronic constipation when simpler, less drastic measures have failed.

Dosage

Contents of one enema (128 ml) are instilled in the rectum as required.

Nursing implications

- Phosphates enema has a brisk and irritant action. It should be used with caution in the elderly or debilitated and avoided in patients with acute inflammatory or ulcerative disease affecting the large bowel.
- Caution is also advised where patients are sodium restricted.

Storage

Store at room temperature but in a cool place.

Specify standard or long tube enemas when ordering from Pharmacy.

PIPERAZINE CITRATE ELIXIR

Pripsen Piperazine Elixir containing 750 mg in 5 ml orange flavoured syrup. Also contains glucose, alcohol and citric acid.

Actions and uses

Piperazine is an anthelmintic or antihelminth. The Helminths in question include threadworms (enterobiasis) and roundworms (ascariasis) which infest the gastrointestinal tract. Piperazine causes reversible muscle paralysis of the helminth which is subsequently dislodged from the gut and excreted in the faeces.

Dosage

To expel threadworms:
Adults and children over 12 years take 15 ml once daily for 1 week.
Children 7–12 years require 10 ml daily for 1 week.
Children 4–6 years require 7.5 ml daily for 1 week.
Children 1–3 years require 5 ml daily for 1 week.

To expel roundworms:
Adults and children over 12 years take 30 ml as a single dose.
Children 9–12 years take 25 ml as a single dose.
Children 6–8 years take 20 ml as a single dose.
Children 4–5 years take 15 ml as a single dose.
Children 1–3 years take 10 ml as a single dose.

Nursing implications

- A repeat course after 7 days is often required to ensure eradication of threadworms.
- A repeat dose after 14 days is often required to ensure eradication of roundworms.
- Avoid in patients with severe liver or kidney disease and in poorly controlled epilepsy.
- Although a cautionary note appears in the product literature, piperazine has been used in pregnancy without problems subsequently arising. It is at least reassuring that the drug has been in use for many years and has a safe track record.
- Nausea, vomiting, diarrhoea and abdominal pain are occasionally reported.
- Other uncommon side effects include headache and urticaria in hypersensitive individuals.

Storage

Store at room temperature. Protect from light.

PIPERAZINE AND SENNA POWDER

Pripsen Piperazine Phosphate Powder containing piperazine phosphate 4 g plus standardized senna pods 15.3 mg (as total sennosides) with flavourings, saccharin and carmine colouring.

Actions and uses

Piperazine is an anthelmintic or antihelminth. The Helminths in question include threadworms (enterobiasis) and roundworms (ascariasis) which infest the gastrointestinal tract. Piperazine causes reversible muscle paralysis of the helminth which is subsequently dislodged from the gut and excreted in the faeces. The inclusion of senna, a stimulant laxative, aids expulsion of the parasite.

Dosage

To expel threadworms and roundworms:
Adults and children over 6 years take contents of one sachet as a single dose.
Children 1–6 years take one level 5 ml spoonful as a single dose.
Younger children take one level 2.5 ml spoonful as a single dose.

Nursing implications
- A repeat course after 7 days is often required to ensure eradication of threadworms.
- A repeat dose after 14 days is often required to ensure eradication of roundworms.
- Avoid in patients with severe liver or kidney disease and in poorly controlled epilepsy.
- Although a cautionary note appears in the product literature, piperazine has been used in pregnancy without problems subsequently arising. It is at least reassuring that the drug has been in use for many years and has a safe track record.
- Nausea, vomiting, diarrhoea and abdominal pain are occasionally reported.
- Other uncommon side effects include headache and urticaria in hypersensitive individuals.

Storage

Store at room temperature. Protect from light.

POVIDONE IODINE SOLUTION

Also known as Povidone-iodine 10% Antiseptic Solution.

Actions and uses

Povidone-iodine is a complex formed between an inactive carrier substance, polyvinylpyrrolidine, and a weak antiseptic, iodine, which is gradually released on contact with an infected surface. Aqueous (Antiseptic) solution is applied pre- and postoperatively for skin disinfection (though alcohol-based solution may be preferred) and has been used in wet soaks applied on a daily basis to disinfect wounds, burns and ulcers in the treatment of established or presumed local infection.

Dosage

Apply once or twice daily, as required.

Nursing implications
- The routine application of disinfectants (including povidone-iodine) to wounds, burns and ulcers is often questioned. While wound surfaces may contain environmental microorganisms it does not follow that active infection is present. On the other hand, povidone iodine may actually impair tissue repair mechanisms so delaying wound healing. If in doubt, seek medical advice.
- A proportion of patients develop hypersensitivity reactions to iodine preparations. Avoid further application of povidone iodine in such cases.
- Avoid regular application to large surfaces in patients with known thyroid disorders.
- Not recommended for regular use in children. Avoid use in neonates.
- Irritant – avoid contact with the eyes.

Storage

Store at room temperature.

SENNA PREPARATIONS

Includes:
Senna Tablets 7.5 mg
Senna Granules 5.5 mg/g
Senna Oral Solution 7.5 mg in 5 ml

Actions and uses

Senna is a naturally occurring substance derived from a plant source and standardized on its laxative constituents (known as the sennosides). Sennosides are anthraquinone derivatives which are released in the colon by the action of colonic bacteria. They have a powerful stimulant action on the bowel wall promoting bowel emptying about 8–12 hours after an oral dose.

Senna is used in the treatment of constipation and in the prevention of constipation associated with prolonged or regular use of analgesics of the opioid class. It is also taken as a single large dose at night to promote bowel clearance before colonoscopy, sigmoidoscopy, barium X-ray or other bowel investigations on the following morning. Similarly, it may be used to empty the bowel prior to bowel surgery.

Dosage

- Constipation in adults: initially 2 tablets (or 10–20 ml oral solution or one to two 5 ml spoonfuls of granules) increasing to double the dose, taken once at bedtime.
- Constipation in children >6 years: Half adult dosage.

Prevention of constipation: 1–2 tablets twice daily for patients taking regular analgesics containing codeine, dihydrocodeine, morphine, diamorphine, etc.

Nursing implications

- In children <6 years, senna preparations should only be prescribed by or used on the instructions of a doctor.
- When treating constipation, give consideration to its type and the likely cause.
- Chronic mild to moderate constipation is best treated by paying attention to diet (high fibre) and/or the use of bran substitutes such as Fybogel or Regulan. More severe constipation may respond to the addition of an osmotic laxative such as magnesium hydroxide.

Only when severe, unresponsive constipation is present should a short course of stimulant laxative be considered.

- Overuse, or indeed misuse, of stimulant laxatives has in the past led to chronic loss of bowel function, especially in the elderly who may be malnourished and are frequently immobilized.
- Despite the above, stimulant laxatives are justified for patients with chronic pain treated with opioid drugs. They are also used short term postoperatively or after myocardial infarction.
- The powerful action of senna on the bowel wall may result in excessive irritation, spasm or colic with typical cramp-like pain. Diarrhoea may result and be associated with salt and water depletion.
- Avoid stimulant laxatives where there is gastrointestinal obstruction and, if possible, in patients with inflammatory bowel disease. Note also, if taken regularly in high dosage, senna may be transferred to breastfeeding infants via mother's milk.

Storage

Store at room temperature.

SODIUM BICARBONATE EAR DROPS

Contains Sodium Bicarbonate 5% + Glycerol in Purified Water.

Actions and uses

Wax is a natural body secretion which has a protective function in the ear but which, on occasion, accumulates and dries out to affect hearing or impede visual inspection of the ear drum. Sodium Bicarbonate Ear Drops are used in conjunction with ear syringing to soften ear wax and so aid its removal. The drops are instilled in the affected ear and left for 5–10 minutes before syringing or, if the wax is excessively dry and impacted, instilled daily for 3–5 days beforehand.

Dosage

Instil 3–4 drops in the affected ear.

Nursing implications

- Patients should be instructed to lie on their side or tilt their head to the side for 5–10 minutes after each instillation.
- Avoid if there is a history of recurrent otitis media, prior ear surgery or perforation of the ear drum.
- In general syringing should proceed with caution if there is deafness in one ear and only the affected ear is functional.

Storage

Store at room temperature.

SODIUM CHLORIDE SOLUTION, STERILE

A sterile aqueous solution of isotonic sodium chloride 0.9%, in bottles, bags and sachets (e.g. Noramasol).

Actions and uses

Sodium chloride 0.9% is a sterile isotonic solution which is used as an irrigation in a variety of situations. Since it is isotonic it is non-irritant, hence its frequent use as a wound irrigation and to aid removal of debris from the eye or to wash out the eye after exposure to irritant substances.

Dosage

Apply liberally to the affected area.

Nursing implications

- Safe, non-toxic, non-irritant.
- NOT FOR INJECTION. Sterile sodium chloride 0.9% injection is prepared so as to exclude particulate contamination (less rigorously controlled otherwise).

Storage

Store at room temperature. Sterile until opened. Significant contamination possible within 24 hours of opening.

SODIUM CITRATE COMPOUND ENEMA

Any Micro-enema containing sodium citrate in combination with other agents (e.g. sodium lauryl sulphate, glycerol) acting locally on the colorectum. Includes Fleet Micro-enema, Micolette Micro-enema, Micralax Micro-enema and Relaxit Micro-enema.

Actions and uses

Sodium citrate exerts its local laxative effect by increasing the accumulation of fluid in the bowel and altering the distribution of fluid with the faeces. The addition of sodium lauryl sulphate, a surfactant, increases fluid uptake by the faeces while glycerol exerts a mildly stimulant action. The result is a rapid evacuation of the bowel soon after instillation of the enema. Sodium Citrate Compound Enema is for occasional use when constipation has developed and early bowel evacuation is required.

Dosage

Single dose in acute constipation.

Nursing implications

- See literature for method of use of individual Micro-enemas.
- Well tolerated but diarrhoea may follow excessive use.

Storage

Store at room temperature.

SODIUM PICCOSULPHATE ELIXIR

Laxoberal or Dulco-Lax Liquid containing 5 mg in 5 ml of a fruit-flavoured (sugar-free) mixture.

Actions and uses

Sodium piccosulphate is a stimulant laxative. It is converted to the active component by the action of colonic bacteria which causes a reflex bowel evacuation secondary to an action on the mucosa of the colon and rectum. Its uses are similar to senna, danthron, and other stimulant laxatives, i.e. in constipation associated with poor bowel motility including that encountered in sedentary elderly patients and in association with chronic use of opioid analgesics.

Dosage

Adults and children over 10 years require 5–10 mg at night.
Children 4–10 years require 2.5–5 mg at night.
Younger children, dose based on 250 microgram (0.25 mg)/kg at night.

Nursing implications

- Avoid use of stimulant laxatives in patients with GI obstruction or active inflammatory disease and soon after GI surgery.
- There is no evidence that sodium piccosulphate is harmful if taken during pregnancy.
- Abdominal discomfort and diarrhoea may occur after overzealous use.

Storage

Store at room temperature.

STERCULIA GRANULES

Normacol gluten-free, coated granules containing 62% sterculia in large tubes or individual sachets.

Actions and uses

Sterculia is the gum which is obtained from the Indian Tragacanth or Karaya plant. It appears as irregular or worm-like pieces of non-digestible material which acts as a bulk-forming laxative similar to Ispaghula Husk. Sterculia Granules is therefore a useful supplement to a low residue diet in patients who develop constipation as a result. Agents of this type are also used as an aid to dieting since they swell substantially on contact with fluid in the bowel so giving a sensation of fullness associated with a blunting of appetite.

Dosage

The usual dose is one or two heaped 5 ml spoonfuls or one tablespoonful or the contents of 1–2 sachets once or twice daily with or after meals. Children should receive half this dose.

Nursing implications

- Sterculia Granules will swell up on contact with water so that each dose must be taken with a generous fluid intake in order to act effectively.
- There are no side effects except occasional bloating which may follow excessive use.

Storage

Store at room temperature.

STERCULIA AND FRANGULA GRANULES

Normacol Plus gluten-free, coated granules containing 62% sterculia + 8% frangula in large tubes or individual sachets.

Actions and uses

Sterculia is the gum which is obtained from the Indian Tragacanth or Karaya plant. It appears as irregular or worm-like pieces of non-digestible material which acts as a bulk-forming laxative similar to Ispaghula Husk. Frangula, which is derived from Buckthorn bark, contains anthraquinone (senna-like) substances. Its stimulant effect on the bowel mucosa therefore supplements the action of sterculia. Sterculia and Frangula Granules are therefore a useful supplement to a low residue diet in patients who develop constipation as a result, especially if there is also poor bowel motility.

Dosage

The usual dose is one or two heaped 5 ml spoonfuls or one tablespoonful or the contents of 1–2 sachets once or twice daily with or after meals.

Nursing implications

- The granules will swell up on contact with water so that each dose must be taken with a generous fluid intake in order to act effectively.
- There are no side effects except occasional bloating and abdominal discomfort (possibly diarrhoea) which may follow excessive use.

Storage

Store at room temperature.

STREPTOKINASE AND STREPTODORNASE TOPICAL POWDER

Varidase Topical containing 125 000 unit per vial composed of Streptokinase 100 000 IU plus Streptodornase 25 000 IU.

Actions and uses

Streptokinase is a plasminogen activator which converts plasminogen to plasmin, the proteolytic enzyme which breaks down fibrin resulting in the lysis of blood clots (thrombolysis). It is most often used in the early thrombolytic treatment of myocardial infarction but in this situation, the application of streptokinase results in the dissolution of blood clots and other fibrinous products within the wound exudate. Streptodornase is a complementary proteolytic enzyme which liquifies the nucleoprotein of dead cells and other wound debris so aiding their removal. Thus Varidase Topical is used to aid the cleansing and desloughing of wounds over which thick, dry eschar has formed, without adversely affecting the healing process.

Dosage

Treat the wound once or twice daily. Continue until health granulation tissue is present, usually within 1–2 weeks.

Nursing implications

- Reconstitute each vial with sterile sodium chloride 0.9% (or water for injections) 20 ml. To avoid frothing, do not shake vigorously but wait until the powder is dissolved and the solution has become clear.
- Apply on presoaked gauze or pour over dry gauze packing then cover with a semi-occlusive dressing to prevent the wound from drying out.
- An alternative method is to inject the solution under the eschar but ensuring that it is introduced into the wound cavity. The volume

must not be excessive since the increased pressure which results will cause wound pain.
- DO NOT use if there is active bleeding within the wound.
- AVOID in patients with known allergy to streptokinase.
- DEFINITELY NOT for injection.

Storage

Store in a refrigerator. Reconstituted solution may be stored for 24 hours in a fridge i.e. sufficient for 2 days treatment per vial.

THYMOL GLYCERIN, COMPOUND

An aqueous mixture of thymol 0.05% and glycerol 10% with added colouring and flavouring.

Actions and uses

Thymol is an antiseptic similar in many respects to phenol. Glycerol (glycerin) attracts water and has a lubricating action when applied topically. The combination provides a convenient antiseptic mouthwash for daily cleansing or refreshment of the oral cavity.

Dosage

10–20 ml as a mouthwash.

Nursing implications

Avoid swallowing. Glycerol has systemic side effects.

Storage

Store at room temperature.

TITANIUM OINTMENT

Metanium containing titanium dioxide 20%, titanium peroxide 5% and titanium salicylate 3% in an ointment base containing dimethicone, liquid paraffin, white soft paraffin and benzoin tincture.

Action and uses

Titanium oxides/salicylate has an action similar to that of zinc oxide. Titanium dioxide is also widely used in sunscreen because of its ability to deflect ultra-violet light but the

Metanium Ointment formulation is used as a barrier agent to protect, in particular, the buttocks and perineum from the irritant action of urine and faeces which classically present as nappy rash (napkin dermatitis).

Dosage
Apply liberally to the affected area.

Nursing implications
Non-special considerations apply.

Storage
Store at room temperature.

ZINC AND CASTOR OIL OINTMENT

Ointment containing – zinc oxide 7.5%, castor oil 50%, cetostearyl alcohol 2%, white beeswax 10% and arachis oil 30.5%.

Action and uses
This product combines the soothing, healing action of zinc oxide (an astringent) with the physical barrier of a thick, durable ointment base. Zinc and Castor Oil Ointment is widely used as a barrier agent to protect, in particular, the buttocks and perineum from the irritant action of urine and faeces which classically present as nappy rash (napkin dermatitis).

Dosage
Apply liberally as required.

Nursing implications
- Note that the product contains arachis oil and may therefore pose a risk for those with peanut allergy.
- No other special considerations apply.

Storage
Store at room temperature.

ZINC OXIDE AND DIMETHICONE SPRAY

Sprilon containing zinc oxide 12.5% plus dimethicone 350 1.04% as a spray on ointment.

Actions and uses
- Zinc oxide is mildly astringent. When applied to an inflamed or irritated skin surface it exerts a soothing and healing action. Zinc itself is thought to promote healing in some inflammatory conditions e.g. eczema, haemorrhoids, etc.
- Dimethicone is water repellant providing a protective, durable and flexible film under which the skin surface is suitably moisturized so that optimum healing may proceed.
- Zinc Oxide and Dimethicone Spray is used in the treatment of pressure sores, excoriations, moist eczema, skin irritation due to faeces/urine and around fistulae and ostomy sites.

Dosage
Spray the affected surface as required.

Nursing implications
- Spray surface at right angle from a distance of around 8 inches to 1 foot for 2–3 seconds.
- Sprilon Spray may rarely cause skin irritation in a sensitized patient.
- Contains wool alcohol. AVOID in patients with known allergy to Lanolin.

Storage
- Store at room temperature.
- DO NOT puncture or incinerate after use.
- Highly inflammable. DO NOT heat.

ZINC OXIDE IMPREGNATED MEDICATED STOCKING

Zipzoc sterile rayon stocking impregnated with zinc oxide 20% ointment.

Actions and uses
Zinc oxide is mildly astringent when applied to an inflamed or irritated surface providing a soothing and protective layer under which healing may take place. Zinc itself is thought

to promote healing in some inflammatory conditions e.g. eczema, excoriations, haemorrhoids, etc. The zinc oxide impregnated medicated stocking provides continuous application of zinc oxide to leg venous ulcers associated with chronic venous insufficiency. It may be a more convenient product than Zinc Paste Bandage.

Dosage

Wear as required for up to 7 days. Duration and frequency of application depends upon the individual case.

Nursing implications

- Medicated stocking can be used as the primary contact layer under a compression bandage or hosiery in chronic venous (but not arterial) insufficiency.
- A suitable outer bandage is required in order to protect clothing.
- Apply so as to cover the leg from the base of the toes to the knee.

Storage

Store at room temperature.

Appendix 2

DRUGS IN PREGNANCY AND LACTATION

The prescription and administration of drugs to pregnant and breastfeeding women presents one of the most difficult challenges facing patients and carers alike. All too often little or nothing is known about the safety or otherwise of drugs in these situations and it is impossible, on ethical grounds alone, to determine this scientifically by clinical trial. As a result it is necessary to draw conclusions from studies in experimental animals during drug development or from anecdotal information reported subsequently once the drug becomes used in practice. It follows that concerns are often increased over the decision to use newer medicines about which little is known in practice and there is a tendency to rely more on established medicines simply because of their long track record. Not surprisingly, perhaps, pharmaceutical manufacturers are unable to advise and unwilling to comment on the safety of their medicines in pregnancy and lactation; the licensing authority does not allow them to do so in their product specifications in the absence of scientific data. Therefore negative comments and unhelpful messages are often published in manufacturer's advisory leaflets including Patient Information Leaflets which simply add to the concerns and uncertainties. Despite the above it is very important that pregnant or breastfeeding mothers be kept informed and are part of any decisions taken about their treatment. This Appendix is intended to provide an overview of the problem and a guide for nurses who have an important role to play in advising patients and allaying fears and providing reassurance when warranted.

DRUGS IN PREGNANCY

At the end of the 1950s and into the early 1960s, thalidomide, a new antiemetic, was widely prescribed for the treatment of nausea and vomiting including nausea and vomiting of pregnancy. Within a few years of its introduction, however, it was apparent that the drug had a devastating effect on the developing fetus and, in particular, that it produced gross limb deformities. The thalidomide disaster was a turning point in medicine.

It raised huge awareness of the potential risks from the use of drugs in pregnancy and gave rise indirectly to modern legislation on drug testing and licensing and adverse reaction monitoring leading eventually to the formation of the present day Committee on Safety of Medicines. Previously it had been thought that the placenta afforded protection to the fetus by filtering out potentially harmful substances in the mother's circulation. However it is now recognized that most substances and indeed most drugs administered to the mother will reach her baby via the placental circulation. The ease with which this occurs and the extent of fetal exposure is dependent on a number of factors including molecular size and relative lipid/water solubility.

The harmful effects of drugs in pregnancy may include the following:

• Death in utero, spontaneous abortion and stillbirth.
• Induction of malformations (embryotoxicity).
• Pharmacological adverse effects on the fetal tissues.
• Organ dysfunction persisting into the neonatal period.
• Drug dependence and withdrawal.

What then can be done to avoid these effects or limit their impact?

Stage of pregnancy

Taking of drugs at different stages of pregnancy may have an important bearing on eventual outcomes.

It is customary to divide pregnancy into three stages or trimesters each of around 3 months duration. The first trimester is a period of rapid cell division during which the groundwork is laid for the development of the fetal tissues and organs. It is at this stage that drugs known to cause malformations and limb deformities (so-called teratogens) are at their most harmful. Teratogenic drugs include many cytotoxic agents, the retinoids (e.g. isotretinoin) and, notably, thalidomide. Such is the devastating nature of their embryotoxic effect that teratogenic drugs are generally well known and the decision to treat a women of childbearing potential with such a drug is only taken after careful counselling. This must be accompanied by advice on the use of reliable contraception throughout the treatment period and often for some time afterwards. The second trimester of pregnancy is a period of organ growth and development during which the immature fetal organs may be affected by the pharmacological action of drugs while drugs taken during the third trimester and close to term can affect organ function and produce prolonged effects into the neonatal period (e.g. neonatal withdrawal, neonatal hypoglycaemia, etc.).

Which drugs are safe ... and what must be avoided?

It is not possible to guarantee the absolute safety of any drug taken during pregnancy and, given that a proportion of pregnancies will not proceed to term or will be associated with an unfavourable outcome (for whatever reason), it would be unwise to do so. However, based on past experience and information gleaned from animal research it is often possible to reassure patients or inform decisions that may eventually be taken about particular treatments. The easy option would be to avoid all drugs but this is often unrealistic and greater harm may befall the fetus if maternal disease or symptoms are allowed to go untreated. This is illustrated in the case of malaria prophylaxis. Antimalarials such as chloroquine and proguanil do cross the placenta and may have potentially adverse effects on the fetus but the use of prophylaxis in high risk areas is mandatory because of the devastating effects of malaria on the fetus and newborn.

In the following Tables 1–3 an indication is given of the perceived safety or potential risks to the fetus and newborn from a number of common drugs or drug groups. Although extensive, the list is far from exhaustive and opinions may differ about the catergorization of individual drugs in this way. The drugs list is therefore intended for guidance only.

Table 1 Drugs which the balance of evidence would suggest can be safely prescribed in pregnancy

Amoxycillin	Indomethacin
Amphotericin	Ipratropium bromide
Aspirin (antiplatelet dosage)	Lactulose
Azithromycin	
Calcitonin	Meropenem
Cephalosporins	Mesalamine
Cimetidine	Methadone
Clarithromycin	Metoclopramide
Clindamycin	Morphine
Clotrimazole	Multivitamins
Co-amoxiclav	Naproxen
Corticosteroids (inhaled, topical)	Nitrofurantoin (preferred treatment
Cyclosporin	of UTI)
Cyclizine	Ondansetron
Diclofenac	Paracetamol
Dicyclomine	Penicillins
Dipyridamole	
Erythromycin	Ranitidine
Folic acid	Salbutamol (inhaled)
Frusemide	Sucralfate
Glyceryl trinitrate	Theophylline
Heparin (including low molecular	Thiamine
weight heparins)	Thyroxine
Ibuprofen	Vaccines (except live vaccines)
	Vitamins

Table 2 Drugs which can be considered neither safe nor uniformly harmful. It is important to carefully weigh the potential benefits against supposed or apparent risks. Use the lowest possible dosage to control symptoms or disease

(a) Benefits likely to outweigh risks

Aciclovir
Amiodarone
Amitriptyline
Antidepressants, tricyclic
Antipsychotics
Carbamazepine (but ↑ risk of spina bifida?)
Corticosteroids (systemic)
Chloroquine (treatment and prophylaxis of malaria)
Digoxin
Fluoxetine
Gabapentin
Gentamicin
HIV treatments (treatment mandatory)
Hydroxychloroquine
Lamotrigine
Lansoprazole

Metronidazole (avoid in 1st trimester)
Nifedipine
Omeprazole
Paroxetine
Prochlorperazine
Rifampicin
Sertraline
Sotalol
Sulphasalazine
Sumatriptan
Tobramycin
Trifluoperazine
Trimethprim
Vancomycin

(b) Benefits may be outweighed by concerns about safety – seek alternatives where possible

Atenolol (intrauterine growth retardation?)
Azathioprine
Carbimazole
Cerivastatin (concern over effect of ↓ physiological lipid levels during pregnancy)
Ciprofloxacin (fetal cartilage damage?)
Diazepam (oral clefts, other malformations?)
Fluconazole
Fluvastatin (concern over effect of ↓ physiological lipid levels during pregnancy)
Gliclazide (insulin preferred)
Glipizide (insulin preferred)
Itraconazole
Lithium
Phenytoin
Pravastatin (concern over effect of ↓ physiological lipid levels during pregnancy)
Propranolol (intrauterine growth retardation?)

Table 2 (*continued*)

Simvastatin (concern over effect of ↓ physiological lipid levels during pregnancy)
Sodium valproate (neural tube defects, spina bifida, malformations well described)

Tamoxifen
Temazepam

Table 3 Drugs known to cause harm or potential harm to the fetus – AVOID!

ACE Inhibitors (major malformations reported in animals)
Acetretin (major teratogen)
Alcohol (in excess causes a fetal alcohol syndrome)

Captopril (an ACE inhibitor, see above)
Cyctotoxic drugs (affect growth – high risk of teratogenicity)

Enalapril (an ACE inhibitor, see above)
Etretinate (major teratogen)

Isotretinoin (major teratogen)

Lisinopril (an ACE inhibitor, see above)

Measles vaccine (live vaccine)
Methotrexate (malformations reported)
Misoprostol (in Arthrotec, causes abortion)
Mumps vaccine (live vaccine)

Oestrogens (but stopping oral contraceptives promptly poses little risk)

Perindopril (an ACE inhibitor, see above)

Ramipril (an ACE inhibitor, see above)
Rubella vaccine (live vaccine)

Tetracyclines (maternal liver toxicity, teratogenic, affects teeth and bones
   in the infant)

Warfarin (fetal warfarin syndrome described)

DRUGS IN LACTATION

Almost any drug present in the mother's blood can also be detected in her milk.

Factors influencing the passage of drugs into breast milk
The actual amount of drug in breast milk will depend upon factors such as the concentration in maternal blood, lipid solubility, the degree of ionization, protein binding, molecular size, etc. Breast milk concentrations are likely to be generally very low but ingestion of even small quantities of some potent drugs can have profound effects on the infant. Other drugs may be harmless because, although present in breast milk, they are either

not absorbed from, or else destroyed in, the infant's gastrointestinal tract. Other considerations are important. The infant's immature liver and kidney function can delay drug inactivation and excretion such that continuous delivery from mother's milk leads to the accumulation of potentially harmful concentrations of some drugs. Furthermore, if the mother's own liver or kidney function is impaired, drugs which would otherwise be present in small amounts may reach much higher concentrations in breast milk. Higher drug levels in milk are also more likely after intravenous administration.

Limiting infant exposure and dosage

The degree of exposure may be difficult to assess. The actual infant ingested dose will not only vary with the concentration of drug in milk but the volume of milk ingested as well as the timing of feeds in relation to maternal drug dosing. It is generally accepted that suckling infants ingest approximately 150 ml of milk per kg body weight in one day. Clearly the concentrations of drugs in breast milk will be lowest (trough levels) just prior to the next dose and it is advisable, if possible, to breastfeed (or express milk) just before the next dose of a drug is due.

In Tables 4–6 the safety or otherwise of specific drugs or drug groups when taken by nursing mothers is indicated. The list is far from exhaustive and opinions may differ about the catergorization of individual drugs in this way. It is intended only as a guide.

Table 4 Drugs thought to present little, if any, risk during lactation – no reason to routinely discourage breastfeeding

Aciclovir	Clarithromycin
Alcohol (moderate amounts)	Clindamycin
Allopurinol	Co-amoxiclav
Amoxycillin	Codeine
Antihistamines (older agents may cause drowsiness)	Corticosteroids (inhaled, topical)
Aspirin (antiplatelet dosage)	Diclofenac
	Digoxin
Baclofen	Diltiazem
Beclomethasone	Dipyridamole
Captopril	Enalapril
Carbamazepine	Epoetin alfa
Carbimazole	Erythromycin
Cephalosporin antibiotics	Ethosuximide
Chloroquine	Famotidine
Cimetidine	Fentanyl

Table 4 (*continued*)

Flecainide	Paracetamol
Fluconazole	Penicillins
Gentamicin (not absorbed but may alter infant's bowel flora – diarrhoea)	Pethidine
	Phenytoin
Heparin (including low molecular weight heparin)	Prednisolone
	Prochlorperazine
	Proguanil
Ibuprofen	Promethazine
Indomethacin	Propranolol
Insulins	Propylthiouracil
Ipratropium bromide	Pseudoephedrine
Isoniazid	Pyridoxine
Lisinopril	Ramipril
Loperamide	Rifampicin
Magnesium salts	Salbutamol
Medroxyprogesterone	Sodium valproate
Mefloquine	Sotalol
Methadone	Spironolactone
Metoclopramide (maximum dose 40 mg/day)	Sucralfate
	Sumatriptan
Morphine (may cause constipation)	Terbutaline
Multivitamins	Theophylline
Nalidixic acid	Thiamine
Naproxen	Thyroxine
Nifedipine	Tobramycin
Nitrofurantoin	Vaccinations
Octreotide	Verapamil
Oestrogens (but they do suppress lactation)	Vitamins
Oral contraceptives (progestogen only may be preferred, oestrogens ↓ lactation)	

Table 5 Drugs for which the evidence is inconclusive – careful assessment of risk versus benefit necessary

Amitriptyline and related antidepressants

Antipsychotics (may stimulate lactation, drowsiness/lethargy possible – monitor)

Barbiturates (but withdrawal symptoms reported after long term exposure)

Beta-blockers (possible bradycardia, monitor infant heart rate)

Diuretics (but they do suppress lactation)

Fluoxetine (some sources consider it a contraindication, little information available, monitor infant for diarrhoea, irritability)

Table 5 (*continued*)

Frusemide (but suppresses lactation)
Mesalamine (monitor for diarrhoea)
Ondansetron
Primidone (but withdrawal symptoms reported after long term exposure)
Sertraline (opinions divided however, little information)

Table 6 Drugs which may pose a risk to the infant – DO NOT BREASTFEED

Amiodarone (may affect thyroid function)
Arthrotec – see Misoprostol
Bromocriptine (suppresses lactation)
Ciprofloxacin (phototoxicity, may also affect infant's joints)
Cytotoxic agents (general precaution because of wide ranging toxicity)
Diazepam (very sedative, long-acting – may accumulate)
Fluvastatin (high concentrations in milk, possible adverse effects)
Gliclazide (infant hypoglycaemia possible)
Glipizide (infant hypoglycaemia possible)
Itraconazole (high levels in milk, may accumulate in infant)
Lamotrigine (potentially severe toxicity, manufacturer's recommendation)
Levofloxacin (phototoxicity, may also affect infant's joints)
Lithium (risk of lithium toxicity)
Methotrexate (potentially severe toxicity)
Metronidazole (potentially mutagenic, delay breastfeeding for 48 hours
   after a course)
Misoprostol (in Arthrotec, may produce severe diarrhoea)
Pravastatin (high concentrations in milk, possible adverse effects)
Simvastatin (high concentrations in milk, possible adverse effects)
Sulphasalazine (bloody diarrhoea in infant reported)
Tamoxifen (inhibits lactation)
Tetracyclines (may affect tooth and bone development)

In summary

When prescribing for a nursing mother the following basic principles apply.

- Never prescribe a drug unless it is absolutely necessary.
- Consider stopping or even temporarily suspending current therapy, if possible.
- Consider safer alternatives wherever possible.

- Use the lowest possible dose for the shortest possible period.
- Advise feeding (or expressing) just prior to dosing to limit the concentration in milk.
- Ensure that mother understands the dosage regimen and is aware of any recognizable effects and she is thus able to monitor the suckling infant for any drug-related effects.

Typical adverse effects which might alert the mother to a possible drug side effect include irritability (especially CNS drugs), poor suckling, excessive drowsiness, colicky pain and altered bowel habit or stool consistency (antibiotics, GI drugs).

Finally, the benefits of breastfeeding to both mother and child are widely recognized. Every effort should be made to encourage the highly motivated mother to breastfeed her child whenever possible. The decision to do so ultimately rests with the mother but she may be informed by careful consideration of the individual case and through the provision of advice and support. The nurse has a key role to play in this respect.

Appendix 3

ANALGESIC AND RELATED DRUG THERAPY

How to prescribe – the analgesic stepladder

1. By mouth
Make adequate use of the oral route. It is frequently abandoned too soon. Remember that the sublingual route provides rapid onset of analgesia and avoids presystemic elimination by the liver (first-pass metabolism).

2. By the clock
The need for regular rather than 'prn' analgesia is again stressed. Remember that most oral analgesics act for 4 hours or less. If 4 hours, prescribe oral analgesia 4-hourly. Pain is increasingly difficult to control if frequent breakthrough is allowed to occur. It is still necessary, therefore, to co-prescribe extra (rescue) doses of 1/6th the total daily dose 'prn' (at any time) in order to treat breakthrough pain should it occur.

3. By the ladder
The WHOs Analgesic Stepladder (see Figure 1) has been previously mentioned. Start at the bottom (Step 1). If one drug on that step does not control pain – move up a step.

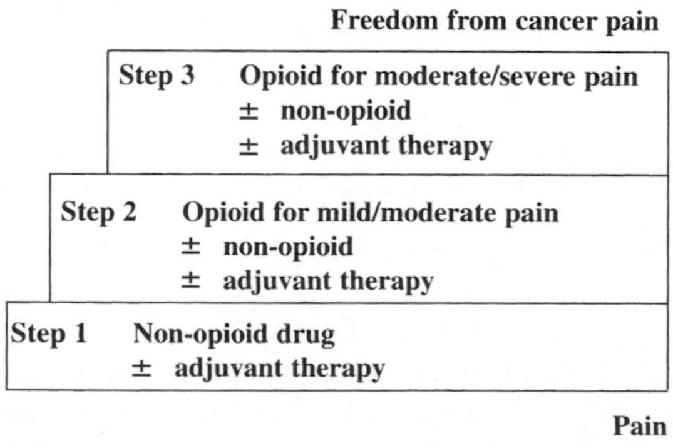

Freedom from cancer pain

Step 3	Opioid for moderate/severe pain ± non-opioid ± adjuvant therapy
Step 2	Opioid for mild/moderate pain ± non-opioid ± adjuvant therapy
Step 1	Non-opioid drug ± adjuvant therapy

Pain

Figure 1

Adjuvant drug therapy
Note that non-steroidal antiinflammatory drugs (NSAIDs) have both analgesic and antiinflammatory properties and may therefore be used as either non-opioid drugs (Step 1) or adjuvant therapy (Steps 1, 2 and 3) in the above scheme.

Opioids used for mild/moderate pain include the opioid *partial agonists* which are so-called because their action at the receptor site is limited within a relatively narrow dosage range. They are therefore *low ceiling* analgesics which have a clearly defined upper dosage limit. In contrast, opioids for moderate/severe pain are *pure agonists* or *high ceiling* analgesics whose action at the receptor site increases with increasing dosage and for which there is effectively no upper dose limit.

What to prescribe – the choice of analgesic

Nociceptive pain

(a) Step 1. Non-opioid analgesic
Although aspirin is often quoted in the textbooks, paracetamol (1 g, 4-hourly up to a maximum of 8 tablets daily) is almost always used for this purpose. It has no antiinflammatory action but acts by inhibition of prostaglandin-mediated pathways in the spinal cord. Its combination with opioids is therefore rational since the latter influence pain transmission elsewhere in the CNS.

(b) Step 2. Opioid for mild/moderate pain
This group includes preparations which contain dextropropoxyphene and codeine in combination with paracetamol. These are respectively *co-proxamol* and *high strength co-codamol 30/500 (but not standard co-codamol which contains only an antitussive dose of 8 mg codeine per tablet)*. All are taken in a dose of 2 tablets, 4-hourly which does however necessitate exceeding the usual recommended maximum dose of paracetamol of 4 g/day. *Dihydrocodeine* as a single agent exists in conventional tablet and liquid form and as controlled release tablets. An injection is also available.

Tramadol (Zydol) is a relatively new drug in the UK but has been around for many years in the US and elsewhere in Europe. It is chemically related to codeine with which it shares weak (low ceiling) opioid activity supplemented by a further analgesic action which affects pain transmission centrally. Its side effect profile largely reflects its opioid action – nausea, vomiting, headache, dizziness, sweating and dry mouth are common occurrences. In particular, its non-opioid activity is associated with the risk of neurotoxicity when used in excessive dosage or in overdosage. For practical purposes tramadol is a Step 2 analgesic and *its use should not delay the introduction of an opioid for moderate/severe pain when warranted.*

Analgesics which are not favoured include pethidine
This is a potent but still low ceiling Step 2 drug which is rarely, if ever, given in doses exceeding 100 mg. The duration of analgesia is only about 1–2 hours which makes pethidine very unsuitable for the treatment of chronic pain.

(c) Step 3. Strong opioid for moderate/severe pain
Morphine is the standard oral agent.

Diamorphine is converted to morphine during first pass and has no advantage by the oral route. Liquid mixtures are unstable, require to be freshly prepared and have a short shelf life. Diamorphine is however the drug of choice by subcutaneous injection.

Although paracetamol, dihydrocodeine and co-proxamol are used in standard dosage, the dose of morphine can be tailored to the individual by careful titration against response. Thus *morphine is a 'high ceiling' drug for which there is no maximum dosage* (a common misconception which often leads to inadequate prescribing).

Initial prescription
When moving to Step 3 on the analgesic ladder it must not be assumed that dosage should initially be very low. Start an *immediate release* (quick-acting) morphine preparation (see Box 1, below) in a suitable dose (e.g. morphine 5–10 mg, or 2.5 mg for elderly or cachectic patients or those in renal failure) 4-hourly and titrate dosage thereafter against the patient's pain until a stable, pain-free state is achieved. Dosage should be reviewed at least daily. A suggested dosage increment scale is given in Figure 2. *Note* also the need to make extra (rescue) dose of 1/6th the total daily dose available 'prn' at any time, to treat breakthrough pain.

Box 1 Available immediate release (quick-acting) oral morphine preparations

Oramorph solution containing morphine sulphate 2 mg in 1 ml

Oramorph Conc solution containing morphine sulphate 20 mg in 1 ml

Oramorph Unit Dose solution containing morphine sulphate 10 mg, 30 mg and 100 mg in 5 ml vial for oral use

Sevredol tablets containing morphine sulphate 10 mg, 20 mg and 50 mg

Sevredol solution containing morphine sulphate 2 mg in 1 ml

Sevredol Conc solution containing morphine sulphate 20 mg in 1 ml

Morphine Hydrochloride Mixture (various strengths) which are still freshly prepared in some pharmacies

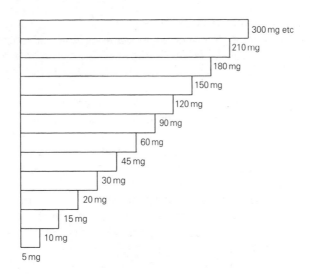

Figure 2 Suggested incremental scale

Once pain control has been achieved and the dosage stabilized, conversion to *controlled release* (prolonged action) morphine is possible. Calculate the required total daily dose of morphine provided by the immediate release preparation (including any breakthrough doses) and administer this once or twice (12-hourly) daily. Remember to continue to make breakthrough medication available. See Box 2 below for available preparations.

Box 2 Available controlled release (prolonged action) oral morphine preparations

– Administered 12-hourly

MST Continus tablets containing morphine sulphate 5 mg, 10 mg, 15 mg, 30 mg, 60 mg, 100 mg and 200 mg

MST Continus suspension containing granules in sachet for reconstitution with water (or sprinkled over food) to give morphine sulphate 20 mg, 30 mg, 60 mg, 100 mg and 200 mg per dose

Oramorph SR tablets containing morphine sulphate 10 mg, 30 mg, 60 mg and 100 mg

Zomorph capsules containing morphine sulphate 10 mg, 30 mg, 60 mg, 100 mg and 200 mg

– Administered once daily

Morcap SR capsules containing morphine sulphate 20 mg, 50 mg and 100 mg

MXL capsules containing morphine sulphate 30 mg, 60 mg, 90 mg, 120 mg, 150 mg and 200 mg

Tolerance and addiction

Addiction to morphine is not seen in patients with advanced cancer. However, psychological dependence is often mistakenly inferred by the patient's 'craving' for the few pain-free periods which may be achieved by inadequate analgesic therapy. Thus, when patients regularly demand medication – rather than assume addiction – a complete review of analgesic therapy would seem more appropriate. Clinical experience has shown that dosages of opioid drugs may be rapidly reduced or even stopped when other (non-drug) methods e.g. cordotomy, are used to achieve pain control, without precipitating withdrawal symptoms. Tolerance to the analgesic effect of the opioids may develop after the first few months of treatment but is easily overcome by relatively small dosage increments. There is evidence that a plateau is reached thereafter when effective analgesia can be maintained for longer periods at fixed dosage. Increased dose may however be necessary where there is an increase in the level of pain due to an extension of the disease. Similarly, tolerance to opioid induced drowsiness and nausea rapidly occurs and is a useful phenomenon.

Effects on ventilatory function

It is uncommon to find clinical (or biochemical) evidence of serious ventilatory failure as a result of pain control therapy. Clinically important respiratory depression is rarely seen in patients with severe pain due to malignant disease even when receiving large doses of opioids. Pain and emotional stress are powerful antagonists of opioid-induced respiratory depression. In fact the slowing effect of morphine on the respiratory rate may be used to good effect in patients with tachypnoea and respiratory distress. Provided the dose is built up by standard increments at correct dosage intervals and the use of other depressant drugs (e.g. the benzodiazepines) is similarly controlled, the drive to respiration will only fall off once the patient is pain-free and calm. Even patients with hypercapnic respiratory failure can and should be prescribed opioids when required for pain control.

Box 3 Alternatives to oral morphine		
Drug/strength	Dose equiv: to 10 mg oral morphine	Comments
Dextromoramide 5 mg tablets	5 mg	Sublingual – rapid onset/brief duration (2–3 hours). Useful for painful procedure (dressing change, bathing, etc) and for breakthrough pain
Phenazocine 5 mg tablets	2.5 mg	Oral or sublingual 4–6 hourly. Less nausea and constipation than with morphine
Rectal morphine 15 mg, 30 mg supps		Use oral morphine dose as a guide. Insert 4-hourly and titrate against pain tolerance

Fentanyl transdermal (Durogesic)
Fentanyl is a strong opioid with a characteristic brief duration of action which is reported to produce less constipation than morphine. As with other opioids, however, the co-prescription of laxative therapy is still required whenever regular doses are prescribed. The formulation of fentanyl in a transdermal patch provides a novel method of delivering continuous analgesia for patients with *stable* chronic pain. Patches which deliver fentanyl from a reservoir contained within at rates of 25, 50, 75 and 100 microgram/hour *at steady state* are an alternative to continuous subcutaneous infusions (CSI) in patients who are unable to take oral medication. For practical purposes a rate of administration of 25 microgram/hour fentanyl is approximately equivalent to diamorphine 30 mg/24 hour by CSI or a total daily dose of oral morphine 90 mg.

The delivery of fentanyl from Durogesic is triphasic. When the patch is first applied, drug is slowly absorbed across the skin surface to establish a subcutaneous depot from which it is subsequently released into the systemic circulation. The onset of action is delayed for up to 12 hours when the patch is first applied and the *steady state* (at which drug release is matched by drug absorption and drug clearance) is only reached after 24–48 hours at which time a smooth plasma concentration profile results. A similar delay also arises when changing from one strength patch to another and the need for *additional* immediate release analgesia should be considered at this time, as well as at the start of treatment. If follows that transdermal fentanyl is suitable only for patients who have relatively stable pain and hence predictable analgesic requirements. It is *inappropriate* for the management of breakthrough pain for which co-prescription of an immediate release opioid is required.

Fentanyl patches will continue to provide a steady state plasma concentration profile for over 48–72 hours while in place. Therefore most patients will require the patch to be changed every 3 days but for some more frequent reapplication may be necessary. Note that once the patch is removed, the skin depot will remain 'active' and continue to deliver a declining quantity/hour of fentanyl to the systemic circulation for up to 24–48 hours. This should be taken into account when reestablishing patients on analgesia by other routes. The fentanyl reservoir is never depleted throughout the period of drug administration and significant quantities of fentanyl remain in the patch after removal.

Note that if pain becomes unstable (particularly likely in the terminal phase) while on a fentanyl patch, it is preferable to leave the patch in situ and to add doses of SC diamorphine (bolus or continuous infusion), or other immediate release analgesia, until pain control is reestablished.

Hydromorphone capsules (Palladone)
Hydromorphone is a hydrogenated ketone derivative of morphine which has been available in the USA for many years but marketed in the UK only

relatively recently. It is available in immediate release and controlled release forms – Palladone capsules (1.3 mg and 2.6 mg) and Palladone SR capsules (2 mg, 4 mg, 8 mg, 16 mg and 24 mg) for 4-hourly and 12-hourly administration respectively. The oral analgesic potency ratio of morphine : hydromorphone is approximately 7.5 : 1. Therefore:

> Controlled release hydromorphone (Palladone SR) 2 mg is approximately equivalent to MST/Oramorph SR 15 mg
> Conventional hydromorphone (Palladone) capsules 1.3 mg is approximately equivalent to standard morphine preparations (e.g. Oramorph mixture, Sevredol tablets) 10 mg

The oral bioavailability of hydromorphone, like that of morphine, is around 50% and in most other respects, hydromorphone appears to resemble morphine. So far, its role appears to be as an alternative for patients in whom morphine is associated with confusion or oversedation, although hydromorphone is nevertheless still a morphine derivative.

Oxycodone tablets (OxyContin)

Oxycodone is a hydroxy derivative of dihydrocodeine ketone which was previously marketed in the UK in rectal form as Pralodone suppositories. It has recently reappeared in the form of controlled release tablets (OxyContin containing 10 mg, 20 mg, 40 mg and 80 mg) and immediate release capsules (OxyNorm containing 5 mg, 10 mg and 20 mg) for 12-hourly and 4-hourly administration respectively. In practice, oxycodone 10 mg is equipotent with morphine 20 mg. Its oral bioavailability is less variable than that of morphine for which it might be substituted. However, it remains to be seen just what its future role will be.

> NB: Important reminder: laxatives must always be co-prescribed with regular opioid therapy – See Adjuvant drug therapy

POTENT ANALGESIA BY INJECTION

Diamorphine is the drug of choice, preferably administered by continuous subcutaneous infusion (CSI)

Subcutaneous injections are generally more comfortable for patients and are easily administered, especially to patients with poor veins or little muscle bulk. Regular analgesia is provided without the discomfort of frequent injections and the dose is readily titrated against the individual's pain tolerance and within narrow therapeutic limits (i.e. any high peak/low trough effect is eliminated). It is also cost effective in terms of nursing time and the overall use of disposables. Modern syringe drivers are relatively inexpensive, non-bulky and readily portable.

When is parenteral therapy required?

CSI is not a universal method of delivering analgesia and it does not replace the oral or sublingual routes. It is an alternative which is available should these first line routes of administration become impractical or impossible. It has been mistakenly assumed in the past that injections are necessary for all patients with severe pain though, in fact, oral analgesics are equally effective in equipotent dosage. Subcutaneous diamorphine should however be considered in the following situations:

(i)   Where patients can no longer tolerate oral therapy due to nausea, vomiting or dysphagia.
(ii) Where patients are very drowsy, comatose or semi-comatose.
(iii) Where patients experience adverse effects related to high peak levels soon after dosing (drowsiness, nausea, hallucinations, etc.) and/or breakthrough pain before the next dose, i.e. to smooth out a high peak/low trough profile.
(iv) For patients whose analgesic requirements would involve the use of excessive numbers of tablets.
(v)   For patients at home, to facilitate the supervision of regular parenteral analgesia. This is easily managed by the community nurse visiting on a daily basis.

The above does not cover all contingencies and there may be other situations where CSI is considered.

The possibility of re-establishing patients on oral therapy once an acute problem necessitating parenteral dosing has resolved should be considered. It is recognized that some derive great psychological benefit from syringe drivers and may be reluctant to return to oral therapy. This is not a sign of drug dependence: it is more likely to indicate the efficacy of the subcutaneous route coupled with a fear of recurring severe pain.

The role of diamorphine

As hydrochloride, diamorphine is fifteen times more soluble than morphine so that very small volumes can be injected at any dosage level. For example, 120 mg diamorphine can be administered in as little as 0.2 ml water and most single doses are soluble in less than 0.1 ml. With morphine, on the other hand, dosage may become a limiting factor due to the volume required to be administered at higher dosage.

Diamorphine is also widely preferred to morphine because of its more favourable pharmacokinetics. Although it is eventually converted to morphine its rate of distribution to the tissues (as 6-O acetylmorphine) is much more rapid so that its onset of action is faster, and more intense, albeit slightly briefer. Thus the potency ratio of diamorphine : morphine is 2 : 3.

Delivery of subcutaneous infusions: use of syringe drivers

Various devices are available and it is not possible to give details of them all here. Most are battery operated and there may be differences in the method of operation, *particularly in setting the delivery rate.* The variable speed Graseby Medical MS16A (Blue) syringe driver is widely used but this does not imply that it is any better than others and it should be noted that the development of syringe drivers is increasing all the time.

Site(s) of administration/choice of giving sets

The subcutaneous tissues of the pectoral region and anterior abdominal wall are most frequently chosen, but a change of site may be required in the event of a local reaction (see adverse effects). An ordinary blue 22 gauge 'butterfly' cannula is selected or, if a longer tube is required, a Graseby Medical Infusion Set (Part No 105-029).

The continuous delivery of drug should be checked at regular intervals, usually during drug administration rounds, by observing the flashing indicator light. Accurate delivery can also be determined by measuring the 'length' of solution remaining.

Dosage of diamorphine by CSI

For any patient, the diamorphine requirement is only established by careful titration of dose against the individual's pain tolerance.

When transferring from oral morphine the '3 : 2 : 1 Rule' (below) is a useful guide:

3 mg morphine = 2 mg oral diamorphine = 1 mg SC diamorphine

Therefore, one-third of the total daily dose of oral morphine is used initially as a guide.

Some examples are given below.

Total daily dose (mg)		
Oral morphine	Subcutaneous diamorphine	Dose of SC diamorphine for breakthrough pain*
90	30	5
120	40	5
150	50	10
180	60	10
240	80	15
300	100	20

*It is important to prescribe additional bolus SC doses of diamorphine, approximately 1/6th of the total daily dose, as required (prn) at any time for breakthrough pain.

Stability of admixtures for subcutaneous infusion

Mixtures of diamorphine and various adjuvant drugs have been administered in a day-to-day practice in response to patient need, although extensive stability data are generally lacking. Nevertheless, experience has shown
that few, if any, problems arise if attention is paid to the following:

(a) Drug combination should normally be used within 24 hours of
     admixture.
(b) Visual inspection of the mixture, to detect signs of flocculation or
     precipitation, particularly when higher doses of diamorphine are
     used, is essential.

The following example illustrates the use of the syringe driver.

It is required to transfer to subcutaneous diamorphine in a patient
developing uncontrollable nausea and vomiting on MST tablets, 120 mg
12-hourly.

(i)   The 3 : 2 : 1 rule gives an equivalent 24 hour dose of 80 mg diamor-
       phine.
(ii)   Dissolve 80 mg diamorphine in 8 ml[†] water for injections.
(iii) Measure the '*length*' of this solution using the '*length scale*' on
       the side of the device. A volume of 8 ml measures 48 mm if a 10 ml
       BD Plastipak syringe is used: thus a daily dose of 48 mm length is
       required and this is delivered at a rate 48 mm/24 hour = 2 mm/hour.
(iv)   Fit the battery in the syringe driver (alkaline batteries will last about
       2 weeks): its activation is confirmed by the bleep which is immedi-
       ately emitted.
(v)   Adjust the '*rate setting dial*' to 2 mm/hour using the plastic key
       provided (or else a paper clip).
(vi)   Place the syringe in the driver, fix in position with the '*securing strap*'
       and advance the '*plunger drive*' to meet the syringe plunger.
(vii) Press the '*start/test button*' to set the infusion running and confirm
       that the '*indicator light*' is flashing at a rate of 1 per second.
(viii) The device may be placed under the pillow or, if the patient is
       ambulant, in a pocket.

In this way effective pain control can be maintained even if, for any reason, pain
increases e.g. as a result of extension of the disease itself or worsening of other signs
or symptoms. Regular need for additional doses is a signal that total analgesic therapy
should be reviewed. Also, remember to give a stat SC bolus (loading) dose, equal to
1/6th the total daily dose, if the patient is in pain when setting up a syringe driver.

[†]8 ml is the standard volume in a 10 ml syringe. Less soluble drugs e.g. dexamethasone,
midazolam, etc. may require larger volumes to deliver the required dosage. Note that
14 ml may be administered in a 20 ml syringe and 17 ml in a 30 ml syringe.

When setting up an infusion, it is necessary to make the first change before the initial 24 hour period has elapsed. This allows solution to take up dead space in the giving set. Change of syringe every 24 hours thereafter is possible.

The frequency of change of cannula/giving set depends upon frequency of skin reactions, but should be changed at least every 72 hours.

Box 4 Adjuvant drugs which may be mixed with diamorphine in the syringe driver (single agents)

Diamorphine and	Single agents	Comments
	Cyclizine (Valoid)	50 mg in 1 ml amps. Crystals formed at concentrations around 20 mg/ml. Incompatible if concentration of cyclizine or diamorphine exceeds 25 mg/ml. Dose: 100–150 mg/24 hours
	Dexamethasone (Decadron)	8 mg in 2 ml vial. Do not mix with cyclizine or methotrimeprazine. Careful inspection of the syringe contents essential with high dose diamorphine (gram quantities). Discard if cloudy. Dose range: 4–16 mg/24 hours
	Glycopyrronium (Robinul)	200 microgram in 1 ml amps. Drying of salivary secretions with less likelihood of effect on heart rate than with atropine or hyoscine. Dose: 1.2 mg/24 hour
	Haloperidol (Haldol, Serenace)	5 mg in 1 ml, 10 mg in 2 ml, 20 mg in 2 ml amps. Do not use oily depot injection. Precipitation occurs if final concentration of haloperidol exceeds 1 mg/ml. Antiemetic with sedative/tranquillizer properties, see text. Dose 5–20 mg/24 hours
	Hyaluronidase (Hyalase)	1500 IU amps. Contents of one amp mixed with diamorphine to reduce local (injection site) reactions, see text
	Hyoscine HCl/HBr	400 microgram in 1 ml amps. For bronchial hypersecretion, see text. Dose: 1.2–2.4 mg/24 hours
	Hyoscine Butylbromide (Buscopan)	20 mg in 1 ml amps. Antispasmodic for use in bowel colic; less effect on secretions. Dose: 60–120 mg/24 hours
	Ketorolac (Toradol)	10 mg in 1 ml, 30 mg in 1 ml amps. Potent NSAID co-analgesia, see text. Dose: 60–90 mg/24 hours

(continued)

Box 4 (*continued*)

Diamorphine and	Single agents	Comments
	Levomepromazine (Nozinan)	25 mg in 1 ml amps. Potent sedative and antiemetic used for agitation/nausea. Sedative dose range: 25–300 mg/24 hours. Antiemetic dose range: 3.125–12.5 mg/24 hours
	Metoclopramide (Maxolon)	10 mg in 2 ml amps. Antiemetic, see text. Compatible with diamorphine at almost any concentration. Dose: 40–80 mg/24 hours
	Midazolam (Hypnovel)	10 mg in 2 ml, 10 mg in 5 ml. Potent anxiolytic/sedative useful for terminal restlessness, see text. Dose range: 10–120 mg/24 hours. Doses exceeding 80 mg should be split and administered over 12 hours
	Octreotide (Sandostatin)	50, 100, 500 microgram in 1 ml in 5 ml multidose vial. Control of symptoms associated with malignant GI obstruction, see text. Dose: 300–900 microgram/24 hours
	Ondansetron (Zofran)	4 mg in 2 ml, 8 mg in 4 ml amps. Versatile antiemetic for difficult nausea and vomiting, associated with a variety of causes, see text. Dose: 16–24 mg/24 hours

---

Box 5 Adjuvant drugs that may be mixed with diamorphine in the syringe driver (multiple agents)

Diamorphine and *Multiple agents*

Cyclizine + Haloperidol	Metoclopramide + Haloperidol
Cyclizine + Hyoscine	Metoclopramide + Midazolam
Cyclizine + Midazolam	Metoclopramide + Octreotide
Dexamethasone + Haloperidol (requires to be well diluted seek advice)	Midazolam + Glycopyrronium
Dexamethasone + Metoclopramide	Midazolam + Hyoscine
Haloperidol + Midazolam	Midazolam + Ketamine
Levomepromazine + Hyoscine	Octreotide + Hyoscine
Levomepromazine + Metoclopramide	Ondansetron + Hyoscine

Note: Hyaluronidase can be mixed with any of the above combinations

Avoid the following admixtures containing diamorphine which are known to be incompatible

Diamorphine and *Multiple agents*

Dexamethasone + Cyclizine	Metoclopramide + Ondansetron
Dexamethasone + Levomepromazine	Octreotide + Cyclizine
Dexamethasone + Midazolam	Octreotide + Dexamethasone
Cyclizine + Metoclopramide	Octreotide + Levomepromazine

Adverse effects of diamorphine administered by CSI

This is generally a well tolerated method of administering analgesia.

In a proportion of patients however, usually those receiving higher doses of diamorphine, the appearance of small areas of redness, induration and swelling at the injection site has been noted, often necessitating resiting of the needle. Biopsies show formation of sterile granulomas and exclude an infective cause. It seems likely therefore that the reaction is due to some property of the solution itself (chemical irritancy, pH, osmolality, etc.) or a degradation product, or perhaps to the needle in situ.

The addition of dexamethasone (an antiinflammatory agent) does not appear to influence the rate of formation of subcutaneous granulomas. However experience has shown that 1500 IU hyaluronidase added to the syringe will reduce the reaction, presumably by hastening removal of drug from its site of administration. So far chemical incompatibility between hyaluronidase and other syringe contents has not been noted.

An alternative method is to infuse the mixture via a 22 gauge Teflon IV cannula which is sited subcutaneously but it is important to note that these may 'kink' and interrupt the flow of drug.

NB: Important reminder: laxatives must always be co-prescribed with regular opioid therapy – see Adjuvant drug therapy.

ADJUVANT DRUG THERAPY

1. Treatment of neuropathic pain

A *tricyclic antidepressant* e.g. *amitriptyline* (10–150 mg at night) is a useful first choice for the treatment of pain due to nerve destruction. An *anticonvulsant* (e.g. *sodium valproate* 200 mg tds, *clonazepam* 0.5–4 mg bd, *gabapentin*, up to 1.8 g daily) may be an effective alternative. Note that antidepressants and anticonvulsants are administered in *low initial dosage* then *carefully titrated upwards* until pain control is achieved in the individual patient.

A *corticosteroid* (e.g. *dexamethasone* 4–16 mg daily) should be considered for pain associated with *raised intracranial pressure, bone metastases, nerve infiltration/compression, pressure due to soft tissue swelling or infiltration and stretched liver capsule.*

(d) Role of ketamine in neuropathic pain

Ketamine (Ketalar) is a non-opioid general anaesthetic agent used in sub-anaesthetic doses in the treatment of neuropathic or 'opioid-resistant' pain. It is a specific inhibitor of the N-methyl-D-aspartate (NMDA) receptor which is activated by glutamate, an excitatory neurotransmitter in the

CNS. There remains controversy over the efficacy of strong (Step 3) opioids in neuropathic pain, with the possible exception of methadone which also inhibits the NMDA receptor. Ketamine is, therefore, used, in addition to a strong opioid, to establish pain control and to reduce the opioid dosage requirement.

Injection vials containing 10 mg/ml and 50 mg/ml are available. Solution can be taken orally, diluted in fruit juice, instilled rectally if the oral route is unavailable, or administered by continuous subcutaneous infusion (CSI) via the syringe driver. The response to ketamine is first established using a test dose, 5 mg orally/rectally or 2.5 mg by subcutaneous bolus. Suggested starting doses are 15 mg, 6-hourly (oral/rectal) or 25 mg/24 hours by CSI titrated, according to response. Breakthrough pain is managed by additional doses based on 10% of the total daily dose. The average oral dose is in the range 75–250 mg daily.

It is important to note that the addition of ketamine is likely to affect the requirement for oral morphine or subcutaneous diamorphine (or other opioid analgesia) such that a *reduction* in opioid dosage, by one-third, is recommended when ketamine is introduced.

2. Treatment of other types of pain

(a) Metastatic bone pain

Radiotherapy is first line treatment for all new, and some previously treated, lesions.

The non-steroidal antiinflammatory drugs (NSAIDs) may be used in an attempt to reduce pain and inflammation associated with bony metastases. Since there is an associated risk of gastroduodenal upset and ulceration, particularly in patients receiving concurrent steroid therapy, the co-administration of misoprostol or proton pump inhibitor (e.g. omeprazole) should be considered. Further, there may be a risk of renal impairment, especially in the elderly who often tolerate NSAIDs poorly. There is no evidence that any one NSAID is more effective than another for this indication. Common examples include Ibuprofen (400 mg tds), naproxen (1 g bd), diclofenac (50 mg tds) and ketoprofen (100 mg bd). Controlled release forms may also be used.

Ketorolac (Toradol) is a very potent drug reported to be effective in the treatment of intractable bone pain which is less responsive to other NSAIDs. It is available in both oral and injectable forms and has been administered by continuous subcutaneous infusion via the syringe driver, either alone or in combination with diamorphine, in a dose of 60–90 mg/24 hours. Note however that ketorolac is not licensed for subcutaneous administration or indeed for treatment exceeding 2 days by injection or 7 days by the oral route. This arises because of concerns over toxicity so that monitoring of renal function and GI tolerance is advised during chronic administration.

(b) Pain associated with smooth muscle spasm

The anticholinergic, antispasmodic *hyoscine butylbromide* (dose: 20 mg qds orally, 60–120 mg daily by SC infusion) may relieve colicky pain in the bowel and ureter.

(c) Pain associated with spinal infiltration and skeletal muscle spasm

Baclofen, an antispasmodic which inhibits reflex voluntary muscle spasm, may be tried. The dose is established by careful titration from a starting dose of 5 mg tds gradually increased (every 3 days) up to a maximum of 20 mg tds, until control is achieved.

(d) Pain associated with soft tissue infection

Cellulitis is treated with an appropriate antibiotic e.g. oral *flucloxacillin* 500 mg qid, *clindamycin* 300 mg qid or *co-amoxiclav* 2 tablets tid.

3. Treatment of nausea and vomiting

There are many causes of nausea and vomiting in patients with cancer. The choice of antiemetic should be made on the basis of cause, and the site of action of specific drugs. Note also that alternative strategies may be more appropriate e.g. prevent constipation, correct hypercalcaemia, reduce anxiety, etc.

Box 6 Some causes of nausea and vomiting in cancer patients

Constipation	Irritation of upper GI tract (e.g. due to candida, sputum in pharynx or drug-induced)
Blood in stomach	GI obstruction
Hepatomegaly	Raised intracranial pressure
Cough	Pain
Anxiety	Hypercalcaemia
Hyponatraemia	Uraemia
Cancer toxicity	Gastric stasis
Nauseating smells, sounds or memories	

Causes of nausea and vomiting related to treatment

Radiotherapy	Chemotherapy
Drugs	antibiotics, aspirin, carbamazepine corticosteroids, digoxin, iron salts, NSAIDs, oestrogens, opioids, theophylline

---

NB: More than one cause of nausea and vomiting may exist and treatment with more than one antiemetic may therefore be necessary.

Choosing an antiemetic drug

First consider the cause(s) of nausea and vomiting then choose the antiemetic accordingly. The vomiting centre (VC) is triggered via several different pathways including:

Chemoreceptor trigger zone (CTZ) – stimulus is presence of emetogenic substance(s) in the circulation or metabolic change. Note that the blood–brain barrier is breached at this site so that substances which do not enter the CNS still influence activity in the CTZ.

Gastrointestinal tract – vagal stimulation by pharyngeal irritation, oesophageal reflux, ureteric or bowel distension. Also gastric stasis due to reduced upper GI motility, squashed stomach syndrome, floppy stomach syndrome or direct mucosal toxicity. Reduced motility in the upper GI tract may be detected as nausea and often precedes emesis.

Box 7

Recommended antiemetic(s)	*Indication(s)*
Cyclizine 50 mg tid Cyclizine 50 mg tid	{ Motion sickness Intestinal obstruction Raised intracranial pressure
GI prokinetic agents	
Metoclopramide 10 mg qid or Domperidone 10 mg qid or Cisapride 10 mg tid or Methotrimeprazine 3.125–12.5 mg at night	{ Oesophageal reflux and Delayed gastric emptying
Dexamethasone 2–4 mg tid	{ Cancer toxicity Visceral organ involvement Stretched liver capsule Raised intracranial pressure
Haloperidol 5–20 mg daily or Ondansetron 8 mg bd/tds	{ Radiotherapy Chemotherapy Other drug induced Uraemia Hypercalcaemia
Hyoscine Hydrobromide 400 microgram 4–6 hourly	– Bronchial hypersecretion

NB: Avoid constipation – it is a frequent cause of nausea and vomiting.

Visceral organs – e.g. liver, heart, testes, etc.

Vestibular apparatus – vomiting induced by movement e.g. motion sickness.

Raised intracranial pressure – associated with intracerebral lesions.

Higher centres – also likely to influence the VC: this may be a factor in anticipatory emesis and nausea caused by smells, sounds, sights or memories.

The choice is based on pharmacology of the drug and its likely site of action.

Metoclopramide and *domperidone* increase upper GI motility and, in addition, block stimulation of the CTZ, probably because they are dopamine antagonists. *Cisapride* may also act at the CTZ but its precise action remains uncertain.

The above is also the basis for the use of *haloperidol* which, as a potent tranquillizer, may have an additional action on higher centres.

Ondansetron, and related 5HT3 antagonists, inhibit emetogenic serotonin at specific sites in the GI tract and at the CTZ.

Cyclizine acts directly on the VC and has some activity at the CTZ. Since it is also anticholinergic, it may be preferred if GI obstruction precludes the use of a prokinetic drug.

Hyoscine is similar but it also possesses marked antisecretory activity which is useful in suppressing respiratory hypersecretion.

Methotrimeprazine in low dosage (range 3.125–12.5 mg daily) is an effective antiemetic without producing marked sedation. It is a member of the phenothiazine group and as such it increases upper GI motility.

The antiemetic action of *dexamethasone* and other corticosteroids is unknown. It is likely that a central action may at least contribute to this by influencing pathways in higher centres.

4. Prevention and treatment of constipation

The need for co-prescription of laxatives, whenever regular opioid analgesia is used, has been stressed throughout the text.

Constipation can be a major problem to the extent that it influences pain tolerance and contributes towards other common problems. For example it is a common cause of disabling nausea and vomiting.

A suggested order of laxative use is:

(i) A stimulant with, or without, a stool softener (*co-danthramer forte* or *co-danthrusate* or *senna* as a single agent). This is usually required to counter the effect of opioids on normal control of bowel function. Also, many elderly patients will have received stimulant laxatives over a prolonged period and are unresponsive to first line measures such as increased, or augmented, dietary fibre intake.

(ii) An osmotically-active agent e.g. *magnesium hydroxide* or *lactulose*, with or without a *fibre supplement*, will increase stool water content and therefore stool bulk and mobility. Such a drug may be tried in addition to a stimulant, if necessary.

(iii) If constipation is established, it is often necessary to evacuate the bowel using locally-acting agents. Thus *bisacodyl suppositories* and/or *Micolette enemas* may be required.

(iv) *Phosphate* enema b.d. plus *arachis oil enema* once daily will usually work in the most difficult cases but treatment should be aimed thereafter at preventing recurrence.

5. Treatment of bronchial hypersecretion

Excessive secretions and inadequate clearance result in a characteristic 'rattle' which may be distressing to patients and relatives. This is particularly noticeable in the last few hours of life. Administration of the anticholinergic, *hyoscine hydrobromide*, via the syringe driver will reduce mucus production and eliminate 'rattle'. Dose: 1.2–2.4 mg per 24 hours by CSI or 200–400 microgram (0.2–0.4 mg) 4-hourly by SC bolus. An alternative is glycopyrronium 1.2 mg per 24 hrs or 200–400 microgram (0.2–0.4 mg) 4 hourly SC.

6. Relief of agitation and terminal restlessness

Levomepromazine (Nozinan), a phenothiazine which is tolerated by the subcutaneous route, and which may be administered via the syringe driver, possesses both antiemetic and marked sedative properties. It is therefore a useful drug for relieving agitation, particularly if control of nausea and vomiting is also required. Dose: 25–300 mg per 24 hours.

Midazolam, a water soluble benzodiazepine derivative is also tolerated by subcutaneous injection. It has been increasingly used, as an alternative to rectal diazepam, to control anxiety and severe restlessness i.e. in patients with myoclonus or parkinsonism, or those in whom seizures may be precipitated by a phenothiazine drug.

Dose: range of 10–120 mg per 24 hours. Maximum of 80 mg in a single syringe: dissolve in 17 ml water for injections in a 30 ml syringe. Doses >80 mg should be split and administered over 12 hours.

Some drugs are *too irritant* for subcutaneous administration. These include chlorpromazine, prochlorperazine, and diazepam. The latter is however very effective in controlling anxiety and restlessness when given in a dose of 10 20 mg rectally as required.

7. Treatment of respiratory symptoms

Many patients develop chronic respiratory symptoms in the end-stages of advanced malignancy, typically, those with pulmonary malignancies, either primary (e.g. carcinoma of the bronchus) or secondary (e.g. carcinoma of the breast, renal carcinoma, etc). Such symptoms may be exacerbated by preexisting conditions such as chronic obstructive pulmonary disease, cor pulmonale, congestive cardiac failure, or anaemia.

The most frequent symptoms are dyspnoea, cough, haemoptysis, and chest pain; stridor, and the choking sensation associated with superior vena caval obstruction are much less common.

(a) Central cough suppression
Morphine and other opioids depress the cough reflex by direct suppression of the cough centre in the medulla.

(b) Local cough suppression
The long acting local anaesthetic *bupivacaine* can be administered over 5–10 minutes as 4 ml of a 0.25% solution, driven by nebulizer or bedside oxygen (rate 6–8 litres/minute). This provides particles of 2–10 micron which suppress cough down to the level of the larger bronchi. Caution: may cause bronchospasm or loss of gag reflex.

(c) Dyspnoea
Consider the following and institute appropriate treatment measures.

(i)   Reversible airways obstruction (*bronchodilators, corticosteroids*)
(ii)   Respiratory infection (*antibiotic therapy*)
(iii)   Pleural effusion (*drain and pleurodesis*)
(iv)   Lobar collapse (*radiotherapy, corticosteroids*)
(v)   SVC obstruction (*corticosteroids and radiotherapy*)
(vi)   Lymphangitis carcinomatosa (*corticosteroids*)
(vii)   Anaemia (*consider transfusion if Hb < 8 g/dl*)
(viii) Haemoptysis (*ethamsylate or tranexamic acid*)

(d) Persistent dyspnoea
In the palliation of dyspnoeic patients, the main benefit comes from suppression of respiratory awareness. Drugs which induce global cerebral sedation also reduce dyspnoea, associated with varying degrees of depression of ventilatory drive. The following, used in carefully titrated dosage, can be described in simple terms as respiratory sedatives and used to palliate dyspnoea.

(i) The use of *opioids* to control breathlessness is controversial. They may reduce the subjective sensation of breathlessness and demand for ventilation without causing clinically significant respiratory depression (discussed earlier in text). They appear to act on medullary chemo-receptors to reduce the tidal volume and response to hypercapnia. The dose should be titrated against response: if the patient is already receiving opioids, increase the dose by 50% and titrate thereafter.

Consider also the nebulized route of delivery which offers certain advantages.

- *Speed of effect*: the lungs present a huge surface area for absorption
- *Compliance*: patients with chronic respiratory disease are used to nebulizer therapy. Its use on an 'as required' basis promotes patient control and autonomy
- *Specificity*: reduced systemic effects and possible additional benefit on the local sensation of breathlessness.

(ii) *Benzodiazepines* e.g. diazepam/lorazepam, reduce associated anxiety.
(iii) *Alcohol* probably 'self-prescribed' by patients more often than is recognized.

(e) Acute respiratory distress and suffering due to respiratory symptoms e.g. associated with SVC obstruction

Although this is an emergency requiring treatment with high dose corti-costeroid and radiotherapy, if the patient is unfit for radiotherapy or unwilling, consider administration of diamorphine 5–20 mg via a nebulizer.

8. Octreotide in the treatment of malignant gastrointestinal obstruction

Bowel obstruction frequently occurs as a complication of advanced abdominal and pelvic malignancies, and with metastatic peritoneal deposits. It causes symptoms of intestinal colic, abdominal pain and distension, vomiting and anorexia. In advanced disease, the decision to proceed to surgical palliation is complex and must take into consideration survival time, general condition, quality of life and surgical risk as well as patients'/relatives' wishes.

The commonly used medical management of nasogastric suction and intravenous fluid replacement may also be considered, but recent studies indicate that pharmacological control can be achieved using octreotide (Sandostatin), an analogue of somatostatin which is a natural hormone having multiple physiological roles including regulation of GI motility and secretory function. Octreotide is currently licensed for use in variceal bleeding, acromegaly and to reduce secretions from neuroendocrine tumours. Octreotide may be a better alternative in patients for whom surgery is not viable, especially those who wish to remain at home.

Octreotide alleviates the predominant symptoms of malignant GI obstruction by the following mechanisms.

- Decreased gut peristalsis from stomach to large bowel
- Slowed gastric emptying
- Suppression of induced increase in lower oesophageal pressure
- Decreased volume of gastrointestinal secretions

Commonly, doses of 600 microgram delivered by continuous subcutaneous infusion over 24 hours result in symptomatic improvement within 2–3 days. Adequate oral fluid intake can usually be maintained but some patients with high intestinal obstruction (e.g. gastric outflow or jejunal obstruction) may still require decompression by nasogastric tube. Octreotide may also be administered in the syringe with the anticholinergic hyoscine butylbromide (Buscopan) where prolonged colicky pain is predominant.

Long term management may be possible using depot preparations including long-acting octreotide injection (Sandostatin LA) or lanreotide (Somatuline) administered by deep intramuscular injection every 2–4 weeks. However these preparations require further evaluation in the treatment of malignant gastrointestinal obstruction.

Appendix 4

METRIC WEIGHTS AND OTHER MEASURES

In recent years the introduction of metrication into medical practice has altered the ways in which drug dosages and concentrations, patient data (including height, weight and body surface area), drug levels in the body and other measurements are expressed. The following are those units of measurements which the nurse will commonly encounter in everyday practice.

1. **Weight.** The unit of weight is the kilogram (kg). This is made up of 1000 grams (g) and each gram is composed of 1000 milligrams (mg). Each milligram in turn is composed of 1000 micrograms (µg or mcg) – hence, 1 kg = 1000 g; 1 g = 1000 mg; 1 mg = 1000 µg or mcg. When converting from or to the imperial system 1 kg = 2.2 lb. NB: Whenever drugs are prescribed in microgram dosages it is good practice to write the units in full i.e., digoxin 250 micrograms, as the use of the contracted terms µg or mcg may in practice be mistaken for mg and as this dose is one thousand times greater, disastrous consequences may follow.

   Drug dosages are often described in terms of unit dose per kg of body weight i.e. mg/kg, µg/kg, etc. This method of dosage is frequently used in paediatric medicine and allows doses to be tailored to the individual patient's size.

2. **Volume.** The unit of volume is the litre which is denoted by the symbol 'l'. One litre comprises 1000 millilitres (ml). Occasionally the term decilitre (dl) is used. 1 l = 10 dl; 1 dl = 100 ml and 1 l = 1000 ml. When converting from or to the imperial system 1 l = 35.2 fluid ounces (fl oz) or 1 ml = 0.0352 fl oz. The symbols 'l' or 'ml' account for almost all measurements expressed in unit volume for the prescription and administration of drugs.

3. **Concentration.** When expressing concentration or dosages of a medicine in liquid form, several methods are available:

   a. **Unit weight per unit volume:** This describes the unit of weight of a drug contained in unit volume, e.g. 1 mg in 1 ml; 2 mg in 1 l; 40 mg in 2 ml; etc. Examples of drugs in common use expressed in these terms: diazepam injection 10 mg in 1 ml; chloral hydrate mixture 1 g in 10 ml; penicillin suspension 250 mg in 5 ml.

b. **Percentage (weight in volume):** This describes the weight of a drug expressed in grams (g) which is contained in 100 ml or 1 dl of solution. Common examples are: lignocaine hydrochloride injection 2%: this contains 2 g in each 100 ml of solution or 0.2 g (200 mg) in each 10 ml of solution or 0.02 g (20 mg) in each 1 ml of solution, etc. Calcium gluconate injection 10%: this contains 10 g in each 100 ml of solution or 1 g in each 10 ml or 0.1 g (100 mg) in each 1 ml, etc.

c. **Percentage (weight in weight):** This describes the weight of a drug expressed in grams (g) which is contained in 100 g of a solid or semi-solid medicament, e.g. ointments and creams. Examples are: Fucidin ointment 2% which contains 2 g of fusidic acid in each 100 g of ointment; Betnovate cream 25% in Aqueous cream which contains 25 g Betnovate cream mixed with 75 g of Aqueous cream (overall weight 100 g).

d. **Volumes containing '1 part':** A few liquids and to a lesser extent gases, particularly those containing drugs in very low concentrations, are often described as containing 1 part per 'x' units of volume. For liquids 'parts' are equivalent to grams and volume to millilitres, e.g. adrenaline injection 1 in 1000 which contains 1 g in 1000 ml or expressed as a percentage (w/v): 0.1%.

e. **Molar concentration:** Only very occasionally are drugs in liquid form expressed in molar concentration. The mole is the molecular weight of a drug expressed in grams and a one molar (1 M) solution contains this weight dissolved in each litre. More often the term millimole (mmol) is used to describe a medicinal product. 1000 mmol = 1 mole, e.g. potassium chloride solution 15 mmol in 10 ml indicates a solution containing the molecular weight of potassium chloride in milligrams × 15 dissolved in 10 ml of solution. Molar concentrations are most commonly seen in the results of biochemical investigations.

4. **Body height and surface area.** Occasionally drug doses are expressed in terms of microgram, milligram or gram per unit of body surface area. This is frequently the case where precise dosages tailored to individual patient's needs are required. Typical examples may be seen in cytotoxic chemotherapy or in drugs used in paediatric problems. Body surface area is expressed as square metres or m^2 and drug dosages as units/m^2 or units per square metre. Examples are: cytarabine injection 100 mg/m^2 (q.v.); dacarbazine injection 250 mg/m^2 (q.v.). The surface area is calculated from the patient's body weight (in kilograms, kg) and height (in centimetres, cm), as follows:

Body surface area of children – nomogram for determination of body surface area from height and weight

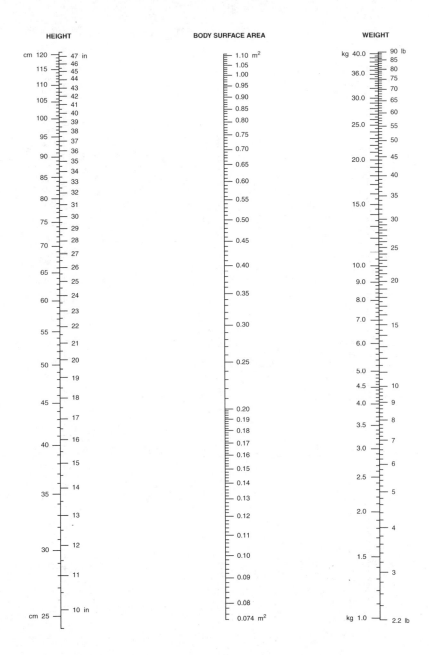

Body surface area of adults – nomogram for determination of body surface area from height and weight

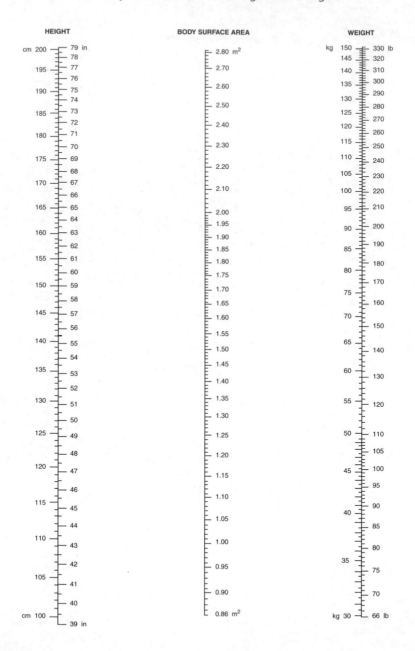

HEIGHT	BODY SURFACE AREA	WEIGHT
cm 200 — 79 in 78 195 — 77 76 190 — 75 74 185 — 73 72 180 — 71 70 175 — 69 68 170 — 67 66 165 — 65 64 160 — 63 62 155 — 61 60 150 — 59 58 145 — 57 56 140 — 55 54 135 — 53 52 130 — 51 50 125 — 49 48 120 — 47 46 115 — 45 44 110 — 43 42 105 — 41 40 cm 100 — 39 in	2.80 m² 2.70 2.60 2.50 2.40 2.30 2.20 2.10 2.00 1.95 1.90 1.85 1.80 1.75 1.70 1.65 1.60 1.55 1.50 1.45 1.40 1.35 1.30 1.25 1.20 1.15 1.10 1.05 1.00 0.95 0.90 0.86 m²	kg 150 — 330 lb 145 — 320 140 — 310 135 — 300 130 — 290 125 — 280 120 — 270 115 — 260 110 — 250 105 — 240 100 — 230 95 — 220 90 — 210 85 — 200 80 — 190 75 — 180 70 — 170 65 — 160 60 — 150 55 — 140 50 — 130 45 — 120 40 — 110 35 — 100 kg 30 — 66 lb

INSTRUCTIONS FOR USE OF TABLE

With a ruler join the points corresponding height and weight. The surface area is then determined by the point at which the central perpendicular line is crossed by the line joining the points on the height and weight perpendicular lines.

(Table reproduced with kind permission of Geigy Pharmaceuticals from Documenta Geigy Scientific Tables, 7th edn. 1970.)

DRUG INDEX

Index: Drugs by proprietary (trade) name